Study Guide for

Pathophysiology

The Biologic Basis for Disease in Adults and Children

Study Guide for

Pathophysiology

The Biologic Basis for Disease in Adults and Children

Sixth Edition

Kathryn L. McCance
Sue E. Huether
Valentina L. Brashers
Neal S. Rote

Prepared by

Clayton F. Parkinson, PhD
Professor Emeritus
College of Health Sciences
Weber State University
Ogden, Utah

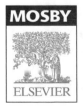

3251 Riverport Lane
Maryland Heights, Missouri 63043

STUDY GUIDE FOR PATHOPHYSIOLOGY: THE BIOLOGIC BASIS
FOR DISEASE IN ADULTS AND CHILDREN   ISBN: 978-0-323-06750-8
Copyright © 2010, 2006, 2002, 1998 by Mosby, Inc., an affiliate of Elsevier Inc. All rights reserved.

Notice

Knowledge and best practice in this field are constantly changing. As new research and experience broaden our understanding, changes in research methods, professional practices, or medical treatment may become necessary.

Practitioners and researchers must always rely on their own experience and knowledge in evaluating and using any information, methods, compounds, or experiments described herein. In using such information or methods they should be mindful of their own safety and the safety of others, including parties for whom they have a professional responsibility.

With respect to any drug or pharmaceutical products identified, readers are advised to check the most current information provided (i) on procedures featured or (ii) by the manufacturer of each product to be administered, to verify the recommended dose or formula, the method and duration of administration, and contraindications. It is the responsibility of practitioners, relying on their own experience and knowledge of their patients, to make diagnoses, to determine dosages and the best treatment for each individual patient, and to take all appropriate safety precautions.

To the fullest extent of the law, neither the Publisher nor the authors, contributors, or editors, assume any liability for any injury and/or damage to persons or property as a matter of products liability, negligence or otherwise, or from any use or operation of any methods, products, instructions, or ideas contained in the material herein.

International Standard Book Number 978-0-323-06750-8

Acquisitions Editor: Sandra Clark
Developmental Editor: Charlene Ketchum
Publishing Services Manager: Anitha Raj
Project Manager: Janaki Srinivasan Kumar

Printed in the United States of America

Last digit is the print number: 9 8 7 6 5 4 3 2

Reviewers

Deborah Dawn Hutchinson Allen, RN, MSN, CNS, FNP-BC, AOCNP
Oncology Clinical Nurse Specialist
Duke Brain Tumor Center Nurse Practitioner
Comprehensive Cancer Center
Duke University Medical Center
Durham, North Carolina

Mandi Counters, RN, MSN, CNRN
Assistant Professor
Nursing Department
Mercy College of Health Sciences
Des Moines, Iowa

David J. Derrico, RN, MSN
Assistant Clinical Professor
Department of Adult and Elderly Nursing
University of Florida College of Nursing
Gainesville, Florida

Jennifer J. Donwerth, MSN, RN, ANP-BC, GNP-BC
Faculty
Department of Nursing
Tarleton State University
Stephenville, Texas

Jo A. Voss, PhD, RN, CNS
Associate Professor
West River Department of Nursing
South Dakota State University
Rapid City, South Dakota

Diane Young, PhD, CNE, RN
Professor
Nursing Department
Allen College
Waterloo, Iowa

Preface

The study of pathophysiology is complex, ever expanding, and challenging. It requires correlation between normal and abnormal anatomy and physiology and the processes resulting in the manifestations of disease.

This study guide is designed for students as an adjunct to *Pathophysiology: The Biologic Basis for Disease in Adults and Children* by Kathryn L. McCance and Sue E. Huether. It is intended to facilitate an understanding of the consequences of pathologic processes on the structure and function of the human body.

The guide has 47 chapters, and each follows the organization of the textbook. The guide's chapters have two different formats—one for normal anatomy and physiology and another for anatomic and physiologic alterations.

For the normal anatomy and physiology chapters, it is assumed that the student possesses knowledge of anatomy and physiology; therefore no supplemental narrative is provided.

- These chapters have prerequisite knowledge objectives that direct review of information, principles, and concepts that are essential for understanding the specific diseases that follow in the next chapter.
- Each chapter has a practice examination to give students an opportunity to assess their understanding of normality.

The alterations chapters direct the learner's study of abnormal anatomy and physiology. Their information is not intended to be all inclusive.

- These chapters have limited, but essential (1) foundational knowledge objectives featuring Memory Checks and (2) learning objectives with concise selective narrative, flow charts, and tables to help students better comprehend the information to be learned.
- Each chapter has a practice examination requiring factual and conceptual knowledge related to disease mechanisms.
- Each chapter has one or two case studies linking fact and concept to reality.

The objectives for all chapters are referenced to corresponding pages in McCance and Huether's textbook. These authors' philosophy that students need to grasp basic laws and principles to understand how alterations occur led them to develop an understandable and conceptually integrated textbook. I enjoyed working with Elsevier, particularly Sandra Clark, Charlene Ketchum, and Joy Moore. All of Elsevier's staff ensured that my efforts were developed into a creative, professional, and pleasing style for student learners.

I wish to dedicate my efforts during the preparation of this study guide to eager students who make teaching pleasurable and inspire me to search for truth and a better way to convey it to students.

Clayton F. Parkinson

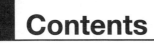

Contents

1 Cellular Biology

PREREQUISITE KNOWLEDGE OBJECTIVES

After reviewing the primary text where referenced, the learner will be able to do the following:

1. **Identify the eight major cellular functions.**
   Review text page 2.
2. **Identify the location of the three principal parts of a typical eukaryotic cell.**
   Refer to Figure 1-1.
3. **Describe the function of the nucleus and the cytoplasmic organelles.**
   Review text pages 2 and 4 through 10; refer to Figures 1-2 through 1-9.
4. **Describe the structure and composition of the plasma membrane.**
   Review text pages 10 through 13 and 15; refer to Figures 1-10 through 1-13.
5. **Categorize plasma membrane functions.**
   Refer to Tables 1-1 and 1-2.
6. **Describe the mechanisms that bind cells together.**
   Review text pages 15, 16, and 18; refer to Figures 1-14 and 1-15.
7. **Describe the primary modes of chemical signaling.**
   Review text pages 18 through 20; refer to Figures 1-16 through 1-21 and Tables 1-3 and 1-4.
8. **Describe cellular metabolism and the transfer of energy to drive other cellular processes.**
   Review text pages 21 through 25; refer to Figures 1-22 through 1-24.
9. **Classify cellular transport as active or passive; give examples of each.**
   Refer to Figures 1-25 through 1-29 and Table 1-5.
10. **Contrast macromolecular transport by endocytosis and exocytosis with micromolecular transport by potocytosis.**
    Review text pages 30 through 32; refer to Figures 1-30 and 1-31.
11. **Describe the changes in the plasma membrane that result in an action potential.**
    Review text pages 32 and 33; refer to Figure 1-32.
12. **Identify the phases of mitosis and cytokinesis; give examples of growth factors.**
    Refer to Figure 1-33 and Table 1-6.
13. **Identify two mechanisms for tissue formation.**
    Review text pages 35 and 36; refer to Figure 1-34.
14. **Identify the location and a major function of each of the following types of tissue: epithelial, connective, muscle, and nervous.**
    Review the tissue summary on text page 43; refer to Tables 1-7 through 1-9.

PRACTICE EXAMINATION

Multiple Choice

Circle the correct answer(s) for each question.

1. Which are principal parts of a eukaryotic cell?
   a. Fat, carbohydrate, and protein
   b. Minerals and water
   c. Organelles
   d. Phospholipids and protein
2. Caveolae:
   a. serve as repositories for some receptors.
   b. provide a route for transport into a cell.
   c. relay signals into cells.
   d. a and b are correct.
   e. a, b, and c are correct.
3. A vault is:
   a. an organelle.
   b. barrel-shaped.
   c. believed to transport mRNA to ribosomes.
   d. a and b are correct.
   e. a, b, and c are correct.
4. For a cell to engage in active transport processes, it requires:
   a. an expenditure of energy.
   b. appropriate fuel.
   c. ATP.
   d. All of the above are correct.
5. Which of the following is *inconsistent* with the others?
   a. Diffusion
   b. Osmosis
   c. Hydrostatic pressure
   d. Phagocytosis

1

6. Which of the following can transport substances against or up the concentration gradient?
   a. Active transport
   b. Osmosis
   c. Dialysis
   d. Facilitated diffusion
   e. None of the above is correct.
7. Imagine that you have an aqueous (water) solution A and an aqueous solution B separated by a membrane that is permeable to the solvent but is not permeable to the solute. If solution A is isotonic to human blood and solution B is hypotonic to human blood, then:
   a. net diffusion of the solute will occur from side B to side A.
   b. net diffusion of the solute will occur from side A to side B.
   c. net osmosis will occur from side B to side A.
   d. net osmosis will occur from side A to side B.
8. Which statement is true about cytoplasm?
   a. It is located outside the nucleus.
   b. It provides support for organelles.
   c. It is mostly water.
   d. All of the above are true.
   e. Only a and b are true.
9. Ribosomes:
   a. are found on smooth endoplasmic reticulum.
   b. are the sites for cellular protein synthesis.
   c. are synthesized in the cytosol.
   d. are made of the protein clathrin.
   e. conduct nerve impulses.
10. Activities occurring in the cytosol include:
    a. intermediary metabolism.
    b. ribosomal protein synthesis.
    c. conversion of glucose to glycogen.
    d. a and b are correct.
    e. a, b, and c are correct.
11. Ligands that bind with membrane receptors include which of the following?
    a. Hormones
    b. Antigens
    c. Neurotransmitters
    d. Drugs
    e. Infectious agents
12. The products from the metabolism of glucose include which of the following?
    a. Kilocalories
    b. CO_2
    c. H_2O
    d. ATP
13. Identify the correct alphabetical sequence of events for initiation and conduction of a nerve impulse.
    a. Sodium moves into cell.
    b. Potassium leaves cell.
    c. Sodium permeability changes.
    d. Resting potential is reestablished.
    e. Potassium permeability changes.
14. Potocytosis:
    a. involves the cellular uptake of small molecules.
    b. opens and closes caveolae.
    c. does not form a membrane-enclosed vesicle.
    d. a and b are correct.
    e. a, b, and c are correct.
15. Cell junctions:
    a. coordinate activities of cells within tissues.
    b. are an impermeable part of the plasma membrane.
    c. hold cells together.
    d. a and c are correct.
    e. b and c are correct.
16. Cells respond to external stimuli by activation of a variety of signal transduction pathways. Signaling molecules cause all of the following *except*:
    a. acceleration/initiation of intracellular protein kinases.
    b. arrest of cellular growth.
    c. apoptosis.
    d. conversion of an intracellular signal into an extracellular response.

Matching

Match the term with its descriptor.

_____ 17. Signal recognition particles

_____ 18. Metaphase

_____ 19. Mitochondria

_____ 20. Gating

_____ 21. Rafts

_____ 22. Paracrine signaling

a. 75% to 90% H_2O, lipids, and protein

b. RNA stored within the nucleus

c. compartmentalizes cellular activity

d. attach to and detach from ribosomes

e. "generation plant" for ATP

f. enables uninjured cells to seal themselves away from injured cells

g. chromatid pair alignment

h. hook cells together

i. acts on nearby cells

j. help organize membrane components

Match the location with its tissue type.

_____ 23. Lines kidney tubules

_____ 24. Lines urinary bladder

_____ 25. Lines upper respiratory tract

a. simple squamous

b. simple cuboidal

c. simple columnar, ciliated

d. stratified squamous

e. transitional

Chapter **1** **Cellular Biology**

2 Altered Cellular and Tissue Biology

FOUNDATIONAL KNOWLEDGE OBJECTIVES

After reviewing the primary text where referenced, the learner will be able to do the following:
a. Describe processes of cellular intake and output.
Review text pages 25 through 32.

MEMORY CHECK!

- The intact, normally functioning plasma membrane is selectively permeable to substances; this means that it allows some substances to pass and excludes others. Water and small, uncharged substances move through pores of the lipid bilayer via passive transport, which requires no expenditure of energy. This process is driven by the forces of osmosis, hydrostatic pressure, and diffusion. Larger molecules and molecular complexes are moved into the cell via active transport, which requires the expenditure of energy, or ATP, by the cell. In active transport, materials move from areas of low concentration to areas of high concentration. The largest molecules and fluids are ingested through endocytosis and expulsed through exocytosis after cellular synthesis of smaller building blocks. When the plasma membrane is injured, it becomes permeable to virtually everything, and substances move into and out of the cells in an unrestricted manner. Notably, such substances may affect (1) the nucleus and its genetic information, or (2) the cytoplasmic organelles and their varied functions; when either of these happens, there is altered cellular physiology and pathology.

b. Identify the relationship among homeostasis, stress, and disease.

MEMORY CHECK!

- Homeostasis is the concept of a dynamic steady state and a turnover of bodily substances that maintains physiologic parameters within narrow limits. Stressors cause reactions that alter this dynamic steady state. Deviations from normal values, which are normally maintained by homeostasis, cause disease.

LEARNING OBJECTIVES

After studying this chapter, the learner will be able to do the following:
1. **Describe the cellular adaptations that occur during atrophy, hypertrophy, hyperplasia, dysplasia, and metaplasia and identify conditions under which each can occur.**
Study text pages 47 through 50; refer to Figures 2-1 through 2-6 and Table 2-1.
When confronted with stresses that disrupt normal structure and function, the cell undergoes adaptive changes that permit survival and maintain function. An adapted cell is neither normal nor injured—it is somewhere between these two states. These changes may lead

to atrophy, hypertrophy, hyperplasia, metaplasia, or dysplasia. These adaptive responses occur in response to need and an appropriate stimulus. Once the need is no longer present, the adaptive response ceases.
Cellular atrophy decreases the cell substance and results in cell shrinkage. The size of all of the structural components of the cell usually decreases as the cell atrophies. Causes of atrophy include disuse, denervation, lack of endocrine stimulation, decreased nutrition, and ischemia. Disuse atrophy is seen in muscles that are not used. Denervation atrophy occurs in the muscles of paralyzed limbs. Lack of endocrine stimulation causes changes that may occur in reproductive structures during menopause. During prolonged periods of malnutrition,

5

the body may undergo a generalized wasting of tissue mass. Ischemia reduces blood flow and delivery of oxygen and nutrients to tissues.

Hypertrophy increases the amount of functioning mass by increasing cell size; this allows the cell to achieve an equilibrium between demand and function. Hypertrophy usually is seen in cardiac and skeletal muscle tissue. These tissues cannot adapt to increased workload by mitotic division to form more cells. The increase in cell components is related to an increased rate of protein synthesis. However, the extent of hypertrophy may be related to limitations in blood flow. Hypertrophy may be either physiologic or pathologic. In myocardial hypertrophy, initial enlargement is caused by dilation of the cardiac chambers in response to valvular disease or hypertension. This adaptation is short-lived and is followed by increased synthesis of cardiac muscle proteins that allows cardiac muscle fibers to do more work. Ultimately, advanced hypertrophy becomes pathologic and can lead to heart failure.

Hyperplasia is an increase in the number of cells of a tissue or an organ. It occurs in tissues in which cells are capable of mitotic division. Hyperplasia is a controlled response to an appropriate stimulus, and it ceases after the stimulus has been removed. Breast and uterine enlargement during pregnancy are examples of a *physiologic* hyperplasia that is hormonally regulated. A *pathologic* hyperplasia occurs when the endometrium enlarges because of excessive estrogen production; in this situation, the abnormally thickened uterine layer may bleed excessively and frequently. *Compensatory* hyperplasia enables certain organs, like the liver, to regenerate after a loss of substance.

Dysplasia (atypical hyperplasia) is deranged cell growth that results in cells that vary in size, shape, and appearance at maturity. Minor degrees of dysplasia occur in association with chronic irritation or inflammation in the uterine cervix, oral cavity, gallbladder, and respiratory passages. Dysplasia is potentially reversible after the irritating cause has been removed. In females, atypical hyperplasia changes may progress to breast neoplastic disease. Importantly, dysplasia does not indicate cancer and may not progress to cancer.

Metaplasia is a reversible conversion from one adult cell type to another adult cell type. It allows for replacement with cells that are better able to tolerate environmental stresses. In metaplasia, one type of cell may be converted to another type of cell within its tissue class (i.e., an epithelial cell cannot change to a connective tissue cell). An example of metaplasia is the substitution of stratified squamous epithelial cells for ciliated columnar epithelial cells in the airways of the person who is a habitual cigarette smoker.

2. **Identify the mechanism of cellular injury for the following causes.**

Hypoxia (study text pages 52 through 55; refer to Figures 2-8 through 2-10 and Tables 2-2 through 2-5); **chemicals** (study text pages 56, 57, and 59 through 62; refer to Figures 2-11 through 2-13 and Table 2-6); **unintentional and intentional injuries** (study text pages 62 through 69; refer to Figures 2-14 through 2-21); **infectious agents** (study text page 69); **immunologic and inflammatory responses** (study text page 69); **genetic factors** (study text page 69); **nutritional imbalances** (study text page 69; refer to Figure 2-22 and Table 2-7); and **physical trauma** (study text pages 71 through 76; refer to Figure 2-23 and Tables 2-8 and 2-9).

Hypoxia deprives the cell of oxygen and interrupts oxidative metabolism and the generation of ATP. As the levels of ATP decline, there is (1) decreased sodium pump activity, and (2) increased glycolysis. One of the earliest effects of reduced ATP is acute cellular swelling caused by failure of the sodium-potassium membrane pump. With impaired function of this pump, intracellular potassium levels decrease, and sodium and water accumulate within the cell. As fluid and ions move into the cell, there is dilation of the endoplasmic reticulum, increased membrane permeability, and decreased mitochondrial function as extracellular calcium accumulates in the mitochondria; all of these lead to decreased protein synthesis, lytic enzyme release, and cellular lysis.

If the oxygen supply is not restored, there is continued loss of essential enzymes, proteins, and ribonucleic acid through the very permeable membrane of the cell. Increased glycolysis decreases the pH, which leads to protein denaturation, nuclear chromatin clumping, and lysosomal swelling with enzyme release and cellular digestion. Hypoxia can result from inadequate oxygen in the air, respiratory disease, decreased blood flow due to circulatory disease, anemia, or inability of the cells to use oxygen.

Restoration of oxygen can cause **reperfusion (reoxygenation) injury.** Reperfusion is a cause of injury in tissue transplantation and in myocardial, hepatic, intestinal, cerebral, renal, and other ischemic syndromes. During reperfusion with oxygen, xanthine oxidase is produced, which makes massive amounts of superoxide, hydrogen peroxide, and the free radical nitric oxide.

Free radicals and reactive oxygen species (ROS), which overwhelm endogenous antioxidant systems, cause membrane damage and mitochondrial overload. A free radical is an atom or group of atoms with an unpaired electron; the unpaired electron makes the atom or group unstable. To gain stability, the radical gives up an electron to another molecule or steals an electron. These radicals can bond with proteins, lipids, and carbohydrates, which are key molecules in membranes and nucleic acids. These reactive species cause injury by (1) lipid peroxidation, which destroys unsaturated fatty acids; (2) fragmentation of polypeptide chains within proteins; and (3) alteration of DNA by breakage of single strands. Free radicals are difficult to control, and they initiate chain reactions. Free radicals may be initiated within cells by the absorption of ultraviolet light or x-rays, oxidative reactions that occur during normal metabolism, and enzymatic metabolism of exogenous chemicals or drugs.

Toxic chemical agents can injure the cell membrane and cell structures, block enzymatic pathways, coagulate cell proteins, and disrupt the osmotic and ionic balance of

6

any cell. Chemicals may injure cells during the process of metabolism or elimination. Carbon tetrachloride, for example, causes little damage until it is metabolized by liver enzymes to a highly reactive free radical, and then it is extremely toxic to liver cells. Carbon monoxide has a special affinity for the hemoglobin molecule, and it reduces the ability of this molecule to carry oxygen.

Lead likely acts on the central nervous system by interference with neurotransmitters; this may cause hyperactive behavior. Manifestations of brain involvement include convulsions and delirium. Peripheral nerve involvement may cause wrist, finger, and foot paralysis. Lead inhibits enzymes that are involved in hemoglobin synthesis; anemia is seen in lead toxicity.

Alcohol (ethanol) is the favorite mood-altering drug in the United States. Liver and nutritional disorders are serious consequences of alcohol abuse. The hepatic changes, which are initiated by ethanol conversion to acetaldehyde, include deposition of fat, enlargement of the liver, interruption of transport of proteins and their secretions, increase in intracellular water, depression of fatty acid oxidation, increased membrane rigidity, and acute liver cell necrosis. In the central nervous system, alcohol is a depressant that initially affects subcortical structures. Consequently, motor and intellectual activities become disoriented. At high blood alcohol levels, respiratory medullary centers become depressed. **Fetal alcohol syndrome (FAS)** caused by prenatal alcohol exposure can lead to growth retardation, cognitive impairment, facial anomalies, and ocular disturbances.

Unintentional and intentional injuries are important health problems in the United States, and death from these causes is more common in men than in women and in blacks and other racial groups than in whites. Injuries by **blunt force** result in tearing, shearing, or crushing of tissues; the most common blunt force injuries are caused by falls and vehicle accidents. A **contusion** is bleeding into the skin or underlying tissues as a consequence of a blow; when blood is contained in an enclosed space, it is called a **hematoma**. An **abrasion** results from the removal of the superficial layers of the skin caused by friction between the skin and an injuring object. A **laceration** occurs when the tensile strength of the skin or tissue is exceeded and a tear or rip results. An **incised wound** is a cut that is longer than it is deep, and a **stab wound** is deeper than it is long. A **gunshot wound** may be penetrating (bullet remains in the body) or perforating (bullet exits the body). **Asphyxial injuries** are caused when cells fail to receive or use oxygen, and they occur as a result of suffocation, strangulation, chemical exposure, or drowning.

Infectious agents produce injury by invading and destroying cells, producing toxins, or inducing hypersensitivity reactions. (Infection is discussed in Chapter 9.)

Immunologic and inflammatory injury are important causes of cellular injury. Cellular membranes are injured by direct contact with cellular and chemical components of the immune and inflammatory responses. Such mediators are lymphocytes and macrophages and chemicals such as histamine, antibodies, lymphokines,

complement, and proteases. Complement, which is a serum protein, is responsible for many of the membrane alterations that occur during immunologic injury. Membrane alterations are associated with the rapid leakage of potassium out of the cell and the rapid influx of water. Antibodies can interfere with membrane function by binding to and occupying receptor molecules on the plasma membrane. (Later chapters deal with these injurious consequences and with hypersensitivity and autoimmune disease.)

Genetic disorders may alter the cell's nucleus and the plasma membrane's structure, shape, receptors, or transport mechanisms. (Mechanisms that cause genetic abnormalities are discussed in Chapters 4 and 5.)

Nutritional imbalances are important because cells require adequate amounts of proteins, carbohydrates, lipids, vitamins, and minerals to function normally. If inadequate or excessive amounts of nutrients are consumed and transported, pathophysiologic cellular effects can develop.

Proteins are the major structural units of the cell, and they participate in many enzymatic and hormonal functions. With lowered plasma proteins, particularly albumin, fluids move into the interstitium and produce edema. Children with protein malnutrition are very susceptible to and often die from infectious diseases.

Glucose is the major carbohydrate obtained from the breakdown of starch. Hyperglycemia (excessive glucose in the blood), if caused by excessive carbohydrate intake, may lead to obesity. Deficiencies of glucose result from starvation or from inadequate use, as in diabetes. In both of these conditions, the body compensates by metabolizing lipids to obtain cellular energy. In lipid deficiency, the body compensates by mobilizing fatty acids from adipose tissue; this causes an increase in the production and circulation of acidic ketone bodies. Severe increases in ketone bodies can cause coma or death. Hyperlipidemia, which is an increase in lipoproteins in the blood, results in deposits of fat in the heart, liver, and muscle.

Vitamins are involved in many reactions, including metabolism of visual pigments (vitamin A), calcium and phosphate metabolism (vitamin D), prothrombin synthesis (vitamin K), and antioxidation reactions (vitamin E). Vitamin B affects amino acid transfer reactions; flavin adenine dinucleotide (FAD), FMN, and nicotinamide adenine dinucleotide (NAD) help transfer electrons. Deficiencies in vitamin C cause poor wound healing and scurvy. Vitamin D deficiency causes rickets and problems with healing of fractures. Folate deficiency is associated with plasma and membrane changes of the red blood cell, and it is particularly a problem in individuals with severe liver dysfunction. Vitamin deficiencies are associated with several other disease states, including cancer.

Injurious physical agents include temperature extremes, changes in atmospheric pressure, radiation, illumination, mechanical factors, noise, and prolonged vibration. Physical injury is often environmental.

The **temperature extremes** of chilling or freezing of cells cause hypothermic injury directly by creating high intracellular sodium concentrations. This results from the formation and dissolution of ice crystals. Indirect forms of injury like vasoconstriction paralyze vasomotor control, and vasodilation follows, with increased membrane permeability; this causes cellular and tissue swelling. Hyperthermic injury from excessive heat varies depending on the nature, intensity, and duration of the heat. Burns cause extensive loss of fluids and plasma proteins. Also, intense heat damages temperature-sensitive enzymes and the vascular endothelium and causes coagulation of the blood vessels.

Sudden increases or decreases in **atmospheric pressure** cause blast injury. In air blast or explosive injuries, tissue injury is caused by compressed waves of air against the body. The pressure changes may collapse the thorax, rupture solid internal organs, or cause widespread hemorrhage. In increased pressure caused by immersion blast, water pressure is applied suddenly to the body, and the body is forced up out of the water. The positive pressure compresses the abdomen and ruptures hollow internal organs such as the spleen, kidneys, and liver. With sudden decreases in pressure, carbon dioxide and nitrogen normally dissolved in the blood leave solution and form tiny bubbles (gas emboli) that obstruct blood vessels; this is seen in rapidly ascending deep sea divers and underwater workers. At low atmospheric pressure (above 15,000 feet), there is a decrease in available oxygen; this causes hypoxic injury. The compensatory vasoconstriction shunts the blood from the peripheral circulation to the visceral organs, including the lungs. The combination of increases in pulmonary blood flow and systemic hypoxia causes pulmonary edema, which is also known as interstitial water excess.

Ionizing radiation is any form of radiation capable of removing orbital electrons from atoms. Ionizing radiation is emitted by x-rays, gamma rays, and the process of radioactive decay. Radiant energy from sunlight can also injure cells. DNA is the most vulnerable target of radiation, particularly the bonds within the DNA molecule. Irradiation during mitosis produces chromosome aberrations, and membrane molecules and enzymes are also damaged by radiation. Radiosensitivity depends on the rate of mitosis and cellular maturity. The more numerous the mitotic figures, the greater is the sensitivity; more maturity equals less sensitivity. Particularly vulnerable cells are embryonic germ cells, which are precursors of ova and sperm. Throughout life, cells of the bone marrow, intestinal mucosa, testicular seminiferous epithelium, and ovarian follicles are susceptible to injury, because they are always undergoing mitosis.

Exposure to x-radiation and gamma radiation is most strongly correlated with leukemia and cancers of the thyroid, breast, and lung. Radiation exposure in children may increase the incidence of lymphomas and melanomas. Radiation exposure is significantly related to cardiovascular disease, hypertension, and elevated cholesterol levels. Studies of late effects in survivors of atomic bombs reveal elevated levels of mediators of inflammation and immune globulins.

The harmful effects of **illumination** in fluorescent lighting include eye strain, obscured vision, and possible cataract formation. Emission of ultraviolet radiation from halogen lamps is thought to be in the range of wavelengths responsible for inducing melanoma, which is a malignant skin growth.

Mechanical injury is caused by physical impact or irritation (e.g., a head injury when a worker is struck by a falling object). Most mechanical stresses, however, are subtle, and they can cause accumulative injuries and disorders over time. Mechanical stimulation of body tissues and cells is constant. When the forces exceed thresholds, injury results. The structural responses to deformation and strain mostly involve the cell membrane. Disruption of cell membranes, or **mechanoporation,** are central to progression of mechanical injury.

Noise is sound that has the potential for inflicting bodily harm. Noise trauma can be caused by acute loud noise or by the cumulative effects of various intensities, frequencies, and durations of noise.

Acoustic trauma is instantaneous damage and can rupture the eardrum, displace the ossicles of the middle ear, or damage the organ of Corti in the inner ear. Structural changes associated with prolonged exposure to loud sounds include intracellular changes in the sensory cells, swelling of the auditory nerve endings, and cochlear blood flow impairment. Noise-induced hearing loss is gradual and painless. Symptoms of noise-induced hearing loss include inability to hear soft sounds and tinnitus.

3. **Identify the various cellular accumulations and their causes and subsequent injuries.**
   Study text pages 76 through 79 and 81; refer to Figures 2-24 through 2-28. See Table on page 9.
4. **Identify systemic manifestations and causes of cellular injury.**
   Refer to Table 2-10. See Table on page 9.
5. **Identify the major types of cellular necrosis, and cite examples of the tissues involved in each type. Compare necrosis to apoptosis.**
   Study text pages 81 through 85; refer to Figures 2-29 through 2-36.

Necrosis is local cell death, and it involves the process of cellular self-digestion known as autodigestion or autolysis. As necrosis progresses, most organelles are disrupted, and **karyolysis**, which is the nuclear dissolution from the action of hydrolytic enzymes, becomes evident. **Pyknosis** is a process wherein the nucleus shrinks and becomes a small, dense mass of genetic material. **Karyorrhexis** is nuclear fragmentation into smaller particles or "nuclear dust." There are four major types of necrosis: coagulative, liquefactive, caseous, and fat. Gangrenous necrosis is not a distinctive type of cell death; rather, it refers to large areas of tissue death.

Coagulative necrosis occurs primarily in the kidneys, heart, and adrenal glands and usually results from hypoxia caused by severe ischemia. Protein denaturation causes coagulation. An increased intracellular level of calcium may be a critical event in coagulation necrosis.

Liquefactive necrosis is common after ischemic injury to neurons and glial cells in the brain. Because brain cells are rich in digestive hydrolytic enzymes and

Cellular Accumulations

Accumulation	Causes	Injury
H₂O	Reduced ATP and ATPase, sodium accumulates in cell, extracellular H₂O shifts into cell	Cellular swelling, vacuolation, hydropic degeneration
Lipids, carbohydrates	Imbalance in production, utilization, or mobilization of lipid or carbohydrates	Vacuolation, displaced nucleus and organelles; leads to fibrosis and scarring
Glycogen	Genetic disorders, diabetes mellitus	Cytoplasmic vacuolation
Proteins	Enzymes digesting cellular organelles, renal disorders, plasma cell tumor	Disrupted function and intracellular communication, displaced cellular organelles
Pigments	Exogenous particle ingestion, UV light stimulating melanin production, malignancy, loss of hormonal feedback, genetic defects, bruising and hemorrhaging increasing hemosiderin, liver dysfunction	Membrane injury
Calcium	Altered membrane permeability, influx of extracellular calcium, excretion of H⁺ leading to more OH⁻ that precipitates Ca⁺⁺, endocrine disturbances	Hardening of cellular structure; interferes with function
Urate	Absence of enzymes	Crystal deposition, inflammation

Systemic Manifestations of Cellular Injury

Manifestation	Cause
Fever	Endogenous pyrogens released by inflammatory response
Increased heart rate	Fever raises the metabolic rate
Pain	Bradykinins released, obstructive pressures
Extracellular fluid (blood) enzymes*	Released from injured cells or tissues

*Specific enzymes, such as creatine kinase (CK), lactic dehydrogenase (LDH), or amylase, are released from injured hearts, kidneys, skeletal muscles, among others.

lipids, the brain cells are digested by their own hydrolases. The brain tissue becomes soft and liquefies, and is walled off from healthy tissue to form cysts. Liquefactive necrosis can also result from bacterial infections. Here, the hydrolases are released from the lysosomes of phagocytic neutrophils that are attracted to the infected area to kill the bacteria; these hydrolases also destroy brain tissue. The accumulation of pus is present in liquefaction necrosis.

Caseous necrosis is commonly seen in tuberculous pulmonary infection and is a combination of coagulative and liquefactive necrosis. The necrotic debris is not digested completely by hydrolases, so tissues appear soft and granular and resemble clumped cheese. A granulomatous inflammatory wall may enclose the central areas of caseous necrosis.

Fat necrosis, found in the breast, pancreas, and other abdominal structures, is a specific cellular dissolution caused by lipases. Lipases break down triglycerides and release free fatty acids that then combine with calcium, magnesium, and sodium ions to create soaps (a process known as saponification). The necrotic tissue appears opaque and chalk white.

Gangrenous necrosis refers to the death of tissue, usually in considerable mass and with putrefaction. It results from severe hypoxic injury subsequent to arteriosclerosis or blockage of major arteries followed by bacterial invasion. Dry gangrene is usually due to a coagulative necrosis, and wet gangrene develops when neutrophils invade the site and cause liquefactive necrosis. Gas gangrene, which is a special type of gangrene, is caused by the bacterial infection of injured tissue by a species of *Clostridium*. These anaerobic bacteria produce hydrolytic enzymes and toxins that destroy connective tissue and the cellular membrane; bubbles of gas likely form in muscle cells.

Apoptosis is an important, distinct type of cell death that differs from necrosis. It is an active process of cellular self-destruction in both normal and pathologic tissue changes. Apoptosis likely plays a role in the deletion of cells during embryonic development and in endocrine-dependent tissues that are undergoing atrophic change. It may occur spontaneously in malignant tumors and in normal, rapidly proliferating cells treated with cancer chemotherapeutic agents and ionizing radiation. The progression of apoptosis depends on specific signaling

9

molecules that interplay among subcellular compartments. Proteases, in response to signals, cleave key proteins in the cell, thereby killing the cell quickly and neatly. Unlike necrosis, apoptosis affects scattered, single cells and results in shrinkage of a cell; whereas in necrosis, cells swell and lyse.

6. Describe theories of aging.

Study text pages 87 through 90; refer to Figure 2-37 and Table 2-11.

There are two general theories of aging: (1) aging is caused by the accumulations of injurious events, which are sometimes called damage-accumulation theories; or (2) aging is the result of a genetically controlled developmental program. In support of these two categories, three mechanisms of aging have emerged: (1) genetic, environmental, and behavioral factors produce cellular aging change; (2) changes in regulatory mechanisms, especially in the cells of the endocrine, immune, and central nervous systems, are responsible for aging; and (3) degenerative extracellular and vascular alterations cause aging.

Regardless of injurious environmental factors, some believe that each cell may have a finite life span during which it can replicate. Fibroblasts have been demonstrated to be limited to 40 to 60 cell doublings. Alternatively, an intrinsic program within the human genome progressively slows or shuts down mitosis.

Alterations of cellular control mechanisms include increased hormonal degradations, decreased hormonal synthesis and secretion, and decreased receptors for hormones and neuromodulators. This suggests that a genetic program for aging is encoded in the brain and relayed through hormonal and neural agents because of shared, common receptors within these systems.

Immune function declines with age and the number of autoantibodies that attack body tissues increases with age; these observations implicate the immune system in the aging process.

A degenerative extracellular change that affects the aging process is collagen cross-linking, which makes collagen more rigid and results in decreased cell permeability to nutrients. Free radicals of oxygen are believed to damage tissues during aging. These reactive species not only permanently damage cells but also may lead to cell death. Damage accumulates over time and reduces the body's ability to maintain a steady state.

Frailty is a wasting syndrome of aging. The syndrome invokes decreased protein synthesis, muscular mass and strength decline, and neuroendocrine and immune dysfunction.

7. Characterize somatic death and its manifestations.

Study text page 90.

Somatic death is death of the entire organism. Unlike the changes that follow cellular death in a viable body, somatic death is diffuse and does not involve components of the inflammatory response, which is a vascular response to injury. The most notable manifestations of somatic death are complete cessation of respiration and circulation, skin surface usually becoming pale and yellowish, and body temperature falling gradually until, after 24 hours,

body temperature equals that of the environment. Within 6 hours after death, depletion of ATP interferes with ATP-dependent detachment of the contractile proteins, and muscle stiffening, or rigor mortis, develops. Within 12 to 14 hours, rigor mortis usually affects the entire body. Rigor mortis gradually diminishes as the body becomes flaccid because of the release of enzymes and lytic dissolution.

PRACTICE EXAMINATION

Multiple Choice

Circle the correct answer(s) for each question.

1. A deranged cellular growth observable in uterine cervical epithelium is:
   a. atrophy.
   b. hyperplasia.
   c. hypertrophy.
   d. dysplasia.
   e. metaplasia.
2. What is the consequence when a cell is forced into anaerobic glycolysis?
   a. Insufficient glucose production
   b. Excessive pyruvic acid retention
   c. Increased lactic acid production
   d. Excessive CO_2 production
3. What is the probable cause of cellular swelling during the early stages of cell injury?
   a. Fat inclusion
   b. Loss of genetic integrity
   c. Hydrolytic enzyme activation
   d. Na^+, K^+ pump fails to remove intracellular Na^+
4. Calcification:
   a. alters membrane permeability.
   b. is the result of low calcium levels in the blood.
   c. is caused by UV light.
   d. is caused by hypoparathyroidism.
5. Cellular swelling is:
   a. reversible.
   b. evident early in all types of cellular injury.
   c. associated with hyperkalemia.
   d. extracellular movement of fluid.
6. Which of the following is irreversible?
   a. Karyolysis
   b. Fatty infiltration
   c. Hydropic degeneration
   d. Glycogen formation
7. Aging:
   a. likely involves autoantibodies.
   b. does not have a genetic relationship.
   c. results from damage accumulation.
   d. decreases hormonal degradation.
8. In the theories of aging, cross-linking implies that:
   a. the life span and number of times a cell can replicate are programmed.
   b. the number of cell doublings is limited.
   c. there is oxygen toxicity.
   d. cell permeability decreases.

Matching

Match the descriptor with its appropriate condition.

_____ 9. Caused by tuberculosis infection

_____ 10. Rigidity of muscles after somatic death

_____ 11. Increased tissue mass because of increased cell numbers

_____ 12. Results from lysosomal release of hydrolytic enzymes

_____ 13. Replacement of one cell type with another, more suitable type

a. liquefactive necrosis

b. rigor mortis

c. caseous necrosis

d. hyperplasia

e. metaplasia

f. cellular swelling

g. coagulation necrosis

Match the circumstance with the appropriate condition.

_____ 14. Disruption of cell membranes

_____ 15. Pancreatic necrosis

_____ 16. Coagulative and liquefactive necrosis

_____ 17. Tissue death

_____ 18. Normal and pathologic cellular self-destruction

a. fatty necrosis

b. gangrene

c. mechanoporation

d. caseous necrosis

e. apoptosis

f. algor mortis

g. hypertrophy

Match the consequence with its cause.

_____ 19. Lipid peroxidation

_____ 20. Neurotransmitter interference

_____ 21. Asphyxiation

_____ 22. Depressed fatty acid oxidation

_____ 23. Depressed protein synthesis

a. carbon monoxide

b. oxygen-derived free radicals

c. ethanol

d. lead

e. detached ribosomes

f. increased lactate

g. lysosomal edema

Fill in the Blanks

Supply the correct response for each statement.

24. During reperfusion with oxygen, _____ is produced, which creates superoxides, hydrogen peroxide, and free radicals.

25. Specific enzymes such as _____ are released into extracellular fluids during muscular injury.

Chapter **2** **Altered Cellular and Tissue Biology**

3 The Cellular Environment: Fluids and Electrolytes, Acids and Bases

FOUNDATIONAL KNOWLEDGE OBJECTIVES

After reviewing the primary text where referenced, the learner will be able to do the following:

a. Describe the different compartments for body fluids, and identify the fluid distribution changes that occur with age.
Review text pages 96 and 97; refer to Tables 3-1 through 3-3.

b. Describe the factors that affect water movement.
Review text pages 97 and 98; refer to Figures 3-1 and 3-2.

MEMORY CHECK!

- Fluid movement is explained by the following formula:

$$Q = (BHP + IFOP) - (IFHP + BOP)$$
$$\text{[from vessel]} \qquad \text{[to vessel]}$$

Q = fluid movement, BHP = blood hydrostatic pressure, IFOP = interstitial fluid osmotic pressure, IFHP = interstitial fluid hydrostatic pressure, and BOP = blood osmotic pressure.

c. Identify the formula for determining the distribution of electrolytes in body compartments.
Refer to Table 3-4.

MEMORY CHECK!

- mEq/L = $\dfrac{\text{milligrams of ion per liter of solution} \times \text{number of charges of one ion}}{\text{atomic weight of ion}}$

- mEq/L expresses chemicals dissolved in body fluids; they relate to chemical activity.

d. Identify the roles of ADH, aldosterone, and natriuretic hormone in water and electrolyte balance.
Review text pages 101 and 102; refer to Figure 3-4.

MEMORY CHECK!

Hormone	Target	Action
Antidiuretic hormone (ADH)	Renal collecting ducts	Water reabsorbed into blood, decreased plasma osmolality, less urine
Aldosterone	Renal distal tubule	Sodium and chloride reabsorbed into blood, potassium excreted into urine, usually more urine
Natriuretic hormone	Renal proximal tubule	Inhibits sodium reabsorption into blood, more urine

13

e. **Identify body mechanisms that buffer excessive hydrogen ion/acid, and explain the mechanics of the most important buffers. Distinguish between short-term and long-term adjustments.**
Review text pages 114 through 117; refer to Figures 3-8 through 3-10 and Table 3-9.

MEMORY CHECK!

- Pulmonary acid-base regulation of blood involves CO_2 and is rapid.

$$CO_2 + H_2O \leftrightarrow H_2CO_3 \leftrightarrow H^+ + HCO_3^-$$

An increase in CO_2 tension liberates hydrogen ions; thus, the pH decreases. A decrease in CO_2 tension results in fewer hydrogen ions; thus, the pH increases.
- Renal acid-base regulation of blood involves HCO_3^- conservation and H^+ and NH_3 excretion and is slow. This process essentially secretes H^+ into the urine and returns HCO_3^- to the blood plasma; thus, the pH increases.

LEARNING OBJECTIVES

After studying this chapter, the learner will be able to do the following:

1. **Identify the mechanisms that cause edema.**
   Study text pages 98 through 101; refer to Figure 3-3. See the following chart.
   Edema is the accumulation of fluid within interstitial spaces. It may be excess or sequestered fluid.
2. **Define isotonic, hypertonic, and hypotonic water and solute alterations.**
   Refer to Table 3-5.
   Tonic refers to the concentration of solutes.
   Isotonic imbalances—Extracellular fluid loss or gain is accompanied by proportional changes of electrolytes or solutes in these alterations. Losses are seen during hemorrhage or excessive sweating. Gains occur during administration of intravenous normal saline or renal retention of sodium and water. Recall that isotonic solutions have the same concentration of solute as another adjacent or related solution. Cells neither shrink nor swell in isotonic fluids.

   Hypertonic imbalances (more solute in relationship to water)—Water loss or solute gain occurs in these changes. These alterations are seen with the administration of hypertonic saline solutions, hyperaldosteronism, Cushing syndrome, diabetes, diarrhea, or insufficient water intake. Cells shrink in hypertonic fluids.

   Hypotonic imbalances (less solute in relationship to water)—Water gain or solute loss occurs in these changes. These alterations may be caused by vomiting, diarrhea, burns, diuretics, excessive sweating, or renal failure to excrete water. Cells swell in hypotonic fluids.

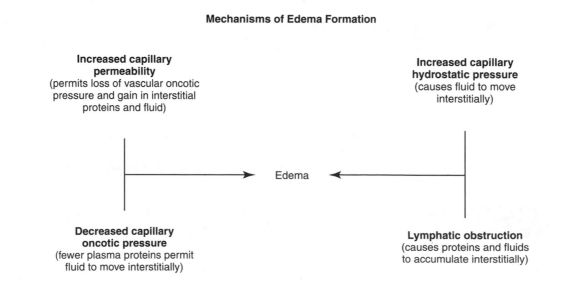

Mechanisms of Edema Formation

Increased capillary permeability
(permits loss of vascular oncotic pressure and gain in interstitial proteins and fluid)

Increased capillary hydrostatic pressure
(causes fluid to move interstitially)

Edema

Decreased capillary oncotic pressure
(fewer plasma proteins permit fluid to move interstitially)

Lymphatic obstruction
(causes proteins and fluids to accumulate interstitially)

NOTE: Fluids move from where there is <u>more</u> to where there is <u>less</u> and to dilute the solutes, or the fluids stay where there are solutes.

3. **Identify the major consequences/manifestations of abnormal levels of water, sodium, potassium, calcium, phosphate, and magnesium. Indicate terms associated with the excess or deficit of each electrolyte.**

Study text pages 102 through 114, refer to Figures 3-5 through 3-7 and Tables 3-6 through 3-8. See the following table.

Water balance is regulated by the secretion of antidiuretic hormone (ADH) and the perception of thirst. Thirst stimulates water-drinking behavior. The secretion of ADH is initiated by an increase in plasma osmolality or a decrease in circulating blood volume and lowered blood pressure. Sodium ions are the most abundant extracellular ions. They are involved in impulse transmission, muscle contraction, and fluid and electrolyte balance. The sodium level is controlled by aldosterone, ADH, and atrial natriuretic peptide. Potassium ions are abundant in intracellular fluid. They are important in the resting membrane potential and the action potential of neurons and muscle fibers; they help maintain intracellular fluid volume; and they contribute to regulation of pH. The potassium level is controlled by aldosterone.

Clinical Manifestations of Excess and Deficit States of Major Electrolytes

Excess	Deficit
Sodium (136 to 145 mEq/L)	
Hypernatremia	Hyponatremia
≥147 mEq/L	≤135 mEq/L
Cellular shrinking may cause central nervous system irritability, tachycardia, dry and flushed skin, hypertension, thirst, elevated temperature, rapid pulse, weight loss, anuria	Cellular swelling may cause cerebral edema, headache, stupor, coma, peripheral edema, polyuria, absence of thirst, decreased body temperature, rapid pulse, hypotension, nausea, vomiting
Potassium (3.5 to 4.5 mEq/L)	
Hyperkalemia	Hypokalemia
≥5.5 mEq/L	≤3.5 mEq/L
Depressed conductivity in heart, muscle cramping, paresthesias, nausea, diarrhea, associated with metabolic acidosis	Cardiac irritability, dysrhythmias, vomiting, paralytic ileus, thirst, associated with metabolic alkalosis, inability to concentrate urine
Calcium (8.6 to 10.5 mg/dl)	
Hypercalcemia	Hypocalcemia
≥12 mg/dl	≤8.5 mg/dl
Decreased neuromuscular excitability, muscle weakness, central nervous system depression, stupor to coma, increased risk of bone fracture, vomiting, constipation, kidney stones	Increased neuromuscular excitability, skeletal cramps, tetany, laryngospasm, asphyxiation, death
Phosphate (2.5 to 4.5 mg/dl)	
Hyperphosphatemia	Hypophosphatemia
≥4.5 mg/dl	≤2.0 mg/dl
See Hypocalcemia	Anorexia, weakness, osteomalacia, muscle weakness, tremors, seizures, coma, anemia, bleeding disorders, leukocytic alterations
Magnesium (1.8 to 2.4 mEq/L)	
Hypermagnesemia	Hypomagnesemia
≥2.5 mEq/L	≤1.5 mEq/L
Skeletal muscle depression, muscle weakness, hypotension, bradycardia, respiratory depression	Hypocalcemia and hypokalemia, neuromuscular irritability, tetany, convulsions, tachycardia, hypertension

4. **Differentiate between metabolic/respiratory acidosis and metabolic/respiratory alkalosis.**

Study text pages 117 through 123; refer to Figures 3-11 through 3-16 and Tables 3-10 and 3-11.

Important normal mean values include the following: pH = 7.35 to 7.45; K^+ = 5 mEq/L; Na^+ = 142 mEq/L; Cl^- = 104 mEq/L; HCO_3^- = 24 mEq/L; Pco_2 = 35 to 45 mmHg, and CO_2 = 28 mEq/L.

Essentially, acidosis causes nervous system depression, and alkalosis causes nervous system irritability. The manifestations vary with the degree of alteration. See the flow charts on pages 16 through 18 of this workbook.

Correction of imbalances requires therapy if the disturbance is severe. For metabolic acidosis, sodium bicarbonate administration is required, and sodium and water deficits must be corrected. For respiratory acidosis, if renal buffer is ineffective, mechanical ventilation may be required. For metabolic alkalosis, chloride or potassium may be required, and for respiratory alkalosis, correction is directed toward alleviation of the underlying disorder. For each imbalance, the underlying condition must be identified and corrected.

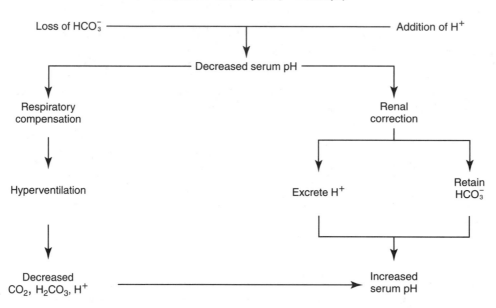

Metabolic Acidosis (HCO_3^- <24 mEq/L)

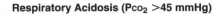

Respiratory Acidosis (Pco$_2$ >45 mmHg)

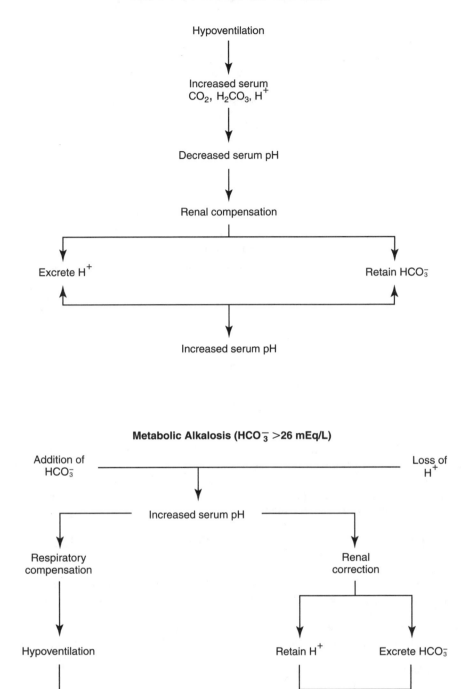

Metabolic Alkalosis (HCO$_3^-$ >26 mEq/L)

Chapter **3** **The Cellular Environment: Fluids and Electrolytes, Acids and Bases**

Respiratory Alkalosis (Pco$_2$ >35 mmHg)

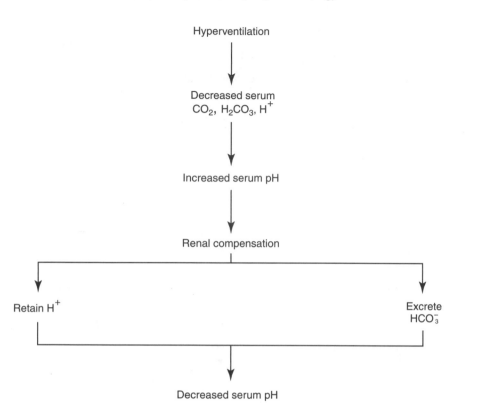

Hyperventilation

↓

Decreased serum
CO$_2$, H$_2$CO$_3$, H$^+$

↓

Increased serum pH

↓

Renal compensation

Retain H$^+$ Excrete
                     HCO$_3^-$

↓

Decreased serum pH

---

5. **Describe what is meant by the "anion gap," and explain the significance of an abnormal anion gap in metabolic acidosis.**

Study text pages 118 and 119; refer to Table 3-11.

The blood and cellular electrolytes must maintain osmotic neutrality (i.e., the number of cations must equal the number of anions present). Routine measurement of serum electrolytes usually involves only Na$^+$ and K$^+$ cations and the anions of Cl$^-$ and HCO$_3^-$ as total CO$_2$. There are about 12 mEq/L of other anions present in the blood that are not routinely measured (e.g., phosphates, sulfates, and protein anions). Therefore, assuming that no abnormal anions are present, an individual's serum sodium and potassium should equal the chloride + the bicarbonate + 12 mEq/L of unmeasured, normal anions. If this is true, then the individual would have a normal **anion gap**. This may be expressed by the following formula:

$$Na^+ + K^+ = Cl^- + HCO_3^- + 12 \text{ mEq/L of}$$
$$\text{unmeasured anions}$$

In metabolic acidosis, a normal anion gap is related to bicarbonate loss and retention of chloride to maintain an ionic balance. This is described as hyperchloremic metabolic acidosis.

The significance of an abnormally large anion gap is that an abnormal anion is present in the blood from substances such as lactic acid, ketone bodies, and salicylates. When this is the case, the individual will have a low bicarbonate level, but there is not a corresponding increase in

chloride. The anion gap will be greater than 12 mEq/L. If the anion gap is normal but the Cl$^-$ has increased and the HCO$_3^-$ is low, the metabolic acidosis may be due to diarrhea, ammonium chloride ingestion, or renal dysfunction.

PRACTICE EXAMINATION

Multiple Choice

Circle the correct answer for each question.

1. The total water loss per day in the adult is approximately:
   a. 0.8 L.
   b. 1.2 L.
   c. 1.8 L.
   d. 2.2 L.
   e. 2.8 L.

2. Of the 60% of the body weight made up of water, about 3 L is:
   a. extracellular water.
   b. intracellular water.
   c. intravascular water.
   d. interstitial water.

3. Sodium is responsible for:
   a. intracellular fluid (ICF) osmotic balance.
   b. extracellular fluid (ECF) osmotic balance.
   c. total body water (TBW) osmolality.
   d. osmotic equilibrium.

18

4. A milliequivalent is a unit of:
   a. mass.
   b. physical activity.
   c. chemical activity.
   d. osmotic concentration.
5. The principle of osmotic neutrality means that:
   a. the number of ions and the number of anions in the body must be equal.
   b. intravascular molecules of protein are without charge.
   c. the sodium ions must be united with the chloride ions.
   d. the positive and negative charges in blood plasma must be equal to each other.
6. Aldosterone controls ECF volume by:
   a. carbohydrate, fat, and protein catabolism.
   b. sodium reabsorption.
   c. potassium reabsorption.
   d. inhibition of chloride reabsorption.
7. The release of ADH is stimulated by:
   a. decreased plasma osmolality.
   b. increased circulating blood volume.
   c. increased blood pressure.
   d. increased plasma osmolality.
   e. decreased plasma volume.
8. Laboratory studies of an adult reveal the following:
   plasma sodium = 110 mEq/L
   plasma chloride = 100 mEq/L
   plasma potassium = 4.8 mEq/L
   plasma calcium = 9 mEq/L
   plasma bicarbonate = 26 mEq/L
   The most likely alteration is:
   a. base bicarbonate deficit (metabolic acidosis).
   b. hypokalemia.
   c. hyponatremia.
   d. base bicarbonate excess (metabolic alkalosis).
   e. calcium deficit.
9. An individual has weakness, dizziness, irritability, and intestinal cramps. Laboratory studies reveal the following:
   plasma sodium = 138 mEq/L
   plasma potassium = 6.8 mEq/L
   blood pH = 7.38
   plasma bicarbonate = 25 mEq/L
   An ECG that has a tall, peaked T wave but is otherwise normal.
   The individual has:
   a. hypernatremia.
   b. hyponatremia.
   c. hypercalcemia.
   d. hyperkalemia.
   e. hypokalemia.
10. An acid is which of the following?
    a. An anion
    b. A cation
    c. A substance/chemical that combines with a hydrogen ion to lower pH
    d. A substance/chemical that donates a hydrogen ion or a proton

11. The most significant consequence of hyperkalemia is:
    a. muscular weakness.
    b. paralytic ileus.
    c. depressed cardiac conductivity or arrest.
    d. metabolic alkalosis.
12. The blood pH is maintained near 7.4 by buffer systems. The sequence from the fastest-acting compensation to the slowest-acting compensation is, respectively:
    a. lungs, kidneys, blood buffers.
    b. blood buffers, lungs, kidneys.
    c. blood buffers, kidneys, lungs.
    d. lungs, blood buffers, kidneys.
13. The pH of saliva is about 7, and the pH of gastric juice is about 2. How many times more concentrated is the hydrogen ion in gastric juice than in saliva?
    a. 5
    b. 50
    c. 100
    d. 10,000
    e. 100,000
14. If a hypotonic solution is infused intravenously into a patient, fluid movement will:
    a. be from vascular to interstitial.
    b. not occur.
    c. be from intracellular to extracellular.
    d. occur from the interstitial to the vascular compartment.
15. A young female became quite agitated and apprehensive and eventually lost consciousness. At the hospital emergency department, the following laboratory values were obtained:
    plasma sodium = 137 mEq/L
    plasma potassium = 5.0 mEq/L
    blood pH = 7.53
    serum CO_2 = 22 mmHg
    plasma bicarbonate = 24 mEq/L
    Her immediate diagnosis was:
    a. hypokalemia.
    b. metabolic acidosis.
    c. metabolic alkalosis.
    d. respiratory acidosis.
    e. respiratory alkalosis.
16. As HCO_3^- shifts from the red blood cell to the blood plasma, it is expected that the plasma:
    a. Na^+ increases.
    b. Cl^- shifts into the red blood cell.
    c. K^+ increases.
    d. pH decreases.
17. An elevated anion gap is associated with an accumulation of:
    a. chloride anions.
    b. lactate anions.
    c. high bicarbonate levels.
    d. sodium cations.

Matching

Match the term with its description.

____ 18. Hydrostatic pressure

____ 19. Oncotic/osmotic pressure

a. water-pulling effect of plasma proteins

b. pressure of blood within the capillaries

c. mechanism to move fluid to lymph glands

d. movement of fluid through semipermeable membrane

Match the acid-base imbalance with its probable cause.

____ 20. Respiratory acidosis

____ 21. Respiratory alkalosis

____ 22. Metabolic alkalosis

a. severe anxiety

b. diabetes

c. chronic diarrhea

d. emphysema

e. excessive baking soda ingestion

Match the acid-base imbalance with its compensatory mechanism.

____ 23. Respiratory acidosis

____ 24. Respiratory alkalosis

____ 25. Metabolic acidosis

a. kidneys retain H^+ and excrete HCO_3^-

b. kidneys excrete H^+ and retain HCO_3^-

c. respirations increase, and more CO_2 is eliminated

d. respirations decrease, and more CO_2 is retained

CASE STUDY

A 70-year-old woman was brought to an urgent care facility complaining of severe muscular weakness and a 3-week history of diarrhea. The on-site clinical laboratory provided the following electrolyte test results:

$Na^+ = 142$ mEq/L

$K^+ = 2.1$ mEq/L

$Cl^- = 94$ mEq/L

$CO_2 = 30$ mEq/L

What electrolyte levels are abnormal?

Is there a medical emergency? If so, what is it, and what should be done?

4 Genes and Genetic Diseases

FOUNDATIONAL KNOWLEDGE OBJECTIVES

After reviewing the primary text where referenced, the learner will be able to do the following:
a. Describe the interrelationships of DNA, RNA, and proteins.
 Review text page 129; refer to Figures 4-1, 4-2, and 4-5 through 4-8.

MEMORY CHECK!

- The gene consists of a particular sequence of nucleotides in the deoxyribonucleic acid (DNA) of the chromosome. The sequence of nucleotides in a gene determines either the structure or the function of a cell. Thus, the genes dictate which proteins are found in a cell, and these proteins determine the form and function of the cell.
- Genetic information flows from DNA to RNA to proteins. Three major processes are involved in the preservation and transmission of genetic information. The first is replication, which is the copying of DNA to form identical daughter molecules. The second is transcription, in which the genetic message encoded within DNA is transcribed into the form of RNA and is carried to the ribosomes, which are the sites of protein synthesis. The third is translation, in which the genetic message is decoded and converted into the 20-letter alphabet of protein structure. Because the sequence of nucleotides in the DNA bears a linear correspondence to the sequence of amino acids in the formed proteins, genetic information is preserved and transmitted to progeny.

b. Define general genetic terms.
 Review text pages 134, 135, 143, 145, and 148 through 150. See the following.

MEMORY CHECK!

Genetic Term	Definition
Progeny	Offspring
Chromosomes	Structures in the nucleus that contain DNA, which transmits genetic information; each chromosome is composed of thousands of genes arranged in linear order
Gene	DNA, the basic unit of heredity, located at a particular site on the chromosome
Allele	One of two or more different genes that contain specific inheritable characteristics (e.g., eye color) and that occupy corresponding positions on paired chromosomes— one gene from each parent; a different version of the same paired gene
Gamete	Mature male or female reproductive cell
Gametogenesis	Development of gametes
Homozygous	Trait of an organism produced by identical or nearly identical alleles

Continued

LEARNING OBJECTIVES

After studying this chapter, the learner will be able to do the following:

1. **Characterize chromosome abnormalities.**

   Study text pages 135 through 143; refer to Figures 4-12, 4-17, and 4-19.

   In **chromosome abnormalities,** the defect is due to an abnormality in **chromosome number** or **structure.** The structure of the genes in chromosome disorders may be normal, but the genes may be present in multiple copies or be situated on a different chromosome.

   Normal somatic cells that have two sets of 23 chromosomes are **diploid** (double) or 2N. Gametes with a single set of 23 chromosomes are **haploid** (single) or N. A cell with an exact multiple of the haploid number is **euploid.** Euploid numbers may be 2N, 3N (triploid), or 4N (tetraploid). Chromosome numbers that are exact multiples of N but that are greater than 2N are called **polyploid.** **Aneuploid** refers to a chromosome complement that is abnormal in number but that is not an exact multiple of N. An aneuploid cell may be **trisomic** (2N + 1 chromosome) or **monosomic** (2N − 1 chromosome). Any cell with a chromosome number that deviates from the characteristic N and 2N is **heteroploid.**

   Disjunction is the normal separation and migration of chromosomes during cell division. Failure of the process, or **nondisjunction,** in a meiotic division results in one daughter cell receiving both homologous chromosomes and the other receiving neither; it is the primary cause of aneuploidy. If this deviation in normal processes occurs during the first meiotic division, half of the gametes will contain 22 chromosomes and half will contain 24. If joined with a normal gamete, a gamete produced in this manner will produce either a monosomic (2N − 1) or trisomic (2N + 1) zygote.

   Deviations in the normal structure of chromosomes result from the chromosome material breaking and reassembling in an abnormal arrangement. These changes in structure may be stable and persist through future cell divisions. Stable types of structural abnormalities include deletion, duplication, inversion, and translocation.

   In **deletion,** which is the loss of a portion of a chromosome, the missing segment may be a terminal portion of the chromosome that results from a single break or an internal section that results from two breaks.

   Duplication is the presence of a repeated gene or gene sequence. A deleted segment of one chromosome may become incorporated into its homologous chromosome.

   Inversion is the reversal of gene order. The linear arrangement of genes on a chromosome is broken, and the order of a portion of the gene complement is reversed in the process of reattachment.

   Translocation is the transfer of part of one chromosome to a nonhomologous chromosome. This occurs when two chromosomes break and the segments are rejoined in an abnormal arrangement.

22

2. Cite examples of chromosome disorders.

Refer to Figures 4-13 through 4-16 and 4-18 through 4-20.

A common example of a disorder that results from an abnormality of chromosome number is trisomy 21, or **Down syndrome.** This disorder can result when nondisjunction of chromosome 21 occurs at meiosis, thereby producing one gamete with an extra chromosome 21 (N + 1 = 24) and one gamete with no chromosome 21 (Ñ − 1 = 22). Union of the 24-chromosome gamete with a normal sperm produces a 47-chromosome zygote, or trisomy 21.

The overall incidence of Down syndrome is 1 per 800 live births; the incidence increases with increasing maternal age. Clinical diagnosis of trisomy 21 is often based on facial appearance. The nose is small, and the facial profile is flat. Mental retardation is consistent in children with Down syndrome, but its degree may vary. The average IQ is approximately 50.

A fragile site located on the long arm of the X chromosome is associated with a disorder known as **fragile X syndrome.** Fragile X syndrome is the most common genetic cause of mental retardation after Down syndrome. Males who inherit the mutation may not express the disease but can pass it to descendants who express the disease, irrespective of gender.

Two other chromosomal disorders are **Turner syndrome** (female) and **Klinefelter syndrome** (male). The most common karyotype showing female phenotype is 45 X; the male karyotype is 47 XXY.

The overall incidence of Turner syndrome is 1 per 3000 female births. The frequency at conception is higher, but 99% of fetuses with this condition spontaneously abort. The diagnosis is suggested in the newborn by the presence of redundant neck skin and peripheral edema. Later, the presence of short stature or primary amenorrhea is suggestive of the condition.

The incidence of Klinefelter syndrome is 1 per 1000 males. This syndrome is the most common cause of hypogonadism and infertility in men; female breasts develops in about 50% of cases.

Cri du chat syndrome is caused by deletion of part of the short arm of chromosome 5. Symptoms include the "cry of the cat" by the affected child, low birth weight, severe mental retardation, small head size, heart defects, and abnormal facial appearance.

3. Characterize single-gene disorders.

Study text pages 145, 146, and 148 through 155; refer to Figures 4-21, 4-22, and 4-28 through 4-30.

Single-gene disorders are caused by the genetic code, which is the sequence of nucleotides, in a single gene. Each gene has a specific site or locus on a specific chromosome. The inherited gene may be present on one or both chromosomes of a pair. The pedigree patterns of inherited traits are dependent on whether the gene is located on an autosomal chromosome, which is any chromosome other than a sex chromosome, or the X chromosome and whether the gene is dominant or recessive. There are no known Y-linked genetic disorders. These factors allow for four basic patterns of inheritance for single-gene traits, whether normal or abnormal: autosomal dominant, autosomal recessive, X-linked dominant, and X-linked recessive.

In **autosomal dominant** inheritance of a genetic defect, the abnormal allele is dominant, and the normal allele is recessive. The phenotype is the same whether the allele is present in a homozygous or a heterozygous state.

Characteristics of autosomal dominant inheritance are that (1) affected people have an affected parent; (2) affected people mating with normal people have affected and unaffected offspring in equal proportion; (3) unaffected children born to affected parents have unaffected children; and (4) males and females are equally affected.

In **autosomal recessive** disorders, the abnormal allele is recessive. For the trait to be expressed, a person must be homozygous for the abnormal allele. Because the dominant or normal allele masks the trait, most people who are heterozygous for an autosomal recessive allele go undetected. When two heterozygous individuals mate and an offspring receives the recessive allele from each parent, the trait is expressed. Procreation by people who are blood relatives may increase the probability of expression.

Characteristics of autosomal recessive inheritance are that (1) the trait usually appears in siblings only, not in the parents; (2) males and females are equally likely to be affected; (3) for parents of one affected child, the recurrence risk is one in four for every subsequent birth; (4) both parents of an affected child carry the recessive allele; and (5) the parents of the affected child may be consanguineous or blood relatives.

Of the 23 pairs of chromosomes that determine the karyotype of the human, 22 are **autosomes** and 1 is the **sex chromosome.** Unlike the 44 autosomes that can be arranged in 22 homologous pairs, the two sex chromosomes in the female are XX, and in the male they are XY. Because the ovum must contain an X chromosome, if it is fertilized by a sperm that contains an X chromosome, the progeny will be a female (XX). If the sperm contributes a Y chromosome, the progeny will be male (XY).

Traits determined by either dominant or recessive **X-linked genes** are expressed in the male. The genes on the X chromosome cannot be transmitted from father to son (fathers contribute a Y chromosome to sons), but they are transmitted from father to all daughters through one X chromosome. Recessive abnormal genes on the X chromosome of a female may not be expressed, because they are matched by normal genes inherited with the other X chromosome.

X-linked dominant disorders are rare. Most X-linked diseases are recessive.

In **X-linked recessive disorders,** the recessive gene located on the one X chromosome of the male is not balanced by the dominant allele on the Y chromosome and is thus expressed. Only matings between an affected male and a carrier (affected) female should result in an affected female.

Males affected with an X-linked recessive disorder cannot transmit the gene to sons, but they transmit it to all daughters. An unaffected female who is heterozygous for the recessive gene transmits it to 50% of her sons and daughters.

Characteristics of the X-linked recessive inheritance are that (1) males are predominantly affected; (2) affected males cannot transmit the gene to sons, but they transmit the gene to all daughters; (3) sons of female carriers have a 50% risk of being affected; and (4) daughters of female carriers have a 50% risk of being carriers.

4. Cite examples of well-known single-gene disorders.
Study text pages 148, 149, 151, 152, and 154; refer to Figures 4-23 through 4-25 and 4-27.

One of the most well-known autosomal dominant diseases is **Huntington disease,** a neurologic disorder that exhibits progressive dementia and increasingly uncontrollable movements of the limbs. One of the key features of this disease is that its symptoms are not usually seen until after age 40. Thus, those who develop the disease often have had children before they are aware that they have the gene.

The severity of an autosomal dominant disease can vary greatly. An example of variable expressivity in an autosomal dominant disease is **type 1 neurofibromatosis,** or von Recklinghausen disease, which has been mapped to the long arm of chromosome 17. The expression of this gene can vary from a few harmless café-au-lait spots on the skin to numerous malignant neurofibromas, scoliosis, seizures, gliomas, neuromas, hypertension, and mental retardation.

The **cystic fibrosis** gene, which is the cause of a lethal autosomal recessive gene, has been mapped to the long arm of chromosome 7. In this disease, defective transport of chloride ions leads to a salt imbalance that results in secretions of abnormally thick, dehydrated mucus. Some of the digestive organs, particularly the pancreas, become obstructed with mucus, and this results in malnutrition. The lung airways tend to become clogged with mucus, thereby making them highly susceptible to bacterial infections.

The most common and severe of all X-linked recessive disorders is **Duchenne muscular dystrophy,** which affects males. This disorder is characterized by progressive muscle degeneration; individuals are usually unable to walk by age 10 or 12 years. If **dystrophin** is not encoded and absent, the muscle cell cannot survive, and muscle deterioration occurs. The disease also affects the heart and respiratory muscles, and death due to respiratory or cardiac failure may occur before age 20; these cases are generally due to frameshift deletions, in which all of the amino acids are altered after the deletion.

PRACTICE EXAMINATION

Multiple Choice

Circle the correct answer(s) for each question.

1. Which genetic disease is caused by an abnormal karyotype?
   a. Down syndrome
   b. Huntington disease
   c. Phenylketonuria
   d. Neurofibromatosis
   e. Cystic fibrosis
2. Down syndrome usually occurs because of:
   a. an abnormal X chromosome.
   b. nondisjunction by older ova.
   c. an autosomal dominant gene.
   d. an autosomal recessive gene.
3. Cri-du-chat syndrome is an abnormality of chromosomal structure that involves:
   a. translocation.
   b. an inversion.
   c. duplication.
   d. deletion.
4. Fragile X syndrome can affect intelligence and behavior in:
   a. males only.
   b. females only.
   c. both males and females.
   d. neither because affected fetuses are aborted.
5. If homologous chromosomes fail to separate during meiosis, the disorder is:
   a. polyploidy.
   b. aneuploidy.
   c. disjunction.
   d. nondisjunction.
   e. translocation.
6. Cystic fibrosis has been mapped to chromosome:
   a. 17.
   b. 7.
   c. X.
   d. 16.
7. In autosomal dominant inherited disorders:
   a. affected individuals do not have an affected parent.
   b. affected individuals who mate with unaffected people have a 50% risk of having an affected offspring.
   c. male offspring are most often affected.
   d. unaffected children born to affected parents will have affected children.

8. In X-linked recessive inherited disorders:
   a. affected males have normal sons.
   b. affected males have affected daughters.
   c. sons of female carriers have a 50% risk of being affected.
   d. the affected male transmits the gene to all daughters, thus, they are carriers.
9. Duchenne muscular dystrophy is:
   a. a sex-linked genetic disease wherein dystrophin is not encoded.
   b. an autosomal recessive disease.
   c. an autosomal dominant disease.
   d. mapped to chromosome 17.
10. If a male inherits an autosomal recessive disorder, he inherited it from his:
   a. mother.
   b. father.
   c. mother and father.
11. Trisomy 21 syndrome is caused by:
   a. paternal disjunction.
   b. maternal disjunction.
   c. maternal translocation.
   d. maternal nondisjunction.

Matching

Match the term with the correct circumstance.

____ 12. Recessive disorder

____ 13. Genotype

____ 14. Aneuploidy

____ 15. Chromosomal aberration

____ 16. Phenotype

____ 17. Pedigree

____ 18. Autosomal recessive inheritance

a. due to numerical or structural aberrations

b. gene combination

c. a cell with fewer or more chromosomes than normal

d. individual homozygous for a gene

e. failure of homologous chromosomes to separate during meiosis or mitosis

f. outward appearance of an individual

g. a probability of 0.25

h. expresses genes

Match the term with the correct circumstance.

____ 19. Expressivity

____ 20. X-linked

____ 21. Inversion

____ 22. Dominant trait

____ 23. Allele

____ 24. 47 XXY

____ 25. Karyotype

a. a probability of 0.5

b. females unlikely to be affected

c. species chromosomal morphology

d. one allele permits expression

e. Turner syndrome

f. different version of the same paired gene

g. Klinefelter syndrome

h. no loss or gain of genetic material

i. extent of phenotypic variation of a particular genotype

Mrs. S.J. is a 42-year-old woman who is pregnant for the first time and who was admitted to the labor and delivery unit. She appears to be in excellent health, and this anticipated delivery is the culmination of an uneventful pregnancy. Her admitting blood pressure and pulse and the fetal heart rate were normal. Eight hours after admission, Mrs. S.J. delivered a 7-pound, 3-ounce baby boy. The baby had low-set ears, a flat facial profile with a small nose, wide epicanthal folds, and simian creases. The parents were told, "Your baby's features are the result of a genetic aberration and your infant son has Down syndrome." The parents ask, "Why did this happen and what is the future for our son?"

Question

How would you answer the parents' questions?

5 Genes, Environment, and Common Diseases

FOUNDATIONAL KNOWLEDGE OBJECTIVE

After reviewing the primary text where referenced, the learner will be able to do the following:
a. Describe inheritance and environmental interactions.
Review text pages 165, 166, and 169 through 171.

MEMORY CHECK!

- The struggle between nature (genetic traits) and nature environment with regard to disease causality continues today. However, good epidemiologic data are now making distinctions and establishing relationships. The relative impact of genes and environments varies with each disease. For example, an extra chromosome 21 is manifested regardless of environment; it has only a genetic basis. However, an individual who is genetically lacking the enzyme to metabolize the amino acid phenylalanine could develop brain damage and mental retardation only if exposed to dietary phenylalanine. This, then, is a disease that requires both an inherited defect and an environmental exposure.

LEARNING OBJECTIVES

After studying this chapter, the learner will be able to do the following:

1. Define terms used to analyze relationships between disease and populations.
Study text pages 164 through 172; refer to Figures 5-1, 5-2, and 5-4 and Tables 5-1 through 5-5. See the table at top of page 28 of this study guide.

2. Identify the criteria used to describe multifactorial disease.
Study text pages 167 through 169.

Several criteria can be used to define multifactorial inheritance. First, the **recurrence risk** becomes higher if more than one family member is affected. If two siblings have the same defect, the recurrence risk is greater than if only one sibling has the defect; the family has more genetic or environmental risk factors and is more likely to produce an affected child. In single-gene diseases, the recurrence risk is the same regardless of the number of affected siblings.

Second, if the disease is expressed in the proband and is severe, the recurrence risk is higher. A more severe expression indicates that the affected individual is at the extreme end of liability distribution and that his or her relatives are at a higher risk of inheriting the disease genes.

Third, the recurrence risk is higher if the proband is of the less commonly affected sex. This is because an affected individual of the less susceptible gender is usually at a more extreme position of the liability distribution.

Fourth, the recurrence risk for the disease usually decreases rapidly in more remotely related relatives. This is because many genes and environmental factors must combine to produce a trait or disease. All risk factors are unlikely to be present in less-closely related family members.

Last, if the **prevalence** of the disease in a population is defined as *f*, the risk for offspring and siblings of probands is approximately equal to the square root of *f*. This is not true of single-gene traits, because their recurrence risks are independent of population prevalence.

Population Incidence and Prevalence Terms

Terms	Definitions
Proband	Individual with whom the pedigree begins
Incidence rate	Number of new cases of a disease divided by the number of individuals in the population in a defined time
Prevalence rate	Proportion of the population affected by a disease at a specific time
Relative risk	Ratio of the frequency of a disease in populations exposed and populations not exposed to a particular factor
Polygenic	Traits or diseases caused by the combined effects of multiple genes
Multifactorial	Type of disease that results from the interaction of many factors, usually polygenes influenced by environmental factors
Liability distribution	Diseases that are present or absent in individuals that do not follow the inheritance patterns of single-gene diseases
Threshold of liability	Present or absent diseases that appear when the threshold is exceeded; below the threshold, the disease is not expressed
Recurrence risk	Ratio of the reappearance of a disease in a diseased population after a period of remission
Empirical risk	Risk based on direct observation of the disease in the siblings of a diseased proband
Concordant	Both members of a twin pair share a disease; identical twins should be concordant
Discordant	Members of a twin pair do not share the disease; fraternal twins are concordant less often than are identical twins
Congenital	Diseases present at birth; genetic information is intact, but intrauterine environment may cause malformations

3. **Describe the relationship between genetics and the environment or lifestyle as causal factors in diseases.**

Study text pages 170 and 171; refer to Figure 5-4 and Table 5-3.

Family members share genes and a common environment. Family resemblance in traits such as blood pressure reflects both genetic and environmental–lifestyle commonality (**"nature"** and **"nurture,"** respectively). Few traits are influenced only by genes or only by environment or lifestyle factors; most are influenced by both. A disease in which the genetic influence is relatively small, such as lung cancer, may be prevented most effectively through emphasis on lifestyle changes (avoidance of tobacco). When a disease has a relatively larger genetic component, as in breast cancer, family history is important in addition to lifestyle modification.

Twin studies and adoption studies are used to estimate the relative influence of genes and environment. **Monozygotic (MZ, or "identical") twins** originate when the developing embryo divides to form two separate but identical embryos. Because they are genetically identical, MZ twins are an example of natural clones. **Dizygotic (DZ, or "fraternal") twins** are the result of a double ovulation followed by the fertilization of each egg by a different sperm.

Because MZ twins are genetically identical, any differences between them should be caused only by environmental effects. MZ twins should thus resemble one another very closely for traits that are strongly influenced by genes. DZ twins provide a convenient comparison, because their environmental differences should be similar to those of MZ twins, but their genetic differences are as great as those between siblings. Twin studies thus usually consist of comparisons between MZ and DZ twins. If both members of a twin pair share a trait, it is said to be a **concordant trait.** If they do not share the trait, it is a **discordant trait.** For a trait determined totally by genes, MZ twins should always be concordant, whereas DZ twins should be concordant less often, because they, like siblings, share only 50% of their genes.

Studies of adopted children also are used to estimate the genetic contribution to a multifactorial trait. Children who are born to parents who have a disease but are adopted by parents lacking the disease can be studied to find out whether they develop the disease. In some cases, such children develop the disease more often than a comparative control population (i.e., adopted children who were born to parents who do not have the disease). This provides some evidence that genes may be involved in the causation of the disease, because the adopted children do not share an environment with their affected natural parents.

Genetic and nongenetic factors usually interact to influence one's likelihood of developing a common disease. In some cases, a genetic predisposition may interact with an environmental factor to increase the risk of disease to a much higher level than would either factor acting alone. A good example of a gene−environment−lifestyle interaction is given by α_1-antitrypsin deficiency, a genetic condition that causes pulmonary emphysema and is greatly exacerbated by cigarette smoking.

Complex Genetic/Environmental Diseases

Disease: Genetic Contributors	Contributing Environmental Factors
Gastrointestinal Disorders	
Colon cancer: mutated APC tumor suppressor genes	High-fat, low-fiber diet
Type 1 diabetes: HLA Class II alleles	Viral infections triggering immune responses
Type 2 diabetes: adipocyte and glucose metabolism genes	Obesity, dietary sugar
Obesity: leptin and its receptor genes control appetite	Excessive caloric intake
Cardiovascular Disorders	
Coronary heart disease: LDL and apolipoprotein genes	Saturated fat intake, minimal exercise, smoking, elevated cholesterol
Hypertension, stroke: angiotensinogen genes	Fat intake, minimal exercise, smoking, stress
Neuromuscular Disorders	
Alzheimer disease: presenilin genes cleave amyloid protein, apolipoprotein E gene precludes cleavage of amyloid	Advancing age
Psychiatric disorders: gene for excitatory neurotransmitter	Fetal neural defects, stressors, traumatic injury
Alcoholism: genes encoding for inhibitory neuro-transmitter GABA	Social reinforcement
Breast Disorder	
Female breast cancer: *BRCA1, BRCA2*, and mutated tumor suppressor genes	High fat intake, alcohol overuse, ionizing radiation

4. **Identify some major system diseases that exhibit familial tendencies; suggest possible contributing environmental or lifestyle factors in these diseases.**
   Study text pages 172 through 180; refer to Figures 5-5 through 5-7 and Table 5-6. See the table above.

5. **State some general principles about complex multifactorial disorders.**
   Study text page 180.

First, the more strongly inherited forms of complex disorders such as Alzheimer and heart disease generally have an earlier age of onset. These complex diseases often represent conditions in which there is single-gene inheritance, so they are experienced early. Second, the bilateral forms (e.g., bilateral rather than unilateral cleft lip) are more likely to cluster strongly in families. Third, although the sex-specific threshold model fits some of the complex disorders, such as pyloric stenosis, cleft lip/palate, autism, and heart disease, it fails to fit others, such as type 1 diabetes. Environmental modifications, such as improved diet, increased exercise, and reduced stress, often significantly reduce the risk for individuals who have a family history of a particular disease. This means that the course of a disease can be altered.

PRACTICE EXAMINATION

True or False

For each statement, write T (true) or F (false) in the blank provided.

_____ 1. Hypertension is a multifactorial disease.

_____ 2. Fat intake is controlled by leptin and its receptor genes.

_____ 3. A multifactorial trait is expressed when multiple genes and environmental influences blend together.

_____ 4. In Down syndrome, the pathology is manifested independent of environment.

_____ 5. It is easy to distinguish between the effect of shared environmental factors and the effects of a common pool of genes.

_____ 6. Psychiatric disorders depend on genes encoding for inhibitor neurotransmitters.

_____ 7. Relative risk is a ratio between incidence and individuals.

_____ 8. Early type 2 diabetes may develop when an individual's diet changes to include heavy carbohydrate consumption.

_____ 9. Finding and understanding environmental factors that affect the penetrance of specific genes are important if chronic familial diseases are to be prevented.

_____ 10. A variation in the phenotype for different genotypes caused by environmental factors is a threshold liability trait.

_____ 11. The frequency of genetic disease in the population depends on phenotypes.

_____ 12. Risk factors, when removed or eliminated, delay or prevent disease.

_____ 13. A proband is the individual who began the pedigree.

_____ 14. The recurrence risk is less when more than one sibling is affected.

_____ 15. The existence of a particular risk factor indicates that an individual will develop a specific disease.

_____ 16. The expression of a disease may require both an inherited defect and environmental exposure.

_____ 17. Multifactorial diseases can change substantially from one population to another because gene frequencies and environments differ.

_____ 18. Dizygotic twins are identical.

_____ 19. Recurrence risk is higher if the disease is more severe in the proband.

_____ 20. The prevalence rate is the number of individuals affected with a disease.

_____ 21. The incidence rate is the number of people who have died from a disease.

Matching

Match the genetic disease with the environmental factor(s).

_____ 22. Type 1 diabetes

_____ 23. Hypertension

_____ 24. Colon cancer

_____ 25. Coronary artery disease

a. wheat gluten

b. high-fat, low-fiber diet

c. minimal exercise

d. iron absorption

e. streptococcal infection

f. pollen exposure

g. viral infections

h. elevated serum cholesterol

30

Mrs. C. is a 58-year-old, recently widowed black woman who was admitted to the emergency department because of shortness of breath and palpitations. She states, "My shortness of breath is worst when I am lying flat or climbing stairs." After climbing stairs, Mrs. C. indicates that her heart "continues to pound" for several minutes.

Physical examination showed Mrs. C. to be well oriented and her mucous membranes and nail beds to be pink. Her skin was cool and dry. Mrs. C.'s blood pressure was 200/120 mmHg, and her heart rate was 110 beats per minute and strong but irregular. Respirations were 30 per minute and labored. The cardiac monitor displayed atrial fibrillations with premature ventricular response. Neither Mrs. C.'s electrocardiograms nor her cardiac enzyme levels indicated myocardial infarction. Appropriate in-hospital intervention reduced Mrs. C.'s blood pressure.

Questions

What is the likely discharge diagnosis?

What are contributors to its development?

31

6 | Innate Immunity: Inflammation

PREREQUISITE KNOWLEDGE OBJECTIVES

After reviewing the primary text where referenced, the learner will be able to do the following:
1. **Identify human defense mechanisms.**
   Review text page 184; refer to Table 6-1.
2. **Describe the first line of defense.**
   Review text pages 184 through 186; refer to Figure 6-1 and Table 6-1.
3. **State the components of the second line of defense: the inflammatory response.**
   Refer to Figure 6-2 and Table 6-2.
   NOTE: Inflammation is considered to be a nonspecific, rapid response by (1) vascularized tissue, (2) plasma protein systems, (3) cellular mediators, and (4) cellular products. These responses are initiated against a wide variety of causes that damage tissue.
4. **Describe the inflammatory changes occurring at the vascular level.**
   Review text pages 186 and 187; refer to Figures 6-2 through 6-4.
5. **Identify the plasma protein systems and their interactions during inflammation.**
   Review text pages 187 through 192; refer to Figures 6-5 through 6-8.
6. **Describe the recognition of biochemical and cellular mediators of inflammation by cellular receptors.**
   Review text pages 192, 194, and 195; refer to Table 6-2.
7. **Identify the causes of mast cell degranulation and the effects of the released preformed granular mediators.**
   Review text pages 195 and 196; refer to Figures 6-9 and 6-10.
8. **State the effects of lipid-derived, synthesized inflammatory mediators of mast cells.**
   Review test pages 196 through 198; refer to Figure 6-12.
9. **Describe the process of phagocytosis.**
   Review text pages 198 through 201; refer to Figures 6-11 through 6-13 and Table 6-3.
10. **Identify a role for neutrophils, monocytes, macrophages, eosinophils, natural killer (NK) cells, and platelets in the inflammatory process.**
    Review text pages 201 through 203; refer to Figure 6-14.

11. **State the roles of the cellular products interleukins, interferons, tumor necrosis factor-alpha, and chemokines.**
    Review text pages 203 through 205; refer to Figures 6-15 and 6-17.
12. **Name and describe the local and systemic signs of acute inflammation.**
    Review text pages 205 and 206; refer to Table 6-4.
13. **Characterize chronic inflammation.**
    Review text pages 206 through 208; refer to Figures 6-17 and 6-18.
14. **Differentiate between resolution and repair processes, and identify factors that promote healing.**
    Review text pages 208 and 210 through 212; refer to Figures 6-19 and 6-20.
15. **Compare pediatric and aging mechanisms of self-defense.**
    Review text pages 212 and 213.

PRACTICE EXAMINATION

Multiple Choice
Circle the correct answer for each question.
1. Innate resistance or immunity:
   a. involves "memory."
   b. is a development of an individual's later years.
   c. is a relatively slow and specific process.
   d. depends on physical, mechanical, and biochemical barriers.
2. Collectins:
   a. are triple-stranded sheets.
   b. protect against respiratory infections.
   c. are produced by monocytes.
   d. are produced by neutrophils.
3. Complement is:
   a. a series of proteins in the blood.
   b. an antibody.
   c. a hormone.
   d. a lymphokine.
4. Diapedesis is a process in which:
   a. neutrophils migrate from the bloodstream to an injured tissue site.
   b. phagocytes stick to capillary and venule walls.
   c. bacteria are "coated" with an opsonin.
   d. there is oxygen-dependent killing of cells.

5. Interferon:
   a. interferes with the ability of bacteria to cause disease.
   b. prevents viruses from infecting healthy host cells.
   c. inhibits macrophage migration from inflamed sites.
   d. increases the phagocytic activity of macrophages.
6. The sequence of inflammatory events within the vasculature is:
   a. slower blood flow, arteriolar vasoconstriction, increased capillary permeability, and site of injury edema.
   b. arteriolar vasoconstriction, vasodilation, increased capillary permeability, plasma leakage, and site of injury edema.
   c. vasodilation, vasoconstriction, decreased local blood flow to injured site, and site of injury edema.
   d. blood becomes more viscous, vasodilation, increased capillary permeability, and site of injury edema.
7. The inflammatory response:
   a. prevents blood from entering the injured tissue.
   b. elevates body temperature to prevent spread of infection.
   c. prevents the formation of abscesses.
   d. minimizes injury and promotes healing.
8. The alternative complement pathway is activated by:
   a. antibodies binding to specific antigens.
   b. certain bacterial carbohydrates.
   c. gram-negative bacterial and fungal cell wall polysaccharides.
   d. a plasma protein called mannose-binding lectin.
9. The C3b subcomponent of complement:
   a. opsonizes microbes to facilitate phagocytosis.
   b. dilates arterioles.
   c. lyses cells.
   d. induces rapid degranulation of mast cells.
10. The activation of Hageman factor impacts all three plasma protein systems by:
    a. activation of the clotting cascade through factor X.
    b. control of clotting by degradation of plasmin.
    c. activation of the kinin system by a fragment of Hageman factor.
    d. activation of C5 in the complement cascade.
11. The sequence for phagocytosis is:
    a. margination or pavementing, recognition of the target, adherence or binding, and fusion with lysosomes inside the phagocyte.
    b. diapedesis, margination or pavementing, phagosome formation, recognition of the target, and fusion with lysosomes inside the phagocyte.
    c. recognition of the target, margination or pavementing, and destruction of the target by lysosomal enzymes.
    d. margination, diapedesis, recognition, adherence, ingestion, fusion with lysosomes inside the phagocyte, and destruction of the target.

12. Swelling during acute inflammation is caused by:
    a. collagenase.
    b. the fluid exudate.
    c. lymphocytic margination.
    d. neutrophilic margination.
    e. anaerobic glycolysis.
13. Recognition of abnormal environmental components so cells can respond to these substances is by binding to cell surface receptors. Cells involved in innate resistance have:
    a. T-cell receptors (TCRs).
    b. B-cell receptors (BCRs).
    c. pathogen-associated molecular patterns (PAMPs).
    d. pattern recognition receptors (PRRs).
14. Mast cell degranulation releases:
    a. histamine, neutrophil chemotactic factor, and leukotrienes.
    b. histamine, IL-4, and eosinophil chemotactic factor of anaphylaxis.
    c. histamine and prostaglandins.
    d. histamine and platelet-activating factor.
15. Interleukin 10:
    a. is a proinflammatory cytokine and an endogenous pyrogen.
    b. increases the number of circulating neutrophils.
    c. suppresses growth of lymphocytes and production of proinflammatory cytokines.
    d. increases lysosomal enzyme activity.
16. Soluble tumor necrosis factor-alpha:
    a. is secreted by neutrophils.
    b. enhances endothelial cell adhesion molecule expression.
    c. induces fever by acting as an exogenous pyrogen.
    d. causes decreased synthesis of inflammatory serum proteins by the liver.
17. Characteristic systemic manifestations of acute inflammation include:
    a. leukopenia.
    b. a "right shift" in the ratio of immature to mature neutrophils.
    c. reduced host susceptibility to the effects of endotoxins.
    d. fever caused by the release of IL-1 by neutrophils and macrophages.
18. Chronic inflammation is characterized by:
    a. hypertrophy.
    b. metaplasia.
    c. neutrophilic infiltration.
    d. lymphocytic and macrophagic infiltration.
19. Scar tissue is:
    a. nonfunctional collagenous and fibrotic tissue.
    b. functional tissue that follows wound healing.
    c. regenerated tissue formed in the area of injury.
    d. fibrinogen that has entrapped phagocytes and neurons.

Fill in the Blanks

Supply the correct response for each statement.

20. _____ are the predominant phagocytes arriving early at inflammatory and infection sites.

21. _____, unlike neutrophils and basophils, function for a longer time and later in the inflammatory response and are involved in the activation of the adaptive immune system.

22. _____ serve as primary defenders against parasites and help regulate vascular mediators released from mast cells by preventing more inflammatory activity than is needed.

23. _____ recognize and eliminate virus-infected cells and cancerous cells.

24. _____ returns injured tissues to an approximation of their original structure and physiologic function.

25. _____ is filled with new capillaries and is surrounded by fibroblasts and macrophages.

7 | Adaptive Immunity

PREREQUISITE KNOWLEDGE OBJECTIVES

After reviewing the the primary text where referenced, the learner will be able to do the following:

1. **Describe antigens, immunoglobulins, and immunocompetent lymphocytes; and list antigenic substances.**
   Review text pages 217 through 219; refer to Figures 7-1 through 7-3 and Table 7-1.

2. **Distinguish between humoral and cell-mediated immunity and between active and passive immunity.**
   Review text pages 219 and 220.

3. **Identify the structures and important roles of each of the five immunoglobulins.**
   Review text pages 222 through 226 and 244 through 247; refer to Figures 7-5 through 7-7 and 7-26 and Tables 7-3 and 7-4.

4. **Characterize antigens and their antigen determinant sites or epitopes and antigen-binding sites or paratopes. Distinguish among the CD, MHC, HLA, BCR, and TCR recognition molecules.**
   Review text pages 221 through 228; refer to Figures 7-5 through 7-9 and Table 7-2.

5. **Identify adhesion molecule pairings that result in intracellular signaling.**
   Refer to Box 7-1.

6. **Characterize the functional relationship between cytokines and their receptors.**
   Review text pages 228 and 229; refer to Table 7-5.

7. **Distinguish generation of clonal diversity from clonal selection.**
   Review text pages 229 through 236; refer to Table 7-6.

8. **Describe T-cell maturation.**
   Review text pages 230 through 233; refer to Figures 7-10 and 7-11.

9. **Describe B-cell maturation.**
   Review text pages 233 through 235; refer to Figures 7-12 and 7-13.

10. **Characterize antigen processing and presentation and the role of helper T cells.**
    Review text pages 235 through 240; refer to Figures 7-14 through 7-17.

11. **Describe the role of the B cell in humoral immunity, distinguish between primary and secondary immunity.**

Review text pages 240 through 243; refer to Figures 7-18 through 7-21.

12. **Describe the roles of various T cells in cell-mediated immunity; identify the role of superantigens.**
    Review text pages 243, 244, and 247 through 250; refer to Figures 7-22, 7-23, 7-27, and 7-28.

13. **Indicate the effects of aging on immune function.**
    Review text page 251; refer to Figures 7-29 and 7-30.

Multiple Choice

Circle the correct answer for each question.

1. Immunogenicity depends on:
   a. host foreignness.
   b. tolerance.
   c. chemical simplicity.
   d. low-molecular-weight molecules.

2. Which of the following are capable of forming clones?
   a. Helper T cells
   b. Cytotoxic T cells
   c. B cells
   d. Both T and B cells

3. Which cells are stimulated by IL-2?
   a. B cells
   b. T cells and NK cells
   c. Mast cells
   d. Thymic epithelial cells

4. Which bind with MHC class I molecules?
   a. helper T cells
   b. cytotoxic T cells
   c. B cells
   d. both B and T cells

5. HLAs:
   a. when dissimilar in transplanted tissue or organs, the more likely the transplant will be successful.
   b. are not found on the surfaces of erythrocytes.
   c. are found on the surfaces of very few human cells.
   d. are not MHC molecules.

6. CD4 markers are associated with:
   a. cytotoxic T cells.
   b. suppressor T cells.
   c. helper T cells.
   d. Antigen presenting cells (APCs).

7. Antibodies are produced by:
   a. B cells.
   b. T cells.
   c. helper cells.
   d. plasma cells.
   e. memory cells.
8. An immunoglobulin contains:
   a. two heavy and two light polypeptide chains.
   b. four heavy and four light polypeptide chains.
   c. two heavy and four light polypeptide chains.
   d. four heavy and two light polypeptide chains.
9. The antibody class that has the highest concentration in the blood is:
   a. IgA.
   b. IgD.
   c. IgE.
   d. IgG.
   e. IgM.
10. Which of the following antibodies is matched with its appropriate role?
    a. IgA/allergic reactions
    b. IgD/found in respiratory secretions
    c. IgE/found in gastric secretions
    d. IgG/first to challenge the antigen
    e. IgM/first to challenge the antigen
11. The primary immune response involves:
    a. a rapid plasma cell response with peak antibody levels by 3 days.
    b. macrophage production of antibodies.
    c. T cell production of antibodies.
    d. a latent period followed by peak antibody production.
12. The B-cell receptor (BCR) complex consists of:
    a. IgG or IgD antibody.
    b. IgE or IgD antibody.
    c. antibody-like transmembrane protein.
    d. antigen-recognition molecules
13. Cytokines and their receptors function:
    a. as intracellular chemical signals.
    b. as chemical signals between cells.
    c. as negative regulators of acquired immune responses.
    d. to decrease the production of proteins.
14. Clonal selection:
    a. occurs primarily in the fetus.
    b. induces central tolerance.
    c. occurs primarily after birth and throughout life.
    d. occurs in central lymphoid organs.
15. Immunologic tolerance develops because:
    a. self-reactive lymphocytes are eliminated in the primary lymphoid organs.
    b. self-reactive lymphocytes are inactivated in the secondary lymphoid organs.
    c. lymphocytes remember their first exposure to the antigen.
    d. T cells may reprogram themselves by receptor editing.
16. Endogenous antigens:
    a. are carried on microorganisms that are phagocytized.
    b. are presented by class II major histocompatibility complex (MHC) molecules.
    c. may be produced by cancerous cells.
    d. are digested in a lysosomal environment.
17. Cytotoxic T cells:
    a. inhibit extracellular viruses.
    b. inhibit virus-infected cells.
    c. inhibit viral protein synthesis.
    d. decrease expression of MHC molecules.
18. Antibody is effective against:
    a. extracellular viruses.
    b. virus-infected cells.
    c. viral protein synthesis.
    d. expression of MHC molecules.
19. Adhesion molecule pairings involve:
    a. cytotoxic T cell CD4 ↔ MHC class II on APC.
    b. cytotoxic T cell CD8 ↔ MHC class I on APC.
    c. helper T cell CD2 ↔ CD58 on APC.
    d. helper T cell CD4OL ↔ MHC class II on APC.
20. Transforming growth factor (TGF) functions to:
    a. increase phagocytosis.
    b. increase expression of MHC class II.
    c. be chemotactic for neutrophils and T cells.
    d. stimulate wound healing

Fill in the Blanks

Supply the correct response for each statement.

21. _____ are necessary to induce both humoral and cellular immune responses.

22. A second challenge by the same, earlier antigen results in an _____ immune response characterized by more antibody production in a shorter time than the initial or first challenge.

23. _____ function to avoid attacking self-antigens or avoid overactivation of immune responses.

24. _____ cause activation of large populations of T lymphocytes irrespective of antigen specificity.

25. The _____ consists of antibodies in bodily secretions that protect the body against antigens yet to penetrate the skin or mucous membranes.

38

8 Alterations in Immunity and Inflammation

FOUNDATIONAL KNOWLEDGE OBJECTIVES

After reviewing the primary text where referenced, the learner will be able to do the following:

a. **Diagram a scheme for the role of complement in the amplification of the immune response. Relate opsonization, inflammation, and cytolysis to the components of complement.**
   Review text pages 188 through 190; refer to Figure 6-5.

MEMORY CHECK!

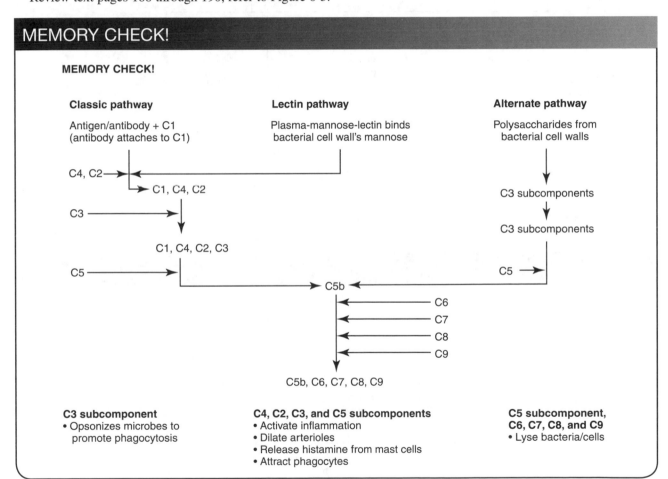

MEMORY CHECK!

Classic pathway

Antigen/antibody + C1
(antibody attaches to C1)

C4, C2 →

→ C1, C4, C2

C3 →

C1, C4, C2, C3

C5 →

Lectin pathway

Plasma-mannose-lectin binds
bacterial cell wall's mannose

Alternate pathway

Polysaccharides from
bacterial cell walls
↓
C3 subcomponents
↓
C3 subcomponents

C5 →

C5b ←

← C6
← C7
← C8
← C9

C5b, C6, C7, C8, C9

C3 subcomponent
• Opsonizes microbes to
  promote phagocytosis

C4, C2, C3, and C5 subcomponents
• Activate inflammation
• Dilate arterioles
• Release histamine from mast cells
• Attract phagocytes

C5 subcomponent, C6, C7, C8, and C9
• Lyse bacteria/cells

b. Diagram the consequences of the acute inflammatory process.
   Review text pages 186 and 187; refer to Figures 6-2 and 6-3.

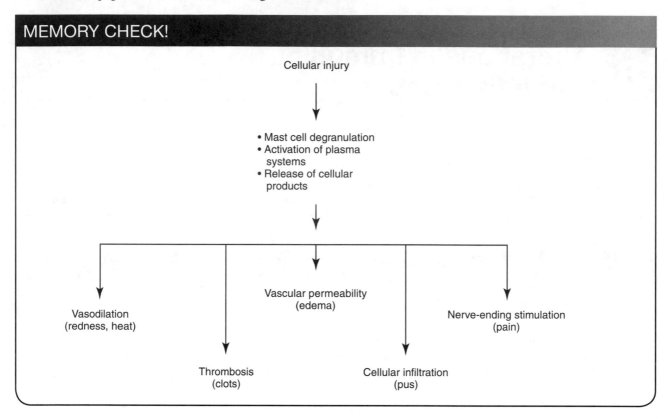

c. Diagram the consequences of the chronic inflammatory process.
   Review text pages 206 through 208; refer to Figure 6-17.

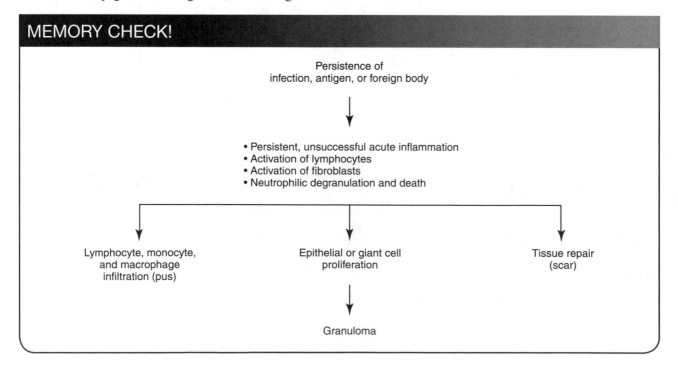

d. Diagram the difference between regeneration (resolution) and repair.
   Review text pages 208 and 210 through 212; refer to Figure 6-19.

MEMORY CHECK!

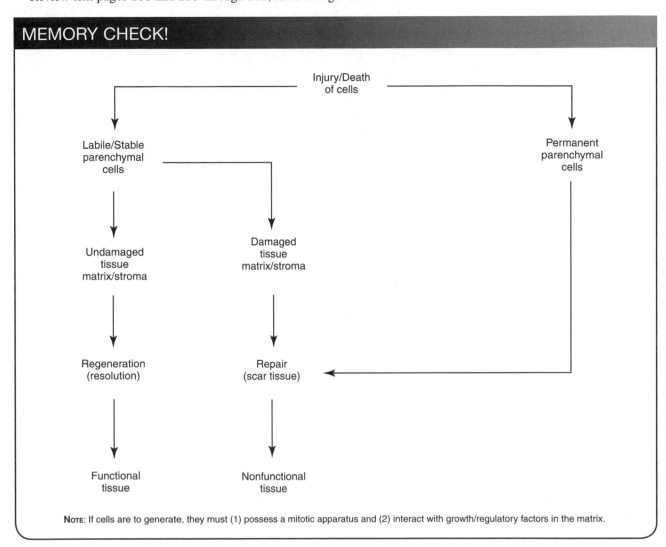

NOTE: If cells are to generate, they must (1) possess a mitotic apparatus and (2) interact with growth/regulatory factors in the matrix.

e. (1) Use a flow chart to compare innate (nonspecific) defenses with adaptive (specific) immunity.
Refer to Table 6-1.

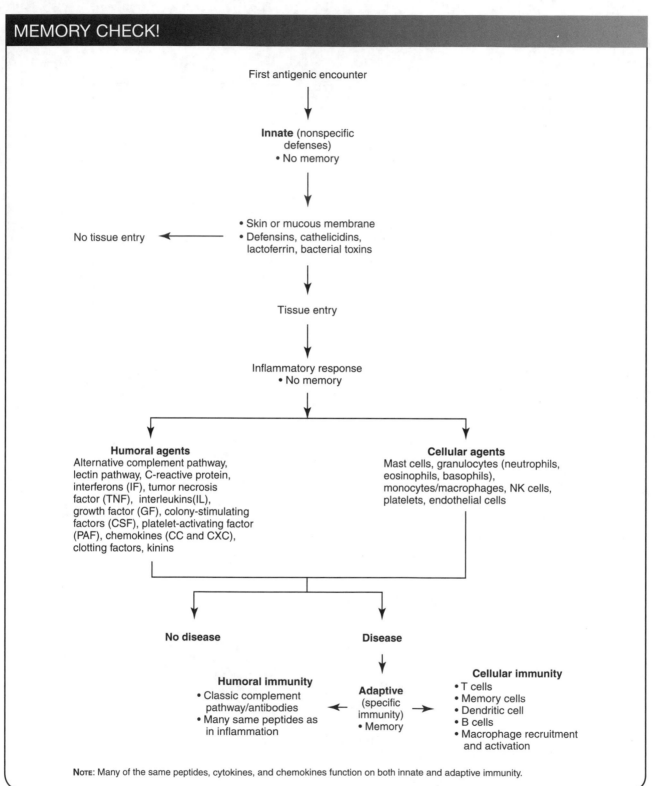

MEMORY CHECK!

First antigenic encounter

↓

Innate (nonspecific defenses)
• No memory

↓

No tissue entry ← • Skin or mucous membrane
• Defensins, cathelicidins, lactoferrin, bacterial toxins

↓

Tissue entry

↓

Inflammatory response
• No memory

↓

Humoral agents
Alternative complement pathway, lectin pathway, C-reactive protein, interferons (IF), tumor necrosis factor (TNF), interleukins(IL), growth factor (GF), colony-stimulating factors (CSF), platelet-activating factor (PAF), chemokines (CC and CXC), clotting factors, kinins

Cellular agents
Mast cells, granulocytes (neutrophils, eosinophils, basophils), monocytes/macrophages, NK cells, platelets, endothelial cells

↓

No disease   **Disease**

↓

Humoral immunity
• Classic complement pathway/antibodies
• Many same peptides as in inflammation

← **Adaptive** (specific immunity)
• Memory →

Cellular immunity
• T cells
• Memory cells
• Dendritic cell
• B cells
• Macrophage recruitment and activation

NOTE: Many of the same peptides, cytokines, and chemokines function on both innate and adaptive immunity.

Chapter **8** **Alterations in Immunity and Inflammation**

e. (2) Diagram the interaction between lymphocytes and phagocytes.
Refer to Figure 7-15.

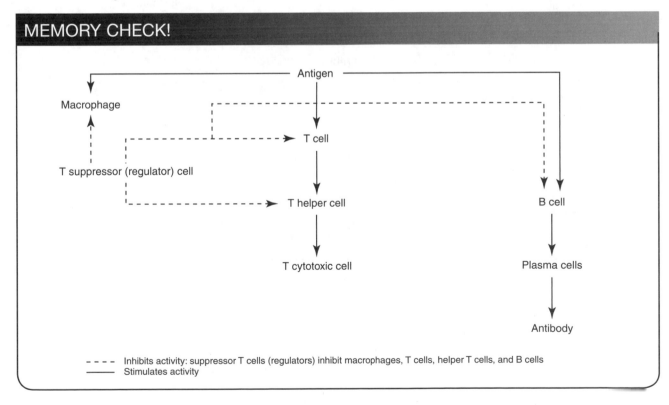

MEMORY CHECK!

NOTE: There is interaction between specific and nonspecific areas of the immune system, The phagocytes cannot specifically recognize antigens but process and present them to the lymphocytes. Lymphocytes specifically recognize and produce antibodies or lymphokines, which help the phagocytes combat the antigen.

e. (3) Diagram the interrelationships between cell-mediated immunity and humoral immunity.
Refer to Figures 7-2 and 7-19 through 7-22.

MEMORY CHECK!

- - - - Inhibits activity: suppressor T cells (regulators) inhibit macrophages, T cells, helper T cells, and B cells
——— Stimulates activity

f. Chart the development and activities of specific immunity.
Refer to Figures 7-2, 7-10, and 7-12 and Table 7-6.

MEMORY CHECK!

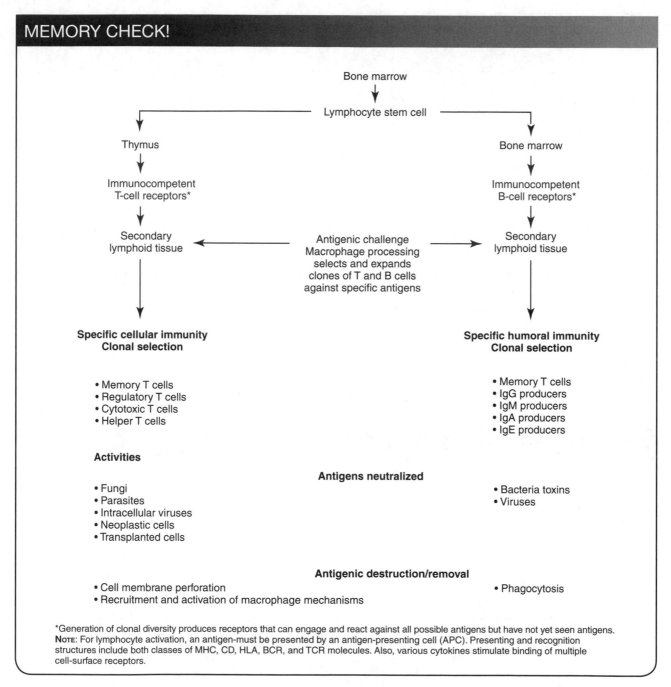

Bone marrow
↓
Lymphocyte stem cell

Thymus
↓
Immunocompetent
T-cell receptors*
↓
Secondary
lymphoid tissue

Antigenic challenge
Macrophage processing
selects and expands
clones of T and B cells
against specific antigens

Bone marrow
↓
Immunocompetent
B-cell receptors*
↓
Secondary
lymphoid tissue

Specific cellular immunity
Clonal selection

- Memory T cells
- Regulatory T cells
- Cytotoxic T cells
- Helper T cells

Specific humoral immunity
Clonal selection

- Memory T cells
- IgG producers
- IgM producers
- IgA producers
- IgE producers

Activities

Antigens neutralized

- Fungi
- Parasites
- Intracellular viruses
- Neoplastic cells
- Transplanted cells

- Bacteria toxins
- Viruses

Antigenic destruction/removal

- Cell membrane perforation
- Recruitment and activation of macrophage mechanisms

- Phagocytosis

*Generation of clonal diversity produces receptors that can engage and react against all possible antigens but have not yet seen antigens.
NOTE: For lymphocyte activation, an antigen-must be presented by an antigen-presenting cell (APC). Presenting and recognition structures include both classes of MHC, CD, HLA, BCR, and TCR molecules. Also, various cytokines stimulate binding of multiple cell-surface receptors.

g. Identify the source and function of some major cytokines.
   Review Table 7-5.

MEMORY CHECK!

Types	Sources	Function
Interleukins (ILs)		
IL-1	Macrophages	Increase inflammatory and immune responses
IL-2	Helper T cells	Increase T cells and NK cells
IL-3	T cells, mast cells, NK cells	Growth factor for immature hematopoietic cells
IL-4	T cells, mast cells	Increase immune and chronic inflammatory responses
IL-5 through IL-17	Various cells	Increase B and T cells; modify activity of other cytokines; elevate inflammatory responses
Interferons (IFNs)	B and T cells, macrophages, fibroblasts, epithelial cells	Antiviral protection; decrease neoplastic growth; regulate interleukins
Tumor necrosis factors (TNFs)	T cells, macrophages	Tumor cytotoxicity; increase inflammatory and immune responses
Colony-stimulating factors (CSFs)	Various cells	Myelocytic stem cell growth factor; macrophage growth factor
Transforming growth factor (TGF)	Lymphocytes, macrophages, platelets, bone	Macrophage chemotaxis; stimulate fibroblasts

LEARNING OBJECTIVES

After studying this chapter, the learner will be able to do the following:

1. Define allergy, autoimmunity, and alloimmunity.
   Study text pages 256 and 258; refer to Tables 8-1 and 8-2.

Hypersensitivity is an altered immunologic reaction to an antigen that results in a disease or damage to the host after reexposure to the same antigen. All hypersensitivity reactions require sensitization to the initial antigenic exposure that results in the primary immune response. Symptoms appear after an adequate secondary immune response. Allergy, autoimmunity, and alloimmunity are hypersensitivity responses; the difference is the source of the antigen to which the hypersensitivity is directed. **Allergy** is a hypersensitivity response to an innocuous environmental antigen that is harmful to the individual. **Autoimmunity** occurs when tolerance to one's self-antigens breaks down and antibody is formed against one's own antigens. Self-antigens are recognized as foreign in autoimmunity, and host tissues are destroyed by autoantibodies. **Alloimmunity** is the development of antibodies against antigens from an individual of the same species. It is observed during immunologic reactions to transfusions, grafted tissue,

or a fetus during pregnancy. Hypersensitivity reactions may be immediate (minutes or hours) or delayed (hours or days) depending on the time required to manifest symptoms after reexposure to the antigen.

2. Compare the four hypersensitivities.
   Study text pages 258 through 261 and 263 and 264; refer to Figures 8-1 through 8-4 and Tables 8-3. See table on page 46.

3. Describe the general characteristics of allergic hypersensitivities.
   Study text pages 264 through 267.

Typical allergens that induce type I hypersensitivity include pollens, molds and fungi, foods, animal danders, cigarette smoke, and house dust. Type II and III are relatively rare, but may include systemic antibiotics and soluble antigens produced by infectious agents such as hepatitis B. Type IV hypersensitivities include plant resins, metals, and chemicals in rubber, cosmetics, detergents, and topical antibiotics. Clinical manifestations of allergic reactions usually are confined to the areas of initial intake or contact with the allergen. Ingested allergens induce gastrointestinal symptoms, airborne allergens induce respiratory or skin manifestations, and contact allergens induce allergic responses at the site of contact. Certain individuals are genetically predisposed to develop allergies, particularly type I allergies, which are called **atopic.** Multiple genes have been associated with the atopic state, including polymorphisms in cytokines that regulate IgE synthesis and cellular receptors.

Several tests to determine allergen sensitivity are available, including food challenges, skin tests with allergens, and laboratory tests for total IgE and allergen-specific IgE in the blood. Clinical **desensitization** can be achieved in some individuals. Minute quantities of the allergen are injected in increasing doses over a prolonged period. This may reduce the severity of the allergic reaction. The mechanisms by which the desensitization occurs may be several; one is the production of large amounts of **blocking antibodies,** which are usually IgE. These antibodies compete in the tissues or in the circulation for binding with antigenic determinants on the allergens so that the allergen is neutralized and unable to bind with IgE on mast cells, thus slowing histamine release. Sublingual desensitization produces IgA and circulating IgG that may prevent the allergen from accessing mast cells. Desensitization injections also may stimulate the generation of clones of regulatory T lymphocytes. This inhibits hypersensitivity by suppressing the production of IgE or modifying the Th1/Th2 interactions in favor of production of anti-inflammatory cytokines.

Comparison of Hypersensitivity Disorders

Hypersensitivity	Immunity/Response Time	Effectors	Examples
Type I			
IgE mediated Anaphylactic	Humoral/immediate	*Antigen* reacts with IgE bound to mast *cells, histamine* release, histamine effects	Allergy: allergic rhinitis, asthma, urticaria, food allergies, anaphylactic shock
Type II Cytotoxic Tissue specific	Humoral/immediate	*IgG or IgM* reacts with *antigen* on a cell's membrane, *complement* via the classic pathway is activated with lysis, opsonization, and phagocytosis by macrophages of cell; incomplete phagocytosis but attracted neutrophils release granules toxic to tissue; non–antigen-specific NK cells release a toxic substance that destroys the target cell; antibody binds to target cell and alters the receptor, causing cells to malfunction	Allergy: immediate drug reaction Autoimmunity: hemolytic anemia, Graves disease Alloimmunity: transfused blood cells, hemolytic disease of the newborn
Type III Immune complex	Humoral/immediate	*IgG or IgM* unite with a soluble *antigen* to form a complex that is deposited in vessel walls or tissues, neutrophil attraction, *complement* activation, *lysosomal enzymes* injure tissue	Allergy: Arthus reaction, allergic alveolitis Autoimmunity: serum sickness, celiac disease, glomerulonephritis, systemic lupus erythematosus
Type IV Cell mediated	Cellular/delayed	Reaction of sensitized *T lymphocytes* with *antigen* leads to *lymphokine* release, recruitment of *macrophages* and *lysosomal release*	Allergy: contact dermatitis Autoimmunity: Hashimoto thyroiditis, rheumatoid arthritis Alloimmunity: graft rejection

Rarely is a particular disorder associated with a single mechanism. Any of the types may cause allergic responses.

4. **Describe the likely causes of autoimmune diseases.**

Study text pages 267 through 270; refer to Table 8-5.

Self-antigens are usually tolerated by the host's own immune system; this immunologic central tolerance develops in humans during the embryonic period. Auto-reactive lymphocytes are either eliminated or suppressed in the primary lymphoid organs during differentiation and proliferation of immature T or B lymphocytes. Peripheral tolerance is maintained in secondary lymphoid organs by regulatory T cells or antigenic-presenting dendritic cells.

Autoimmunity is a breakdown of tolerance in which the body's immune system begins to recognize self-antigens as foreign. The mechanisms of breakdown are varied and often unknown. Some of the mechanisms implicated in the development of autoimmunity include (1) exposure within the body of a previously sequestered antigen, (2) the complications of an infectious disease, (3) the development of a neoantigen, (4) forbidden clones of lymphocytes reactive against self-antigen that did not mature nor proliferate later in life, and (5) an alteration of suppressor T cells.

To be tolerated after birth, a self-antigen must be present in the fetus and exposed to the developing fetal immune system. Some self-antigens never encounter antigen-processing cells in the draining lymph nodes or other lymphoid organs; they are **sequestered** or hidden from the immune system. Later, the immune system will recognize these antigens as foreign if the structure of a site that has sequestered antigen is disturbed and the previously sequestered antigens are released from the damaged tissue and enter the lymphatics. A primary immune response against these antigens occurs, and this can inflict extensive immunologic damage to other, similarly antigenic, nontraumatized sites.

Foreign antigens from infectious microorganisms can initiate autoimmune disease. They do so either by forming immune complexes that precipitate in host tissues and causing inflammatory disease or by closely resembling or mimicking a particular self-antigen. The antibodies produced against the similar antigenic sites of the infectious agent also recognize the self-antigen as foreign; thus there is an immune response against self. Group A streptococci are capable of initiating both of these mechanisms, usually as sequelae to streptococcal pharyngitis.

Many **neoantigens** are haptens that become immunogenic after binding to host proteins. The immune reaction against the neoantigen may lead to an immunologic reaction to unaltered host protein.

One of the roles of **suppressor T cells** is to suppress the immune responses against self-antigens; therefore, suppressor T cell dysfunction could result in autoimmune disease. This constitutes ineffective peripheral tolerance. If a single antigen-specific population of suppressor cells is affected, a tissue-specific autoimmune disease could result. A generalized autoimmune reaction could occur if many suppressor cell populations were dysfunctional. Systemic lupus erythematosus (SLE) may be caused by a general breakdown in the suppressor cell network.

It is fairly well established that autoimmune diseases can be familial. Particular autoimmune diseases have been identified for a variety of major histocompatibility complex (MHC) alleles or non-MHC genes. It is possible that particular human leukocyte antigen (HLA) molecules present antigen or use particular HLAs as receptors for disease-causing microorganisms. Non-MHC genes encode for inflammatory cytokines or co-stimulatory molecules found on cell surfaces.

5. **Characterize alloimmunity; cite examples of alloimmunity and autoimmunity disorders between mother and child; describe transplantation and transfusion complications.**

Study text pages 270 through 275; refer to Figures 8-7 through 8-10.

Alloimmunity occurs when an individual's immune system reacts against antigens on the tissues of other members of the same species. The two clinically relevant examples of this reactivity are (1) several transient neonatal diseases in which the maternal immune system becomes sensitized against antigens expressed by the fetus, and (2) transplant rejection and transfusion reactions when the immune system of a recipient of an organ transplant or blood transfusion reacts against antigens on the donor cells.

Because the fetus has antigens from both the mother and father, it expresses paternal antigens that are not found in the mother. Occasionally, these fetal antigens cross the placenta and elicit an immune response in the mother by the production of alloantibodies against the fetal antigens. The maternal alloantibody may be transported across the placenta into the fetal circulation, bind to the fetal cells, and produce alloimmune disease in the fetus and neonate. The mother's immune system produces the antibody, but because her cells do not express the target antigen, she has no symptoms of the disease.

Neonatal alloimmune disease may be secondary to maternal autoimmune diseases in which the mother produces an IgG autoantibody specific for maternal self-antigens that are found on fetal cells as well. Therefore, symptoms of the same autoimmune disease may affect both mother and child, even though the autoantibody is being produced only by the mother's immune system. This form of disease usually occurs only in association with type II (tissue-specific) hypersensitivity reactions.

At birth, maternal circulating antibody can no longer enter the child. Symptoms of the alloimmune disease may be present in utero or immediately after birth and may be fatal to the fetus or neonate. If symptoms are successfully treated at birth, the disease will disappear as the maternal antibody is catabolized.

At least one alloimmune disease is transported through breast milk. Human breast milk contains antibodies of the secretory immune system, primarily IgA. The gut of the human newborn will not transport antibody from the ingested milk into the circulation after about 24 hours after delivery; therefore, the antibody in breast milk protects the newborn against gastrointestinal infections. In some mothers with pernicious anemia, the breast milk contains IgA against intrinsic factor, which is normally

47

secreted into the gut to bind and transport dietary vitamin B$_{12}$ into the child. The presence of IgA anti-intrinsic factor may prevent its interaction with B$_{12}$, leading to symptoms of B$_{12}$ deficiency from an alloimmune pernicious anemia in the child.

Examples of maternal autoimmune or alloimmune hypersensitivity diseases in which the child can be affected include the following antibody-mediated diseases:

1. *Graves disease:* an autoimmune disease in which maternal antibody against the receptor for thyroid-stimulating hormone (TSH) causes neonatal hyperthyroidism
2. *Myasthenia gravis:* an autoimmune disease in which maternal antibody binds with receptors for neurotransmitters on muscle cells (acetylcholine receptors), causing neonatal muscular weakness
3. *Immune thrombocytopenic purpura:* both autoimmune and alloimmune variants in which maternal antiplatelet antibody destroys platelets in the fetus and neonate
4. *Alloimmune neutropenia:* in which maternal antibody against neutrophils destroys neutrophils in the neonate
5. *Systemic lupus erythematosus:* autoimmune disease in which diverse maternal autoantibodies induce anomalies in the fetus or cause pregnancy loss
6. *Rh and ABO alloimmunization (e.g., erythroblastosis fetalis):* in which maternal antibody against erythrocyte antigens induces anemia in the child.

Transplantation of organs is commonly complicated by an alloimmune response to donor antigens. The primary mechanism of the rejection of transplanted organs is a type IV, cell-mediated reaction. Because HLA antigens are the principal targets of the rejection reaction, HLA matching of donor and recipient greatly enhances the possibility of a successful graft.

Transplant rejection is classified as hyperacute, acute, or chronic depending on the amount of time that elapses between transplantation and rejection. **Hyperacute rejection** usually occurs in recipients who have pre-existing IgG or IgM antibody to antigens in the graft. As circulation to the graft is reestablished, antibody binds to the grafted tissue and activates the inflammatory response; this response initiates the coagulation (blood clotting) cascade that results in the cessation of blood flow into the graft.

Acute rejection is a cell-mediated immune response that occurs within days to a month after transplantation. The recipient develops an immune response to unmatched HLA antigens and shows an infiltration of lymphocytes and macrophages that are characteristic of type IV hypersensitivity reaction. The Th1 cells release cytokines that activate the infiltrating macrophages, and the Tc cells directly attack the endothelial cells in the transplanted tissue.

Chronic rejection may occur after months or years of normal function. It is characterized by slow, progressive organ failure. Chronic rejection may be caused by inflammatory damage to endothelial cells that line the blood vessels; it is likely a result of a weak immunologic reaction against minor histocompatibility antigens on the grafted tissue.

Red blood cells (erythrocytes) express several important surface antigens, known collectively as the **blood group antigens**, which can be targets of alloimmune reactions during transfusions. More than 80 different red cell antigens are grouped into several dozen blood group systems, each determined by a different locus or set of loci. The most important of these, because they provoke the strongest humoral alloimmune response, are the ABO and Rh systems.

The **ABO blood group** consists of two major carbohydrate antigens, labeled A and B. These two carbohydrate antigens are codominant, which means that both A and B can be simultaneously expressed, resulting in an individual having any one of four different blood types. The erythrocytes of persons with blood type A carry the type A carbohydrate antigen, those with blood type B carry the B antigen, those with blood type AB carry both A and B antigens, and those with blood type O carry neither the A nor the B antigen. A person with type A blood also has circulating plasma antibodies to the B carbohydrate antigen. If this person receives blood containing B antigens from a type AB or B individual, a severe transfusion reaction occurs and the transfused erythrocytes will be destroyed by agglutination or complement-mediated lysis.

Similarly, a type B individual whose blood contains anti-A antibodies cannot receive blood from a type A or AB donor. Type O individuals, who have neither antigen but have both anti-A and anti-B antibodies, cannot accept blood from any of the other three types. These naturally occurring antibodies, called isohemagglutinins, are immunoglobulins of the IgM class and are induced by similar antigens expressed on naturally occurring bacteria in the intestinal tract.

Because individuals with type O blood lack both types of antigens, they are considered **universal donors,** meaning that anyone can accept their red blood cells. Similarly, type AB individuals are considered **universal recipients** because they lack both anti-A and anti-B antibodies and can be transfused with any ABO blood type. Agglutination and lysis cause harmful transfusion reactions and can be prevented only by complete and careful ABO matching between donor and recipient.

The **Rh blood group** (inaccurately named after the Rhesus monkey in which a similar antigen system was first described) is the most polymorphic system of red cell antigens, consisting of at least 45 separate antigens. At least five major antigens and a large number of rare variants have been identified and are expressed only on erythrocytes. The major antigens are contained on two proteins. The RhD protein expresses the dominant antigen, which determines whether an individual is Rh positive or Rh negative. Individuals who express the D antigen on the RhD protein are Rh positive, whereas individuals who do not express the D antigen are Rh negative. Anti-D antibody produced by an Rh-negative mothers against erythrocytes of their Rh-positive fetuses is the primary cause of Rh maternal-fetal incompatibility and the resulting hemolytic disease of the newborn.

6. **Characterize immunodeficiencies; describe examples of primary immune diseases.**

Study text pages 275 and 278 through 284; refer to Figures 8-11 through 8-14 and Table 8-6.

Immune deficiencies occur because of impaired function of one or more components of the immune or inflammatory response: B cells, T cells, phagocytic cells, or complement. The clinical manifestation of immune deficiency is a tendency to develop unusual or recurrent severe infections. Deficiencies in T-cell immune responses are suspected when recurrent infections are caused by certain viruses, fungi, yeasts, or certain atypical organisms. B-cell deficiencies are suspected if the individual has recurrent infections with encapsulated bacteria or viruses against which humoral immunity is normally effective.

Most **primary immune deficiencies** are the result of a single gene defect. Generally, the mutations are sporadic and are not inherited—there is a family history in only about 25% of individuals.

Di George syndrome is the complete or partial absence of T-cell immunity. It is also characterized by severe congenital structural defects of the heart and low levels of calcium, which may result in seizures. This syndrome exhibits a congenital thymic aplasia or hypoplasia because of deletions on chromosome 22.

Bruton's agammaglobulinemia is caused by failure of B-cell precursors to become mature B cells. This condition results from mutations in the gene for Bruton's tyrosine kinase that is involved in intracellular signaling for several B-cell receptors. Infective signaling results in the arrest of development in the bursal-equivalent tissue (bone marrow) into mature B cells.

Several **defective class-switch deficiencies** cause genetic rearrangement of the genes for the antibody variable region resulting in decreased or absent production of IgA and IgG, poor development of memory B cells, and overproduction of IgM, which does not require class-switch. T-cell immunity is not affected.

IgG subclass deficiency reflects a switch to a subclass constant region. Low levels of IgG2 may be responsible for recurrent pneumonias because of encapsulated bacteria.

Another common defect in which a particular class of antibody is affected is **selective IgA deficiency.** Individuals with selective IgA deficiency are able to produce other classes of immunoglobulin but fail to produce IgA. Individuals with IgA deficiency frequently present with chronic intestinal candidiasis. IgA may normally prevent the uptake of allergens from the environment; therefore IgA deficiency may lead to increased allergen uptake and a more intense challenge to the immune system because of prolonged exposure to environmental antigens.

Severe combined immune deficiencies (SCIDs) occur when a common stem cell for all white blood cells is absent. Therefore, T cells, B cells, and phagocytic cells never develop. Most children with SCID caused by reticular dysgenesis, which is the most severe form of SCID, die in utero or very soon after birth. Many individuals with SCID are deficient only in a stem cell for lymphocyte development rather than for all white blood cells, as is the case with reticular dysgenesis, and therefore they have normal numbers of all other white cells. T and B lymphocytes are few or absent in the circulation, the spleen, and the lymph nodes. The thymus is usually underdeveloped. IgM and IgA immunoglobulin levels are absent or greatly reduced; however, IgG levels may be almost normal because of the presence of maternal antibodies. Other forms of SCID are caused by autosomal recessive enzymatic defects that result in the accumulation of toxic metabolites to rapidly dividing lymphocytes.

In general, the most common infections in individuals with defects of cell-mediated immune responses are fungal and viral; whereas, infections in individuals with defects of the humoral immune response or complement function are primarily bacterial. The most severe defect in complement involves C3 deficiency, resulting in recurrent bacterial infections. **Defects in phagocyte function,** which include insufficient numbers of phagocytes or defects of chemotaxis, can result in recurrent, life-threatening infections, such as septicemia and disseminated pyogenic lesions.

7. **Cite causes and consequences of acquired or secondary immune deficiencies.**

Study text pages 284 through 286.

Acquired or secondary immune and inflammatory deficiency develops after birth and is caused by other illnesses. These diseases are not related to genetic defects but are more common than primary deficiencies. Nutritional deficits in calorie or protein intake can lead to deficiencies in T-cell function and numbers. The humoral immune response is less affected by starvation, although complement activity, neutrophilic chemotaxis, and bacterial killing by neutrophils are frequently depressed. Enzyme cofactors such as zinc and vitamins may result in severe depressions of both B- and T-cell function.

Acquired immunodeficiencies are caused by superimposed conditions. A relationship between **emotional stress** and depressed immune function seems to exist. Many lymphoid organs are innervated and can be affected by nerve stimulation. Also, lymphocytes have receptors for many hormones, such as neurotransmitters, and can respond to changing levels of these chemicals with increased or decreased function.

Malignancies of lymphoid tissue result in depletion of normal lymphocytes and their replacement by malignant cells. Response to infection is depleted. Many malignancies produce cytokines that suppress immune responses. Cancer chemotherapeutic agents suppress blood cell formation in the bone marrow. Immunosuppressive corticosteroids for the treatment of individuals with transplants or autoimmune diseases depress B- and T-cell formation. The consequence of these therapies for cancer and immunosuppression is manifested as a progressive increase in infections with opportunistic microorganisms.

Traumatized burn victims are susceptible to severe bacterial infections because of decreased neutrophil function and complement levels. Burn victims also have increased regulatory T-cell function, which may increase antigen-specific suppression.

8. Describe some therapies for immune deficiencies.

Study text pages 286 through 288; refer to Table 8-7.

Individuals with hypogammaglobulinemia or agammaglobulinemia can usually be treated successfully with the administration of **gamma globulin**. Administration of fresh frozen plasma can be successful in individuals who require larger amounts of IgM or IgA.

In immune deficiencies caused by lack of lymphoid cells, stem cells can be transplanted from HLA-matched bone marrow, umbilical cord cells, or cell populations rich in stem cells. Graft-versus-host (GVH) disease must be avoided; an HLA match is essential. GVH disease occurs when immunocompetent T lymphocytes in the grafted material recognize foreign antigens in the recipient.

Thymus deficiency diseases can be treated by transplanting fetal thymus tissue, which lacks immunocompetent T cells. Also, thymic epithelial cells that produce the thymic hormones from which mature T cells have been removed can be transplanted. The administration of **soluble materials** that affect lymphocytic function can restore T cell function. The use of transfer factor, a low-molecular-weight nucleoprotein, can confer specific reactivity against certain antigens.

The **therapeutic replacement of defective genes** may be possible when there is immunologic deficiency. The normal gene could be cloned and inserted into a retroviral vector. Such a gene replaces some of the retroviral genes and results in a virus that carries the normal human gene but that will not cause disease. The virus infects defective cells and then inserts the normal gene into the patient's genetic material. The genetically altered cells may then be infused into the individual to reconstitute the immune system.

PRACTICE EXAMINATION

Multiple Choice

Circle the correct answer(s) for each question.

1. Which of the following is *not* characteristic of hypersensitivity?
   a. Specificity
   b. Immunologic mechanisms
   c. Inappropriate or injurious response
   d. Prior contact unnecessary to elicit a response
2. When the body produces antibodies against its own tissue, it is:
   a. hypersensitivity/autoimmunity.
   b. an immunologic reaction/cell-mediated immunity.
   c. alloimmunity/hypersensitivity.
   d. hypersensitivity/cell-mediated immunity.

3. Damage in glomerulonephritis is due to the formation of antigen/antibody complexes mediated by:
   a. IgE.
   b. mast cells.
   c. the cell-mediated immune system.
   d. the humoral immune system.
   e. lymphokines.
4. Which of the following is an alloimmune disorder?
   a. Graft rejection
   b. Insulin-dependent diabetes
   c. Myxedema
   d. All of the above are correct.
   e. None of the above is correct.
5. The most frequently observed selective antibody-dependent immunodeficiency is a deficit of:
   a. IgA.
   b. IgD.
   c. IgE.
   d. IgG.
   e. IgM.
6. An infusion of plasma may be used to treat:
   a. SCID.
   b. thymus deficiencies.
   c. hypogammaglobulinemia.
   d. enzymatic defects.
7. Deficiencies in B-cell immune responses are suspected when unusual or recurrent severe infections are caused by:
   a. fungi.
   b. yeasts.
   c. encapsulated bacteria.
   d. viruses.
8. C6, C7, C8, and C9:
   a. lyse bacteria.
   b. activate inflammation.
   c. attract phagocytes.
   d. opsonize microbes.
9. Cellular immunity neutralizes:
   a. bacterial toxins.
   b. viruses.
   c. bacteria.
   d. intracellular viruses.
10. Which is characteristic of hypersensitivity?
    a. Sensitization required
    b. Occur on initial antigenic exposure
    c. Intolerance to self antigens
    d. Reactions may be immediate or delayed
11. When the body produces antibodies against antigens of the same species, it is a/an:
    a. hypersensitivity.
    b. antibody reaction.
    c. cell-mediated immunity.
    d. alloimmune disease.
    e. opsonization.

50

Matching

Match the condition with the immunologic mechanism(s).

_____12. Graves disease

a. IgE mediated

_____13. Serum sickness

b. cytotoxic/tissue specific

_____14. Allergic rhinitis

c. immune complex

_____ 15. Systemic lupus erythematosus

d. cell mediated

_____16. Contact dermatitis

_____17. Hemolytic anemia

_____18. Graft rejection

Match the term with the circumstance.

_____19. Sequestered antigen

a. lymphocytic clones are prevented from maturing

_____20. Neoantigen

b. suppressor T cells become dysfunctional

c. traumatized tissue releases antigens

d. integration of drug into plasma membrane of a cell

Match the condition with the hypersensitivity.

_____21. Maternal antibody destroys platelets in the fetus and neonate

a. autoimmunity

b. alloimmunity

_____22. Antibody binds with receptors for neural transmitters on muscle cells

c. both autoimmunity and alloimmunity

Match the class of primary immunodeficiency with its consequence.

_____23. B-cell receptor signaling defect

a. lack of white blood cells

_____24. SCID:TCR defect

b. little or no B-cell maturation or antibody

_____25. Alternative complement pathway defect cells

c. defective switch to an IgG subclass

d. incomplete T-cell maturation, normal B and NK

e. secondary C3 deficiency

A 23-year-old male financial advisor seeks relief from itchy eyes, repetitive sneezing, and nasal congestion that worsens at night. He says "If I could only sleep at night, I could handle this."

His history revealed that these symptoms occur every spring/summer and last for 6 to 8 weeks. As a teenager, he worked in his father's hay fields. His mother had asthma as a child. The physical examination showed that his internal nares were swollen and moist and there was a clear discharge without purulence. There was no wheezing and the lungs were clear to auscultation and percussion.

Questions

What is your diagnosis?

What do you recommend?

9 | Infection

FOUNDATIONAL KNOWLEDGE OBJECTIVE

a. **Very carefully review all Foundational Knowledge Objectives in Chapter 8.**

LEARNING OBJECTIVES

After studying this chapter, the learner will be able to do the following:

1. **Identify the reasons that the incidence and spread of infectious disease have increased in recent years.**
   Study text pages 293 and 294; refer to Table 9-2.

   Infection is the third leading cause of death in the United States after heart disease and cancer, although many individuals with cancer die of infection. However, it is the leading cause of death worldwide. The reversal of earlier declining death rates from infection occurred because of the emergence of previously unknown infections, the reemergence of old infections that were thought to be controlled, and the development of infectious agents resistant to multiple antibiotics. The reasons for this are numerous and include the following:

   - Vast and rapid urbanization in many areas of the world, resulting in a breakdown in public health programs and a more rapid spread of infection;
   - Poverty and social inequality;
   - War and famine;
   - Global travel, allowing more rapid spread of disease from isolated areas to virtually any point around the world in a few hours;
   - Globalization of the food supply;
   - Human encroachment into wilderness areas, resulting in contact with previously sequestered infectious agents;
   - Antibiotics that are prescribed excessively, that are not taken for a complete course of therapy, or that, even when appropriately used, result in the selection of antibiotic-resistant microorganisms;
   - Decreases in federal research budgets to study infectious disease;
   - Denial of a problem by governments, allowing infections to spread in an uncontrolled way;
   - Diminished use of effective insecticides; and
   - Increased global warming allowing insect vectors to spread into and breed in areas that were previously too cool for them.

2. **Describe the relationships between microorganisms and humans; note specific infectious processes.**
   Study text pages 295 and 296.

   To many microorganisms, the human body is a hospitable site in which to grow and flourish; it provides sufficient nutrients and appropriate conditions of temperature and humidity. In many cases, a **symbiotic relationship** exists, in which both humans and microorganisms benefit. These microorganisms make up the **normal flora** and reside in different parts of the body, including the skin, mouth, gastrointestinal tract, respiratory tract, and genital tract. For instance, the normal bacterial flora of the human gut are provided with nutrients from ingested food and in exchange produce enzymes that facilitate the digestion and use of many of the more complex molecules found in the human diet, produce antibacterial factors that prevent colonization by pathogenic microorganisms, and produce usable metabolites such as vitamin K and B vitamins.

   The symbiotic relationship with the normal flora can be breached as a result of injury that compromises the physical protective barriers. Damage to the intestinal tract releases intestinal bacteria into the bloodstream, potentially leading to sepsis, shock, and death. Cuts in the skin may allow normally noninfectious bacteria such as *Staphylococcus aureus* to cause local infections and potentially invade further and infect various organs. Symbiosis is also maintained by the immune and inflammatory systems. If those systems are compromised, many microorganisms will leave their normal sites and cause infection elsewhere in the body. Individuals with immune deficiencies easily become infected with microorganisms that normally would not cause disease but seize the opportunity to do so when a person's defensive systems are weakened.

   Unlike **opportunistic infectious agents,** true pathogens have devised means to circumvent the individual's defenses and directly cause infection. Successful infection with theses agents is usually dependent on adequate numbers of microorganisms rather than compromise of the host's defenses.

3. **Describe the stages of clinical infection and their clinical manifestations.**
   Study text pages 296 and 297.

   The clinical infectious process occurs in four distinct stages:
   - The **incubation** period is from initial exposure to the infectious agent and the onset of the first symptoms.

53

The microorganism has entered the individual, undergone initial colonization, and begun multiplying, but is in insufficient numbers to cause symptoms. This period may last from several hours to years;

- The **prodromal** stage begins with the occurrence of initial symptoms, which are often very mild and include a feeling of discomfort and tiredness;

- During the **invasion** period, the pathogen is multiplying rapidly, invading further, affecting the tissues at the site of initial colonization, and invading other areas. The immune and inflammatory responses are being triggered with development of specific responses related to the pathogen; symptoms are related to the ongoing protective inflammatory response;

- With **convalescence**, in most instances, the individual's immune and inflammatory systems have successfully removed the infectious agent and symptoms decline. Alternatively, the disease may be fatal or may enter a latency phase with resolution of symptoms until reactivation at a later time.

Effects of infection may be acute, chronic, secondary to the immune and inflammatory responses, or a consequence of bacterial toxins. Manifestations can arise directly from the infecting microorganism or its products; however, the majority of manifestations result from the host's inflammatory and immune responses. The hallmark of most infectious diseases is **fever.**

Fever is not failure of the body to regulate temperature; rather, body temperature is being regulated at a higher level than normal. Body temperature is regulated by nervous system feedback to the hypothalamus, which functions as a central thermostat. A large number of pyrogenic agents can produce fever. Pyrogens derived from outside the host are termed **exogenous pyrogens** and those produced by the individual are termed **endogenous pyrogens.** There is little evidence that exogenous pyrogens cause fever directly. Such pyrogens indirectly affect the hypothalamus through endogenous pyrogens released by cells of the host. A number of cytokines have been identified as endogenous pyrogens. They are interleukins 1 and 6 (IL- I and IL-6), interferon (IFN), and tumor necrosis factor (TNF). These cytokines seem to raise the thermoregulatory set point through stimulation of prostaglandin synthesis. Many investigators consider fever as an adaptive host-defense response.

4. Identify the general factors influencing microbial pathogenicity.

Study text page 297.

Several factors influence the capacity of a pathogen to cause disease:

- **Communicability** allows the disease to spread from one individual to others.

- **Immunogenicity** is the ability of pathogens to induce an immune response.

- **Infectivity** is the ability of the pathogen to invade and multiply in the host.

- **Mechanism of action** is how the microorganism damages tissue.

- **Pathogenicity** is the ability of an agent to produce disease; success depends on communicability, infectivity, extent of tissue damage, and virulence.

- **Portal of entry** is the route by which a pathogenic microorganism infects the host. It can be by direct contact, inhalation, ingestion, or bites of an animal or insect.

- **Toxigenicity** is the ability to produce soluble toxins or endotoxins; these agents greatly influence the pathogen's degree of virulence.

- **Virulence** indicates the capacity of a pathogen to cause severe disease; for example, measles virus is of low virulence, whereas rabies virus is highly virulent.

Infectious diseases are also classified by their prevalence and spread within the community. **Endemic** diseases have relatively high, but constant, rates of infection in a particular population. In **epidemic** diseases, the number of new infections in a particular population greatly exceeds the number usually observed. **Pandemic** disease is an epidemic that spreads over a large area, either a continent or worldwide.

5. Characterize bacteria and their specific defensive mechanisms against host inflammation and immunity.

Study text pages 297, 298, and 300 through 309; refer to Figures 9-1 through 9-6 and Tables 9-4 through 9-7.

Bacteria are prokaryotic unicellular microorganisms with no nuclei, mitochondria, or membrane-bound organelles. They are generally divided into several groups:

- **"True bacteria"** divide by binary fission and may have a variety of morphologies, including cocci (spherical), bacilli (rod shaped), vibrios (comma shaped rods), or spirilla (twisted rod shaped). Most disease-causing bacteria fall into this classification.

- **Filamentous bacteria** may have branching, mycelium-like structures that resemble fungi. Examples include the mycobacteria, *Mycobacterium tuberculosis* and *Mycobacterium leprae,* that cause tuberculosis and leprosy, respectively.

- **Spirochetes** are flexible spiral filaments that are motile. Most are anaerobic. Pertinent examples include *Borrelia recurrentis* (relapsing fever), *Treponema pallidum* (syphilis), and *Borrelia burgdorferi* (Lyme disease).

- **Mycoplasma** lack a rigid cell wall and are small and pleomorphic. They are the smallest and most simple members of the bacteria. *Mycoplasma pneumoniae* causes atypical pneumonia and *Mycoplasma genitalium* is a suspected cause of urethritis and pelvic inflammatory disease.

- **Rickettsia** are strict intracellular parasites that can be rod shaped, spherical, or pleomorphic. They are typically spread by insect vectors and cause Rocky Mountain spotted fever *(Rickettsia rickettsii)* and typhus *(Rickettsia prowazekii).*

- **Chlamydia** are also strict intracellular parasites, but with more complex intracellular lifecycles. The primary chlamydial pathogen is *Chlamydia trachomatis,* which causes bacterial sexually transmitted infection (pelvic inflammatory disease) and eye infections (conjunctivitis).

The establishment of a stable **colonization** requires adhesion. Many bacteria attach through **pili,** also called fimbriae, which are thin rodlike projections from the bacterial surface. Pathogenic strains of *Escherichia coli* involved in urinary tract infections have a variety of different pili-associated adhesion molecules capable of binding with glycoproteins specifically expressed on the bladder epithelium. The particular adhesin may vary depending on growth conditions under which bacteria may undergo a "phase change" and shift from one type to another. *Neisseria* spp. bind to urinary tract epithelial cell membrane–associated cofactor protein (CD46), which is a receptor that regulates complement and protects cells by helping inactivate C3b and C4b. A variety of proteins and carbohydrates not associated with pili function as adhesion molecules. Flagella, used for motion, act as adhesions in *Vibrio cholerae.* Hemagglutinins on *Bordetella pertussis, Salmonella* spp., and *Helicobacter pylori* bind to erythrocyte surface molecules.

Fibronectin is a common component of mucosal cell surfaces and is frequently used as a receptor. Several bacteria, *Streptococcus pyogenes, S. aureus,* and *T. pallidum,* have developed specific adhesion molecules that recognize a particular amino acid sequence in fibronectin. Many other bacteria have developed adhesion molecules that bind to collagen, laminin, and vitronectin, which are plentiful in connective tissue.

Invasion results in direct confrontation with the individual's primary defense mechanisms against bacteria, which include the complement system, antibodies, and phagocytes. Bacterial survival and growth depend on the effectiveness of the body's defenses and on the bacterium's capacity to resist those defenses and obtain nutrients and multiply. **Evasion** of the body's defense mechanisms may result in infectious microorganisms being transported in the blood (**bacteremia**) to infect other organs or even multiply in the blood (**sepsis**).

Exotoxins are proteins released during bacterial growth. They are usually enzymes and have highly specific effects; they include cytotoxins, neurotoxins, pneumotoxins, enterotoxins, and hemolysins. Exotoxins can damage cell membranes, activate second messengers, and inhibit protein synthesis. For instance, a key component of invasion by *Neisseria meningitidis* is a toxin that weakens intercellular adhesion between epithelial cells, thus allowing penetration into the underlying tissue. Pathogenic strains of streptococci and staphylococci produce hyaluronidase, lipases, and hemolysins that break down cells and intercellular matrix.

Endotoxins are **lipopolysaccharides (LPSs)** contained in the cell walls of gram-negative bacteria that are released during lysis of the bacteria. **Endotoxin** also may be released from the membrane of the bacteria either during bacterial growth or during treatment with antibiotics. As the antibiotic destroys the bacteria, the endotoxin still exerts its effects. Bacteria that produce endotoxins are called **pyrogenic** bacteria, because they activate the inflammatory process and produce fever. The innermost part of the lipopolysaccharide, *lipid A,* is made of polysaccharides and fatty acids and is responsible for the substance's toxic effects.

Because the primary immune response may take 3 to 5 days to reach protective levels, some pathogens **divide** rapidly and proliferate at rates that surpass the development of the immune system. Cholera develops within 2 to 3 days of ingestion of the bacteria and has a mortality rate of 60%. Some strains of toxin-producing group A streptococci cause destructive skin infections and pneumonia that may kill an individual within 2 days.

Intracellular survival is possible as bacteria may hide from the immune response by growing in sites that are poorly protected by immune cells; for example, *Salmonella typhi* in the intestinal tract and gall bladder. Even asymptomatic people may undergo prolonged local colonization and shed infectious microorganisms in urine and feces, thus creating **a carrier state.**

Many **intracellular** bacteria, such as *Brucella, Listeria,* and *M. tuberculosis,* can survive and even multiply in macrophages. A second means is escape from the phagosome. Several bacteria secrete lysins that break down the phagosome membrane; the bacteria are released into the cytoplasm where they multiply. The third means is by prevention of phagosome-lysosome fusion. *M. tuberculosis* and *Toxoplasma gondii* produce toxins that prevent fusion, so that the environment in the phagosome remains relatively nontoxic.

Protection against phagocytosis is possible because some bacteria produce a large variety of toxins and extracellular enzymes that kill phagocytic cells. Streptococcal products, such as streptolysin O, bind to cholesterol in the phagocyte's plasma membrane and initiate destruction through the internal release of enzymes in lysosomal granules.

Antiphagocytic **capsules** are expressed by most bacterial pathogens involved in pneumonia and meningitis. Such coatings inhibit phagocytosis and include the thick polysaccharide covering of the *Streptococcus pneumoniae,* the waxy capsule surrounding *M. tuberculosis,* the polysaccharide "slime" capsule of *Pseudomonas aeruginosa,* and the M protein of *S. pyogenes.* The M protein binds fibrinogen and fibrin and also functions as an adhesin.

Some bacterial surface proteins, such as protein A of *S. aureus* and protein G of *S. pyogenes,* bind the Fc portion of the individual's antibody, thus forming a **protective coat** of **self protein.** Binding through the Fc holds the antibody in an orientation that does not allow complement activation or phagocytosis.

Antigenic variation allows the pathogen to alter surface molecules that express antigens that are the targets of protective immune responses. Thus, as the individual develops protective levels of antibodies, the pathogen responds by changing antigens and becoming resistant. The three primary mechanisms of antigenic variation are mutation, recombination, and gene switching.

Protection is afforded by the **degradation of molecules** of the immune or inflammatory system. An **IgA** protease produced by *Neisseria gonorrhoeae, N. meningitidis, Haemophilus influenzae,* and *S. pneumoniae* cleaves IgA at hinge region into ineffective Fc and Fab regions. A staphylokinase produced by *Staphylococcus* spp. activates plasmin resulting in the breakdown of clots and degrades IgG and C3b of the complement system.

55

Pseudomonas produces elastase which breaks down C3 of the complement system and a protease which breaks down C5a. Bacteria may spontaneously release surface molecules that bind to and neutralize antibody. These include endotoxin from gram-negative bacteria, capsular antigens from *Streptococcus pneumoniae* and *Neisseria meningitidis,* and Protein A from *S. aureus.*

Complement evasion is another bacterial protective mechanism. Teichoic acid in the gram-positive cell wall provides resistance against complement-mediated lysis. *Staphylococcus* produces proteins that inhibit complement activity, including C3 and C5 convertases, C5, C2, and the C5a receptor that mediates complement-induced chemotaxis.

Immune suppression, although more prominent in viral infections, some bacterial pathogens can broadly suppress immune responses against their own antigens as well as other antigens unrelated to the infectious agent. Chronic bacterial infections, like *M. leprae* and *M. tuberculosis,* induce suppressed response to multiple antigens in infected hosts. *H. pylori* can release LPSs that bind to dendritic cells and block development of Th1 cells, as well as produce toxins that block the T-cell IL-2 receptor signaling pathway. This inhibits maturation of Th cells.

Antibiotic resistance has become a major problem with *S. aureus.* For several decades pathogenic strains have commonly produced **lactamase,** an enzyme that destroys penicillin. More recently, staphylococci such as *S. aureus* have developed resistance to broad-spectrum antibiotics, including methicillin-like antibiotics, which were widely used to treat penicillin-resistant microorganisms.

6. Characterize fungi and their specific defensive mechanisms against host inflammation and immunity.
Study text pages 309 and 310; refer to Figure 9-7.
Fungi are eukaryotic microorganisms with thick, rigid cell walls and the capacity to form a variety of complex structures. Fungi may grow as a **mold** with branched filaments and a mesh work mycelium structure, a **yeast** with ovoid or spherical shapes, or **dimorphic** with a yeast-like appearance in tissue and mycelium in culture. The cell wall is composed of polysaccharides that differ from the peptidoglycans of bacteria and thus are resistant to bacterial cell wall inhibitors, such as penicillin and cephalosporin. In contrast to bacteria, the cytosol of fungi contains mitochondria, Golgi apparatus, microtubules, microvesicles, endoplasmic reticulum, and nuclei. Molds are aerobic, and yeasts are facultative anaerobes.

The majority of medically relevant fungi either exist as human commensals or cause relatively mild infections of the skin, nails, hair, and mucous membranes of the mouth and vagina. Human-to-human transmission is only a concern with dermatophytic infections. Systemic mycosis caused by pathogenic fungi generally results from inhalation of spores present in a contaminated environment and initially occurs as a pulmonary infection. Infection that disseminates to other organs can be life threatening. Systemic mycosis caused by opportunistic fungi is usually secondary to immunosuppression caused by genetic defects, infections such as HIV, cancer, and drugs used to prevent transplant rejection. Specific

adherence to epithelium is provided by several polysaccharides on the fungal surface that adhere to host receptors. A cell wall adhesion molecule on several fungi such as *Candida albicans* promotes adherence to epithelial cells as well as silicone, thus facilitating infection of implants and other medical devices.

The more virulent morphologies allow fungi to survive in macrophages after phagocytosis. After phagocytosis by macrophages, the yeast form of *Histoplasma* replicates in phagosomes and phagolysosomes. Some yeast may produce proteins that inhibit the activity of lysosomal proteases. The cryptococcal polysaccharide capsule is antiphagocytic by blocking recognition by macrophages and may also be immunosuppressive by inhibiting migration of leukocytes into the site of fungal infection. *Aspergillus* spp. and many other fungi produce toxic metabolites that inhibit macrophage and neutrophil phagocytosis. Molecules like gliotoxin may also be immunosuppressive by suppressing mast cell activation, degranulation, and secretion of leukotrienes and cytokines.

Several yeasts stimulate the production of immunosuppressive cytokines, resulting in down-regulation of some aspects of the host's immune response. The yeast *Cryptococcus neoformans* suppresses inflammation by inhibiting production of the proinflammatory cytokines tumor necrosis factor-alpha (TNF-α) and IL-12 and inducing production of the anti-inflammatory cytokine IL-10. The overall result is suppression of macrophage function.

Secreted enzymes, such as proteases, phospholipases, and elastases, damage cells and intercellular matrix, leading to necrosis. Many molds secrete mycotoxins when grown on nuts, beans, and grains. Ingestion of this toxin affects muscle coordination, causes tremors, and may be fatal. Some fungal toxins may cause cancer; aflatoxins produced by some *Aspergillus* spp. are especially carcinogenic.

In healthy individuals, particularly those whose normal flora has been disturbed by antibiotic therapy, Candida overgrowth may result in vaginitis or oropharyngeal infection. In those with an intact immune system, the infection remains localized. In immunocompromised individuals, particularly those with diminished levels of neutrophils, disseminated infection may occur. Candida is the most common fungal infection in people with cancer, particularly leukemia and other hematologic cancers, transplantation, and HIV/AIDS.

7. Characterize parasites and protozoa and their specific defensive mechanisms against host inflammation and immunity.
Study text pages 310 through 313; refer to Figure 9-8 and Table 9-8.
Parasitic organisms establish a symbiosis with another species in which the parasite benefits at the expense of the other species. Parasites range from unicellular protozoans to large worms. Parasitic worms include intestinal and tissue nematodes, flukes, and tapeworms. A protozoan is a eukaryotic, unicellular microorganism with a nucleus and cytoplasm. The initial attachment depends on whether the microorganism is injected into the blood-stream

56

by a vector or whether entrance is through the gastrointestinal tract. Those in the bloodstream frequently have surface lectins that react with carbohydrates on specific cells.

Leishmania spp. are obligative intracellular parasites of monocytes and macrophages They are protected from killing in the phagosome and phagolysosome in which they multiply. Protection may be afforded by a surface protein that inhibits fusion of lysosomes to the phagosome, thus decreasing the amount of degradative enzymes within the phagolysosome. *Toxoplasma* spp. may be protected by entrance into a variety of cells including macrophages. *Trypanosoma cruzi* bypasses the effects of macrophage activation by escaping from the phagosome and growing in the macrophage cytoplasm. Some organisms produce toxins to protect themselves against phagocytosis; *Entamoeba histolytica* releases phospholipase and pore-forming proteins that disrupt the phagocyte's plasma membrane.

Pathogens that coat themselves with human proteins may be disguised and "fool" the immune system. Schistosomes and trypanosomes mask their antigens by absorbing IgG by the Fc portion of the molecule. Schistosomes secrete an enzyme that diminishes the effectiveness of IgG by specifically removing a critical peptide. *Entamoeba histolytica* secretes a protease that can degrade IgG and IgA. In general, those organisms that undergo part of their life cycle in humans or those assuming multiple morphologic forms will also undergo antigenic changes related to the stage in the life cycle or morphology.

Echinococcus spp. and *Leishmania* spp. produce complement regulatory proteins that affect complement function by destabilizing C3 convertase or promoting degradation of C3b. *E. histolytica* produces complement regulatory factors that inactivate C3a and C5a and thus inhibit phagocyte chemotaxis activity.

The release of large amounts of soluble antigen may induce specific tolerance to the pathogen and induce dysfunctional macrophage antigen processing. The function of immune cells is directly blocked by secretion of cytotoxic molecules by *Trichinella spiralis,* selective inhibitors of T-cell function by schistosomes, or inducers of polyclonal B-cell mitogen released by trypanosomes.

Tissue damage may result directly by parasitic infestation in the tissue or be secondary to the individual's immune and inflammatory responses. The particular process depends a great deal on burden of parasites infesting the site and sensitivity of the particular site to damage. Large infestations may lead to physical loss of function in a tissue or organ. A large number of intestinal parasites such as the roundworm *Ascaris lumbricoides* and the tapeworms compete for and prevent uptake of nutrients, leading to various forms of malabsorption, blocked uptake of fats, or anemia from malabsorption of vitamin B_{12} or from large amount of blood loss. Filarial parasites block the lymphatics and cause accumulation of lymph in tissues. The larva of tapeworm, *Taenia solium,* encysts in and prevent normal function of organs, which is particularly dangerous in human brain.

Toxins released from the parasite may cause significant irreversible organ damage. Proteolytic enzymes from *E. histolytica* are very cytolytic, leading to ulceration of intestinal walls, bloody diarrhea, amoebic dysentery, dehydration, and death in infants and young children. *T. cruzi* secretes a neurotoxin that affects the nervous system, a low-molecular-weight toxin that causes fever, and proteases and phospholipases leading to tissue destruction.

Malaria is one of the most common infections worldwide and can cause cardiovascular collapse, shock, coma, and death. Transmission is through the bite of an infected female anopheles mosquito. The infectious form enters the bloodstream, exits in the liver, and invades parenchyma cells. After several rounds of division, the liver cells rupture and several thousand parasites enter the blood where they infect red blood cells. Multiplication occurs in red blood cells (RBCs), resulting in the release of daughter parasites that re-infect other erythrocytes. The parasite in the blood avoids destruction by phagocytes in the spleen by expressing adhesion proteins that cause adherence and sequestration along the walls of the small vessels. Malaria induces a form of immune suppression. CD4 and CD8 T cells are diminished and lymphocytes likely do not proliferate.

8. **Characterize viruses and their specific defensive mechanisms against host inflammation and immunity.**
   Study text pages 313 and 315 through 318; refer to Figures 9-9 through 9-11 and Table 9-9.

   Viruses are extremely simple microorganisms and do not possess any of the metabolic organelles found in prokaryotes or eukaryotes cells. The basic viral structure (virion) consists of nucleic acid protected by a protein shell, the capsid. The capsid may take many characteristic shapes: helical, icosahedral, or large pleiomorphic shape. Some viruses also have a protective envelope surrounding the capsid, which consists of the plasma membrane from the previously infected cell.

   Viruses are obligatory intracellular parasites. Transmission is usually from one infected individual to an uninfected individual or from an animal reservoir. Transmission may be direct or through a vector, such as mosquitoes. Human-to-human transmission may take many forms including aerosols of respiratory fluids, contact with infected blood, or sexual contact.

   Attachment involves specific interactions between surface proteins on the virus and receptors on the cell to be infected. The specificity of the virus for these receptors and the distribution of receptors throughout the individual's tissues dictate the range of host cells that a particular virus can infect. For example, HIV has a glycoprotein that attaches to the CD4 molecule expressed on helper T cells.

   Once bound, the virion penetrates the plasma membrane by receptor-mediated endocytosis, by envelope fusion with the plasma membrane, or by direct entry through the plasma membrane. Within the cytoplasm, the virus uncoats the protective nucleocapsid and releases viral genetic information. Most RNA viruses directly

57

produce messenger RNA, which is translated into viral proteins and genomic RNA, which is eventually packaged into new viruses. Retroviruses, notably HIV, carry an enzyme **reverse transcriptase** that creates a double-stranded DNA version of the virus. The DNA "provirus" enters the cell's nucleus where it becomes integrated into the host cell's chromosomal DNA. DNA viruses also enter the nucleus and are transcribed into messenger RNA before protein translation. Some DNA viruses also may integrate into the infected cell's chromosomal DNA.

The translation of viral-specific mRNA results in viral proteins that self-assemble. New virions are released from the cell for transmission of the viral infection to neighboring uninfected cells. Enveloped viruses are released through *budding,* in which shed viral particles are enveloped in the plasma membrane from the surface of the infected cell. Nonenveloped viruses commonly are released in large numbers concurrent with the destruction of the cell. Viral DNA that has become integrated with host DNA is transmitted to the daughter cells during mitosis. By this process, viral genes can become part of the genetic information of the cell and its progeny.

Some viruses, particularly those with small genomes, rapidly divide and proliferate after the initial infection and by doing so produce a large number of virions more quickly than the immune system can develop. By the time an effective adaptive immune response develops, which requires 4 or 5 days, the virus has spread and caused severe clinical disease.

Many viral defensive mechanisms are similar to those of intracellular bacteria. As obligative intracellular pathogens, viruses hide within cells and away from normal inflammatory or immune responses. Viral agents that spread from cell to cell after the initial infection must encounter the immune response, which in most cases cures the infection. Thus most viral infections are self-limiting.

If a symbiotic relationship is maintained between the host cell and the virus, persistent unapparent infection may result; this is known as latency. The infected cell will be functional, and the virus persists until it is activated to replicate; an example is the recurrent cold sores of herpes simplex virus infection. Latent viruses usually possess latency-associated transcript (LAT) genes that control persistence indefinitely. Reactivation usually results from expression of lytic genes that lead to increased viral expression and destruction of the infected cell. Latency is characteristic of several chronic viral infections.

Enveloped viruses are the prime examples of how coating with self proteins may succeed. The viral capsid is completely surrounded by a cellular plasma membrane that is highly similar to that of an uninfected cell.

One of the classic examples of antigenic variation is influenza. This virus undergoes frequent antigen shifts and drifts. Some viral enzymes are designed to create small errors in reading mRNA leading to minor changes in the viral proteins. In a manner similar to bacteria, some viruses have multiple stable antigenic serotypes. A person who recovers from an infection with one serotype may not have protective immunity against other serotypes of the same virus

As with other pathogens, the secretion of large amounts of soluble viral antigen may lead to neutralization of antibody and formation of immune complexes. In infection such as hepatitis B, significant levels of circulating immune complexes may form and be deposited in target tissues such as the kidneys. Some viruses also have the capacity to neutralize cytokines, such as IL-1 and TNF-α. Cells infected with vaccinia virus produce a protein that can bind to IL-1. These molecules are frequently called cytokine decoys.

Several viruses induce expression of regulators of complement activation. Cellular complement inhibitors are incorporated into the envelope of some viruses. Cytomegalovirus (CMV) induces complement inhibitors on the surface of infected cells. Herpes simplex virus expresses a cell surface protein that binds and inhibits C3b and blocks the membrane attack complex.

HIV and other viruses have developed the capacity to infect and kill immune cells, thus protecting themselves, but also leading to a broad immunosuppression against other antigens. Some viruses have developed mechanisms for interfering with antigen processing and presentation by MHC class I molecules.

Once inside the infected cell, viruses may have many harmful effects, including the following:

- Cytopathic effects resulting from inhibition of cellular DNA, RNA, or protein synthesis; disruption of lysosomal membranes, resulting in release of digestive lysosomal enzymes that can kill the cell;
- Promotion of apoptosis of the cell;
- Fusion of infected, adjacent cells, thereby producing multinucleated **giant** cells, as seen with herpes viruses, measles virus, mumps virus, and respiratory syncytial virus;
- Transformation of infected cells into cancerous cells, resulting in uninhibited and unregulated growth; and
- Alteration of the antigenic properties, or identity, of the infected cell, causing the immune system to attack the cell as if it were foreign.

9. Describe acquired immunodeficiency syndrome (AIDS).

Study text pages 318, 319, and 321 through 325; refer to Figures 9-12 through 9-16.

The most notable form of secondary or acquired immune deficiency caused by an infectious agent is **acquired immunodeficiency syndrome (AIDS).** AIDS is a viral disease caused by the human immunodeficiency virus (HIV). HIV infects and depletes a portion of the immune system, Th cells, making individuals extremely susceptible to life-threatening infections and malignancies.

HIV is a blood-borne pathogen present in body fluids, such as blood, vaginal fluid, semen, and breast milk. Transmission is by blood or blood products, intravenous drug abuse, both heterosexual and homosexual activity, and mother-to-child transmission before or during birth.

HIV is a member of the retrovirus family, which carries genetic information in the form of two copies of

58

RNA. Retroviruses use a viral enzyme, **reverse transcriptase,** to convert RNA into double-stranded DNA. Using a second viral enzyme, an **integrase,** the new DNA is inserted into the infected cell's genetic material where it may remain dormant. If the cell is activated, translation of the viral information may be initiated and result in the formation of new virions, lysis and death of the infected cell, and shedding of infectious HIV particles. If, however, the cell remains relatively dormant, the viral genetic material may remain latent for years; it is probably present for the life of the individual.

The primary surface receptor on HIV is the envelope glycoprotein gp 120, which binds to the molecule CD4, which is found primarily on the surface of T helper cells. Several other necessary co-receptors have been identified on the target cells, primarily the chemokine receptors CXCR4 and CCR5. Different strains of HIV are selective for the CXCR4 or CCR5 co-receptors, which influences the tropism for different target cells. Strains that prefer the CXCR4 co-receptor tend to be T-cell tropic and usually are found later in an infection, which cause infected cells to fuse and form a multinucleate **syncytium.** Strains that react better with the co-receptor CCR5 are macrophage-tropic and usually cause the primary HIV infection, but not syncytium formation. The primary cellular targets for HIV include CD4+ T helper lymphocytes, dendritic cells, macrophages, CD8+ Tc cells, thymic cells expressing both CD4 and CD8 simultaneously, NK cells, and neural cells of monocyte origin.

Initially, the lymphoid areas of the mucosal surfaces are the primary sites of infection. Dendritic cells and mucosal T cells probably spread the infection to other peripheral lymphoid organs, especially follicular dendritic cells in the lymph nodes, which then infect T cells. Infection also may involve the thymus and bone marrow including the bone marrow stromal cells. Cells in the central nervous system (CNS) may act as a reservoir in which HIV can be relatively protected from antiviral drugs. The virus is also found in T cells and macrophages in semen and in the renal epithelium.

The major immunologic finding in AIDS is the striking decrease in the number of CD4+ T helper lymphocytes. The decrease in CD4+ cell numbers results in a reversal of the normal CD4/CD8 T-cell ratio, which is normally about 1.9, to lower than 0.9 and often near zero.

HIV causes destruction of T helper cells by a variety of means. Production of new HIV virions can be directly cytopathic to the infected cell, causing breakdown of the cell or inducing apoptosis. Additionally, HIV infected cells express new surface antigens and are targets for Tc-mediated lysis. HIV-infected cells shed soluble viral envelope protein, gp 120, which can induce apoptotic cell death of uninfected T lymphocytes, neurons, and monocytes through interaction with cell surface receptors. The interaction between viral envelope protein on the surface of infected cells and its receptors on neighboring uninfected cells also can result in intercellular fusion and syncytium formation. The syncytia undergo apoptosis after a phase of latency.

Envelope protein present on the surface of HIV infected cells also can create partial fusion that results in death of the uninfected cell. The presence of HIV virions and soluble viral antigen can result in a chronic activation of uninfected T cells with HIV-specific T-cell receptors (TCRs). Because activated T cells more efficiently support HIV replication, the most susceptible cells are those with TCRs against HIV.

At the time of diagnosis, the individual may manifest one of several different conditions: serologically negative (no detectable antibody), serologically positive (positive for antibody against HIV) but asymptomatic, early stages of HIV disease, or AIDS. The presence of circulating antibody against HIV indicates infection by the virus, although many of these individuals are asymptomatic. Antibody appears rather rapidly after infection through blood products, usually within 4 to 7 weeks. After sexual transmission, the individual can be infected yet seronegative for 6 to 14 months or, in at least one case, for years. In addition, in the late stages of the disease, some individuals become seronegative because of a deficient immune system.

The period between infection and the appearance of antibody is referred to as the **window period.** Although the individual may not have antibody, he or she may have virus growing, have virus in the blood and body fluids, and be infectious to others. Early symptoms are relatively nonspecific to HIV and include fatigue, fever, muscle aches, and headaches.

Those with the early stages of HIV disease are usually asymptomatic. The early stage may last as long as 10 years in untreated people, during which viral load increases and numbers of CD4+ cells progressively decrease. Some estimates are that approximately 99% of untreated HIV-infected individuals will eventually progress to AIDS.

The current regimen for treatment of HIV infection is a combination of drugs, termed **highly active antiretroviral therapy (HAART).** The combination includes at least three drugs from at least two classes of antiretroviral agents, including nucleoside **reverse transcriptase inhibitors** combined with a viral **protease inhibitor** or a nonnucleoside reverse transcriptase inhibitor. Death from AIDS-related diseases has been reduced significantly since the introduction of HAART; without treatment, an individual may live only 9 to 10 months after diagnosis of AIDS, whereas those who respond well to HAART may survive for several decades. Many people do not respond to HAART therapy. Those who do respond are not "cured," and resistant variants to these drugs have been identified.

Drug therapy for AIDS is difficult because, like most retroviruses, the AIDS virus incorporates into the genetic material of the host and may never be removed by antimicrobial therapy. Therefore drug administration to control the virus may have to continue for the lifetime of the individual. Additionally, HIV may persist in regions where the antiviral drugs are not as effective, such as the CNS. Inhibitors of the initial viral entrance into the target cell, **entrance inhibitors,** may benefit those who do not respond to HAART. Entrance inhibitors include the

59

natural or modified ligands for the co-receptors, CXCR4 and CCR5, and can block infection and inhibit cell membrane fusion. Inhibitors of the viral integrase, **integrase inhibitors,** have undergone clinical trials and eventually may be added to the combination.

10. Describe countermeasures against pathogens.

Study text pages 326 through 332; refer to Figure 9-17 and Tables 9-10 through 9-12.

Infection control measures include routine trash collection and disposal of garbage by incineration or in landfills. Previously successful programs designed to control the breeding of insect vectors have been reversed. Despite an international emphasis on draining standing water that provides breeding grounds for mosquitoes, large unmanaged areas still abound. Since the international ban on DDT for agricultural work and limitation of its use for control of disease vectors, mosquitoes and mosquito-related diseases have rebounded in previously disease-free areas.

Numerous chemicals or **antimicrobials** have been identified that either prevent the growth of microorganisms or directly destroy them. Antibiotics generally act by preventing the function of enzymes or cell structures that are unique to the infecting agent. Because viruses use the enzymes of the host's cells, there has been far less success in developing antiviral antibiotics.

Immediately after antibiotics became widely used, microorganisms mutated and developed resistance. Strains of *S. aureus* have become penicillin resistant. Over the past few decades, healthcare providers have observed increasing incidences of drug-resistant malaria, tuberculosis, gonorrhea, salmonellosis, shigellosis, and staphylococcal infections. *S. pneumoniae,* which causes pneumonia, meningitis, and acute ear infections, was once routinely susceptible to penicillin. Since the 1980s, however, the incidence of penicillin-resistant microorganisms has risen.

Some antibacterial antibiotics are **bactericidal,** or kill the organism; whereas others are **bacteriostatic,** or inhibit growth until the organism is destroyed by the individual's own protective mechanisms. The mechanisms of action of most antibiotics are (1) inhibition of the function or production of the cell wall, (2) prevention of protein synthesis, (3) blockage of DNA replication, or (4) interference with folic acid metabolism.

Antibiotic resistance is usually a result of genetic mutations that can be transmitted directly to neighboring microorganisms by plasmid exchange. Microorganisms commonly develop the capacity to inactive antibiotics. Penicillin resistance, for example, results from the production of lactamase that breaks down the structure of the antibiotic. Other forms of resistance result from modification of the target molecule. Azidothymidine (AZT) is a family of antivirals that suppresses the enzymatic activity of reverse transcriptase. HIV frequently mutates and produces an AZT-resistant reverse transcriptase. Another mechanism of resistance is mediated by multidrug transporters in the microorganism's membrane. These transporters affect the rate of intracellular accumulation of the antimicrobial by preventing entrance or, more commonly, increasing active efflux of the antibiotic. Antibiotic-resistant strains of *Mycobacterium*

tuberculosis are protected from aminoglycosides and tetracycline by the multidrug efflux pump.

Methicillin-resistant *S. aureus* (MRSA) incorporates several different mechanisms of resistance. MRSA produce a penicillinase that destroys penicillin. Penicillinase-resistant antibiotics, methicillins, can be used as a substitute, but MRSA carrying the gene *mecA* are also methicillin-resistant because of a lower affinity for lactams. Resistance to the glycopeptide antibiotic vancomycin is controlled by a gene, *vanA,* that results in alterations in peptidoglycans and loss of the vancomycin binding site. After treatment with the antibiotic clindamycin, the normal intestinal flora can become compromised, allowing the overgrowth of *Clostridium difficile* and the development of pseudomembranous colitis. *C. difficile* is a frequent cause of hospital-acquired infections. Also, lack of compliance concerning the necessity of completing the therapeutic antibiotic regimen allows the selective resurgence of microorganisms that are more relatively resistant to the antibiotic.

Contracting and surviving an infectious disease is the most effective means of developing lifelong immunity against a particular pathogen. However, some infections cause a great deal of morbidity and mortality. The purpose of **vaccination** is to induce **active immunologic protection** before exposure to the infectious agent. For each vaccine an initial immunization protocol is developed to produce large numbers of memory cells and a sustained protective **secondary immune response** in the greatest number of individuals. In general, vaccine-induced protection does not persist as long as infection-induced immunity; thus, booster injections may be necessary to maintain protection throughout life.

Most vaccines against viral infections contain live viruses that are weakened, or **attenuated;** they continue expressing the appropriate antigens yet are unable to establish more than a limited and easily controlled infection. The limited proliferative capacity of attenuated live viruses appears to afford better long-term protection than using purified viral antigen. Even attenuated viruses can establish life-threatening infections in a vaccine recipient whose immune system is congenitally deficient or suppressed.

Some common bacterial vaccines are killed microorganisms or extracts of bacterial antigens. The vaccine against pneumococcal pneumonia consists of a mixture of capsular polysaccharides from 10 strains of *Streptococcus pneumoniae.* Only these 10 cause the most severe illnesses. However, the capsular vaccine is not very immunogenic in young children. A "conjugated" vaccine is available that contains capsular polysaccharides from 7 strains that are conjugated to carrier proteins to increase immunogenicity. A similar vaccine is available for *H. influenzae* type b (Hib).

Some bacterial diseases are caused by potent toxins that act locally or systemically. These include diphtheria, cholera, and tetanus. Vaccination against the toxins is achieved using **toxoid-purified** toxins that have been chemically detoxified without loss of their immunogenicity. Whooping

60

cough vaccine recently was changed from a killed whole cell vaccine to an acellular vaccine that contained the pertussis toxin and additional bacterial antigens.

Passive immunotherapy is a form of countermeasure against pathogens in which preformed antibodies are given to the individual. This form of therapy has been used for decades. Horse serum–containing antibodies were given to treat diphtheria, pneumococcal pneumonia, tetanus, and other diseases in the early twentieth century. Passive immunotherapy with **human immune globulins** has been approved for several infections including hepatitis B and hepatitis A. Treatment of potential rabies infection after a bite combines both passive and active immunization. The rabies virus proliferates very slowly. Individuals who have been bitten receive a one-time injection with human rabies immune globulin to slow down viral proliferation, which is followed by multiple injections with a killed viral vaccine to induce greater protective immunity. For several diseases, more specific therapy with monoclonal antibodies is being evaluated. A monoclonal antibody against respiratory syncytial virus has been approved for therapy.

PRACTICE EXAMINATION

Multiple Choice

Circle the correct answer(s) for each question.
1. Normal flora describes:
   a. microorganisms usually present on body surfaces.
   b. microorganisms causing disease.
   c. secondary disease producers.
   d. pathogens transmitted by carriers.
2. The ability of a microbe to cause disease is called:
   a. colonization.
   b. infectivity
   c. pathogenicity.
   d. virulence.
3. An opportunistic infection is:
   a. a primary infection by a pathogen.
   b. a secondary infection by an additional pathogen.
   c. an infection by a weak pathogen or normal flora when the immune system is compromised.
   d. infection by a virulent pathogen when the immune system is compromised.
4. During convalescence:
   a. symptoms develop.
   b. the pathogens multiply rapidly.
   c. the inflammatory and immune responses are triggered.
   d. the individual's inflammory and immune responses have succeeded.
5. When bacteria overcome the body's defenses and enter the blood, it is called:
   a. septicemia.
   b. pathogenicity.
   c. toxemia.
   d. asepsis.

6. Colonization requires:
   a. rapid division.
   b. adhesion.
   c. streptolysin O.
   d. phagosome-lysosome fusion.
7. Lack of permanent immunity against a virus is due to:
   a. small doses of virus that are insufficient to elicit an immune response.
   b. deficient response by an individual's immune system.
   c. the immune system being unable to provide immunity for viruses.
   d. antigenic drift of the same virus that is not recognized at a later time by the immune system as foreign.
8. Antigenic drift:
   a. occurs from genome recombination.
   b. results from mutations.
   c. occurs from gene switching.
   d. allows immunity to persist once it has developed.
9. Endotoxins:
   a. are proteins.
   b. have highly specific effects.
   c. are immunogenic.
   d. activate the inflammatory process and cause fever.
10. Which of the following is true of AIDS?
    a. The T4/T8 is greater than 1:1.
    b. The individual will have decreased numbers of CD4 cells or helper cells.
    c. The individual will likely be seronegative.
    d. The individual will unlikely develop cancer.
11. Fungi:
    a. can be treated with vaccines.
    b. have peptidoglycans in their walls.
    c. contain no nuclei.
    d. can adapt to the host's environment and low oxygen environments.
12. The hallmark of most infectious disease is fever. Characteristics of fever include:
    a. the body's inability to regulate temperature.
    b. direct causation by exogenous pyrogens.
    c. an indirect effect of endogenous pyrogen from the host's cells on the hypothalamus.
    d. a hypersensitivity response.
13. The primary immune response from vaccination:
    a. is generally long-lasting.
    b. is increased by booster injections to increase the number of memory cells and sustain protective levels of both antibodies and T cells.
    c. develops in response to repeated antigenic exposure.
    d. destroys the pathogen once the disease has started.
14. Antibiotics:
    a. are synthetic products from bacteria.
    b. are effective against virus because the virus uses the enzymes of the host's cells.
    c. cause intercellular fusion between the host's cells.
    d. may inhibit the synthesis of bacterial cell walls.

61

15. Antibiotic-sensitive microbes mutate and develop resistance to particular antibiotics. Resistance occurs because of:
    a. alteration of bacterial cell membranes so that the antibiotic no longer enters the bacterial cell.
    b. activation of inhibitor enzymes produced by the resistant microbe.
    c. decreased synthesis of an essential metabolite that is antagonistic for the drug.
    d. the lipid-containing outer membrane of gram-positive bacteria.

16. As the body is bombarded by foreign invaders, the immune system's sequential response is which of the following?
    1. Macrophages engulf foreign matter.
    2. Helper T cells multiply and activate B cells.
    3. Complement attaches to the invader.
    4. B cells form plasma cells to produce antibodies.
    5. Macrophages present antigens from ingested invaders to the host's cells.
    6. Neutrophils arrive at the invasion site.
    7. Some B cells and T cells become memory cells.
    8. Suppressor T cells slow or stop immune responses.
    9. Killer T cells form and destroy the invader.
       a. 1, 2, 3, 4, and 5
       b. 6, 3, 1, 5, and 2
       c. 1, 3, 4, 9, and 8
       d. 6, 4, 8, 2, and 7

17. The sequence of viral host cell infection is which of the following?
    1. Penetration
    2. Insertion of viral genome into the host cell
    3. Adsorption
    4. Uncoating
    5. Viral genome replication
    6. Viral protein synthesis
    7. Maturation
    8. Budding
    9. Release of new infective virions
       a. 2, 4, 3, 6, and 7
       b. 3, 1, 4, 2, and 9
       c. 3, 4, 2, 6, and 9
       d. 3, 4, 1, 2, and 7

Matching

Match the pathogen to its diseases or characteristics.

18. _____ Staphylococcus

19. _____ *Neisseria gonorrhoeae*

20. _____ Group A streptococci

21. _____ *Mycoplasma pneumoniae*

22. _____ Chlamydia

23. _____ Hepatitis B virus

a. variola

b. fever blisters

c. cause Sexually Transmitted Diseases (STIs)

d. common cold

e. Intracellular parasite

f. produces proteins that inhibit complement

g. infects urethra and produces a protease that digests IgA

h. antigen resembles human myocardial tissue

i. causes atypical pneumonia

Match the evasive strategy with its defensive mechanism.

24. _____ Coating with self

25. _____ Neutralization of immune molecules

a. adsorption of fibronectin or IgG

b. degradation of complement

c. multiple in phagosomes

d. shedding surface antigens

C.E., a 27-year-old man, was admitted to the emergency department with shortness of breath and a productive cough. He said, "I have had pneumonia several times in the last two years." He volunteered information about his homosexual practices. On physical examination, perianal vesicular and ulcerative lesions of herpes simplex infection were present. Fine crackles on the lower half of his lung fields with inspiratory and expiratory rhonchi were present.

Questions

Considering the circumstances, what laboratory tests would you consider appropriate?

What test results would you expect?

63

10 Stress and Disease

FOUNDATIONAL KNOWLEDGE OJECTIVE

After reviewing the primary text where referenced, the learner will be able to do the following:
a. Identify the function of biochemicals that regulate the stress response.
   Refer to Figures 10-1 through 10-6 and Tables 10-2 through 10-6.

MEMORY CHECK!

- There is a relationship between the nervous, endocrine, and immune systems that involves the common usage of molecules and receptors in each system. Central nervous system and autonomic nervous system neuropeptides affect immune cells. Endocrine products influence immune and neuroimmune cell function. The immune cell cytokines affect both nervous and endocrine cell function.
   These intersystem effectors and their actions include the following:
- Corticotropin-releasing factor (CRH) is a hypothalamic hormone that regulates many stress-induced alterations. It activates the pituitary gland and the sympathetic nervous system. Also, direct suppressive effects of CRH occur on two immune cell types possessing CRH receptor: the monocyte-macrophage and the helper T lymphocyte.
- Adrenocorticotropic hormone (ACTH) controls the production and secretion of glucocorticoids by the cortex of the adrenal glands. ACTH is produced by the anterior pituitary and in small amounts by lymphocytes.
- Cortisol is secreted by the adrenal cortex, and it then circulates in the blood plasma. It elevates blood glucose and is anabolic for liver RNA and protein but catabolic for muscle and lymphoid tissue. When excessive, it stimulates gastric secretion. Cortisol is immunosuppressive for immunoglobulins and reduces eosinophils, macrophages, and lymphocytes; it is generally anti-inflammatory.
- Growth hormone (GH) is secreted by the anterior pituitary; it elevates blood glucose and promotes protein anabolism, tissue repair, and antibody production by plasma cells. Prolonged stress suppresses growth hormone.
- Interleukin-1 (IL-1) and interleukin-6 (IL-6) are substances produced by macrophages that stimulate the release of ACTH through CRH. These factors affect B-cell and T-cell proliferation and body temperature.
- Interleukin-2 (IL-2) is produced by T cells and potentiates B cells and T cells, monocyte, and natural killer cell activity and increases pituitary ACTH levels. Prolactin acts as a second messenger for IL-2 and has a positive influence on B-cell activation and differentiation.
- Interferon (IFN) is produced by lymphocytes, macrophages, and fibroblasts. These proteins are antiviral; they enhance phagocytic activity, suppress neoplastic growth, and stimulate the hypothalamus, pituitary, and adrenal pathway.
- Tumor necrosis factor (TNF) is produced mostly by macrophages. It stimulates inflammatory and immune mediators.
- Substance P is found in sensory nerves, spinal cord pathways, and parts of the brain; it stimulates the perception of pain.
- Endorphins are concentrated in the pituitary gland and inhibit pain by blocking the release of substance P; they may inhibit CRH secretion and inhibit or delay blood pressure increases.
- Epinephrine and norepinephrine levels are controlled by sympathetic preganglionic neurons that stimulate their secretion by the adrenal medulla. Both increase heart rate, blood pressure, and blood glucose. Epinephrine dilates skeletal muscle blood vessels. Lymphoid tissue is innervated and, therefore, influenced by these substances.
- Neuropeptide Y (NPY) is a neurotransmitter and neurohormone released from the sympathetic nerves and the adrenal medulla. NPY increases vasoconstriction and increases the action of catecholamines.
- Histamine and serotonin are both vasoactive amines that participate in inflammation. Serotonin is found in the brain stem and in blood platelets. Histamine is found in basophils, mast cells, and platelets.
- Testosterone is immunosuppressive, whereas estrogen enhances resistance to infection but increases risk for autoimmune disease
- Oxytocin likely is associated with reduced hypothalamic-pituitary-adrenal (HPA) axis activation and reduced anxiety, so it has antistress properties.

LEARNING OBJECTIVES

After studying this chapter, the learner will be able to do the following:

1. Define stress, identify stressors, and state the effects of stress.

Study text page 337.

Stress arises when a person interacts or transacts with situations in certain ways. People are not disturbed by situations as they exist but by the ways they individually appraise and react to situations. Stress is a condition in which a demand exceeds a person's coping abilities. Stress reactions may include disturbance of cognition, emotion, and behavior that can adversely affect an individual's well-being. Stressors, such as infection, noise, decreased oxygen supply, pain, heat, cold, trauma, and radiation; prolonged exertional responses to life's events, which include anxiety, depression, anger, old age, fear, excitement, and obesity associated with disease, drugs, surgery, and medical treatment can all elicit the stress response. The effects of stress on inflammatory and immune processes influence the course of cardiovascular disease, autoimmune disorders, and cancer.

2. Describe Selye's original general adaptation syndrome; cite its stages.

Study text page 338.

While attempting to discover a new sex hormone, Selye injected crude ovarian extracts into rats. Repeatedly, he found the following triad of structural changes: (1) enlargement of the cortex of the adrenal gland, (2) atrophy of the thymus gland and other lymphoid structures, and (3) development of bleeding ulcers of the stomach and duodenal lining. Selye discovered that this triad of manifestations was not specific for his ovarian extracts but also occurred after he exposed the rats to other noxious stimuli such as cold, surgical injury, and restraint. Selye concluded that this triad or syndrome of manifestations represented a nonspecific response to noxious stimuli. Because many diverse agents caused the same syndrome, Selye suggested that it be called the **general adaptation syndrome (GAS).**

Selye later defined three successive stages in the development of the GAS: (1) the alarm stage, (2) the stage of resistance or adaptation, and (3) the stage of exhaustion. The nonspecific physiologic response identified by Selye consists of interaction among the sympathetic branch of the autonomic nervous system and two glands, the pituitary gland and the adrenal gland; hence, the interaction was known as the **hypothalamic-pituitary-adrenal (HPA) axis** system.

The alarm phase of the GAS begins when a stressor triggers the actions of the pituitary gland and the sympathetic nervous system. The resistance or adaptation phase begins with the actions of cortisol, norepinephrine, and epinephrine. Exhaustion occurs if stress continues and adaptation is not successful. The ultimate signs of exhaustion are impairment of the immune response, heart failure, and kidney failure, leading to death. Selye identified three components of the physiologic stress: (1) the exogenous or endogenous stressor initiating the disturbance, (2) the chemical or physical disturbance produced by the stressor, and (3) the body's counteracting (adaptational) response to the disturbance.

3. Identify current concepts that modify Selye's work.

Study text pages 338 and 339.

Selye believed that stressors cause a general or nonspecific but purely physiologic response. However, research has shown the remarkable sensitivity of the central nervous system and endocrine system to psychological influences. As with a physically mediated stress response, psychological stressors can elicit a reactive stress response. The **reactive response** is a physiologic response derived from psychological stressors. For example, the stress of an examination may produce an increased heart rate and dry mouth in the unprepared student. Although there is no physical stressor, the psychological stress of an examination elicits a reactive physiologic response.

Another type of psychologically mediated stress response is the **anticipatory response**. Rather than reacting to an obvious stressor, the body mounts a physiologic stress response in anticipation of disruption of the optimal steady state, also known as **homeostasis.** These anticipatory responses can be generated either by species-specific innate programs, such as predators and unfamiliar situations, or by experience-dependent memory programs created by **conditioning.** Under some circumstances these memory programs may become so strong that psychological disorders, such as phobias, develop. Some individuals develop **posttraumatic stress disorders** in response to the memory of traumatic events. These memories are characterized by flashback memories, sleep disturbances, depression, and other symptoms that render the victim incapable of employment or maintaining personal relationships.

Stressors also cause **psychoneuroimmunology responses.** Psychoneuroimmunology assumes that all immune-related disease is multifactorial, or the result of interrelationships among psychosocial, emotional, genetic, neurologic, endocrine, and immune systems and behavioral factors.

Specifically, **corticotropin-releasing hormone (CRH)** is released from the hypothalamus, the sympathetic nervous system, the pituitary gland, and the adrenal gland. CRH is also released peripherally at inflammatory sites and is called **peripheral** or **immune CRH.** Sufficient data now exist to conclude that immune modulation by psychosocial stressors or interventions leads directly to health outcomes, with the strongest data in studies of infectious disease and wound healing.

4. Summarize the major interactions of the nervous, endocrine, and immune systems in the stress response and develop an abbreviated flow chart showing these relationships.

Study the stress response in the summary review on text pages 355 and 356; refer to Figure 10-2.

CRH is the primary mediator of many stress-induced alterations to immune functions because of its role as an initiator of biologic brain responses to stress. It activates the HPA axis, which regulates many stress-induced

66

responses by the anterior pituitary, the LC-NE system and the adrenal medulla, and the posterior pituitary. However, direct suppressive effects of CRH have also been reported on two immune cell types that process CRH receptors: the monocyte-macrophage and the CD4 (T helper) lymphocyte. The production of CRH is initiated by a high level of IL-1. Production of IL-1 by activated macrophages and monocytes is inhibited by circulating glucocorticoids. The stimulation of CRH production in the hypothalamus by IL-1 demonstrates immune-induced regulation of the CNS and the cytokines (TNF and IFN). The T-cell growth factor IL-2 can increase pituitary ACTH as well.

The following flow chart summarizes the interaction of the three systems.

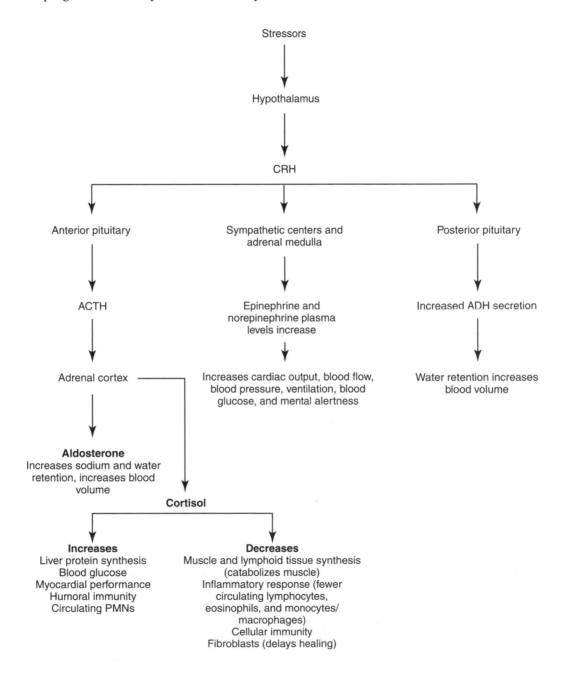

Communication among these three systems involves the common use of signal molecules and their similarly designed receptors. These signal/receptor interactions then regulate cellular behavior in each system, thereby linking each to the other(s).

5. **Distinguish between ineffective and effective methods of coping with stress.**
Study text pages 352 through 355; refer to Figure 10-7.
Stress is not an independent entity but rather a system of interdependent processes that are moderated by the

nature, intensity, and duration of the stressor. The perception, appraisal, and coping efficacy of the affected individual mediate the psychological and physiologic responses to stress. Coping is managing the stressful demands that exceed the individual's resources.

Periods of depression and emotional upheaval with ineffective coping place the affected individual at risk for immunologic deficits.

Adverse life events that have the most negative effect on immunity have been characterized as those events that are uncontrollable and undesirable and that overtax the individual's ability to cope. Those individuals unable to cope may develop immune dysfunction.

Factors that may influence stress susceptibility or resilience include age, socioeconomic status, gender, social support status, personality, self-esteem, genetics, life events, past experiences, and current health status.

Problem-focused and social support coping processes have a beneficial influence during stressful experiences. An individual who is experiencing distress may draw upon internal and external resources to meet the demands. Social support groups can improve psychological coping and immune function by increasing natural killer cell activity.

Stress-Related Diseases

Organ or System	Disease or Condition
Cardiovascular	Coronary artery disease, hypertension, stroke, arrhythmia
Muscles	Tension headaches, backache
Connective tissues	Rheumatoid arthritis
Pulmonary	Asthma, hay fever
Immune	Immunosuppression, deficiency, autoimmunity
Gastrointestinal	Ulcer, irritable bowel syndrome, diarrhea, nausea and vomiting, ulcerative colitis
Genitourinary	Diuresis, impotence, frigidity
Integumentary	Eczema, neurodermatitis, acne
Endocrine	Type 2 diabetes mellitus, amenorrhea
Central nervous	Fatigue and lethargy, type A behavior, overeating, depression, insomnia

6. Cite examples of stress-related diseases.

Refer to Table 10-1. See the table above.

The previous table includes an abbreviated grouping of stress-related disease. However, there is convincing evidence linking cancer with psychological distress with three possible mechanisms involved. First, natural killer cell activity is inhibited in stressed or depressed people. Stress and depression are also associated with poorer repair of damaged DNA and alterations in the rates of apoptosis of immune and cancer cells.

New evidence is showing a relationship among immune stimulation, infections, and heart disease. The relationship between stress and cardiovascular health may be mediated by stress-induced changes in immune function, which may potentiate proinflammatory processes and permit infections that lead to heart disease.

PRACTICE EXAMINATION

Multiple Choice

Circle the correct answer for each question.

1. Which of the following is a characteristic of Selye's stress syndrome?
   a. Adrenocortical enlargement
   b. Thymus enlargement
   c. It is a specific response to stress
   d. Lymphatic organs enlarge
2. Which of the following characterizes the alarm stage?
   a. Increased lymphocytes
   b. Increased sympathetic activity
   c. Increased parasympathetic activity
   d. Increased eosinophils
3. In stressed or depressed individuals:
   a. natural killer cells are stimulated.
   b. damaged DNA is repaired properly.
   c. apoptosis of immune and cancer cells is altered.
   d. cellular immunity is increased and humoral immunity is decreased.
4. Which is the correct sequence of Selye's hypothesis for stress?
   a. Increased ACTH secretion, alarm
   b. Increased ACTH in the blood, hypertrophy of the adrenal cortex
   c. Stimulation of the sympathetic centers, alarm
   d. Increased secretion of epinephrine, increased ACTH in the blood
5. Corticotropin-releasing hormone (CRH) is released by the:
   a. adrenal medulla.
   b. adrenal cortex.
   c. anterior pituitary.
   d. hypothalamus.
6. Stress may be defined as any factor that stimulates the:
   a. posterior pituitary.
   b. anterior pituitary.
   c. hypothalamus to release CRH.
   d. hypothalamus to release ADH.
7. Which of the following is true?
   a. Stressors initially stimulate the adrenal cortex.
   b. Stressors stimulate immunity.
   c. The emotions of fear, anxiety, and grief can act as stressors.
   d. Stressors are the same for all individuals.

8. Glucocorticoids are highest during the stage of:
   a. exhaustion.
   b. alarm.
   c. resistance.
9. The physiologic response to the stress of a student's final exam may be:
   a. reactive.
   b. a conditioned behavior.
   c. anticipatory.
   d. caused by a physical stressor.
10. The production of cortisol in response to stress can be initiated by:
    a. the hypothalamus, anterior pituitary, and adrenal cortex.
    b. the hypothalamus, posterior pituitary, and adrenal cortex.
    c. the hypothalamus, sympathetic nerve fibers, and adrenal cortex.
    d. the hypothalamus, sympathetic nerve fibers, and adrenal medulla.
11. Cortisol:
    a. affects protein catabolism.
    b. decreases blood sugar.
    c. increases immune response.
    d. increases allergic reactions.
12. Which of the following would occur in response to stress?
    a. Increased systolic blood pressure
    b. Decreased epinephrine
    c. Constriction of the pupils
    d. Decreased adrenocorticoids
13. Which of the following would be least useful in the assessment of stress?
    a. Total blood cholesterol
    b. Eosinophil count
    c. Lymphocyte count
    d. Adrenocorticoid levels
14. In response to stress, the adrenal cortex secretes:
    a. norepinephrine.
    b. norepinephrine and cortisol.
    c. cortisol and aldosterone.
    d. norepinephrine and aldosterone.
15. Coping:
    a. slows natural killer cell activity.
    b. best involves solving the stress circumstance by oneself.
    c. effectively leads to immune dysfunction.
    d. manages stressful demands exceeding an individual's resources.

Fill in the Blanks

Supply the correct response for each statement.

16. Biochemicals secreted by the adrenal cortex in response to stress are _____.

17. _____ cause disturbances in cognition, emotion, and behavior.

18. The bodily changes initiated by noxious stimuli cause the _____.

19. The stage of GAS wherein the immunity of an individual is most impaired is the _____.

20. The stage of GAS that triggers the sympathetic nervous system is the _____.

21. The cytokine produced by macrophages stimulating release of CRH is _____.

22. An interleukin that increases ACTH levels is _____.

23. A neurotransmitter augmenting the action of catecholamines is _____.

24. A substance produced by lymphocytes, macrophages, and fibroblasts that enhances phagocytic activity is _____.

25. _____ inhibit pain, CRH secretion, and blood pressure increases.

11 Biology, Clinical Manifestations, and Treatment of Cancer

FOUNDATIONAL KNOWLEDGE OBJECTIVES

After reviewing the primary text where referenced, the learner will be able to do the following:
a. **Describe the phases of cellular mitosis and cytokinesis.**
   Review text page 35 and Figure 1-33.

MEMORY CHECK!

- The reproduction or division of somatic cells involves two sequential phases: mitosis (nuclear division) and cytokinesis (cytoplasmic division). These phases occur in close succession, with cytokinesis beginning toward the end of mitosis. Before a cell can divide, it must double its mass and duplicate all of its contents. Most of the preparation for division occurs during the growth phase, which is also called interphase. The alteration between mitosis and interphase in all tissues that have cellular turnover is known as the cell cycle.
- There are four designated phases of the cell cycle: (1) the S phase (synthesis), in which DNA is synthesized in the cell nucleus; (2) the G2 phase, in which RNA and protein synthesis occur; (3) the M phase (mitosis), which includes both nuclear and cytoplasmic division; and (4) the G1 phase, which is the period between the M phase and the start of DNA synthesis. Interphase, which consists of the G1, S, and G2 phases, is the longest phase of the cell cycle.
- The M phase of the cell cycle, which is made up of mitosis and cytokinesis, begins with prophase, which is the first appearance of chromosomes. Each chromosome has two identical halves called chromatids that lie side by side and are attached together at a site called a centromere. The nuclear membrane disappears in this phase. Spindle fibers are microtubules formed in the cytoplasm that radiate from two centrioles located at opposite poles of the cell.
- During metaphase, which is the next phase of mitosis and cytokinesis, the spindle fibers pull the centromeres until they are aligned in the middle of the spindle or at the equatorial plate.
- Anaphase begins when the centromeres separate and the genetically identical chromatids are pulled apart. The chromatids are pulled, centromeres first, toward opposite sides of the cell. When the identical chromatids are separated, each is considered to be a chromosome. The cell has 92 chromosomes during this stage, but by the end of anaphase, there are 46 chromosomes at each side of the identical cell. Each of the two groups of 46 chromosomes should be identical to the original 46 chromosomes present at the start of the cell cycle.
- During telophase, a new nuclear membrane is formed around each group of 46 chromosomes, the spindle fibers disappear, and the chromosomes begin to uncoil. Cytokinesis causes the cytoplasm to divide into roughly equal parts during this phase. At the end of telophase, two identical diploid cells, called daughter cells, have been formed from the original cell.
- The difference between slowly and rapidly dividing cells is the length of time spent in the G1 phase of the cell cycle. Some cells that divide very slowly can remain in the G1 phase for years. Once the S phase begins, progression through mitosis requires a relatively constant amount of time. After a cell has progressed out of the G1 phase, it must complete the S, G2, and M phases.

b. Identify mechanisms that control cell division.

Review text page 35; refer to Table 1-6.

MEMORY CHECK!

- Gene and protein growth factors govern the proliferation of different cell types within tissues. It is likely that some genes code for growth factors, some for growth factor receptors, some for intracellular regulatory proteins involved in cell adhesion, and some for proteins that help relay signals for cell division to the cell nucleus.
- Cells require highly specific proteins to stimulate cell division. These growth factors are present in the serum in very low concentrations. For example, platelet-derived growth factor stimulates the production of connective tissue cells. Another important growth factor is interleukin, which stimulates the proliferation of T cells. Cells that respond to a particular growth factor have specific receptors for the specific growth factor in their plasma membrane. Some growth factors are also regulators of cellular differentiation.

c. Describe mechanisms that confine cells and tissues to specific anatomic sites.

Review text pages 35 and 36; refer to Figure 1-34.

MEMORY CHECK!

- All cells are within a network of extracellular macromolecules known as the extracellular matrix. The extracellular matrix holds cells and tissues together and provides an organized framework in which cells can interact with each other.
- To confine themselves and form tissues, cells must have intercellular recognition and adhesion. Specialized cells are likely to form a tissue in one of two ways. The first way is mitosis of one or more founder cells. Founder cells, which are basic precursor cells, are prevented from "wandering away" by macromolecules in the extracellular matrix and by adherence to one another at specialized junctions on their plasma membranes. The second way for specialized cells to form tissues involves their migration to and subsequent accumulation at the site of tissue formation. Migrant cells are thought to arrive at the specific site of tissue formation through chemotaxis or contact guidance. Cells at the migrant cells' destination secrete a chemical known as chemotactic factor that attracts specific migrant cells. Contact guidance is movement along a pathway or "pavement" within the extracellular matrix. To stay together in groups, cells must recognize each other and remain distinct from the cells of surrounding tissues.
- Cells in direct physical contact with neighboring cells are often linked together at specialized regions of their plasma membranes; these regions are known as cell junctions. Cell junctions hold cells together and allow small molecules to pass from cell to cell; this coordinates the activities of cells that form tissues. There are three main types of cell junctions: (1) desmosomes, (2) tight junctions, and (3) gap junctions. Desmosomes hold cells together by forming either continuous bands of epithelial sheets or buttonlike points of contact. Desmosomes also provide a system of braces to maintain structural stability. Tight junctions act as a barrier to diffusion, prevent movement of substances through transport.

LEARNING OBJECTIVES

After studying this chapter, the learner will be able to do the following:

1. Define neoplasia and cancer.

Study text pages 360 and 361.

The word **tumor** originally referred to any swelling, for example, due to inflammation, but is now generally reserved for a new growth, or **neoplasm.** Not all tumors or neoplasms, however, are cancer. The term **cancer** refers to a *malignant tumor* and is not used to refer to *benign* growths such as lipomas or hypertrophy of an organ.

2. Cite the method for naming and classifying tumors; provide examples.

Study text pages 361 and 362; refer to Figures 11-1 and 11-2 and Tables 11-1 and 11-2. See the table on page 73.

Tumors are named according to the tissue of origin with the suffix "-oma" added. Cancers having an epithelial tissue origin are identified as carcinomas, whereas those with a connective tissue origin are sarcomas. Lymphomas arise from lymphatic tissue, gliomas arise from glial cells of the central nervous system, and leukemias arise from the bone marrow. **Carcinoma in situ** (often abbreviated CIS) refers to preinvasive epithelial tumors of glandular or squamous cell origin. These early stage tumors have not broken through basement membranes of the epithelium. The time that such preinvasive lesions remain in situ before becoming invasive is unknown. However, some carcinomas remain in situ several years before they progress to carcinoma and metastatic tumors. The classification of cancers was originally based on gross and light microscopic appearance, but now this is aided by additional immunohistochemical analysis of protein expression. Sometimes, a single gene is examined or a panel of genes and proteins are examined.

3. **Identify some changes that occur in cancerous cells and their functional significance.**

   Study text pages 362 through 367; refer to Figures 11-3 through 11-6. See the table below.

4. **Describe tumor cell markers; cite marker examples that suggest the existence of cancer.**

   Study text page 367; refer to Table 11-3. See the table on page 74.

   Tumor cell markers are substances that are produced by cancer cells and found on tumor plasma membranes or in the blood, spinal fluid, or urine. They include hormones, enzymes, genes, antigens, and antibodies.

Tumor cell markers can be used in three ways: (1) to identify individuals at high risk for cancer, (2) to help diagnose the specific type of tumor in individuals with clinical manifestations of cancer, and (3) to observe the clinical course of cancer. The presence of a tumor marker may increase the probability of cancer, but it is not used alone as a diagnostic test.

5. **Postulate a model for the causes and sequence of carcinogenesis.**

   Study text pages 367 through 375, 377, and 378; refer to Figures 11-7 through 11-20 and Tables 11-4 through 11-6. See the flow chart on page 74.

   Oncogenes are genes that can transform a normal cell into a cancerous cell when inherited or activated by oncogenic viruses. Oncogenes can develop from normal

Common Benign and Malignant Tumors

Tissue	Benign Tumor	Malignant Tumor
Connective Tissue		
Fibrous	Fibroma	Fibrosarcoma
Cartilage	Chondroma	Chondrosarcoma
Bone	Osteoma	Osteosarcoma
Fat	Lipoma	Liposarcoma
Smooth muscle	Leiomyoma	Leiomyosarcoma
Striated muscle	Rhabdomyoma	Rhabdomyosarcoma
Blood vessels	Hemangioma	Hemangiosarcoma
Hematopoietic		
Lymphoid tissue	Infectious mononucleosis	Lymphosarcoma (lymphoma)
Plasma cells		Multiple myeloma
Leukocytes		Leukemia
Nerve Tissue		
Nerve cell	Neuroma	
Nerve sheath	Neurilemmoma	Neurogenic sarcoma
Glial tissue		Glioma
Retina		Retinoblastoma
Epithelial Tissue		
Squamous epithelium	Papilloma	Squamous carcinoma
Glandular epithelium	Adenoma	Adenocarcinoma

Cancerous Cell Changes and Their Significance

Change	Significance
Transformation (autonomy)	Independence from normal cellular controls
Anchorage-independent (fewer anchoring junctions)	Continue to grow and divide when not attached to firm surface, favors growth in new area
Immortal	Unlimited life span, continue to divide
Defective differentiation	More immature cells, acquire specialized function
Anaplasia	Loss of differentiation or specialization, loses ability to function and control its growth and division
Pleomorphism	Variable size and shape

NOTE: The most malignant tumors have the most anaplasia.

73

Examples of Tumor Markers

Marker	Name	Type of Cancer Suggested
AFP	α-fetoprotein	Hepatic, germ cell
CEA	Carcinoembryonic antigen	GI, pancreas, lung, breast
β-hCG	Human chorionic gonadotropin	Germ cell
PSA	Prostate-specific antigen	Prostate
Catecholamines (epinephrine)		Pheochromocytoma (adrenal medulla)
Urinary Bence-Jones protein		Multiple myeloma
ACTH	Adrenocorticotropic hormone	Pituitary adenomas

genes (**proto-oncogenes**) that regulate growth and development by encoding for growth factors and growth factor receptors. These genes may undergo some change that either causes them to produce an abnormal product or disrupts their control so that they are expressed inappropriately and accelerate proliferation.

Some cancers are not caused by oncogenes but rather by genes called **tumor suppressor genes** that have mutated. These genes produce proteins that normally oppose the action of an oncogene or inhibit cell division. Carcinogenesis inactivates tumor suppressor genes by loss of **heterozygosity** (loss of one gene copy), which unmasks mutations in recessive genes, or by **silencing** (in which methylation of DNA shuts off genes without mutation) and activates oncogenes.

Cells have a self-destruct mechanism, known as **apoptosis,** triggered by normal development and excessive growth. The most common mutations causing resistance to apoptosis occur in the *p53* gene.

Other than germ cells, cells in the body can divide only a limited number of times. **Telomeres** are at the ends of each chromosome and block unlimited cell division. **Telomerase** maintains telomeres. Cancer cells activate telomerase to restore and maintain telomeres so cells can divide over and over again.

Whenever normal DNA integrity is disrupted during mitosis or by external mutagens, multiple mechanisms have evolved to protect and repair the genome. These repair mechanisms are directed by **caretaker genes.** These genes encode proteins that repair damaged DNA, and loss of caretaker genes leads to increased mutation rates.

6. Identify some oncogenic viruses; characterize an oncogenic bacterium.

Study text pages 379 through 381; refer to Table 11-7.

Viruses implicated in human cancers are called oncogenic viruses. Viruses alter the genome of the infected cell, which then alters the progeny of the host cell. Up to 80% of worldwide liver cancer is associated with chronic hepatitis caused by hepatitis B or C virus. Chronic liver inflammation predisposes to the development of hepatic carcinoma. Virtually all human cervical cancer is caused by specific subtypes of human papillomavirus (HPV). This virus infects basal skin cells and causes warts. When the virus is integrated into the DNA of the basal cell of the cervix, it produces viral oncogenes. Human T-cell leukemia/lymphoma virus is linked to developing adult

T-cell leukemia and lymphoma. It can be inherited by children and transmitted by breast-feeding, sexual intercourse, and blood transfusions.

Helicobacter pylori infects more than half of the world's population. This **bacterium** is now accepted as

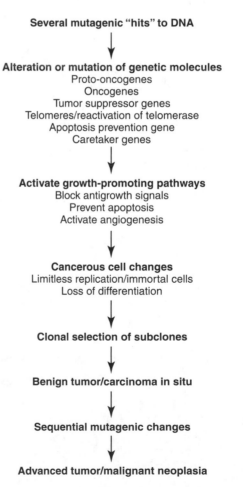

Causes and Sequence of Carcinogenesis

Several mutagenic "hits" to DNA

↓

Alteration or mutation of genetic molecules
Proto-oncogenes
Oncogenes
Tumor suppressor genes
Telomeres/reactivation of telomerase
Apoptosis prevention gene
Caretaker genes

↓

Activate growth-promoting pathways
Block antigrowth signals
Prevent apoptosis
Activate angiogenesis

↓

Cancerous cell changes
Limitless replication/immortal cells
Loss of differentiation

↓

Clonal selection of subclones

↓

Benign tumor/carcinoma in situ

↓

Sequential mutagenic changes

↓

Advanced tumor/malignant neoplasia

NOTE: Genetic mutations can occur in response to exposure to a large number of environmental agents. See Chapter 12 for agent exposures related to cancer. Epigenetic changes in genes by DNA methylation and covalent histone modification can mimic mutation by heritably turning off tumor suppressor genes.

the most common cause of gastric infection, and it is responsible for the majority of individuals with peptic ulcer disease, gastric lymphomas, and gastric carcinomas. It is also associated with a less common gastric mucosa-associated lymphoid tissue (MALT) lymphoma.

7. Describe the mechanisms involved in metastasis.

Study text pages 381 through 383; refer to Figures 11-21 through 11-24 and Table 11-8.

Most cancer cells are unable to cause metastases. The reason lies both in the "seed" and the "soil." Cancer cells (the seeds) must overcome multiple physical and physiologic barriers to spread, survive, and proliferate in distant locations (the soil), which must be receptive to the cancer cells As cancers grow, they develop increasing **heterogeneity.** As this diversity increases, the number of cells in the cancer mass increases with new abilities that facilitate metastasis.

For cells to move from their normal, original niche, they must **detach** from the stroma and migrate. To spread, many tumors and their associated inflammatory cells secrete proteases and protease activators. Proteases digest the extracellular matrix and basement membranes and thus create pathways through which cancer cells move. These cells release bioactive peptides as digestion products that stimulate tumor growth and mobility. Another mediator of cell detachment is the down-regulation in the cancer cell of specific adhesion molcules, such as E-cadherin and integrins. When E-cadherin is lost, cells are able to detach from their extracellular attachments and migrate more readily.

After detachment, the cancer cell must **survive** and **spread within the circulation.** These detached cells have already adapted to a hypoxic environment and already have been selected to resist apopotosis because they have lost their interggrins. They then access the circulation through new tumor-associated blood vessel growth or angiogenesis, also known as **neovascularization.** Mobile tumor cells enter the circulation because of chemoattractive mediators coming from these new vessels. Once in the circulation, metastatic cells must withstand the stresses of travel in the blood and lymphatic vessels as well as exposure to immune cells. One survival mechanism is for the tumor cells to bind to blood platelets. This provides a protective coat that shields the cell and creates a small tumor embolus able to move to a distant site through veins and lymphatics for **escape** from the **circulation.** Lymphatic and venous blood flow enable colon cancer to spread to the liver, liver cancers to spread to the lungs, lung cancers to spread to the brain, and breast cancers to spread to axillary lymph nodes. There is a major selectivity of different cancers for different sites. This **site selectivity** is likely caused by specific interactions between the cancer cells and specific receptors on the small blood vessels.

Cancer cells may arrive in a new location and survive but not proliferate to form a clinically revelant metastasis nor **develop a new microenvironment.** This dormancy may account for the observation that solitary tumor cells can be detected in the blood for years after a clinical remission in individuals; many individuals with detectable micrometastases will not develop clinically obvious metastases. It is possible that successful metastatic tumor cells secrete factors that recruit circulating mesenchymal stem cells to the metastatic site. These newly recruited stem cells then differentiate into tumor-supporting stroma and new blood vessels.

8. Describe the diagnosis and staging of cancer.

Study text pages 383, 386, and 387; refer to Figure 11-25 and Tables 11-9 and 11-10

The diagnostic symptoms a cancer produces are as diverse as the types of cancer. The location of the cancer can determine symptoms by physical pressure, obstruction, and loss of normal function. Cancer can cause problems far away from its source by pressing on nerves or secreting bioactive compounds. Once the diagnosis of cancer is suspected or identified, tumor tissue must be obtained to establish a **definitive diagnosis** and correctly classify the disease. The classification of cancer can be further facilitated by other available tests, including immunohistochemical stains, flow cytometry, electron microscopy, chromosome analysis, and nucleic acid–based molecular studies.

If cancer exists, it is critical to know the extent of its spread, or its **stage.** Staging the tumor is an important component of cancer diagnosis. In general, a four-stage

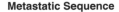

Metastatic Sequence

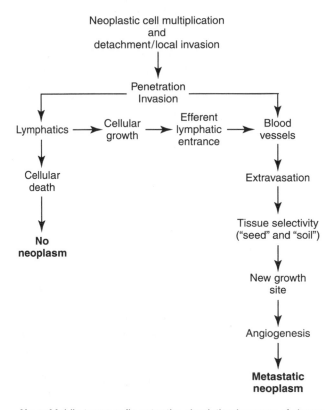

NOTE: Mobile tumor cells enter the circulation because of chemo-attractive mediators released from neovascularization. Specific interactions between the cancer cells and receptors on small blood vessels create the microenvironment ("soil").

75

system is used, with carcinoma in situ regarded as a special case. Cancer confined to the site of origin is stage 1, cancer that is locally invasive is stage 2, cancer that has spread to regional structures such as lymph nodes is stage 3, and cancer that has spread to distant sites is stage 4. In general, the lower the stage, the more amenable the cancer is to treatment. Also, staging alters the choice of therapy; more aggressive therapy is delivered to more invasive disease.

9. Compare the treatment modalities for neoplasms.

Study text pages 387 and 388; refer to Table 11-11.

Cancer is treated with chemotherapy, radiotherapy, surgery, immunotherapy, and combinations of these modalities. The mechanism by which **chemotherapy** acts to eradicate tumor cells depends largely on its effect on the cell cycle. The goal of chemotherapy is to kill cells that are undergoing mitosis and cytokinesis and those in interphase. To be effective, chemotherapy must eliminate enough neoplastic cells so that the body's own defenses can eradicate the remaining cells. **Combination chemotherapy** is the synergistic use of several agents, each with an effect against a certain cancer, used to avoid single-agent resistance and acquired drug resistance. Also, lower doses of each agent may be used, causing fewer side effects. Faster growing neoplasms are generally more sensitive to chemotherapy. **Induction chemotherapy** seeks to cause shrinkage or disappearance of tumor. **Adjuvant chemotherapy** is given after surgical excision of a cancerous lesion with the goal of eliminating micrometastases. **Neoadjuvant chemotherapy** is given prior to localized surgery or radiation.

Radiation or ionizing radiation is a common approach to the treatment of malignant disease. To eradicate neoplastic cells without producing excessive toxicity and to avoid damage to normal structures are the challenges of radiation therapy. Ionizing radiation damages important macromolecules, especially DNA. Rapidly renewing and dividing cells are generally more radiosensitive than other cells. Because radiation produces irreversible changes in normal tissue, there is a maximum lifetime dose that tissue can tolerate. Radiation is well suited to treat localized disease in areas that are difficult to reach surgically. Radioactive iodine capsules can be placed temporarily into body cavities for treatment of cervical, prostate, and head and neck cancers; this delivery method is termed **brachytherapy.**

Surgical therapy is useful and definitive when the neoplasm is accessible and has not yet spread beyond the limits of surgical excision. If there is any chance of regional lymph node involvement and no evidence of distant disease, the lymph nodes should also be removed. Debulking surgery in which the majority of a tumor is removed can allow greater success with adjuvant chemotherapy or irradiation. Palliative surgery (alleviation without cure) may be used to relieve or avoid symptoms of malignancy. Surgery is also indicated for benign tumors and tumors that could become malignant. The key principle that applies to cancer surgery includes obtaining adequate surgical margins during resection to prevent local recurrences and scrupulous avoidance of the spread of cancer cells during the surgical procedures.

10. Describe the complications of cancer and the side effects of treatment.

Study text pages 388 through 392; refer to Figures 11-26 and 11-27 and Tables 11-12 and 11-13.

Paraneoplastic syndromes are symptom complexes triggered by cancer. They are caused by biologic substances released from the tumor such as hormones and immune modifiers. These syndromes may be the earliest symptoms of cancer and may be life threatening.

Usually little or no **pain** is associated with the early stages of malignant disease, but pain will affect individuals who are terminally ill with cancer. Cancer-associated pain arises from multiple sources. Direct pressure, obstruction, invasion of sensitive structures, stretching of visceral surfaces, tissue destruction, infection, and inflammation all can cause pain. Pain can occur at the site of the primary tumor or from a metastatic lesion. Furthermore, it can be referred from the any involved site.

Fatigue is the most frequently reported symptom of cancer and cancer treatment. Likely causes of fatigue include sleep disturbance, biochemical changes, psychologic factors, altered nutritional status, and level of activity. Decreased muscle contractibility and function are observed in individuals with cancer. Muscle loss may result from cancer treatment or from circulating tumor necrosis factor and IL-1.

Cachexia is a wasting, emaciation manifesting symptoms of anorexia; early satiety; anemia; marked weakness; taste alteration; and altered protein, lipid, and carbohydrate metabolism, which is a loss of appetite, contributes to the syndrome of cachexia. Individuals show hyperinsulinemia, insulin resistance, hyperglycemia, and abnormal blood glucose tests. In cancer, protein is used to meet energy needs rather than spared to protect vital tissues. Cytokines including IL-6, TNF, and an interferon appear to cause the metabolic alterations associated with tissue loss in cancer wasting.

Anemia is also commonly associated with malignancy. The majority of individuals with cancer have a mild anemia, although 20% may have hemoglobin concentrations below 9 g/dl or more than 40%. Chronic bleeding, severe malnutrition, medical therapies, or malignancy in blood-forming organs may cause anemia by depleting erythrocyte building blocks or destroying the site for synthesis of erythrocytes.

Direct tumor invasion into the bone marrow causes **leukopenia** and **thrombocytopenia.** Many chemotherapeutic drugs are toxic to the bone marrow and cause **granulocytopenia** as well as thrombocytopenia. Radiation therapy that involves the bone marrow also may cause granulocytopenia.

Infection is the most significant cause of complications and death in individuals with malignant disease. Individuals with cancer are very susceptible to infection because of reductions in immunologic functions, debility from advanced disease, and immunosuppression from radiotherapy and chemotherapy. Surgery can create favorable sites for infection. The incidence of hospital-related or nosocomial infections for cancer patients is increased because of indwelling medical devices, compromised wound care, and the introduction of microorganisms from visitors and other patients.

Most side effects accompanying cancer treatment are directly related to the targeting of rapidly growing cells. In the gastrointestinal tract, both chemotherapy and irradiation may cause decreased cell turnover leading to **oral ulcers, malabsorption,** and **diarrhea.** Also, disruption of barrier defenses increases the risk of **gastrointestinal tract infection. Nausea** may occur because of the agent's direct action on the vomiting center.

The **reproductive tract** may be affected by irradiation and chemotherapy causing decreased fertility and premature menopause. Prepubertal gonads seem more resistant to damage. In craniospinal irradiation, the hypothalamus or pituitary gland may be affected and result in gonadal failure.

PRACTICE EXAMINATION

Multiple Choice

Circle the correct answer for each question.

1. Which of the following characterizes cancer cells?
   a. Highly differentiated
   b. Unlimited life span
   c. Mature cellular organization
   d. Extensive anchoring junction
2. Anaplasia refers to:
   a. atypical mitosis.
   b. lack of cellular differentiation.
   c. tendency to develop necrosis.
   d. uncontrolled cell growth.
3. Carcinoma in situ:
   a. has a connective tissue origin.
   b. arises from lymphatic tissue.
   c. arises from bone marrow.
   d. refers to preinvasive epithelial tumors.
   e. tumors break through basement membranes of the epithelium.
4. An adenoma is:
   a. malignant.
   b. a glandular epithelial neoplasm.
   c. a teratoma.
   d. an epithelial tumor.
5. Infectious mononucleosis arises from:
   a. glandular epithelium.
   b. blood vessels
   c. glial tissue.
   d. lymphoid tissue.
6. Tumor-suppressor genes:
   a. have the ability to transform a normal cell into a cancerous cell.
   b. regulate growth and development.
   c. produce proteins that inhibit cellular division.
   d. can develop from proto-oncogenes.

7. Malignant tumors:
   a. resemble their tissue of origin.
   b. exhibit cellular cohesiveness.
   c. have expansive growth modes.
   d. have infiltrative growth modes.
8. Tumor-suppressor genes are inactivated by:
   a. cellular self-destruction.
   b. loss of heterozygosity.
   c. demethylation of DNA.
   d. apoptosis.

Fill in the Blanks

Supply the correct response for each statement.

9. The cause of the majority of gastric lymphomas is _____.

10. _____ is involved whenever a normal cell becomes cancerous.

11. Insulin-like growth factor regulates cell proliferation and inhibits_____.

12. The variable size and shape of cancerous cells is _____.

13. The tumor marker ACTH suggests the possibility of a _____ tumor.

14. Other than germ cells, body cells do not possess the ability to divide an unlimited number of times. Cancer cells activate _____ to maintain and restore _____ so cells can divide over and over again.

Circle the correct answer for each question.

15. Tumor spread depends on:
    a. the growth rate of tumor and its degree of differentiation.
    b. unknown factors.
    c. the presence or absence of anatomic barriers.
    d. All of the above are correct.
16. Which of the following is the correct sequence during the process of metastasis?
    a. Vascularization, adherence of neoplastic cells, invasion into lymph and vascular systems
    b. Transport, vascularization, adherence of neoplastic cells
    c. Cell detachment, invasion into lymph and vascular systems, migration
    d. Vascularization, extravasation, transport
17. For metastasis to occur, local invasive factors require all of the following *except*:
    a. cellular loss from tumor.
    b. fingerlike projections.
    c. lytic enzyme release.
    d. increased cellular adhesion.
    e. increased individual tumor cells.

77

18. Known routes for metastasis of malignant cells include:
    a. continuous extension.
    b. lymphatic spread.
    c. bloodstream dissemination.
    d. All of the above are correct.
19. A malignant cell that becomes lodged in a lymph node may:
    a. die.
    b. divide.
    c. become dormant.
    d. enter the efferent lymphatics.
    e. All of the above are correct.
20. The process by which tumors develop new vascular networks is:
    a. heparinization.
    b. angiogenesis.
    c. anaplasia.
    d. autonomy.
    e. differentiation.
21. The pain experienced with cancer:
    a. affects the individual in the early stages of malignancy.
    b. occurs in bone metastasis.
    c. results from tissue necrosis.
    d. Both b and c are correct.
    e. a, b, and c are correct.
22. The anorexia or loss of appetite seen in the syndrome of cancer cachexia may occur because of:
    a. elevated blood serum levels of glucose and amino acids.
    b. hyperinsulinism.
    c. late satiety.
    d. hypoproteinemia.
23. The anemia associated with malignancy can be:
    a. due to the depletion of hemoglobin building blocks.
    b. severe in the majority of cases.
    c. caused by the destruction of bone marrow.
    d. All of the above are correct.
    e. Both a and c are correct.
24. Chemotherapy kills cancerous cells:
    a. during interphase
    b. during mitosis and cytokinesis.
    c. Both a and b are correct.
    d. that have left the cell cycle.
25. Which is correct about the *p53* gene?
    a. Low oxygen environments decrease its products.
    b. It normally activates apoptosis.
    c. Mutations in it may permit the tumor cells to be less aggressive.
    d. It deactivates the "emergency brake" against uncontrolled growth.

Chapter **11** **Biology, Clinical Manifestations, and Treatment of Cancer**

12 Cancer Epidemiology

FOUNDATIONAL KNOWLEDGE OBJECTIVE

a. **Review the Foundational Knowledge Objective "a" in Chapter 5.**

LEARNING OBJECTIVES

After studying this chapter, the learner will be able to do the following:

1. **Generalize gene-environment-lifestyle interactions.**

   Study text pages 396 and 401; refer to Table 12-1.

   Cancer arises from a complicated and an interacting web of multiple causes. At the cellular level, cancer is genetic. Preventing exposures to **individual carcinogens,** or cancer-causing substances, can prevent many cancers. Widespread general exposures of pollutants from water, air, and the work environment; personal lifestyle choices, such as smoking, excessive alcohol, and poor diet; and involuntary or unknowing exposures in air, water, and the occupation environments are major contributors to cancer.

   It appears that the majority of excess cancer in populations exposed to carcinogens is from the exposure itself and not from rare genetic predispositions. For example, in women who have mutated cancer susceptibility genes, *BRCA1* or *BRCA2,* the risk of having breast cancer at age 50 is 24% for those born before 1940 but 67% for those born later. The implication is related to lifestyle factors that have changed since 1940, including most notably, hormone therapy, later age of first pregnancy, and increased nulliparity.

   Compelling is the role for **environment-lifestyle** contributions to cancer from studies comparing different populations around the world. Breast cancer, for example, is prevalent among northern Europeans and Americans but is relatively rare among women in developing countries. If ethnicity played a major role, then immigrants should retain the cancer incidence rates of their country of origin. Instead, immigrants acquire the same cancer rates of where they move within one to two generations.

   Elevated cancer rates are more common in cities, in farming locations, near hazardous waste sites, downwind of industrial and radiation activities, and near contaminated water wells. In addition, cancers are associated with areas of high pesticide use, toxic work exposures, waste incinerators, and other sources of pollution.

Susceptibility to disease is set **in utero** or **neonatally** as the result of nutrition and exposures to environmental toxins or stressors, or both. Children also may be affected by prenatal exposures, parental exposures prior to conception, and breast milk. Epidemiologic studies have linked higher risks of childhood leukemia and brain and CNS cancers with parental and childhood exposure to particular solvents, pesticides, petrochemicals, dioxins, and polycyclic aromatic hydrocarbons.

2. **Describe the relationship between epigenetics and genetics.**

   Study text pages 401 and 403.

   It is clear that inherited variation in DNA sequence influences individual risk of cancer; however, it constitutes a small percentage of the population. An explosion of data now indicates the importance of epigenetic processes, especially those with resultant gene silencing of *key* regulatory genes. Epigenetic changes collaborate with genetic changes with environmental-lifestyle factors to cause the development of cancer. These changes are mitotically and meiotically heritable.

   The three major areas of **epigenetics** are (1) **methylation** (the addition of methyl group [CH_3] to cytosine ring); this aberrant methylation can lead to silencing of tumor-suppressor genes; (2) **histone modifications** (histone acetylation, alterations in chromatin); and (3) **microRNAs** (miRNAs), small RNA molecules that can target gene expression posttranscriptionally. The expression of miRNAs has recently been linked to carcinogenesis because they can act as either oncogenes or tumor-suppressor genes. An important feature of epigenetic mechanisms and their role in development and disease is that epigenetic processes can be modified by lifestyle, particularly diet and the environment or pharmacological interventions, or both. **Environmental-lifestyle** factors act on individuals through life, changing **gene** expression through epigenetic mechanisms with subsequent implications for health or disease.

   Biologically active food components modify DNA methylation directly. Nutrition influences metabolic effects associated with energy balance. Because adipose tissue is endocrine tissue, obese individuals accumulate macrophages that secrete various proinflammatory signaling molecules and cytokines. Inflammation is strongly associated with cancer development and inflammatory bowel disease is related to methylation in the colon.

79

3. **Indicate the role of in utero and early-life conditions in cancer development.**

Study text pages 403 and 404; refer to Figure 12-1.

It is widely accepted that a **long latency period** precedes the onset of adult cancers. Early life events influence later susceptibility to certain chronic diseases. **Developmental plasticity** is the ability to develop in particular ways depending on the environment or setting. It requires stable gene expression, which appears to be modulated by epigenetic processes, such as DNA methylation and histone modification. Sensitivity to environmental-lifestyle factors influences the mature phenotype and is dependent on the interactions of both the genome and epigenome.

Perhaps one of the best examples of early life events and future cancer was the chemical exposure to **diethylstilbestrol** (DES), a synthetic estrogen. More recent studies have revealed that daughters of women who took DES during pregnancy may have a slightly increased risk of breast cancer before age 40. Epigenetic mechanisms are responsible for tissue-specific gene expression during cellular differentiation and these mechanisms modulate developmental phenotypic changes. The phenotypic effects of epigenetic modifications during development may need long latency periods, such as in cancer, thus manifesting later in life.

4. **Describe tobacco use as a carcinogenic agent.**

Study text pages 404 and 405.

Cigarette smoking is carcinogenic and remains the most important cause of cancer. The risk is greatest in those who begin to smoke when young and continue throughout life. Cigarette smoking accounts for 1 of every 5 deaths each year in the United States. Tobacco use also is associated with squamous and small cell adenocarcinomas. In addition, smoking causes even more deaths from vascular, respiratory, and other diseases than from cancer. Smoking tobacco is linked to cancers of the lower urinary tract, upper digestive tract, paranasal sinuses, liver, kidney, pancreas, cervix, uterus, and myeloid leukemia.

Secondhand smoke, also called **environmental tobacco smoke (ETS),** is the combination of sidestream smoke (burning end of a cigarette, cigar, or pipe) and mainstream smoke (exhaled by the smoker). More than 4000 chemicals have been identified in mainstream tobacco smoke (250 chemicals as toxic), of which 60 are considered carcinogenic. Nonsmokers who live with smokers are at greatest risk for lung cancer as well as numerous noncancerous conditions.

5. **Relate diet and obesity to carcinogenesis.**

Study text pages 405 through 407; refer to Figures 12-2 through 12-6 and Tables 12-3 through 12-5.

People are constantly exposed to a variety of compounds termed **xenobiotics** that include toxic, mutagenic, and carcinogenic chemicals. Many of these chemicals are found in the human **diet.** These chemicals can react with cellular macromolecules, such as proteins and DNA, or can react directly with cell structures to cause cell damage. The body has two defense systems for counteracting these effects: (1) detoxification enzymes and (2) antioxidant systems. Enzymes that activate xenobiotics are called **phase I activation enzymes** and are represented by the multigene cytochrome P450 family, aldehyde oxidase, xanthine oxidases, and peroxidases. **Phase II detoxification enzymes** then protect further against a large array of reactive intermediates and nonactivated xenobiotics. These enzymes are located predominantly in the liver and provide clearance of compounds through the portal circulation, thereby preventing the potentially carcinogenic agent(s) from entering the body through the gastrointestinal tract and portal circulation.

The most relevant carcinogens produced by cooking are the **polycyclic aromatic hydrocarbons** and **heterocyclic aromatic amines** generated by meat protein. The greatest levels are found in well-done, charbroiled beef. People also ingest xenobiotics that are found in environmental or industrial contaminants such as particulate matter of diesel exhaust, contaminating pesticides in food and water supplies, and in certain prescribed and over-the-counter medicines.

Specific nutrients may directly affect the **phenotype** or expression of key genes, for example, epigenetically through abnormalities of methylation of the promoter regions of genes or histones. DNA also can be hypomethylated. **Hypomethylation** can cause overexpression of transcription of proto-oncogenes, increased recombination and mutation as well as loss of imprinting. These alterations can all promote cancer. Aberrant DNA methylation patterns occur in colon, lung, prostate, and breast cancers. Dietary factors may be related to DNA methylation in four ways: (1) dietary factors may influence the supply of methyl groups; (2) factors may modify the use of methyl groups; (3) dietary factors may reduce methyl groups called demethylation; and (4) DNA methylation patterns may influence the response to a dietary factor.

Because **obesity** is associated with other chronic diseases, such as cardiovascular and diabetes, it can increase overall mortality; however, it may not be the causal factor involved in cancer mortality. Yet, obesity is related to increased incidence of several cancer types. Compared with men whose **body mass index** (BMI) was in the normal range (18.5 to 24.9), men with substantial obesity (BMI > 40.0) had significant increases in cancer mortality. In men with higher BMI, there were higher rates of death from esophageal, stomach, colorectal, liver, gallbladder, pancreatic, prostate, and kidney cancers and non-Hodgkin lymphoma, multiple myeloma, and leukemia. Among women, high BMI was correlated with greater morbidity from colorectal, liver, gallbladder, pancreatic, breast, uterine, cervical, ovarian, and kidney cancers and from non-Hodgkin lymphoma and multiple myeloma.

Abdominal obesity, as defined by waist circumference or waist/hip ratio, has been shown to be more strongly related to some tumor types than obesity as defined by BMI. Possible associated mechanisms include insulin resistance and resultant chronic hyperinsulinemia, increased insulin-like growth factors, or increased steroid hormones, increased tissue-derived hormones, and cytokines (adipokines) or inflammatory mediators.

80

Adiposity influences the synthesis and bioavailability of **endogenous sex steroids,** the estrogens, progesterone, and androgens. Three mechanisms are involved: (1) Adipose tissue expresses various sex-steroid metabolizing enzymes that promote the formation of estrogens from androgenic precursors secreted by the gonads and adrenal glands. (2) Adipose cells increase the circulating levels of insulin and increase insulin-like growth factor (IGF) biologic activity. (3) High insulin levels can increase ovarian and, possibly, adrenal androgen synthesis and in some genetically susceptible, premenopausal women cause the development of polycystic ovary syndrome. Adiposity-induced alterations in blood levels of sex steroids explain the correlation noted between indices of excess weight and risks of postmenopausal breast cancer and endometrial cancer.

For breast and endometrial cancers, a central role of estrogens and progesterone is established from a large body of experimental and clinical evidence. These sex steroids are important regulators of cellular proliferation, differentiation, and apoptosis. Among men, prostate carcinogenesis is thought to be related to endogenous hormone metabolism.

Chronically increased insulin levels have been correlated with the pathogenesis of colon, breast, pancreatic, and endometrial cancers. These cancer-causing effects of insulin might be mediated by insulin receptors in the preneoplastic or neoplastic target cells or could be due to alterations in endogenous hormone metabolism secondary to hyperinsulinemia. Excess body weight and a high plasma level of C-peptide both predispose men to prostate cancer and to an increased likelihood of dying from their disease.

6. Relate alcohol consumption to carcinogenesis.

Study text page 416.

Chronic **alcohol consumption** is a strong risk factor for cancer of the oral cavity, pharynx, hypopharynx, larynx, esophagus, and liver. Breast carcinogenesis can be enhanced with relatively low daily amounts of alcohol. Alcohol interacts with smoke, increasing the risk of malignant tumors, possibly by acting as a solvent for the carcinogenic chemicals in smoke products. The strongest genetic associations to alcoholism are those with alcohol dehydrogenase (ADH) and mitochondrial aldehyde dehydrogenase (ALDH2).

7. Identify the carcinogenic risks to individuals of ionizing, ultraviolet, and electromagnetic radiation exposure.

Study text pages 416 through 425; refer to Figures 12-7 through 12-12 and Tables 12-6 through 12-8.

Ionizing radiation (IR) is a mutagen and carcinogen and can penetrate cells and tissues and deposit energy in tissues at random in the form of ionizations which excites or remove an electron from the target atom. These ionizations can lead to irreversible damage or indirect damage from formation and attack by water-based free radicals. IR affects many cell processes, including gene expression, disruption of mitochondrial function, cell cycle arrest, and cell death. IR is a potent DNA damaging agent causing cross-linking, nucleotide base damage, and single- and double-strand breaks. Damage to DNA and disrupted cellular regulation processes can lead to carcinogenesis. The double-strand break (DSB) is considered the characteristic lesion observed for the effects of IR. DSBs are mostly repaired by the nonhomologous end joining (NHEJ) pathway. This pathway is efficient for joining the DNA broken ends; however, errors can occur. Irradiated human cells unable to execute the NHEJ are supersensitive to the introduction of large-scale mutations and chromosomal aberrations.

It is known that radiation may induce a type of genomic instability to the progeny of the directly irradiated cells over many generations of cell radiation. This leads to an increased rate at which mutations/chromosomal aberrations arise in these distant progeny. This is called **transgeneration effects.** In addition, the directly irradiated cells can lead to genetic effects in **bystander cells** or innocent cells, even though these cells received no direct radiation exposure. The bystander and genomic instability effects also have been termed **nontargeted effects**. Although bystander and transgeneration IR effects are associated with induced genomic instability leading to chromosome aberrations, gene mutations, late cell death, and aneupoloidy, all of these effects may be epigenetically mediated. The epigenetic changes include DNA methylation, histone modification, and RNA-associated silencing. Mutations, however, provide a critical hit or induce genetic instability that make cells more susceptible to accumulation of genetic alterations caused by other spontaneous or induced mutations. It is known that the progeny of irradiated cells can exhibit an increased death rate and loss of reproductive potential that continues for several generations and, possibly, indefinitely. This delayed cell death phenotype is known as "lethal mutation" and "delayed reproductive death." Significant is that various genetic alterations are demonstrated in cells that are not, themselves, irradiated but are direct descendents of cells exposed to ionizing radiation. These so-called innocent cells are referred to as bystander effects and are considered manifestations of a radiation-induced genomic instability. Oxidative-stress mediators also have been implicated in the cytotoxic effects observed in solid tumors located at distinct sites away from those receiving radiation.

Exposure to **ultraviolet radiation** (UVR) can emanate from both natural and artificial sources; however, the principal source of exposure for most people is sunlight. UV radiation is now known to cause specific gene mutations; for example, squamous cell carcinoma involves mutation in the *p53* gene, basal cell carcinoma in the *patched* gene, and melanoma in the *p16* gene. In addition, UV light induces the release of tumor necrosis factor (TNF) in the epidermis, which may reduce immune surveillance against skin cancer. Skin exposure to UVR and ionizing radiation, as well as xenobiotic agents or drugs, produces **reactive oxygen species** (ROS) in large quantities that can overwhelm tissue antioxidants and other oxygen-degrading pathways.

Antioxidants decrease ROS and oxidative stress and other protective mechanisms, including DNA repair and

81

apoptosis. With oxidative stress, DNA damage occurs and calcium-dependent enzymes (endonucleases) are activated that produce DNA strand breaks. In addition, ROS are involved in the activation of procarcinogens, such as polycyclic aromatic hydrocarbons.

Health risks associated with **electromagnetic radiation** (EMR) are controversial. Exposure to electric and magnetic fields is widespread. EMRs are a type of non-ionizing radiation, low frequency radiation without enough energy to break off electrons from their orbits around atoms and ionize the atoms. Microwaves, radar, and power frequency radiation associated with electricity and radio waves, fluorescent lights, computers, and other electric equipment all create EMRs of varying strength. Some studies, but not all, linked high EMR exposure with a significantly higher risk of childhood leukemia. Also, cordless and cellular phone use appears to increase lymphomas, benign and malignant brain tumors, and female breast cancer.

Increasing evidence has indicated that the mechanism of harm from EMR is induction of cell stress and damage of intracellular components, free radical formation and altered protein conformation, Adverse EMR has been reported to affect DNA synthesis and alter cell division, electrical charge of ions, and molecules within cells. Interference with cellular electrical charges may modify ionic structures disturbing movement of ions across the membrane, including calcium ions.

8. **Identify behaviors and environment agent exposures associated with carcinogenesis.**
   Study text pages 425 through 428.

Sexually transmitted infection with carcinogenic types of human papillomavirus (HPV), referred to as high-risk types of HPV, causes most cervical cancers. In addition, HPV is a newly identified causal factor for squamous cell carcinoma of the head and neck. HPV infections, however, are very common in sexually active women, and the majority of these infections will resolve or only cause transient, minor problems. Eighty HPV types have been sequenced and 30 of these types infect both the female and male genital tract and two thirds of these are classified as high-risk types. **HPV-16,** in most countries, accounts for 50% to 60% of cervical cancer cases. HPV types correlated with genital warts, HPV-6 and HPV-11, are called low-risk because they are rarely associated with cancer.

For colon cancer, **physical activity** increases gut motility, which reduces the length of time (transit time) that the bowel lining is exposed to potential mutagens. For breast cancer, vigorous physical activity may decrease exposure of breast tissue to ovarian hormones, insulin, and insulin-like factor. A recent, randomized trial found after 12 months of moderate-intensity exercise, postmenopausal women had significantly decreased serum estrogens. Physical activity also helps prevent type 2 diabetes that has been associated with risk of cancer of the colon and pancreas.

One notable **occupational factor** is **asbestos,** which increases the risk of mesothelioma and lung cancer.

Carcinoma of the bladder has been linked with the manufacture of dyes, rubber, paint, and aromatic amines. **Benzol inhalation** is linked to leukemia in shoemakers and in workers in the rubber cement, explosives, and dyeing industries. Other notable occupational hazards include high-nickel alloy, chromium VI compounds, inorganic arsenic, silica, polycyclic aromatic hydrocarbons, sulfuric acid, and chloromethyl ether. Studies of occupational exposure to **diesel exhaust** indicate an increased risk of lung cancer.

Air pollution can be carcinogenic. A person inhales about 20,000 L of air in 1 day; thus even modest contamination of the atmosphere can result in inhalation of appreciable doses of pollutants. Contaminants include outdoor and indoor air pollutants. Concerns include industrial emissions, including arsenicals, benzene, chloroform, formaldehyde, sulfuric acid, mustard gas, vinyl chloride, and acrylamide. Living close to certain industries is a recognized cancer risk factor. Indoor pollution generally is considered worse than outdoor pollution, partly because of cigarette smoke. Environmental tobacco smoke (ETS) can cause the formation of reactive oxygen free radicals and, thus, DNA damage. **Radon** is a natural radioactive gas derived from the radioactive decay of uranium that is ubiquitous in rock and soil; it can become trapped in houses and gives rise to radioactive decay products known to be carcinogenic to humans. The most hazardous houses can be identified by testing and then modified to prevent further radon contamination. Exposure levels are greater from underground mines than from houses. Most of the lung cancers associated with radon are bronchogenic; however, small cell carcinoma does occur with greater frequency in underground miners. Strong evidence indicates an increased risk of bladder, skin, and lung cancers following consumption of water with high levels of **arsenic.**

PRACTICE EXAMINATION

Fill in the Blanks

1. Preventing exposure to _____ can prevent many cancers.

2. The expression of _____ are linked to carcinogenesis because they can act as either oncogenes or tumor-suppressor genes.

3. _____ is the ability to develop in a particular way depending on the environment.

4. _____ is a combination of sidestream and mainstream smoke.

5. _____ include toxic, mutagenic, and carcinogenic chemicals.

6. The most relevant carcinogens produced by cooking are generated by _____ proteins.

7. _____ can cause loss of imprinting.

8. _____ increase the circulating levels of insulin.

9. Exposure to asbestos increases the risk for _____.

10. Prolonged exposure to UVR increases the risk for _____.

11. An inhaled chemical within the dyeing industry linked to leukemia is _____.

12. At the cellular level, cancer is _____.

13. Ionizing radiation causes mutation to clonal progeny and to _____.

14. UVR induces the release of _____, which may reduce immune surveillance.

15. Enzymes that activate xenobiotics are known as _____.

16. Among men, prostate carcinogenesis is related to production of _____.

17. Higher _____ is associated with gastrointestinal, reproductive, renal, and lymphoid cancers.

18. _____ changes are mitotically and meiotically heritable.

19. Estrogen and progesterone play a central role in _____ and _____ cancers.

20. The double-strand break is considered the characteristic affected by_____.

21. ROS in large quantities can overwhelm _____ and _____ pathways.

22. _____ can silence tumor-suppressor genes.

23. The phenotypic effects of epigenetic modification during development require _____ before manifesting in later life.

24. _____ accounts for 50% to 60% of cervical cancer.

25. _____ is derived from radioactive decay of uranium, can be trapped in homes, and is carcinogenic to humans.

13 Cancer in Children

FOUNDATIONAL KNOWLEDGE OBJECTIVE

After reviewing the primary text where referenced, the learner will be able to do the following:
a. Describe the mechanisms that confine cells and tissues to specific anatomic sites.
Review text pages 35 through 36; refer to Figure 1-34.

MEMORY CHECK!

- See this study guide's narrative for Foundational Knowledge Objective "a" in Chapter 12.

LEARNING OBJECTIVES

After studying this chapter, the learner will be able to do the following:
1. Compare childhood neoplasms to adult cancers.
Refer to Table 13-1.

Comparison of Childhood and Adult Cancers

Characteristic	Childhood Cancers	Adult Cancers
Incidence	2% of *all* cancers	98% of *all* cancers
Environmental causation	Weak relationship to environmental exposures and lifestyle	Strong relationship to environmental exposures and lifestyle
Latency (from initiation to diagnosis)	Short	Long
Sites involved	Mesodermal germ layer	Organs
Cells involved	Nonepithelial: sarcomas, embryonal, leukemia, lymphoma	Epithelial: carcinomas
Prevention	Few strategies to prevent	80% may be preventable
Early detection	Generally accidental	Possible by early detection screening test/examinations
Stage at diagnosis	80% have metastasized	Local or regional spread
Treatment/side effects	Less difficulty with acute toxicity but more significant long-term consequences	More difficulty with acute toxicity but fewer long-term consequences
Response to treatment	Very responsive to chemotherapy	Less responsive to chemotherapy
Prognosis	>70% cure	<60% cure, highly variable

2. Identify the most common childhood cancers.

Study text pages 436 and 437.

Most childhood cancers originate from the **mesodermal germ layer** that gives rise to connective tissue, bone, cartilage, muscle, blood, blood vessels, the gonads, the kidneys, and the lymphatic system. Thus the more common childhood cancers are leukemia, sarcomas, and embryonic tumors. **Embryonic tumors** originate during intrauterine life and are diagnosed early in life. These tumors contain abnormal cells unable to mature or differentiate into fully functional cells and are diagnosed usually before 5 years of age. Embryonic tumors often contain the term in their name referring to the immature nature of the cells.

The most common cancers among the 15- to 19-year-old population in the United States are Hodgkin lymphoma, germ cell tumors, central nervous system tumors, non-Hodgkin lymphoma, thyroid cancer, malignant melanomas, and acute lymphocytic leukemia (ALL). Central nervous system (CNS) tumors are the most common types of solid tumors in children. Not all are malignant by histology, but even the benign tumor can be devastating. The treatment of childhood brain tumors often presents difficulties, because treatment, such as radiation, may have debilitating effects on the developing brain.

3. Describe the genetic factors associated with childhood cancers.

Study text pages 438 and 439; refer to Table 13-2.

Both oncogenes and tumor-suppressor genes are associated with childhood malignancies. **Proto-oncogenes** are involves in normal cell division and growth through a signaling process that controls the cell cycle. If they are mutated, these genes become carcinogenic oncogenes, which cause the cell cycle to go out of control. **Tumor-suppressor** genes normally suppress cancer formation but lose their suppressor function, leading to uncontrolled growth and cancers.

Other genetic factors involve chromosome aberrations. For example, the Philadelphia chromosome is associated with myelogenous leukemia, and the deletion of chromosome 13q is observed with retinoblastoma and osteosarcoma. There is an association of trisomy 21 (Down syndrome) with an increased susceptibility to acute leukemia. For children with Down syndrome, the risk of developing leukemia is 10 to 20 times greater during the first 4 years of life than it is in healthy children. Wilms tumor is particularly recognized for its association with a number of congenital anomalies, including absences of the iris of the eye, mental retardation, and neurofibromatosis. Retinoblastoma, which is a malignant embryonic tumor of the eye, occurs as an inherited defect or as an acquired mutation.

Fanconi anemia and Bloom syndrome, two autosomal recessive conditions involving chromosomal fragility, are risk factors for the development of myelogenous leukemia. A genetic defect involving the *p53* tumor-suppressor gene found in families with Li-Fraumeni syndrome increases the risk for developing tumors.

4. Cite the environmental risk factors associated with childhood cancers.

Study text page 439; refer to Table 13-3.

Few childhood tumors have a strong association with environmental factors. Because of the lengthy latency period required between the exposure and development of cancer, early exposure to carcinogens does not result in a tumor until the child is an adult.

Prenatal exposure to some drugs and to ionizing radiation has been linked to subsequent cancers. Perhaps the most well-known such drug is diethylstilbestrol (DES), a drug taken to avert early abortion. Adenocarcinomas of the vagina have developed in a small percentage of the daughters of mothers who took DES while pregnant. Childhood exposure to ionizing radiation is a risk for cancer development. Retrospective research has shown a correlation between radiation-induced malignancies from radiotherapy or from radiation exposure during diagnostic imaging.

Anabolic androgenic steroids, which are used in the treatment of aplastic anemia or illegally by teenage athletes for body development, have been associated with subsequent hepatocellular carcinoma. Cytotoxic agents used in the treatment of pediatric cancers may predispose the child to leukemia in later years. Immunosuppressive agents, particularly those used for transplant surgeries, have been shown to increase the risk of lymphomas.

In children, a strong carcinogenic relationship has been shown between the **Epstein-Barr virus** and **Burkitt lymphoma.** Children with AIDS have an increased risk of developing **non-Hodgkin lymphoma** and **Kaposi sarcoma.**

PRACTICE EXAMINATION

Fill in the Blanks

Supply the correct response for each statement.

1. The unique feature of childhood cancer is its _____ time.

2. Embryonic tumors are unable to differentiate into _____ cells.

3. Approximately 80% of childhood tumors have _____ at the time of diagnosis.

4. Children with Down syndrome have a 10 to 20 times greater risk for _____ during their first 4 years of life.

5. Childhood cancers are very responsive to _____.

6. The treatment of pediatric cancer with _____ may predispose the child to leukemia in later years.

7. By age 20, male-to-female ratio for cancer in the United States is _____.

8. Cancers in children are categorized by their _____.

9. Cancers in adults are categorized by the _____ of the primary tumor.

Matching

Match the syndrome/disorder with the risk factor/cause.

_____ 10. Brain tumors

_____ 11. Congenital absence of the iris of the eye

_____ 12. Retinoblastoma

_____ 13. Fanconi anemia

_____ 14. Vaginal adenocarcinoma

_____ 15. Hepatocellular carcinoma

a. *RBI* gene

b. DES

c. anabolic steroids

d. nonlymphocytic leukemia

e. *p53* gene

f. Wilms tumor

Match each characteristic with the type of cancer.

_____ 16. Less curable

_____ 17. Organ involvement

_____ 18. Likely preventable

_____ 19. Generally detected accidentally

_____ 20. Epithelial origin

_____ 21. High incidence

_____ 22. Fewer long-term consequences to treatment

_____ 23. Mesenchymal origin

_____ 24. Host factors are especially important

_____ 25. Embryonic tumors

a. childhood cancers

b. adult cancers

14 Structure and Function of the Neurologic System

PREREQUISITE KNOWLEDGE OBJECTIVES

After reviewing the primary text where referenced, the learner will be able to do the following:

1. **Identify the structural and functional subdivisions of the nervous system.**
   Review text pages 442 and 443.
2. **Compare the functions of neurons and neuroglia; identify the parts and configurations of neurons.**
   Review text pages 443 through 445; refer to Figures 14-1 through 14-3 and Table 14-1.
3. **Describe the circumstances under which a peripheral nerve fiber can regenerate.**
   Review text page 445; refer to Figure 14-4.
4. **Describe the transmission of nerve impulses by neurotransmitters.**
   Review text pages 446 through 449; refer to Figures 1-32 and 14-5 and Table 14-2.
5. **Identify the three main regions of the brain; characterize their associated structures and functions.**
   Review text pages 449, 450, 452, 453, 455, 456; refer to Figures 14-6 through 14-8 and Table 14-3.
6. **Identify the significance of the decussation of motor fibers.**
   Review text page 452; refer to Figure 14-9.
7. **Describe the location, structure, and function of the spinal cord; define a reflex arc.**
   Review text pages 456 through 459; refer to Figures 14-10 through 14-14.
8. **Identify the structures that are responsible for maintaining and protecting the central nervous system.**
   Review text pages 459 through 462; refer to Figures 14-15 through 14-17 and Table 14-4.
9. **Identify the route of blood circulation within the central nervous system; note the significance of the circle of Willis.**
   Review text pages 462, 463, and 465; refer to Figures 14-18 through 14-22 and Table 14-5.
10. **Describe the structure of a spinal nerve; locate the plexuses.**
    Review text pages 465 and 467; refer to Figure 14-23.
11. **Name the cranial nerves, and state the functions of each.**
    Refer to Table 14-6.
12. **Identify the subdivisions of the autonomic nervous system, their origins, and their general functions.**
    Review text pages 467 and 469 through 471; refer to Figures 14-24 and 14-25.
13. **Identify the type of neurotransmitter secreted by preganglionic and postganglionic fibers in the autonomic nervous system.**
    Refer to Figures 14-26 and 14-27 and Table 14-7.
14. **Identify the structural, cellular, and functional changes that occur with aging.**
    Review pages 471 and 474; refer to Table 14-8.
15. **Identify the tests of neural function.**
    Review text pages 474 through 476; refer to Table 14-9.

PRACTICE EXAMINATION

Multiple Choice

Circle the correct answer for each question.

1. Which is a function of the somatic nervous system?
   a. The conduction of impulses to involuntary muscles and glands
   b. The conduction of impulses to the central nervous system
   c. The conduction of impulses regulating voluntary control of skeletal muscles
   d. The conduction of impulses between the brain and spinal cord
2. A neuron with a single dendrite at one end of the cell body and a single axon at the other end of the cell body would be classified as:
   a. unipolar.
   b. multipolar.
   c. monopolar.
   d. bipolar.
3. Neurons that carry impulses away from the CNS are called:
   a. afferent neurons.
   b. sensory neurons.
   c. efferent neurons.
   d. association neurons.

89

4. Neurons are specialized for the conduction of impulses, whereas neuroglia:
   a. support nerve tissue.
   b. serve as motor end plates.
   c. synthesize acetylcholine and cholinesterase.
   d. initiate responses maintaining homeostasis.
5. There is one-way conduction at a synapse because:
   a. only postsynaptic neurons contain synaptic vesicles.
   b. acetylcholine prevents nerve impulses from traveling in both directions.
   c. only the presynaptic neuron contains neurotransmitters.
   d. only dendrites release neurotransmitters.
6. Which of the following contains the thalamus and hypothalamus?
   a. The diencephalon
   b. The cerebrum
   c. The medulla oblongata
   d. The brainstem
7. The reticular activating system:
   a. programs for fine repetitive motor movements.
   b. maintains wakefulness.
   c. maintains constant internal environments.
   d. affects the positioning of the head to improve hearing.
8. Which of the following statements best describes the spinal cord?
   a. It descends inferior to the lumbar vertebrae.
   b. It conducts motor impulses from the brain.
   c. It descends to the fourth lumbar vertebra.
   d. It conducts sensory impulses from the brain.

9. Which of the following is a protective covering of the CNS?
   a. CSF
   b. Dura mater
   c. Precentral gyrus
   d. Cauda equina
10. The composition of cerebrospinal fluid is:
    a. the same as blood.
    b. distilled H_2O with dissolved salts.
    c. a plasmalike liquid with glucose, salts, proteins, and urea.
    d. a heavy mucous solution with dissolved salts, glucose, and urea.
11. An autonomic ganglion can be described as:
    a. the site of synapses between visceral efferent neurons.
    b. a site where spinal reflexes occur.
    c. a point of synapse between parasympathetic and sympathetic neurons.
    d. the place where unconscious sensations occur.
12. Clusters of nerve cell bodies and dendrites located within the peripheral nervous system are called:
    a. nuclei.
    b. tracts.
    c. nerves.
    d. ganglia.
13. A mass of nerve cell bodies and dendrites located within the central nervous system is a:
    a. sulcus.
    b. ganglion.
    c. nucleus.
    d. tract.

Matching

Match the structures with the sympathetic nerve–stimulating effect.

_____ 14. Breathing passageways

_____ 15. Intestines

_____ 16. Liver

a. increases diameter

b. decreases diameter

c. increases metabolic activity

d. decreases metabolic activity

Match the structure with the most appropriate function/description.

_____ 17. Schwann cell

_____ 18. Dendrite

a. the outer, nucleated layer of a certain cell

b. produces myelin sheaths

c. carries impulses away from perikaryon

d. a covering over neuron fibers

e. conducts impulses to cell body

Match the component of a reflex arc with the descriptor.

_____ 19. Sensory neuron

_____ 20. Effector

a. carries impulses to the central nervous system

b. carries impulses to a responding organ

c. responds to motor impulse

d. stimulated by one neuron and passes impulse onto another neuron

e. responds directly to changes in environment

Match the function with the cranial nerve.

_____ 21. Tasting

_____ 22. Balance maintenance

a. facial

b. olfactory

c. vestibulocochlear

d. hypoglossal

e. optic

Match the characteristic with the appropriate division of the autonomic nervous system.

_____ 23. More extensive use of norepinephrine

_____ 24. Effects are more widespread and long-lasting

_____ 25. Elicits energy conservation and restoration

a. sympathetic

b. parasympathetic

Chapter **14** **Structure and Function of the Neurologic System**

15 Pain, Temperature Regulation, Sleep, and Sensory Function

FOUNDATIONAL KNOWLEDGE OBJECTIVES

a. Characterize nociceptors.
   Review text pages 482 and 483; refer to Figure 15-1 and Table 15-1.

MEMORY CHECK!

- Over the past 20 years, exceptional progress has been made in strengthening the **gate control theory** of pain by elucidating the neuroanatomy and neuropharmacology of pain pathways in the peripheral and central nervous systems. According to this theory, **nociceptive** (pain perception) impulses arising from the skin, muscles, joints, arteries, and viscera are transmitted from nonspecialized, bare sensory nerve endings called nociceptors, which respond to chemical, mechanical, and thermal stimuli. The tips of the fingers have more **nociceptors** than the skin of the back, and all of the skin has many more nociceptors than the internal organs.
- Nociceptors are equipped with a variety of transduction channels that can sense different forms of noxious stimulation and at different intensities. Other types of transmembrane receptors (called transient receptor potential channels, or TRP channels) reside on "naked nerve endings" and respond to a variety of physical, chemical, and thermal stimuli. Nociceptors are categorized according to (1) the stimulus to which they respond and (2) the properties of the axons associated with them. Receptors for severe mechanical deformation and temperature extreme are associated with lightly myelinated, medium-sized A-delta (Aδ) fibers. Other types of mechanical, thermal, and chemical nociception are transmitted by excitation of polymodal nociceptors and are carried on small, unmyelinated C fibers.
- The nerve action potentials generated by excitation of any of these nociceptors travel along these two fiber types to reach the spinal cord. Nociceptive transmission through the Aδ fibers occurs more quickly than through C fibers. **Aδ fibers** carry well-localized, sharp pain sensations and are important in initiating rapid reactions to stimuli (fast pain). The small **unmyelinated C polymodal nociceptors** are responsible for the transmission of the diffuse burning or aching sensations that follow (slow pain).

b. **Describe pathways of nociceptors to the brain**.
   Review text pages 483 and 484; refer to Figures 15-2 and 15-3.

MEMORY CHECK!

- Once the axons of the *primary afferents* (Aδ and C fibers) enter the cord, they may branch into ascending or descending collaterals for one or two cord segments in neuronal projections called the dorsolateral tract of Lissauer. Eventually, all of the primary afferents terminate in the gray matter of the dorsal horn in distinctive layers or *laminae*. Many of the primary afferents carrying nociceptive information were originally found to terminate in a layer that was given the name substantia gelatinosa.
- Three classes of second-order cell bodies are found in the dorsal horn: (1) *projection cells,* which relay information to higher brain areas (cephalad); (2) *excitatory interneurons,* which relay nociceptive transmissions to projection cells, other interneurons, or to motor cells concerned with local reflexes; and (3) *inhibitory interneurons,* which modulate nociceptive transmission. The synaptic connections between cells of primary and second-order neurons located in the substantia gelatinosa and other lamina function as a "pain gate." This "gate" in the spinal cord regulates the transmission of pain impulses that proceed cephalad for further processing and interpretation in the brain.
- Most nociceptive information travels cephalad by means of ascending columns in the lateral spinothalamic tract. Other bits of nociceptive signals travel in the posterior columns of the cord to the dorsal column nuclei of the medulla, and from there ascend in the medial lemniscus to the lateral thalamus. Other spinal cord projection systems convey nociceptive information directly or indirectly to the reticular formation of the brainstem and the periaqueductal gray (PAG) matter of the midbrain.
- The principal target for nociceptive afferents is the thalamus (which is the major relay station of sensory information in general). The thalamus is primarily divided into medial and lateral groups by a band of fibers called the internal medullary lamina. The ventral posterior lateral (VPL) and ventral posterior medial (VPM) nuclei of the thalamus facilitate the localization of pain and integrate these perceptions into a neuroendocrine response.
- From the thalamus, brainstem, and midbrain, third-order neurons project to portions of the CNS involved in the processing and interpretation of pain, the chief areas being the cerebral cortex, and the reticular and limbic systems.

c. **Describe the processing of pain by the brain.**
   Review text pages 484 and 486.

MEMORY CHECK!

- The third-order neurons of the ventral posterior nuclear complex of the thalamus project in a highly organized manner to the primary and secondary somatosensory cortex (Brodmann areas). On the post-central gyrus of the parietal lobe is a topographically organized representation of the body mirroring the concentration of peripheral sensory receptors known as the sensory homunculus. This area of the brain is thought to be involved in the discriminative and cognitive aspects of pain: that is, what we *think* about the pain.
- The frontal lobe of the cerebral cortex receives diffuse projections from the medial thalamic nuclei, which are thought to subserve the affective expression (how your pain looks to an observer) of pain through their frontal-limbic connections.
- The limbic and reticular tracts are involved in alerting the body to danger, initiating arousal of the organism, and emotionally processing the afferent signals now perceived, not just as stimuli, but as pain. The **limbic system** consists of a ring of cortex on the medial aspect of each cerebral hemisphere, the subcortical nuclei, parts of the thalamus and midbrain, and the hypothalamus. The **reticular system** is composed of a number of vaguely defined nuclei situated in the core of the brain stem extending throughout its rostrocaudal extent. Many reticular neurons respond to noxious stimulation by initiating escape behaviors. The limbic system and the reticular system regulate the complex emotional responses to pain: that is, what we *feel* about the pain. Pain signals to these areas serve to arouse the whole organism to ongoing tissue damage, activating protective neuroendocrine and autonomic reflexes such as the "fight or flight" response, the release of stress hormones, and beneficial cardiovascular changes.

Chapter **15**   **Pain, Temperature Regulation, Sleep, and Sensory Function**

d. Describe pain neuromodulation.
   Review text pages 486 through 490; refer to Figures 15-4 and 15-5.

MEMORY CHECK!

- By the mid-1970s and into the 1980s, two other developments played key roles in extending the theory to explain how, under certain stressful conditions, significant traumatic injuries can be completely painless in awake, neurologically intact patients. The first was the discovery of specific descending pathways from the brain to the spinal cord that could produce significant and selective analgesia in those experiencing pain. The second event was the identification of ubiquitous opioid receptors found throughout the body and, shortly thereafter, the isolation, purification, and sequencing of endogenous opioid peptides.
- Segmental inhibition was quickly verified when research into peripheral nerve anatomy demonstrated that stimulation of a group of large, fast, heavily myelinated Aβ fibers (which synapse in the dorsal horn along with their nociceptive Aδ and C fiber counterparts) can close the pain gates. These afferent Aβ fibers carry nonnoxious, low-threshold mechanical information of touch, vibration, and pressure.
- The vast body of work completed since the inauguration of the gate control theory has highlighted the complexity of inhibitory modulation beyond the segmental level (i.e., heterosegmental), emphasizing a functional basis for pain control outside the dorsal horn emphasis of the original gate control hypothesis. Over the past three decades, a wealth of information has added to our understanding of heterosegmental, supraspinal mechanisms elicited by noxious and nonnoxious stimuli. Powerful *heterosegmental control of nociception* probably originates from the cortex, because almost all nociceptive relays within the CNS are under so-called corticofugal (top-down) modulation, which often occurs even in the absence of painful stimuli. Further down, the caudal medulla participates in widespread inhibitory phenomena, called **diffuse noxious inhibitory controls** (DNIC). There are several ascending and descending bulbospinal pathways that respond simultaneously to a noxious stimulus and participate in DNIC. The net effect of these supraspinal structures is to precisely encode the intensity of the noxious stimulus and transmit descending feedback, mainly to the deep dorsal horn neurons. The result is to modify, dampen, or augment nociceptive transmission, depending on the many factors existing both within and without the individual.
- Many neurotransmitters mediate the transmission of pain in the periphery, the spinal cord, and the brain. In the periphery, local injury can result in direct or indirect excitation of nociceptors. Neurotransmitters can be classified as inflammatory, pain excitatory, or pain inhibitory or as modulators of pain.
- *Direct excitation* occurs when nociceptors respond to a threshold depolarization by the application of heat, radiation, toxic chemicals, or tissue trauma. *Indirect excitation* occurs via the release of inflammatory mediators after the tissue is injured.
- Activity in the nociceptors themselves causes them to release peptides and neurotransmitters such as substance P, neurokinin A, calcitonin gene–related peptide (CGRP), and ATP that promote the spread of pain locally and further contribute to vasodilation, increased vascular permeability, and degranulation of even more mast cell cytokines. The resultant "inflammatory soup" serves to lower the threshold for nociceptive depolarization, resulting in peripheral sensitization and pain augmentation.
- In the spinal cord and brain, a wide variety of biogenic amines and other neurotransmitters act to modulate control over the transmission of pain impulses. Serotonin, norepinephrine, glutamate, aspartate, glycine, GABA, and an array of endogenous opioids have been found to stimulate or inhibit interneurons in the CNS. This, in turn, may serve to stimulate or inhibit the gate and the primary nociceptive tracts.
- **Glutamate** and **aspartate,** amino acid precursors, are the most common excitatory neurotransmitters in the brain and spinal cord. High levels of glutamate and aspartate have been found in the PAG as well as at the synapses of first-order nociceptors with ascending spinothalamic tract neurons. High levels of activity in the nociceptive afferents may result in an activity-dependent increase in the excitability of neurons in the dorsal horn of the cord and open the gate.
- **GABA** and **glycine** have major inhibitory effects in the spinal cord and brain and function to inhibit pain by synapsing with neurons containing substance P (a major algogenic chemical found in the dorsal horn and elsewhere). Norepinephrine and 5-hydroxytryptamine (serotonin) contribute to pain modulation (inhibition) in the medulla and pons.
- **Endogenous opioids** are a family of morphine-like neuropeptides that inhibit transmission of pain impulses in the spinal cord and brain. There are four types of opioid neuropeptides: (1) *enkephalins,* (2) *endorphins,* (3) *dynorphins,* and the newest to be discovered, (4) *endomorphins.* These substances are neurohormones that act as neurotransmitters by binding to one or more opioid receptors. Three distinct types of opioid receptors are found in the body: mu (with subtypes mu-1 and mu-2), kappa, and delta. Each receptor type binds differently with the various types of opioids.
- Agonist activity at the opioid receptors by endogenous opioids inhibits the release of excitatory neurotransmitters like substance P in the dorsal horn (blocking the transmission of the painful stimulus) or in other areas of the brain such as the PAG or the rostral ventromedial nuclei in the brainstem. Opioids from the midbrain release adrenergic and serotonergic descending pathways from GABAergic inhibition and decrease pain.

e. **Describe thermoregulation**.
   Review text pages 496 through 498.

MEMORY CHECK!

- The control of body temperature is a function of centers located in the hypothalamus. Thermoreceptors provide the hypothalamus with information about peripheral and core temperatures. If the temperature is low, the body initiates heat conservation measures by a series of hormonal mechanisms. Heat production begins with the hypothalamic release of TSH-RH, which stimulates the release of thyroid-stimulating hormone (TSH) from the anterior pituitary. The TSH causes the release of thyroxine from the thyroid gland. This hormone causes the release of epinephrine from the adrenal medulla. Epinephrine causes vasoconstriction, glycolysis, and increased metabolic rates, which increase heat production. Warmer peripheral and core temperatures reverse the process. Decreasing the sympathetic pathway produces vasodilation, decreased muscle tone, and increased perspiration.
- Because of their greater body surface/mass ratio and decreased subcutaneous fat, infants do not conserve heat well. Elderly individuals have poor responses to environmental temperature extremes as a result of slowed blood circulation, changes in the skin, and an overall decrease in heat-producing activities.

f. **Identify the normal sleep stages; describe nervous system control of sleep**.
   Review text pages 502 through 504; refer to Figures 15-9 and 15-10.

MEMORY CHECK!

- Several areas of the brain process are associated with sleep and sleep-awake cycles. A small group of hypothalamic nerve cells, the **suprachiasmatic nucleus (SCN),** controls the timing of the sleep-wake cycle and coordinates this cycle with the circadian rhythms (24 hours rhythm cycles) in other areas of the brain and other tissues. Normal sleep has two phases that can be documented by electroencephalography (EEG): rapid eye movement (REM) sleep and non-REM (NREM; slow-wave) sleep.
- REM and NREM sleep succeed each other in 90- to 120-minute intervals. Four to six cycles occur during a normal sleep period based on changes in the EEG pattern. NREM sleep is initiated by the withdrawal of neurotransmitters from the reticular formation and by the inhibition of arousal mechanisms. The restorative, reparative, and growth processes occur during slow-wave sleep. Altering periods of REM and NREM occur through the night, with lengthening intervals of REM and fewer intervals of the deeper stages of NREM toward the morning. Many neurotransmitters are associated with excitatory and inhibitory sleep patterns. Sleep-promoting neurotransmitters include prostaglandin D, L-tryptophan, serotonin, adenosine, melatonin, GABA, and growth hormones. Awake-promoting neurotransmitters include hypocreatin, acetylcholine and glutamate. The pontine reticular formation is primarily responsible for generating REM sleep. Projections from the reticular formation and other areas of the mesencephalon and brainstem produce NREM sleep. The sleep patterns of the newborn and young child vary from those of the adult in total sleep time, cycle length, and percentage of time spent in each sleep cycle. Sleep for infants and children is important for growth and neurocognitive development. Elderly individuals experience a total decrease in sleep time.

g. **Describe the eye and its structure**.
   Review text pages 506 through 508; refer to Figures 15-11 through 15-14 and Table 15-5.

MEMORY CHECK!

- The wall of the eye is made up of three layers: sclera, choroid, and retina. It becomes transparent at the cornea in the central anterior region, which allows light to enter the eye. The choroid is the pigmented middle layer that prevents light from scattering inside the eye. The iris, which is part of the choroid, has a round opening, called the pupil, through which light passes.
- The innermost layer of the eye, called the retina, contains the rods and cones. These photoreceptors convert light energy into nerve impulses.
- Nerve impulses pass through the optic chiasm. Nerves from the nasal halves of the retinas cross and join fibers from the temporal halves of the retinas to form the optic tracts. The optic tracts connect to the primary visual cortex in the occipital lobe of the brain. Light entering the eye is focused on the retina by the lens, which is a flexible, biconvex, crystal-like structure. The lens separates the anterior cavity from the vitreous chamber. The aqueous humor of the anterior chamber helps maintain pressure inside the eye and provides nutrients to the lens and the cornea. The vitreous chamber is filled with a gel-like vitreous humor that prevents the eyeball from collapsing inward.
- Six extrinsic eye muscles allow gross eye movement and permit the eyes to follow a moving object. The external structures that protect the eye include the eyelids, the conjunctiva, and the lacrimal apparatus.

h. **Describe the parts of the ear**.
   Review text pages 512 and 514; refer to Figures 15-18 and 15-19.

MEMORY CHECK!

- The ear is divided into three areas: the external ear, which is involved only with hearing; the middle ear, which is involved only with hearing; and the inner ear, which is involved with both hearing and equilibrium.
- The external ear is composed of the pinna, which is visible, and the external auditory canal, which leads to the middle ear. Sound waves entering the external auditory canal hit the tympanic membrane and cause it to vibrate; this membrane separates the external ear from the middle ear.
- The middle ear is composed of the tympanic cavity within the temporal bone. Three ossicles transmit the vibration of the tympanic membrane to the inner ear and set the fluids of the inner ear in motion.
- The inner ear is a system of osseous labyrinths filled with perilymph. The bony labyrinth is divided into the cochlea, the vestibule, and the semicircular canals.
- Sound waves that reach the cochlea through vibrations of the tympanic membrane, the ossicles, and the oval window set the cochlear fluids in motion. Receptor cells on the basilar membrane are stimulated and transmit impulses along the cochlear nerve, which is a division of the vestibulocochlear nerve, to the auditory cortex of the temporal lobe for sound interpretation.
- The semicircular canals and vestibule of the inner ear contain equilibrium receptors. In the semicircular canals, the dynamic equilibrium receptors respond to changes in direction of movement. The vestibule in the inner ear contains receptors that are essential to the body's sense of static equilibrium. Both of these impulses are transmitted through the vestibular nerve, which is a division of the vestibulocochlear nerve, to the cerebellum.

LEARNING OBJECTIVES

After studying this chapter, the learner will be able to do the following:

1. **Classify pain**.
   Study text pages 490 through 495; refer to Figure 15-6 and Tables 15-2 and 15-3.

   Classifications of pain include nociceptor pain (known physiologic cause), nonnociceptor pain (neuropathic pain), acute pain (signals harmful state), and chronic pain (persistence of pain from unknown cause or a therapeutic response).

   Acute pain may be somatic, visceral, or referred. **Somatic pain** comes from the skin or close to the surface of the body and is sharp and localized. **Visceral pain** occurs in internal organs, the abdomen, or the skeleton. It is poorly localized because there are fewer mechanoreceptors in the visceral structures. It is associated with nausea and vomiting, hypotension, restlessness, and possible shock. Visceral pain often radiates or is referred. **Referred pain** is present in an area removed or distant from its point of origin. The area of referred pain is supplied by the same spinal segment as the actual site of injury. Impulses from many cutaneous and visceral neurons converge on the same ascending neuron, and the brain cannot distinguish between the origin of the two.

   Acute pain is a warning of actual or impending tissue injury. Physiologic responses include increased heart rate, increased respiratory rate, elevated blood pressure, pallor or flushing, dilated pupils, and diaphoresis.

   Psychologically, individuals often respond to acute pain with fear, anxiety, and a general sense of unpleasantness or uneasiness. The stress of fear may subsequently contribute to the physiologic signs of pain.

   Chronic pain is prolonged; it may last longer than 3 months and may either persist or be intermittent. Chronic pain may be a result of decreased levels of endorphins or the predominance of C-neuron stimulation.

   Physiologic responses to chronic pain depend on the persistent or intermittent nature of the pain. **Intermittent pain** produces physiologic responses similar to acute pain, whereas **persistent pain** permits physiologic adaptation. Individuals with chronic pain often are depressed, have difficulty sleeping and eating, and may become preoccupied with their pain.

   Low back pain results from poor muscular tone, inactivity, muscle strain, or sudden vigorous activity. **Myofascial pain syndromes** are common causes of chronic pain. These conditions involve injury to the muscles and fascia. The pain from muscles and fascia results from muscle spasm, tenderness, and stiffness. **Chronic postoperative pain** occurs in individuals after thoracotomy, radical mastectomy, radical neck dissection, and surgical amputation.

   The **pain experienced in cancer** is attributed to the advance of the disease; it is associated with the treatment of the disease and attributed to coexisting entities such as osteoarthritis. As cancer advances, pain can be caused by infection and inflammation, increasing pressure of a growing tumor on nerve endings, stretching of visceral surfaces, and/or obstruction of ducts and intestines.

   Neuropathic pain results from nerve trauma or disease and leads to abnormal peripheral and central pain processing. Types of neuropathic pain include deafferentation pain, sympathetically maintained pain, central pain, and phantom pain.

   Deafferentation pain results from tumor infiltration of nerve tissue; trauma or chemical injury to the nerve; or damage from radiation, chemotherapy, or surgical sectioning of the nerve. It is poorly controlled by analgesics and manifests as constant, dull, viselike, or burning. **Sympathetically maintained pain** occurs after peripheral

97

nerve injury and is characterized as severe continuous burning. It is often associated with vasospasm and vasomotor changes in the affected limbs. **Central pain** is caused by a lesion or dysfunction in the CNS. The lesions include infarction, hemorrhage, abscess, degeneration, tumors, and trauma. The pain is either diffuse or localized and is constant and irritating. **Phantom limb pain** is pain that an individual feels in an amputated limb after the residual stump has completely healed. If the neuronal pathway from the amputated limb is stimulated at any point along its pathway, action potentials are transmitted toward the cortex, where CNS integration results in the perception of pain.

2. **Contrast pediatric perception of pain with that of older individuals.**

Study text page 495; refer to Figure 15-7.

The nociceptor system is functional in fetuses by 24 weeks of gestation. Repetitive painful experiences and prolonged exposure to analgesics in infants during the neonatal period may permanently alter synaptic and neuronal organization, and fetuses may remember pain with an enduring effect on behavior and pain perception. Changes in facial expression, crying, and body movements are expressions of pain in infants. Children between the ages of 5 and 18 years tend to have lower pain thresholds than do adults. Older individuals tend to have a slightly higher pain threshold, and women appear to be more sensitive to pain than are men. Pain in the elderly is also influenced by liver and renal function with alterations in the metabolism of drugs and metabolites.

3. **Describe the alterations that occur in fever, hyperthermia, and hypothermia.**

Study text pages 498 and 500 through 502; refer to Figure 15-8 and Table 15-4.

Fever is not the failure of the normal thermoregulatory mechanism. Instead, it is considered "a resetting of the hypothalamic thermostat" to a higher level. The normal thermoregulatory mechanisms are raised so that the thermoregulatory center adjusts heat production, conservation, and loss to maintain the core temperature at a new, higher set-point temperature.

The pathophysiology of fever begins with the introduction of exogenous pyrogens or endotoxins. The production and release of interleukin-1 (IL-1), tumor necrosis factor, interleukin-6, and interferons occur as exogenous bacteria are destroyed and absorbed by phagocytic cells within the host. As the set point is raised, the hypothalamus signals an increase in heat production and conservation to raise body temperature to the new level as described in Foundational Knowledge Objective "e" (see p. 96 of this Study guide). During fever, arginine vasopressin (AVP), alpha-melanocyte-stimulating hormone, and corticotropin-releasing factor are released and act as endogenous antipyretics to help diminish the febrile response. During this antipyretic effect, as fever breaks, the set point is returned to normal. The hypothalamus signals a decrease in heat production and an increase in heat reduction.

Fever can be beneficial. Elevated body temperature kills many microorganisms and has adverse effects on the growth and replication of others. Increased temperature causes lysosomal breakdown with autodestruction of cells; this prevents viral replication in infected cells. Heat increases the lymphocytic transformation and motility of polymorphonuclear neutrophils, which facilitates the immune response.

Hyperthermia can produce nerve damage, coagulation of cell proteins, and death. At 41° C (106° F), nerve damage produces convulsions in the adult. At 43° C (109° F), death follows. In hyperthermia, there is no resetting of the hypothalamic set point. Forms of accidental hyperthermia are heat cramps, heat exhaustion, and heat stroke.

Heat cramps are severe, spasmodic cramps in the abdomen and extremities subsequent to prolonged sweating and associated sodium loss. Heat cramps usually appear in individuals who are unaccustomed to heat or in those who are performing strenuous work in very warm climates. Fever, rapid pulse, and increased blood pressure often accompany the cramps.

Heat exhaustion or collapse results from prolonged high body core or environmental temperatures. These high temperatures cause the hypothalamic inducement of profound vasodilation and profuse sweating. Over a prolonged period of elevated temperatures, the hypothalamic responses produce dehydration, decreased plasma volumes, hypotension, decreased cardiac output, and tachycardia.

Heatstroke is a potentially lethal consequence of a breakdown in control of an overstressed thermoregulatory center. The brain cannot tolerate temperatures of more than 40.5° C (105° F). In cases of very high core temperatures, the regulatory center may cease to function appropriately. Sweating ceases, and the skin becomes dry and flushed. The individual may become irritable, confused, stuporous, or comatose. As evaporation of perspiration ceases, core temperatures rise rapidly. High core temperatures and vascular collapse produce cerebral edema, degeneration of the central nervous system, and renal tubular necrosis. Death results unless immediate, effective treatment is initiated.

Treatment requires more than the fluid and electrolyte replacement required in heat cramps and exhaustion. Removing the person from the warm environment, if possible, and surface cooling are required. Too-rapid surface cooling may cause peripheral vasoconstriction, which would prevent core cooling. Children are more susceptible to heat stroke than adults are. They produce more metabolic heat when exercising, they have a greater ratio of surface area to mass, and their perspiring capacity is less than that of adults.

Malignant hyperthermia is a potentially lethal complication of an inherited muscle disorder. The condition is precipitated by the administration of volatile anesthetics and neuromuscular blocking agents. The risk of this muscle disorder may be about 1 in 200 individuals. Malignant hyperthermia causes intracellular calcium levels to rise, thereby producing sustained, uncoordinated muscle contractions. As a result of these contractions, acidosis develops and body temperature may rise 1° C (1.8° F)

98

every 5 minutes. Approximately 20% of those who develop malignant hyperthermia do not survive.

Treatment is withdrawal of the provoking agents and administration of skeletal muscle relaxants to inhibit calcium release during muscle contraction, treatment of cardiac arrhythmias, sodium bicarbonate administration, and cooling of the body.

Hypothermia slows chemical reactions, increases blood viscosity, slows blood flow, facilitates blood coagulation, and stimulates profound vasoconstriction. Accidental hypothermia, which is a body temperature below 35° C (95° F), is generally the result of sudden immersion in cold water or prolonged exposure to cold environments. The young and the elderly are at risk because of their less-effective thermoregulatory mechanisms. Individuals with conditions that diminish their ability to generate heat (e.g., hypothyroidism, hypopituitarism, malnutrition, Parkinson disease, rheumatoid arthritis) are also at risk.

The hypothalamic center stimulates shivering in an effort to increase heat production at a core temperature of 35° C and continues until core temperature drops between 30° and 32° C. Thinking becomes sluggish and coordination is decreased at 34° C. At 30° C, the individual becomes stuporous, heart rate and respiratory rates decline, and cardiac output is diminished. In severe hypothermia, which is when the core temperature reaches 20° to 28° C, pulse and respirations may be undetectable. Acidosis becomes moderate to severe. Ventricular fibrillation and asystole are common.

Depending on the severity of the hypothermia, rewarming of the peripheral tissues may be the only treatment required. Core rewarming is performed when core temperatures have dropped below 30° C or when severe cardiovascular abnormalities appear. Core rewarming may require the administration of warm intravenous solutions, gastric or peritoneal lavage, or inhalation of warmed gases. Rewarming generally should proceed at no faster than a few degrees per hour.

4. Describe sleep disorders; cite examples.

Study text pages 504 through 506.

Sleep disorders can be categorized by signs and symptoms. Disorders of initiating sleep are classified as **insomnia,** which is the inability to fall or stay asleep. Insomnia may be transient and related to travel across time zones, or it may be caused by acute stress. Long-term insomnia is associated with drug or alcohol abuse, chronic pain disorders, or chronic depression.

Obstructive sleep apnea syndrome (OSAS) is a disorder of breathing during sleep related to upper airway obstruction that is associated with reduced blood oxygen saturation and hypercapnia. Risk factors are obesity, male gender, and age. OSAS is characterized by repetitive increases in resistance to airflow in the upper airway with loud snoring, gasping, intervals of apnea lasting from 10 to 30 seconds, fragmented sleep, and daytime sleepiness. The obstruction is caused by the soft palate or the base of the tongue, or both, collapsing against the pharyngeal walls because of decreased muscle tone during REM sleep.

Restless leg syndrome (RLS) is a sensorimotor disorder associated with prickling, tingling, and crawling occurring at rest In the evening or at night. There also may be an iron deficiency in women and the elderly. There is a familial tendency and an association with circadian fluctuation of dopamine levels.

Hypersomnia is excessive daytime sleepiness associated with voluntary sleep deprivation. There also may be an underlying sleep disorder such as OSAS or narcolepsy

Narcolepsy is characterized by hypersomnia, brief spells of muscle weakness, hallucinations, and sleep paralysis. The disorder is associated with hypothalamic deficiency of hypocretin, which promotes wakefulness.

Circadian rhythm sleep disorder includes rapid time-zone change or "jet-lag syndrome," which is an altered sleep schedule with an advance or a delay of 3 hours or more in sleep time or a change in total sleep time from day to day. Vigilance of psychomotor performance and arousal are markedly depressed after alterations in the sleep-wake schedule. Individuals affected by disorders of the sleep-wake schedule require several days to synchronize circadian rhythm, adjust the body temperature cycle, and adjust cortisol secretion.

Three types of **parasomnias** include *arousal disorders,* such as sleepwalking (somnambulism), night terrors, and sleep enuresis; *sleep-wake transition disorders,* such as sleep talking or nocturnal leg cramps; and *REM sleep disorders,* such as sleep paralysis, nightmares, and sudden infant death syndrome (SIDS).

5. Identify common diseases, their etiology, and manifestations that are associated with the special senses.

Study text pages 509 through 512 and 514 through 517; refer to Figures 15-15 through 15-20 and Tables 15-6 and 15-7.

Vision

Blepharitis is an inflammation of the eyelids caused by staphylococcal infections or seborrheic dermatitis. Redness, edema, and itching occur.

Conjunctivitis is an inflammation of the conjunctiva, which is the mucous membrane that covers the front part of the eyeball. It may be caused by bacteria, viruses, allergies, or chemical irritations. The inflammatory response produces redness, pain, and lacrimation.

Keratitis is an infection of the cornea that is usually caused by bacteria or viruses. Bacterial infections often cause corneal ulceration and require extensive antibiotic treatment. Type I herpes virus usually infects the cornea and conjunctiva. Common symptoms include photophobia, pain, and lacrimation.

Strabismus is the deviation of one eye from the other when the person is looking directly at an object. It is due to a weak or hypertonic muscle in one of the eyes. The deviation may be upward, downward, inward, or outward. The primary symptom of strabismus is diplopia (double vision).

Amblyopia is a vision reduction or dimness for unknown reasons. Amblyopia is associated with diabetes mellitus, renal failure, malaria, and toxic substances such as alcohol and tobacco.

99

A *scotoma* is a circumscribed defect of the central field of vision. It is most often a sequela to an inflammatory lesion of the optic nerve, and it is frequently associated with multiple sclerosis.

A *cataract* is a cloudy or opaque ocular lens. Although the most common form of cataract is degenerative, cataracts may also occur as a result of infection, radiation, trauma, drugs, or diabetes mellitus. Cataracts cause decreased visual acuity, blurred vision, glare, and decreased color perception.

Papilledema is edema and inflammation of the optic nerve at its point of entrance into the eyeball. Generally, papilledema is caused by obstruction to the venous return of the retina. An early symptom is distention of the retinal vein.

Dark adaptation affects visual acuity. An average 80-year-old individual needs over twice as much light as a 20-year-old to see equally well. Changes in rhodopsin, which is a substance found in the rods and responsible for low-light vision, are likely responsible for reduced dark adaptation in older adults. Vitamin A deficiencies can cause the same disorder in individuals of any age.

Glaucoma is characterized by intraocular pressures above the normal range of 12 to 20 mmHg maintained by the aqueous fluid in homeostasis. Intraocular fluid accumulation obstructs aqueous humor outflow. Chronic increased intraocular pressure first causes a loss of peripheral vision, which is followed by central vision impairment and blindness.

Loss of accommodation in the elderly is termed *presbyopia,* a condition in which the ocular lens becomes larger, firmer, and less elastic. The major symptom is reduced near vision, which causes the need for reading material to be held at arm's length.

In *myopia* (nearsightedness), light rays are focused in front of the retina when the person is looking at a distant object. In *hyperopia* (farsightedness), light rays are focused behind the retina when the person is looking at a near object. *Astigmatism* is caused by an unequal curvature of the cornea; light rays are bent unevenly and do not come to a single focus on the retina. Blurred vision and headache develop in all three of these conditions.

Hearing

A *conductive hearing* loss occurs when a change in the outer or middle ear or both impairs sound conduction from the outer to the inner ear. Conditions that commonly cause a conductive hearing loss include impacted cerumen, foreign bodies lodged in the ear canal, neoplasms of the external auditory canal and/or middle ear, eustachian tube dysfunction, infectious otitis media, cholesteatoma, and otosclerosis. Symptoms of conductive hearing loss include diminished hearing and a soft speaking voice. The voice is soft because the individual may hear his or her voice conducted by bone ossicles.

Acute otitis media (AOM) is associated with ear pain, fever, irritability, an inflamed tympanic membrane, and fluid in the middle ear. The tympanic membrane progresses from erythema to opaqueness with bulging as fluid accumulates. There is an increasing prevalence of AOM caused by penicillin-resistant microorganisms. Treatment includes antimicrobial therapy for AOM and placement of tympanotomy tubes when there is bilateral effusion persistent for 3 months and significant hearing loss.

A *sensorineural hearing loss* is due to impairment of the organ of Corti and its hearing receptors or its central connections. Conditions that commonly cause sensorineural hearing loss include congenital and hereditary factors, noise exposure, aging, ototoxicity, and systemic diseases. Congenital and neonatal sensorineural hearing loss may be caused by maternal rubella, premature birth, traumatic delivery, or erythroblastosis fetalis.

Olfaction

Hyposmia is an impaired sense of smell; *anosmia* is a complete loss of smell. When hyposmia or anosmia occurs bilaterally, it is usually the result of inflammation of the nasal mucosa, severe head colds, or excessive smoking. Unilateral hyposmia or anosmia may indicate tumor compression of one olfactory bulb or nerve tract. *Olfactory hallucinations* arise from hyperactivity in cortical neurons and involve the smelling of odors that are not actually present; they are mostly associated with temporal lobe seizures. *Parosmia*, which is an abnormal or perverted sense of smell, may occur in severely depressed individuals.

Taste

Hypogeusia is decreased taste sensation; *ageusia* is the absence of the sense of taste. Ageusia that affects the entire tongue may follow head injury. Damage to the glossopharyngeal nerve causes the inability to detect bitterness; damage to the facial nerve causes inability to detect sour, sweet, and salty tastes. *Parageusia* is a perversion of taste in which substances possess an unpleasant flavor. Parageusia is common in individuals who are receiving chemotherapy for cancer, and it often leads to anorexia.

Touch

Any impairment of reception, transmission, perception, or interpretation of touch alters tactile sensation. Trauma, tumor, infection, metabolic changes, vascular changes, and degenerative disease may cause tactile dysfunction. Sedative drugs and prefrontal injury that interrupt connections between the prefrontal cortex and subcortical centers diminish the interpretation of the sensations.

Proprioception

Proprioception is the perception and awareness of the position of the body and its parts. It depends on impulses from the inner ear and from receptors in joints and ligaments. *Proprioceptive dysfunction* may be caused by alterations at any level of the nervous system; this is similar to that observed in tactile dysfunction.

Vestibular nystagmus is the constant, involuntary movement of the eyeball that is caused when the semicircular canal system is overstimulated. *Vertigo* is the sensation of spinning that occurs with inflammation of the semicircular canals in the ear.

Ménière disease is a vestibular disorder that can cause proprioceptive dysfunction. The pathologic basis of this disease is unclear. The individual with acute Ménière disease may experience a loss of proprioception and become unable to stand or walk.

Peripheral neuropathies are probably caused by metabolic disturbances of the neuron itself. The result is a diminished or absent sense of body position or position of body parts. Gait changes often occur.

PRACTICE EXAMINATION

Multiple Choice

Circle the correct answer for each question.

1. Endorphins:
   a. increase pain sensations.
   b. decrease pain sensations.
   c. may increase or decrease pain sensations.
   d. have no effect on pain sensations.
2. Referred pain from upper abdominal diseases involves:
   a. the sacral region.
   b. L2 to L4.
   c. T8, L1, and L2.
   d. the gluteal regions, the posterior thighs, and the calves.
3. In the gate control theory of pain:
   a. a "closed gate" increases pain perception.
   b. stimulation of large A fibers "closes the gate."
   c. Both a and b are correct.
   d. Neither a nor b is correct.
4. Norepinephrine:
   a. inhibits pain in the spinal cord and brain.
   b. increases excitability of neurons in the dorsal horn of the cord.
   c. contributes to pain inhibition in the pons and medulla.
   d. has major inhibitory effects in the spinal cord.
5. Interleukin-1:
   a. lowers the hypothalamic set point.
   b. is an exogenous pyrogen.
   c. is stimulated by exogenous pyrogens.
   d. None of the above is correct.
6. Increased serum levels of epinephrine increase body temperature by:
   a. increasing vasodilation.
   b. decreasing muscle tone.
   c. increasing heat production by causing glycolysis and increasing metabolic rates.
   d. decreasing basal metabolic rate.
7. In heat stroke:
   a. core temperature usually does not exceed 101° F.
   b. sodium loss follows sweating.
   c. core temperature increases as the regulatory center falls.
   d. Both b and c are correct.

8. Unmyelinated C nociceptors:
   a. are responsible for transmission of the diffuse, burning sensations.
   b. transmit fast pain sensations.
   c. carry well-localized, sharp pain sensations.
   d. terminate in the white matter of the dorsal horn.
9. In hypothermia:
   a. the viscosity of blood is decreased.
   b. acidosis can develop.
   c. the hypothalamic center prevents shivering.
   d. All of the above are correct.
10. Although non-REM and REM sleep are defined by electrical recordings, they are characterized by physiologic events. Which of the following occurs?
    a. During NREM sleep, muscle tone increases.
    b. NREM sleep is initiated by the withdrawal of neurotransmitters from the reticular formation.
    c. During NREM sleep, cerebral blood flow to the cortex is increased.
    d. During NREM sleep, levels of corticosteroids are increased.
11. Sleep apnea:
    a. increases blood oxygen saturation.
    b. results from airway obstruction during sleep.
    c. is associated with "jet-lag syndrome."
    d. produces pulmonary hypotension.
12. Endogenous opioids inhibit:
    a. substance P.
    b. TNF.
    c. prostaglandin E.
    d. arginine vasopressin.
13. Glaucoma is _____ and results from _____.
    a. clouding of the lens; increased aqueous humor formation
    b. decreased intraocular pressure; decreased aqueous humor formation
    c. increased intraocular pressure; decreased aqueous humor drainage
    d. clouding of the lens; decreased aqueous humor drainage
14. Keratitis may cause:
    a. ulcers of the cornea.
    b. conjunctival pus.
    c. a hordeolum.
    d. neither a, b, nor c.
15. Ménière disease:
    a. is a complication of chronic middle ear disease.
    b. affects cochlear function, hence equilibrium.
    c. decreases endolymphatic pressure within the cochlea.
    d. is a genetic cause of vertigo.
16. Which is *neither* an activator *nor* a depolarizer of primary or first-order afferents?
    a. Bradykinin
    b. Prostaglandins
    c. Leukotrienes
    d. Substance P

101

17. Third-order neurons:
    a. terminate in the dorsal horn.
    b. project to the postcentral gyrus of the parietal lobe.
    c. project to the thalamus.
    d. are concerned with reflexes.

18. Deafferentation pain results from:
    a. surgical resection of a nerve.
    b. muscle strain.
    c. infected nerves.
    d. decreased levels of endorphins.

Matching

Match the pain characteristic with the responsible nervous system component.

_____ 19. Basic sensation of pain

_____ 20. Initiation of pain stimulus

_____ 21. Discrimination and precision given

a. nociceptive receptors

b. thalamus

c. brainstem

d. A fibers

e. cortex

Match the circumstance with the sleep disorder.

_____ 22. Drug or alcohol abuse

_____ 23. Obstructive apnea

_____ 24. Depressed vigilance

_____ 25. Insomnia

a. sleep initiation disorder

b. sleep breathing disorder

c. sleep-wake schedule disorder

CASE STUDY

Mrs. D. is a 45-year-old woman who sought care for chronic insomnia of 15 months' duration. She was pleasant and well-informed and responded appropriately during the recording of the health history.

Her history revealed that about 18 months earlier, some important life changes occurred. Her only child, a daughter, left for an out-of-state university. A lifelong friend, who was a confidante, moved to another community. Her husband, a successful dentist, had become more involved in various men's organizations than he had been in the past. She stated, "I wake up 15 to 20 times a night and rarely sleep for more than 4 hours." Various hypnotics had been unsuccessful. A sedating antidepressant was prescribed, and a second appointment was made for 10 days later.

On the second appointment, she noted her sleep pattern had improved. She was able to articulate that she felt unneeded, incompetent, and old.

Question

As an allied health caregiver, how do you assess Mrs. D.'s case?

16 Alterations in Cognitive Systems, Cerebral Hemodynamics, and Motor Function

FOUNDATIONAL KNOWLEDGE OBJECTIVES

a. Identify the structural modulators of consciousness.
   Review text page 450; refer to Figure 14-6

MEMORY CHECK!

- The reticular activating system (RAS) affects many central nervous system (CNS) activities, including sleep and wakefulness. It ascends from the lower brainstem through the midbrain and thalamus and projects throughout the cerebral cortex. Following prolonged wakefulness, the neurons in the RAS gradually fatigue and become less excitable. When this occurs, neuronal mechanisms revert to lower-level functioning and sleep. The ability to respond to stimuli or arousal depends on an intact RAS in the brainstem and the ability to respond to the environment. Cognition relies on an intact cerebral cortex. Therefore, consciousness or responsiveness to impressions made by the senses requires functioning along the reticular formation in the brainstem to the cerebral cortex.

b. Identify the structure and functional components of the brain.
   Review text pages 449, 450, 452, 453, 455, and 456; refer to Figures 14-6 through 14-8 and Table 14-3.

MEMORY CHECK!

- The CNS consists of the brain and spinal cord, which are encased within the meninges and bathed in cerebrospinal fluid (CSF). The brain is divided into several areas, including the cerebrum, the diencephalon, and the cerebellum. The midbrain, the medulla oblongata, and the pons comprise the brainstem.
- The outer covering of the cerebrum is the cortex. The entire cerebrum is divided into two halves (hemispheres) connected by a neural bridge called the corpus callosum. The cortex is involved with thinking and sensory perception. Emotional responses and control of body temperature, water and food intake, and sex drive have their origin in the midbrain area. The cerebellum primarily integrates muscular movements to produce coordination in walking, talking, and other complex muscular activities. The medulla oblongata controls vital functions such as respiration, heart rate, and blood pressure, although these are modified by higher brain centers.
- Within the cerebral hemispheres are subdivisions called lobes. The frontal lobe is located in the anterior portion of each hemisphere. The temporal lobe is located in the lower, middle region of each hemisphere. The parietal lobe is the upper rear portion. The occipital lobe is the lower rear portion.
- The basal ganglia are a collection of cell bodies in several areas of the gray matter of the brain, including the caudate nucleus, the globus pallidus, the putamen, and the substantia nigra. The function of the basal ganglia is thought to involve the planning and programming of movement.
- The functional unit of all CNS tissue is the neuron. The neuron exhibits properties of excitability and electrical transmission. An excitable membrane has electrical activity generated by ion fluxes that enable transmission.

103

c. Identify the parts of the CNS that control voluntary muscle movement.

Review text page 452; refer to Figure 14-8.

MEMORY CHECK!

- The cerebral cortex plays a major role in controlling precise, voluntary muscular movements, whereas other brain regions provide integration for the regulation of automatic movements such as arm swinging during walking. Motor output to skeletal muscles travels down the spinal cord in two types of descending tracts: the pyramidal tracts and the extrapyramidal tracts. The pyramidal tracts originate in the motor cortex and terminate in the brainstem; they cross to the opposite side at the medulla–spinal cord junction. The pyramidal tracts, also known as upper motor neurons, consist of lateral corticospinal, anterior corticospinal, and corticobulbar tracts that convey impulses that cause precise, voluntary movements of skeletal muscles. The extrapyramidal tracts, which are the lower motor neurons, arise from the cortex and project to the cerebellum and basal ganglia before they descend to innervate the motor neurons; they do not cross to the opposite side. Extrapyramidal tracts consist of rubrospinal, tectospinal, and vestibulospinal tracts. They convey nerve impulses that program automatic movements, help coordinate body movements with visual stimuli, maintain skeletal muscle tone and posture, and play a major role in equilibrium by regulating muscle tone in response to movements of the head.

LEARNING OBJECTIVES

After studying this chapter, the learner will be able to do the following:

1. Identify sites and causes for alterations in arousal.

Study text pages 525 and 526; refer to Figure 14-6.

Possible causes of an **altered level of arousal** may be separated into three major groups: structural, metabolic, and psychogenic. Structural causes are divided according to five locations of the pathology: (1) supratentorial, which means above the tentorium cerebella; (2) infratentorial, which means below the tentorium cerebella; (3) subdural; (4) extracerebral; and (5) intracerebral.

Supratentorial processes produce a decreased level of consciousness because of encephalitis, brainstem trauma, or cerebral vascular accident or by impairing function of the thalamic or hypothalamic activating systems. **Infratentorial processes** produce a reduction in arousal by cerebrovascular disease, demyelinating disease, neoplasms, granulomas, abscesses, and head injuries that destroy the brainstem. A decreased level of consciousness may also be caused by compression of the reticular activating system. Specific causes of compression of the brainstem include hematomas, hemorrhages, and aneurysms; cerebellar hemorrhage, infarcts, abscesses, and neoplasms; and demyelinating disorders. **Extracerebral disorders** include neoplasms, closed-head trauma with subsequent bleeding, and subdural accumulation of pus. **Intracerebral disorders** manifest as masses; these disorders include bleeding, infarcts, emboli, and tumors.

A wide spectrum of diseases may produce a metabolically induced alteration in arousal. In these disorders, there is widespread direct or indirect interference with neuronal metabolism throughout much of the brain.

Psychogenic unresponsiveness may develop in general psychiatric disorders. Despite apparent unconsciousness, the person is actually physiologically awake.

2. Summarize the changes in levels of consciousness, pupillary response, muscle tone, and respiratory activity as nonresponsiveness progresses from the cerebrum/diencephalon through the medulla.

Study text pages 528, 529, 531, 532; refer to Figures 16-1 through 16-6 and Tables 16-2 through 16-8. See table on page 105.

Consciousness is alertness with orientation to person, place, and time; the conscious individual has normal speech, voluntary movement, and oculomotor activity. **Confusion** is an alteration in the perception of stimuli. First, there is disorientation to time, then to place, and eventually to person. The attention span is shortened. The individual with **lethargy** exhibits orientation to person, place, and time. However, slow vocalization, decreased motor skills, and oculomotor activity are present. **Obtundation** is awakening in response to stimulation; continuous stimulation is needed for arousal, and the eyes are usually closed. **Stupor** is vocalization only in response to painful stimuli. Markedly decreased spontaneous movement with eyes closed is seen. A person in a **coma** displays no vocalization, no spontaneous eye movement, and no arousal to any stimulus; however, brainstem reflexes are intact.

104

Rostral-Caudal Progression of Nonresponsiveness

Area Involved	Level of Consciousness	Pupils	Muscle Tone	Breathing Pattern
Diencephalon (thalamus/ hypothalamus)	Decreased concentration, agitation, dullness, lethargy, obtundation	Respond to light briskly; full-range eye movements only on "doll's eyes"—none in direction of rotation or after injection of hot or cold water in ear canal (caloric posturing)	Some purposeful movement in response to pain, combative movement Decorticate: flexion in upper extremities and extension in lower extremities	Yawning and sighing to Cheyne-Stokes
Midbrain	Stupor to coma	Midposition fixed (MPF)	Decerebrate: arms rigid, palms turned away from body	Neurogenic hyperventilation
Pons	Coma	MPF	Decerebrate	Apneustic: prolonged inspiration and expiration
Medulla	Coma	MPF	Flaccid	Ataxic: uncoordinated and irregular

3. Distinguish between brain death and cerebral death.

Study text pages 533 and 534; refer to Table 16-8.

Brain death (brainstem death) occurs when irreversible brain damage is so extensive that the brain has no potential for recovery and can no longer maintain the body's internal respiratory and cardiac vascular functions. There is destruction of the brainstem and cerebellum.

Cerebral death, or irreversible coma, is death of the cerebral hemispheres exclusive of the brainstem and cerebellum. The individual is permanently unable to respond in any significant way to the environment. The brain may continue to maintain normal respiratory and cardiovascular functions, normal temperature control, and normal gastrointestinal function.

4. Describe characteristics of seizure disorders.

Study text pages 536 through 539 and 542; refer to Figure 16-7 and Tables 16-9 through 16-12.

A **seizure** is caused by abnormal excessive hypersynchronous discharges of CNS neurons and is characterized by a sudden, transient alteration in brain function. It usually involves motor, sensory, autonomic, or psychological clinical manifestations and an alteration in the level of arousal. The alteration in level of arousal is temporary. The term **convulsion** refers to the clonic-tonic (jerky, contract-relax) movement associated with seizures. **Generalized seizures** involve neurons bilaterally, often do not have a local onset, and usually originate from a subcortical or deeper brain focus. With these seizures, consciousness always is impaired or lost. **Partial seizures** involve neurons only unilaterally, often have a focal onset, and originate from discrete areas usually associated with cortical brain tissue. Partial seizures may become generalized involving neurons of the other hemisphere and deeper brain nuclei. This process is **secondary generalization.** Consciousness is lost at the point of generalization.

Status epilepticus is the occurrence of a second, third, or multiple seizures before the person has fully regained consciousness from the preceding seizure. Status epilepticus most frequently results from abrupt discontinuation of seizure medications, but it may also occur in untreated or inadequately treated individuals with seizure disorders. The individual is still in a **postictal state,** a state that follows a seizure, when the next seizure begins. The situation is serious because of developing cerebral hypoxia.

Etiologic factors in seizures include cerebral lesions, biochemical disorders, cerebral trauma, and epilepsy. Among the causes of seizure activity are:

Metabolic defects	Motor syndromes
Congenital malformations	Infections
Genetic predisposition	Brain tumors
Perinatal injury	Vascular diseases
Postnatal trauma	Fever

Epilepsy is a term that is applied to conditions in which no correctable cause for the seizures is found, so the seizure activity recurs without treatment. Epilepsies may manifest as partial or generalized seizures. Any condition that alters cerebral structure or function or disrupts the biochemistry of the body causes seizures.

In seizures, the primary abnormality may be membrane instability in resting potential, defects of the GABA inhibitory system, abnormalities of potassium conductance or calcium channels, or an abnormality in excitatory transmission of the N-methyl-D-aspartate type. The maintenance of seizure activity demands increased ATP and increased cerebral oxygen consumption. As available serum glucose is depleted, lactate accumulates in the brain and produces acidosis, leading to cerebral injury and destruction.

An **epileptogenic focus** appears to be a group of neurons that is chronically hyperexcitable. If a seizure focus is active for a prolonged time, a secondary focus, called a **mirror focus,** may develop in normal tissue.

105

The brainstem initiates the phase of muscle contraction (**tonic phase**) that is followed by increased muscle tone and loss of consciousness. The phase of alternating contraction and relaxation of muscles (**clonic phase**) starts as inhibitory neurons in the cortex, anterior thalamus, and basal ganglia begin to inhibit the cortical excitation. This inhibition interrupts seizure discharge and produces an intermittent contract-relax pattern of muscle contractions. Two types of symptoms often signal an impending generalized tonic-clonic seizure: an **aura**, a partial seizure that immediately precedes the onset of a generalized tonic-clonic seizure; and a **prodroma**, an early manifestation that may occur hours to days before a seizure.

5. Define descriptive terms of alterations in awareness.

Refer to Figure 16-8 through 16-11 and Table 16-13.

Selective attention deficit refers to the inability to select appropriately from available competing environmental stimuli for conscious processing.

Dysmnesia is the loss of past memories and the inability to form new memories.

Retrograde amnesia is the loss of past memories.

Anterograde amnesia is an inability to form new memories.

Memory is the recording, retention, and retrieval of knowledge. An individual holds and manipulates information in working memory.

Declarative memory involves events and facts.

Nondeclarative memory is a motor memory of how to behave.

A **vigilance deficit** is the inability to concentrate over time or to maintain sustained attention.

In a **detection deficit**, the person is unmotivated and unable to use feedback.

Generally, the primary pathophysiologic mechanism that operates in cognitive system disorders is due directly to ischemia and hypoxia or indirectly to compression, toxins, and chemicals.

6. Define terms used to describe processing deficits.

Study text pages 546, 548, and 551 through 553; refer to Tables 16-14 through 16-19.

Agnosia is a deficit of recognition of the form and nature of objects. Although it most commonly is associated with cerebrovascular accidents, it may arise from any pathologic process that injures specific areas of the brain.

Dysphasia is the impairment of comprehension or production of language. Comprehension or use of symbols in either written or verbal language is disturbed or lost. **Aphasia** is the loss of the comprehension or production of language. Dysphasias usually are associated with cerebrovascular accidents that involve the middle cerebral artery or one of its many branches. Dysphasia results from dysfunction in the left cerebral hemisphere and usually involves the frontotemporal region. Dysphasia may be nonfluent, which means that the individual cannot find words for expression and exhibits difficulty in writing. Dysphasia may also be fluent, which means that verbal language is produced, but it is meaningless and made up of inappropriate words.

Acute confusional states result from cerebral dysfunction secondary to drug intoxication or nervous system disease. These states may begin either suddenly or gradually, depending on the amount of toxin exposure. The predominant feature of an acute confusional state is impaired or lost vigilance. The individual is unable to concentrate on incoming sensory information or on any one particular mental or motor task.

The **dementias** are characterized by the loss of more than one cognitive or intellectual function. There may be a decrease in orientation, general knowledge and information, vigilance, recent memory, remote memory, concept formation, abstraction, reasoning, or language. Memory is the most common cognitive ability lost, with advancing age the greatest risk factor. Causes of dementia include degeneration, cerebrovascular accidents, compression, toxins, metabolic disorders, biochemical imbalances, demyelinization, and infections. Symptoms of dementia may be grouped according to type of memory deficit: amnestic dementia (loss of recent memory), cognitive dementia (loss of remote memory), or intentional dementia (loss of vigilance and executive function), and altered behavior.

7. Describe Alzheimer disease.

Study text pages 553, 554, and 556, 557; refer to Figures 16-12 through 16-15 and Table 16-20.

Alzheimer disease (AD) is one of the most common causes of severe cognitive dysfunction in older people. Its prevalent forms are late-onset familial Alzheimer dementia (FAD) and nonhereditary late-onset AD.

The exact cause of AD is unknown. Several possible theories are notable, including the loss of neurotransmitter stimulation by choline acetyltransferase; a mutation for encoding amyloid precursor protein; an alteration in apolipoprotein E (apoE), which binds beta amyloid; and pathologic activation of N-methyl-D-aspartate receptors, resulting in an influx of excess calcium. Early-onset FAD includes gene defects on chromosomes 21, 14, and 1. Late-onset FAD is linked to a defect on chromosome 19.

Pathogenic mechanisms may be linked to aggregation and precipitation of insoluble amyloid or senile plaques in brain tissue and blood vessels. AD has also been linked to a lysosomal pathway in the breakdown of amyloid precursor protein to yield amyloid beta (AB) peptide. The initial accumulation of AB results in **senile plaques.** This accumulation is followed by other AB depositions along with tau protein, activated glia, and eventually **neurofibrillary tangles.**

Microscopically, the tau protein in the neurons becomes distorted and twisted, forming a tangle called a **neurofibrillary tangle.** These abnormal protein fibers accumulate within the neurons. Groups of nerve cells, especially terminal axons, degenerate and coalesce around an amyloid core. These areas appear like plaques and are called **senile plaques.** These plaques disrupt nerve impulse transmission. Senile plaques and neurofibrillary tangles are more concentrated in the cerebral cortex and hippocampus. The greater the number of senile plaques and neurofibrillary tangles, the more dysfunction and disturbances are found in the blood flow.

106

In addition to cognitive dysfunctions, **dyspraxias**, or the inability to perform coordinated acts, may appear. Motor changes may occur if the posterior frontal lobes are involved. The individual may exhibit rigidity with flexion posturing, propulsion, and retropulsion. There is great variability in age of onset, intensity and sequence of symptoms, and in the location and extent of brain pathology among individuals with the disease.

Pharmacotherapy includes cholinesterase inhibitors to enhance cholinergic transmission. Drugs are available that block the activity of glutamate and function as uncompetitive Methyle aspartate (NMDA) receptor antagonists. Treatment of AD also is directed to decreasing the need for cognitive function by using memory aids, maintaining cognitive functions that are not impaired, and improving the general state of hygiene, nutrition, and health.

8. **Characterize cerebral hemodynamics and the stages of increased intracranial pressure.**
   Study text pages 557 through 559; refer to Figure 16-16, Table 16-21, and Box 16-4.
   When brain tissue is injured, management of increased intracranial pressure and cerebral oxygenation are issues; cerebral oxygenation is most critical. Cerebral oxygenation depends on cerebral blood volume, blood flow, and perfusion pressure. **Increased intracranial pressure** may result from an increase in intracranial content that occurs with tumor growth, edema, excess cerebrospinal fluid (CSF), or hemorrhage. Because the cranial vault is a nonflexible encasement around the brain and its extracellular fluid, a rise in intracranial pressure from one component requires an equal reduction in volume of other components. The most readily displaced content of the cranial vault is CSF.

In stage 1 of intracranial hypertension, vasoconstriction and external compression of the venous system occur in an attempt to further decrease the intracranial pressure following CSF displacement from the cranial vault. Clinical manifestations at this stage are subtle and transient and include confusion, drowsiness, and slight pupillary and breathing changes.

With continued expansion of the intracranial content, the resulting increase in intracranial pressure may exceed the brain's compensatory capacity to adjust to the increasing pressure. This is stage 2, and the pressure begins to compromise neuronal oxygenation. Systemic arterial vasoconstriction occurs to elevate the systemic blood pressure sufficiently to overcome the increased intracranial pressure.

Intracranial pressure begins to approach arterial pressure, and the brain tissues begin to experience hypoxia and hypercapnia. Cheyne-Stokes respiration occurs, the pupils become sluggish and dilated, pulse pressure widens, and bradycardia develops. Accumulating CO_2 causes vasodilation at the local tissue level. The hydrostatic pressure in the vessels drops, and blood volume increases. The brain volume increases, and intracranial pressure continues to rise. This is stage 3 of intracranial hypertension. Cerebral perfusion pressure falls, and cerebral perfusion slows dramatically; the brain tissues experience severe hypoxia and acidosis.

In the last stage of intracranial hypertension, stage 4, brain tissue shifts or **herniates** from the compartment of greater pressure to a compartment of lesser pressure. The herniated brain tissues increase the content volume within the lower pressure compartment, thereby exerting pressure on the brain tissue that normally occupies that compartment; now, both the herniated and lower, displaced tissue blood supply are impaired. Mean systolic arterial pressure soon equals intracranial pressure, and cerebral blood flow ceases.

9. **Describe herniation syndromes.**
   Study text page 559.
   Two types of herniation syndromes exist: **supratentorial** and **infratentorial**; the type is based on whether the affected area is located above or below the tentorium. The tentorium divides the cerebrum from the cerebellum.
   Uncal, central, and cingulate are the types of supratentorial herniation that occurs when brain tissue shifts through the tentorial notch into the posterior fossa. **Uncal** herniation manifests as decreasing consciousness, sluggish pupils before they fix and dilate, Cheyne-Stokes respirations, decorticate and then decerebrate posturing, and hemiplegia. The individual experiencing **central** herniation rapidly passes to an unconscious state; from Cheyne-Stokes respirations to apnea; from small reactive pupils to dilated and fixed pupils; and from decorticate to decerebrate posturing. The signs of **cingulate gyrus** herniation are those of increased intracranial pressure.
   Infratentorial herniation occurs as cerebellar tonsils shift inferiorly through the foramen magnum because of increased pressure within the posterior fossa. The clinical manifestations are an arched, stiff neck; paresthesias in the shoulder area; decreased consciousness; respiratory abnormalities; and varied pulse rates.

10. **Describe the pathogenesis of cerebral edema.**
    Study text pages 559 and 560; refer to Figures 16-17 and 16-18.
    Cerebral edema is an increase of extracellular or intracellular fluid within the brain after brain insult from trauma, infection, hemorrhage, tumor, ischemia, infarct, or hypoxia. Cerebral edema will distort blood vessels, displace brain tissues, and eventually herniate brain tissue from one brain compartment to another. The four types of cerebral edema are (1) vasogenic edema, (2) cytotoxic (metabolic) edema, (3) ischemic edema, and (4) interstitial edema.
    Vasogenic edema is clinically the most important type. It is caused by the increased permeability of the capillary endothelium of the brain after injury to the vascular structure. Plasma proteins leak into the extracellular spaces, thereby drawing water to them, and the water content of the brain parenchyma increases. Vasogenic edema starts in the area of injury and spreads with preferential accumulation into the white matter of the ipsilateral side, because the parallel myelinated fibers separate more easily.
    In **cytotoxic (metabolic) edema**, toxic factors directly affect the neuronal, glial, and endothelial cells, thereby causing failure of the active transport systems. The cells

107

lose their potassium and gain larger amounts of sodium. Water follows by osmosis into the cell and causes the cells to swell. Cytotoxic edema principally occurs in the gray matter.

Ischemic edema follows cerebral infarction. Soon after the onset of ischemia, the initial edema is confined to the intracellular compartment. Later in the process, brain cells begin to undergo necrosis and die. The released lysosomes increase the blood-brain barrier's permeability by lysing it.

Interstitial edema is caused by the movement of cerebrospinal fluid (CSF) from the ventricles into the extracellular spaces of the brain tissues. The brain fluid volume is mostly increased around the ventricles.

11. Describe hydrocephalus.

Study text pages 560 and 561; refer to Figure 16-19.

Hydrocephalus refers to various conditions characterized by excess fluid in the cranial vault, subarachnoid space, or both. It occurs because of interference with CSF flow caused by increased fluid production, obstruction within the ventricular system, or defective reabsorption of the fluid.

Hydrocephalus may develop from infancy through adulthood. Congenital hydrocephalus is rare. **Noncommunicating**, or internal, hydrocephalus in which the flow from the ventricles is obstructed is seen more often in children, and the **communicating** type without obstruction is seen more often in adults.

Obstructed CSF is under pressure and causes atrophy of the cerebral cortex and degeneration of the white matter tracts. There is selective preservation of gray matter.

Acute hydrocephalus manifests signs of rapidly developing increased intracranial pressure. If not promptly treated, the individual quickly becomes comatose. Normal pressure hydrocephalus develops slowly, showing declining memory and cognitive function. In infancy, head enlargement is predominant before cranial suture closure.

The diagnosis is based on physical examination, computed tomography scanning, and magnetic resonance imaging. Hydrocephalus can be treated by surgery to resect cysts, neoplasms, or hematomas. Ventricular bypass into the normal intracranial channel or into an extracranial compartment by a shunt is also used therapeutically.

12. Define common terms that describe alterations in motor functions.

Study text pages 561 through 572, and 575 through 577; refer to Figures 16-20 through 16-26 and 16-33 and Tables 16-22 through 16-29.

Movements are influenced by the cerebral cortex, the pyramidal system, the extrapyramidal system, and the motor units. Dysfunction in any of these areas may cause motor disorders.

Hypotonia is decreased muscle tone shown by passive movement of a muscle against resistance. It is thought to be due to decreased muscle spindle activity secondary to decreased excitability of neurons. Hypotonia is caused by cerebellar damage or, in rare cases, by pyramidal tract damage.

Hypertonia is increased muscle tone shown by passive movement of a muscle with resistance. Spasticity, which is a type of hypertonia, results from hyperexcitability of the stretch reflexes. Rigidity, another hypertonia, is produced by tonic reflex activity. The involved muscles are firm and tense; the increase in muscle movement is even and uniform throughout the range of passive motion.

Hyperkinesia is excessive movement; dyskinesias are abnormal, involuntary movements. Hypokinesia, which is decreased movement, is a loss of voluntary movement despite consciousness and normal peripheral nerve and muscle function. Types of hypokinesia include paresis/paralysis, akinesia, bradykinesia, and loss of associated movement.

Akinesia is a decrease in associated and voluntary movements. It is related to dysfunction of the extrapyramidal system. Pathogenesis is related to either a deficiency of dopamine or a defect of the postsynaptic dopamine receptors. **Bradykinesia** is a slowness of voluntary movements.

Hemiparesis/hemiplegia is paresis/paralysis of the upper and lower extremity on one side. **Diplegia** is the paralysis of both the upper and lower extremities due to cerebral hemisphere injuries. **Paraparesis/paraplegia** refers to weakness/paralysis of the lower extremities. **Quadriparesis/quadriplegia** refers to paresis/paralysis of all four extremities. Both paraparesis/paraplegia and quadriparesis/quadriplegia may be caused by dysfunction of the spinal cord.

Spinal shock is the complete cessation of spinal cord functions below a lesion. It is characterized by complete flaccid paralysis, absence of reflexes, and marked disturbances in bowel and bladder function.

Disturbances that originate in the anterior horn cells or the motor nuclei of the cranial nerves are called **amyotrophies.** Paralytic poliomyelitis is the prototype of these disorders. In the amyotrophies, muscle strength, muscle tone, and muscle bulk are affected in the muscles that are innervated by the involved motor neurons. Several brainstem syndromes involve damage to one or more of the cranial nerve nuclei. These are called **nuclear palsies** and may be caused by vascular occlusion, tumor, aneurysm, tuberculosis, or hemorrhage. **Bulbar palsies** involve cranial nerves IX, X, and XII.

Dystonia is the maintenance of abnormal posture through muscular contractions. **Decorticate posture** is characterized by upper extremities flexed at the elbows and held closely to the body and lower extremities that are externally rotated and extended. Decorticate posture is thought to occur when the brainstem is not inhibited by the motor function of the cerebral cortex. **Decerebrate posture** refers to increased tone in extensor muscles and trunk muscles with active tonic neck reflexes. The decerebrate posture is caused by severe injury to the brain and brainstem. **Basal ganglion** posture refers to a stooped, hyperflexed posture with a narrow-based, short-stepped gait. **Senile posture** is characterized by an increasingly flexed posture similar to a basal ganglion posture. The posture is associated with frontal lobe dysfunction.

108

A **spastic gait** is associated with unilateral, pyramidal injury and is manifested by a shuffling gait with the leg extended and held stiff. This gait causes a scraping over the walking surface. A **scissors gait** is associated with bilateral pyramidal injury and spasticity. The legs are abducted, so they touch each other. A **cerebellar gait** manifests as a wide-based gait with the feet apart and often turned outward and inward for greater stability. Cerebellar dysfunction accounts for this particular gait. A **basal ganglion gait** is a broad-based gait. Small steps are taken, and there is a decreased arm swing when walking. The individual's head and body are flexed and the arms are semiflexed and abducted, whereas the legs are flexed and rigid in more advanced states. Basal ganglion and frontal lobe dysfunction, respectively, account for these two gaits.

Hypermimesia is most commonly manifested as pathologic laughter or crying. Pathologic laughter is associated with right hemisphere injury, whereas pathologic crying is associated with left hemisphere injury. **Hypomimesia** is manifested as aprosodias, which is the loss of emotional language. Aprosodias involve an inability to understand emotion in speech and facial expression. Aprosodias are associated with right hemisphere damage.

Dyspraxia/apraxia is the inability to perform purposeful or skilled motor acts in the absence of paralysis, sensory loss, abnormal posture and tone, abnormal involuntary movement, incoordination, or inattentiveness. Dyspraxias arise when the connecting pathways between the left and right cortical areas are interrupted; conceptualization and execution of a complex motor act are impaired.

Extrapyramidal/motor syndromes include two types. **Basal ganglia disorders** manifest by alterations in muscle tone and posture, including rigidity, involuntary movements, and loss of postural reflexes. **Cerebellar motor syndromes** result in loss of muscle tone, difficulty with coordination and disorders of equilibrium and gait.

13. **Compare Huntington disease with Parkinson disease.**

Study text pages 570, 571, and 572 through 575; refer to Figures 16-27 through 16-32.

Multiple Choice

Circle the correct answer for each question.

1. Obtundation:
   a. is altered perception of stimuli.
   b. exhibits no spontaneous eye movement.
   c. is advanced sleep.
   d. requires continuous stimulation for arousal.

2. An individual shows flexion in upper extremities and extensions in lower extremities. This is:
   a. decorticate posturing.
   b. decerebrate posturing.
   c. excitation posturing.
   d. caloric posturing.

3. Cerebral death:
   a. is the death of the cerebellum.
   b. permits normal respiratory and cardiovascular functions.
   c. no longer maintains respiratory and cardiovascular functions.
   d. is the death of the brainstem.

4. The likely site of injury when central neurogenic hyperventilation appears is:
   a. the midbrain.
   b. the medulla.
   c. cerebral structure.
   d. diencephalic structure.

5. Which epileptic seizure is characterized by automatism?
   a. Autonomic
   b. Status epilepticus
   c. Absence
   d. Jacksonian
   e. Psychomotor

6. Postictal sleeping can be seen in which of the following types of seizures?
   a. Partial
   b. Unilateral
   c. Absence
   d. Grand mal
   e. Psychomotor

Comparison of Parkinson and Huntington Disease

	Parkinson	Huntington
Lesion site	Basal ganglia, degeneration of dopaminergic receptors	Basal ganglia, frontal cortex
Etiology	Imbalance between dopaminergic and cholinergic activity, dopamine deficiency, trauma, viral infection, neoplasms, drugs, toxins	Autosomal dominant, chromosome 4, GABA depletion
Onset	>40 years, peak in 60s	30s and 50s
Manifestations	Resting tremor, stiffness, akinesis, flexed forward leaning, no paralysis, depression, possible late-stage dementia	Dementia, delusions, depression, chorea-type movements
Treatment	Symptomatic, dopaminergic drugs, possible fetal cell transplant	No known treatment, possible recombinant genes

7. Late-onset familial Alzheimer disease is linked to a deficit on chromosome:
   a. 14.
   b. 19.
   c. 21.
   d. 23.
8. The senile plaques and neurofibrillary tangles of Alzheimer disease are mostly concentrated in the:
   a. cerebral cortex and hippocampus.
   b. thalamus.
   c. cerebellum.
   d. basal ganglia.
9. An individual with increased intracranial pressure from a head injury has mean systolic pressure equal to intracranial pressure. Which stage of intracranial pressure is being exhibited?
   a. Stage 1
   b. Stage 2
   c. Stage 3
   d. Stage 4
10. Infratentorial herniation occurs in shifting of the:
    a. mesencephalon.
    b. diencephalon.
    c. cerebellar tonsils.
    d. metencephalon.
11. In cerebral vasogenic edema:
    a. active transport fails.
    b. there is autodigestion.
    c. plasma proteins leak into extracellular spaces.
    d. cerebrospinal fluid leaves the ventricles.
12. Cheyne-Stokes respiration is observed in:
    a. blunt head trauma.
    b. supratentorial injury.
    c. infarction of the pons.
    d. hypoglycemia and meningitis.
13. Parkinson disease exhibits:
    a. akinesia.
    b. muscle flaccidity.
    c. early-stage dementia.
    d. paralysis.
14. Huntington disease is characterized by:
    a. dopamine insufficiency.
    b. depletion of GABA.
    c. resting tremors.
    d. rigidity.
15. In stage 3 of increasing intracranial pressure:
    a. vasoconstriction occurs.
    b. external compression of the venous system occurs.
    c. brain tissue shifts to lower pressure compartment.
    d. accumulating CO_2 causes local vasodilation.
16. Hydrocephalus occurs because of:
    a. reabsorption of CSF.
    b. obstruction within the ventricular system.
    c. excess fluid in the subdural space.
    d. reabsorption into the venous circulation.
17. Central herniation exhibits:
    a. decerebration to decortication.
    b. hemiplegia.
    c. pupil change from small, reactive to dilated and fixed.
    d. sluggish pupils before they dilate and fix.
18. Which stage of intracranial pressure exists when mean systemic blood pressure overcomes intracranial pressure?
    a. Stage 1
    b. Stage 2
    c. Stage 3
    d. Stage 4
19. An epileptogenic focus has:
    a. impermeable plasma membranes.
    b. a depolarized state.
    c. neural excitation during the clonic phase.
    d. neural inhibition during the toxic phase.
20. Extrapyramidal motor syndrome is manifested by:
    a. paralysis of voluntary movement.
    b. increased tendon reflexes.
    c. absence of involuntary movements.
    d. loss of postural reflexes.

Fill in the Blanks

Supply the correct response for each statement.

21. _____ is impaired conceptualization and execution of complex acts.

22. Cerebellar damage can manifest as _____.

23. _____ is characterized by flaccid paralysis, no reflexes, and disturbances in bowel and bladder function.

24. _____ is the inability to form new memories.

25. The inability to concentrate or sustain attention is _____.

A 12-year-old male complained to his mother, "I am seeing blue, flashing lights. Do you see them? I feel funny!" He then lost consciousness and had a major tonic-clonic seizure. His parents rushed him to the emergency department of a local hospital. On arrival at the hospital, he appeared to be asleep.

Studies at the hospital showed routine laboratory work within normal limits (WNL), lumbar puncture (CSF) was WNL, no evidence of skull fracture on x-ray study was revealed, and an electroencephalogram (EEG) showed no abnormalities.

Question

How would you interpret the episode and findings?

L.B. is a 78-year-old widow living in her own home with a caretaker and is regularly visited by her son who resides 300 miles away. He has been aware of his mother's progressing signs of cognitive/perceptual dysfunction since his father's death 2 years earlier, and he believes she has Alzheimer disease. On a Sunday morning visit, his mother offered to take him to lunch at McDonald's. She insisted on paying for both lunches at the ordering counter. When the cashier stated the cost, she objected saying, "I have been overcharged 23 cents." Her son told it was all right; she insisted she was correct. L.B. had summed the cost of the items in her head, multiplied that sum by the tax rate, and added the tax to the sum for a new total bill, and became angry at the young lady for overcharging her. The manager and her son concluded that L.B. was correct. When mother and son arrived home, L.B. was anxious, confused, and asked her son, "When are you going to take me home?" When told she was home, she said, "It is all right and I will stay here tonight but I must go home tomorrow." The next day, Monday, her son took her to a trusted physician who knew that L.B. had asthma and had been treated with an inhaler and low dose steroid for more than forty years. The son's question was "Will medication help mother?"

Question

What do you expect the physician to do?

Disorders of the Central and Peripheral Nervous Systems and the Neuromuscular Junction

17

FOUNDATIONAL KNOWLEDGE OBJECTIVES

a. Cite some examples of neurotransmitters.
Refer to Table 14-2.

MEMORY CHECK!

Neurotransmitter	Location	Function
Acetylcholine	Junctions with motor effectors, many parts of brain	Excitatory or inhibitory memory
Amines		
Serotonin	CNS	Mostly inhibitory; moods and emotions; sleep
Histamine	Brain	Mostly inhibitory; emotions; body temperature; water balance
Dopamine	Brain in autonomic system	Mostly excitatory; emotions/moods; motor control
Epinephrine	CNS, sympathetic division of autonomic nervous system	Excitatory or inhibitory
Norepinephrine	CNS, sympathetic division of autonomic nervous system	Excitatory or inhibitory
Amino acids		
Glutamate (glutamic acid)	CNS	Excitatory
Gamma-aminobutyric acid (GABA)	Brain	Inhibitory
Glycine	Spinal cord	Inhibitory
Neuropeptides		
Substance P	Brain, spinal cord, sensory pain pathways, gastrointestinal tract	Mostly excitatory; transmits pain information
Enkephalins	Several regions of CNS, retina, intestinal tract	Mostly inhibitory; blocks pain
Endorphins	Several regions of CNS, retina, intestinal tract	Mostly inhibitory; blocks pain

NOTE: These are examples only; most of the neurotransmitters are also found in other locations, and many have additional functions.

113

b. State the functions of the parts and associated structures of the brain.
Review text pages 449, 450, and 452 through 456; refer to Figures 14-6 through 14-8 and Table 14-3.

MEMORY CHECK!

Structural Functions of the Brain

Structure	Function
Brainstem	Performs sensory, motor, and reflex functions; controls cardiac, vasomotor, and respiratory centers; cranial nerve reflex
Cerebellum	Coordinates the activities of groups of muscles; maintains equilibrium; controls posture
Diencephalon	
Thalamus	Conscious recognition of crude pain, temperature, and touch; relays sensory impulses (except smell) to cerebrum; emotions; arousal mechanism; complex reflex movements
Hypothalamus	Links nervous system to endocrine system; coordinates autonomic nervous system; controls body temperature, hunger, thirst, and sleep
Cerebrum	
Cerebral cortex lobes	
Frontal	Voluntary control of skeletal muscles; unconscious skeletal muscle movement; speaking and writing
Temporal	Interpretation of odor and sound
Parietal	General body sensations
Occipital	Interpretation of sight
All lobes	Memory; emotions; reasoning; intelligence
Left hemisphere	Language; numeric skills; controls right side of body
Right hemisphere	Musical and artistic awareness; space and pattern perception; insight; controls left side of body

c. Identify the protective structures of the central nervous system.
Review text pages 459 through 462; refer to Figures 14-15 through 14-19 and Table 14-4.

MEMORY CHECK!

- The cranium is composed of eight bones that fuse early in childhood. The cranial vault encloses and protects the brain and its associated structures. The floor of the cranial vault is irregular and contains many foramina, which are openings through which cranial nerves, blood vessels, and the spinal cord exit. The foramen magnum is large enough for the spinal cord to exit. Surrounding the brain and spinal cord are three protective membranes collectively called the meninges: the dura mater, the arachnoid membrane, and the pia mater.
- The dura mater is composed of two layers, and there are venous sinuses between the layers. The outermost dural layer forms the periosteum of the skull; the inner dural meningeal layer forms the rigid plates that support and separate various brain structures.
- One of these membranous plates, the falx cerebri, transverses between the two cerebral hemispheres and anchors the base of the brain to the ethmoid bone. The tentorium cerebelli is a membrane that surrounds the brainstem and separates the cerebellum from the cerebral structures.
- Below the dura mater lies the arachnoid membrane, which is characterized by its spongy, weblike structure. The space between the dura and arachnoid membrane is the subdural space. Many small bridging veins traverse the subdural space. The subarachnoid space between the arachnoid membrane and the pia mater contains cerebrospinal fluid (CSF). The delicate pia mater provides support for the blood vessels that serve the brain tissue. The choroid plexuses, which are structures that produce CSF, arise from the pial membrane. The spinal cord is anchored to the vertebrae by an extension of the meninges. Between the dura mater and skull is a potential space called the epidural space.
- CSF is a clear, colorless fluid that is similar to blood plasma and interstitial fluid. It cushions the soft tissues in the central nervous system (CNS) from traumatic jolts and blows as a result of its buoyant properties. The choroid plexuses in the lateral, third, and fourth ventricles produce the major portion of CSF.

d. Describe the blood supply to the brain.

Review text page 462, 463, and 465; refer to Figures 14-18 through 14-22 and Table 14-5.

MEMORY CHECK!

- The brain receives approximately 20% of the cardiac output (800 to 1000 ml of blood flow) per minute. Carbon dioxide is a potent vasodilator in the CNS and ensures an adequate cerebral blood supply. The brain derives its arterial supply from two systems: the internal carotid arteries and the vertebral arteries.
- The internal carotid arteries originate from the common carotid arteries, enter the cranium through the base of the skull, and pass through the cavernous sinus. After giving off some small branches, they divide into the anterior and middle cerebral arteries. The vertebral arteries originate at the subclavian arteries, pass through the transverse foramina of the cervical vertebrae, and enter the cranium through the foramen magnum; they join to form the basilar artery. The basilar artery divides at the level of the midbrain to form paired posterior cerebral arteries. Superficial arteries supply small branches that project into the brain. The circle of Willis is a structure that has the ability to provide collateral blood flow; it is formed by many communicating arteries that extend to various brain structures.
- The venous drainage of the brainstem and cerebellum parallels the arterial supply; the venous drainage of the cerebrum does not. The cerebral veins are classified as superficial and deep. The veins drain into venous plexuses and dural sinuses and eventually drain into the internal jugular veins at the base of the skull. The blood-brain barrier selectively inhibits certain substances in the blood from entering the interstitial spaces of the brain or CSF. It is believed that the supporting cells and tight junctions between endothelial cells are involved in the formation of the blood-brain barrier and are responsible for its impermeability.

LEARNING OJECTIVES

After studying this chapter, the learner will be able to do the following:

1. Differentiate between focal and diffuse brain injury.

Study text pages 583 through 591; refer to Figures 17-1 through 17-8 and Table 17-1.

Traumatic brain injuries are broadly categorized into blunt (closed) trauma and open (penetrating) trauma. In blunt trauma, the head strikes a hard surface or a rapidly moving object strikes the head. The dura remains intact, and brain tissues are not exposed to the environment. Blunt trauma may result in both focal brain injuries and diffuse axonal injuries. When a break in the dura exposes the cranial contents to the environment, open trauma has occurred. Open trauma results in focal brain injuries.

Focal brain injury involves the specific, grossly observable brain lesions that are seen in cortical contusions, epidural hemorrhage, subdural hematoma, intracerebral hematoma, and open-head trauma. The force of impact typically produces **contusions** (bruises) on the brain. The contusion, in turn, produces epidural hemorrhage, subdural hematomas, and intracerebral hematomas. Contusion and bleeding occur because of small tears in blood vessels as a result of these forces. The smaller the area of impact, the greater is the severity of injury, because the force is concentrated in a smaller area. The focal injury may be coup or contrecoup. **Coup** is the direct impact area; **contrecoup** is the area that lies opposite the line of force: the lesions occur where the brain strikes hard tissue on the opposite side.

The clinical manifestations of a contusion may include an immediate loss of consciousness, a loss of reflexes, a transient cessation of respiration, a brief period of bradycardia, and drop in blood pressure. Vital signs may

stabilize in a few seconds; reflexes return next, and the person begins to regain consciousness. Returning to full alertness takes variable periods of time, from minutes to days. Large contusions and lacerations with hemorrhage may be surgically excised; otherwise, treatment is directed at controlling intracranial pressure and managing symptoms.

Extradural hematomas, which are also called epidural hematomas or epidural hemorrhages, most often have an artery as the source of bleeding. Extradural hemorrhages may result in herniation through the foramen magnum.

Individuals with classic temporal extradural hematomas lose consciousness at the time of injury; some lucid periods follow. As the hematoma mass accumulates, a headache of increasing severity, vomiting, drowsiness, confusion, seizure, and hemiparesis may develop. The level of consciousness declines rapidly as the temporal lobe herniation begins. Clinical manifestations of temporal lobe herniation also include ipsilateral pupillary dilation and contralateral hemiparesis. Surgical therapy evacuates the hematoma through burr holes followed by ligation of the bleeding vessel(s).

Tearing of the bridging veins is the major cause of rapidly developing and subacutely developing **subdural hematomas.** However, torn cortical veins or venous sinuses and contused tissue may be the source of the bleeding. The subdural space gradually fills with blood, and herniation can result.

An acute subdural hematoma classically begins with headache, drowsiness, restlessness or agitation, slowed cognition, and confusion. These symptoms worsen over time and progress to loss of consciousness, respiratory pattern changes, and pupillary dilation. Most people with chronic subdural hematomas appear to have a progressive

115

dementia accompanied by generalized rigidity. Chronic subdural hematomas require a craniotomy to evacuate the gelatinous blood.

In **intracerebral hematomas** (intraparenchymal hemorrhages), small blood vessels are traumatized by shearing forces. The intracerebral hematoma expands, increases intracranial pressure, and compresses brain tissues.

In individuals with intracerebral hematomas, as the intracranial pressure rises, clinical manifestations of temporal lobe herniation may appear. Delayed intracerebral hematoma results in sudden, rapidly progressive decreased levels of consciousness with pupillary dilation, breathing pattern changes, hemiplegia, and bilateral positive Babinski reflexes. Evacuation of a singular intracerebral hematoma is occasionally helpful for subcortical white matter hematomas. Otherwise, treatment is directed at reducing the intracranial pressure and allowing the hematoma to reabsorb slowly.

Diffuse brain injury or **diffuse axonal injury (DAI)** results from the inertial force to the head; it is associated with high levels of acceleration and deceleration. Severity of the diffuse injury correlates with how much shearing force is applied to the brainstem. In DAI, increased intravascular blood within the brain, vasodilation, and increased cerebral blood volume are frequently seen. Several categories of diffuse brain injury exist: mild concussion, classic concussion, mild DAI, moderate, and severe DAI.

Mild concussion involves temporary axonal disturbances. Cerebral cortical dysfunction related to attention and memory systems results, and consciousness is not lost. Amnesia is transient. Classic cerebral concussion causes reflexes to fail transiently. It may exist with or without focal injury. Confusional states last for hours or days. Loss of consciousness is immediate and lasts less than 6 hours. Also, reflexes are lost.

In **mild DAI,** individuals display decerebrate or decorticate posturing; they may experience prolonged stupor or restlessness. In **moderate DAI,** prolonged coma (unconsciousness) lasts days or weeks, and recovery is often incomplete in surviving individuals. In **severe DAI,** the individual experiences immediate autonomic dysfunction (brainstem signs) that resolves in a few weeks. Increased ICP appears 4 to 6 days after injury. Pulmonary complications occur frequently. Severely compromised coordinated movements and verbal and written communication, inability to learn and reason, and inability to modulate behavior also are found.

2. **Discuss the pathogenesis and manifestations of spinal cord injuries.**

Study text pages 591 through 596; refer to Figures 17-9 through 17-13 and Tables 17-2 through 17-5.

Spinal cord injuries mostly occur because of vertebral injuries. Traumatic forces injure the vertebral and/or neural tissues by compressing the tissues, pulling or exerting a traction on the tissues, or shearing tissues so that they slide into one another.

Vertebral injuries occur mostly at the first to second cervical, fourth to seventh cervical, and twelfth thoracic to second lumbar vertebrae; these are the most mobile portions of the vertebral column. The cord occupies most of the vertebral canal in these areas, and its size makes it more easily injured. Within a few minutes following injury, microscopic hemorrhages appear in the central gray matter and pia arachnoid. Edema progresses into the white matter, thereby impairing the microcirculation of the cord, with reduced vascular perfusion and development of metabolic changes in spinal cord tissues that produce further ischemia and necrosis of tissue. Cord swelling increases the individual's degree of dysfunction. In the cervical region of the cord, swelling may be life threatening because of impairment of diaphragm function. The traumatized cord is replaced by acellular collagenous tissue, usually in 3 to 4 weeks. Meninges thicken as part of the scarring process.

Normal activity of the spinal cord cells at and below the level of injury ceases because of the lack of continuous tonic discharges from the brain or brainstem and the inhibition of suprasegmental impulses immediately after cord injury; this causes **spinal shock,** which is characterized by a complete loss of reflex function in all segments below the level of the lesion. This condition involves all skeletal muscles; bladder, bowel, and sexual function; and autonomic control.

Spinal shock may last for 7 to 20 days following onset; in some severe cases, it may persist for as long as 3 months. Loss of motor and sensory function depends on the level and degree of injury. Paraplegia or quadriplegia can result. Return of spinal neuron excitability occurs slowly. Either motor, sensory, reflex, and autonomic functions return to normal or autonomic neural activity in the isolated segment develops.

Autonomic hyperreflexia is a syndrome that may occur at any time after spinal shock resolves. The syndrome is associated with a massive, uncompensated cardiovascular response to stimulation of the sympathetic nervous system. Individuals most likely to be affected have lesions at the T6 level or above. Hyperreflexia involves the stimulation of sensory receptors below the level of the cord injury. The intact autonomic nervous system reflexively responds with an arteriolar spasm that increases blood pressure. Baroreceptors in the cerebral vessels, the carotid sinus, and the aorta sense the hypertension and stimulate the parasympathetic system. The heart rate decreases, but the visceral and peripheral vessels do not dilate, because efferent impulses cannot pass through the cord, and cardiovascular compensation is incomplete. The most common precipitating cause is a distended bladder or rectum, but any sensory stimulation can elicit autonomic hyperreflexia.

For a suspected or confirmed vertebral fracture or dislocation, the immediate intervention is immobilization of the spine to prevent further injury. Decompression and surgical fixation may be necessary. Corticosteroids are given to decrease secondary cord injury. In cases of autonomic hyperreflexia, intervention must be prompt, because cerebrovascular accident is possible. The head of the bed should be elevated, and the injurious stimulus should be found and removed. Medications may be

116

used if these measures do not effectively reduce blood pressure.

3. Describe degenerative disk disease, low back pain, and herniated intervertebral disks.

Study text pages 596 through 600; refer to Figures 17-14 and 17-15.

The etiology for **degenerative disk disease** (DDD) includes biochemical and biomechanical alterations of the tissue that comprise the intervertebral disk. Fibrocartilage replaces the gelatinous mucoid material of the nucleus pulposus as the disk changes with aging; the narrowing disk results in variable segmental instability. The pathologic findings in DDD include disk protrusion, spondylolysis, and/or subluxation and degeneration of vertebrae (spondylolisthesis) and spinal stenosis.

Spondylolysis is a structural defect that involves the lamina (neural arch of the vertebra). The most common site where this occurs is the lumbar spine. Heredity plays a significant role, and spondylolysis is associated with other congenital spinal defects. As a result of torsional and rotational stress, microfractures occur at the affected site and eventually cause dissolution of the pars interarticularis. **Spondylolisthesis** is caused when a vertebra slides forward in relation to an inferior vertebra; this commonly occurs at L5-S1. Spinal stenosis may represent several conditions ranging from entrapment of a single nerve root in the lateral recess to diffuse central stenosis involving many roots.

The local processes involved in **low back pain** arise from tension caused by tumors or disk prolapse, bursitis, synovitis, degenerative joint disease, abnormal bone pressures, spinal immobility, and inflammation caused by osteomyelitis, bony fractures, or ligamentous strains. Pain may be referred from viscera or the posterior peritoneum. General processes that result in low back pain include bone diseases such as osteoporosis or osteomalacia seen in hyperparathyroidism.

Most individuals that have acute low back pain benefit from analgesic medications, exercises, physical therapy, and education. Surgical treatments include diskectomy and spinal fusions. Individuals with chronic low back pain can be treated with anti-inflammatory and muscle relaxant medications and exercise programs. Spinal surgery has a limited role in curing chronic low back pain.

Herniation of an intervertebral disk is a protrusion of part of the nucleus pulposus through a tear in the fibrous capsule that encloses the gelatinous center of the disk. Rupture of intervertebral disks is usually caused by trauma, degenerative disease, or both. Lifting with the trunk flexed and sudden straining when the back is in an unstable position are the most common causes; males are more often affected than are females. Most commonly affected are the lumbosacral disks; disk herniation occasionally occurs in the cervical area. The symptoms may be immediate or occur within a few hours, or they may take months to years to develop. The pain of a herniated disc in the lumbosacral area radiates along the sciatic nerve over the buttocks and into the calf or ankle. With the herniation of a lower cervical disk, paresthesia and pain are present in the upper arm, the forearm, and the hand according to the affected nerve root distribution.

The conservative therapeutic approach involves traction, bed rest, heat, and ice to the affected areas and an effective analgesic regimen. The surgical approach is indicated if there is weakness, decreased deep tendon reflexes, and bladder/bowel reflexes or if the conservative approach is unsuccessful.

4. Compare and contrast cerebrovascular accidents (CVAs).

Study text pages 600 through 603 and 606; refer to Figures 17-16 and 17-17 and Table 17-6. See table below.

Any abnormality of the brain caused by blood vessel pathology is a cerebrovascular disorder. The mildest outcome of CVA is minimal and may be unnoticed. The severe outcomes are hemiplegia, coma, or death. CVAs are classified as ischemic (thrombotic or embolic), global hypoperfusion, or hemorrhagic. The accidents are vascular in origin, but they are manifested neurologically.

The risk factors for cerebrovascular disease include the following:

- Hypertension
- Cigarette smoking
- Elevated blood lipoprotein(a)
- Diabetes mellitus
- Insulin resistance

Cerebrovascular Accidents (Stroke Syndromes)

	Thrombotic	Embolic	Hemorrhagic
History of earlier transient ischemia attacks (TIAs)	Frequent	Occasional	Infrequent
Onset	Acute, hours to days	Acute	Acute, progressive, worsening
Associated headache	Occasional, not severe	Often moderately severe	Frequent, severe
Stiff neck	Rare	Rare	Frequent
Loss of consciousness	Occasional, not at onset	Occasional, brief	Frequent
Blood in CSF	Rare	Rare	Frequent

117

- Hyperhomocysteinemia
- Impaired cardiac function
- Nonrheumatic atrial fibrillation
- Polycythemia and thrombocythemia
- *Chlamydia pneumoniae*

The development of a **thrombotic stroke** is caused by arteries supplying the brain and is most frequently attributed to atherosclerosis and inflammatory disease processes that damage arterial walls. Atheromatous plaques tend to form at branchings and curves in the cerebral circulation. Degeneration or bleeding into the vessel wall may cause endothelial damage. Platelets and fibrin adhere to the damaged wall, and delicate thrombi form. Small thrombi collect over time; gradual occlusion of the artery occurs. Once the artery is occluded, the thrombus may enlarge lengthwise in the vessel.

In thrombotic strokes, treatment is directed at supportive management to control cerebral edema and increased intracranial pressure. Intervention to restore blood supply may be indicated. Arresting the disease process by controlling risk factors is critical. Drugs that achieve defibrinogenation to permit local blood flow are useful.

Transient ischemic attacks (TIAs) represent thrombotic particles that cause an intermittent blockage of circulation. In a true TIA, neurologic deficits are caused by a focal disturbance of brain or retinal ischemic lasting less than an hour without an infarction.

An **embolic stroke** involves fragments that break from a thrombus that was formed outside the brain. Common sites are in the heart, aorta, common carotid artery, or thorax. The embolus usually involves small vessels and obstructs a bifurcation or other narrowing to cause ischemia. Conditions associated with an embolic stroke include atrial fibrillation, myocardial infarction, endocarditis, rheumatic heart disease, valvular prostheses, atrial septal defects, and disorders of the aorta, carotid arteries, or vertebral-basilar circulation. In individuals who experience an embolic stroke, usually a second stroke follows at some point, because the source of emboli continues to exist. Emboli usually lodge in the distribution of the middle cerebral artery.

In embolic strokes, treatment is directed at preventing further embolization by instituting anticoagulation therapy and correcting the primary problem. Rehabilitation is indicated in both thrombotic and embolic strokes.

The most common causes of **hemorrhagic stroke** are hypertension, ruptured aneurysms, arteriovenous malformation, and hemorrhage associated with bleeding disorders. Hypertensive hemorrhage is associated with a significant increase in systolic-diastolic pressure over several years and usually occurs within the brain tissue. A mass of blood forms as its volume increases; adjacent brain tissue is displaced and compressed. Rupture or seepage into the ventricular system occurs in many of the cases. The most common sites for hypertensive hemorrhages are in the putamen of the basal ganglia and the hypothalamus.

Lacunar strokes (lacunar infarcts) are very small and involve the small arteries, predominantly in the basal ganglia, internal capsules, and brainstem. Because of the subcortical location and small area of infarction, these strokes may cause motor and sensory deficits.

Treatment of an intracranial stroke, regardless of cause, is focused on stopping or reducing the bleeding, controlling the increased intracranial pressure, preventing another hemorrhagic episode, and preventing vasospasm. At times, an attempt is made to evacuate or aspirate the blood.

Cerebral infarction results when an area of the brain loses blood. The symptoms depend on the blood vessel involved. Essentially, if the internal carotid artery branches are involved, there is confusion, inability to plan, aphasia, perception disorders, paralysis, or blindness. If the vertebral artery branches are involved, there is diplopia, ataxia, vertigo, dysphagia, and dysphonia.

Aspirin, systemic anticoagulation, and thrombolysis improve outcomes in individuals with ischemic stroke. Antiplatelet therapy and statins decrease reoccurrence. Endarterectomy is effective if carotid stenosis is greater than 50%.

5. **Describe intracranial aneurysms and vascular malformations.**

Study text pages 606 through 609; refer to Figures 17-18 through 17-21 and Table 17-7.

Intracranial aneurysms may result from arteriosclerosis, congenital abnormality, trauma, inflammation, or infection. Cocaine has also been linked to aneurysm formation. Aneurysm development is attributed to hemodynamic stress and is believed to be exacerbated by hypertension and certain connective tissue disorders.

Aneurysms may be classified on the basis of shape and form. **Saccular aneurysms** (berry aneurysms) occur in approximately 2% of the population and are probably the result of congenital abnormalities in the media of the arterial wall. **Fusiform aneurysms** (giant aneurysms) are larger than 25 mm in diameter and occur as a result of diffuse arteriosclerotic changes. They are found most commonly in the basilar arteries or terminal portions of the internal carotid arteries. **Mycotic aneurysms** result from arteritis caused by bacterial emboli; these aneurysms are uncommon. **Traumatic aneurysms** are caused by a weakening of the arterial wall by a fracture line, by a penetrating missile, or after neurosurgical or imaging (e.g., angiography) procedures.

Aneurysms are frequently asymptomatic. Clinical manifestations may arise from cranial nerve compression, but the signs vary depending on the location and size of the aneurysm. The treatment of choice for an aneurysm is surgical management before rupture occurs. The location and size of the aneurysm and the person's clinical status determine whether invasive therapy is feasible.

Four types of **vascular malformation** exist: arteriovenous malformation (AVM), cavernous angioma, capillary telangiectasis, and venous angioma. An AVM is a tangled mass of dilated blood vessels. Although sometimes present at birth, AVM exhibits a delayed age of onset, most commonly occurring before 30 years of age. Fifty percent of individuals with this condition experience a hemorrhage. Clinical manifestations of AVM range from

118

headache and dementia to seizures and intracerebral or subarachnoid hemorrhage.

A **subarachnoid hemorrhage** occurs when blood escapes from defective or injured vasculature into the subarachnoid space. Individuals at risk are those with aneurysm, vascular malformations, and head injuries. When a vessel tears, blood under pressure is pumped into the subarachnoid space and produces an inflammatory reaction in these tissues.

Clinical manifestations of a subarachnoid hemorrhage include headache, changes in mental status, transient motor weakness, nausea or vomiting, visual or speech disturbances, cranial nerve palsies, or stiff neck. A **Kernig sign** produces pain in the back and neck when the knee is straigthened with hip and hip in flexed position. The **Brudzinski sign** occurs when passive flexion of the neck produces neck pain and increased rigidity. Vasospasm and delayed cerebral ischemia are serious complications. Treatment of vasospasm includes use of calcium channel blockers and augmenting cerebral perfusion by volume expansion and hemodilution.

6. Describe chronic, recurring headaches.

Study text pages 609 through 611; refer to Tables 17-8.

Headache is a common neurologic disorder and is usually a benign symptom. However, it can be associated with brain tumors, meningitis, and giant cell arteritis. Migraine, cluster, paroxysmal hemicrania, and tension headaches are chronic, recurring types that are not associated with structural abnormalities or systemic disease.

Migraine headache prevalence is higher in women and is highest at 25 to 55 years of age, and the rate in women remains higher than that in men into older age. Migraine headaches are episodic and repeating and last 4 to 72 hours. It is diagnosed when any two of the following occur: unilateral pain, movement worsens, photophobia or phonophobia exist, and throbbing, moderate to severe nausea, and vomiting. Migraines are caused by multiple genetic and Environmental factors. Trigger factors may include stress, hunger, weather changes, sunlight, noise, jet lag, menstruation, and alcohol or nitrates. The pathogenesis of migraine headaches includes a vascular theory, cortical spreading depression, and serotonergic and other neurotransmitter alterations.

Avoidance of triggers, adequate sleep, regular eating habits, and daily relaxation and meditation can create a headache-protective environment. With the onset of acute migraine, a dark room, ice, and sleep can provide relief. Drug considerations include antiemetics, ergotamine and dihydroergotamine, and 5-HT antagonists.

Cluster headaches occur primarily in men (8:1 ratio to women) between 20 and 50 years of age. Several attacks can occur during the day for a period of days followed by long periods of remission. Cluster headache has an episodic and chronic form.

The headache attack usually begins without warning and is characterized by severe, burning, periorbital, and retrobulbar or temporal pain that lasts 30 minutes to 2 hours. The same side is affected in subsequent episodes. Associated symptoms include lacrimation, reddening of the eye, nasal stuffiness, eyelid ptosis, and nausea. Pain often is referred to the midface and the teeth. If the attacks occur more frequently without sustained spontaneous remission, they are classified as chronic cluster headaches. Alcohol can stimulate an attack in about 50% to 70% of cases, but it is not a triggering factor during remission.

Pathogenic mechanisms may include vascular alterations, neurogenic or neuroimmunologic dysregulation of the hypothalamus, dysregulation of the parasympathetic ganglia, sympathetic deficit, and stimulation of the trigeminal nucleus. The rhythmicity of attacks probably is related to disorders of the hypothalamus.

Prophylactic drugs are used to treat cluster headaches. The most effective ones are prednisone, lithium, methysergide, calcium channel antagonists, and valproate. Acute attacks are managed with oxygen inhalation, sumatriptan, and inhaled ergotamine.

Chronic paroxysmal hemicrania is a cluster type of headache that occurs with more daily frequency but with shorter duration. The attacks are more common in women, usually after pregnancy. The pathophysiology involves a disorder of sympathetic hyperactivity, but the mechanism is different from cluster headache, because there is effective relief of symptoms with indomethacin.

Tension headache is the most common type of headache, and it occurs in 69% of men and 88% of women. It is a mild to moderate bilateral headache with a sensation of a tight band or pressure around the head. The onset of pain is usually gradual. The headache occurs in episodes and may last for several hours or several days. It is not aggravated by physical activity.

Both a central mechanism and a peripheral mechanism cause tension headaches. The central mechanism probably involves hypersensitivity of pain fibers from the trigeminal nerve. The peripheral mechanism is probably related to contraction of jaw and neck muscles.

Mild headaches are treated with ice, and more severe forms are treated with aspirin or nonsteroidal anti-inflammatory drugs. Chronic tension headaches are best managed with a tricyclic antidepressant.

7. Describe the pathophysiology, manifestations, and treatment of CNS tumors; classify common brain tumors.

Study text pages 611 and 613 through 620; refer to Figures 17-22 through 17-31 and Table 17-9. See Table on page 120.

Cranial tumors can be either primary or metastatic. Primary intracerebral tumors originate from brain substance, neuroglia, neurons, cells of the blood vessels, and connective tissue. **Primary extracerebral tumors** originate outside the brain substance and include meningiomas, acoustic nerve tumors, and tumors of the pituitary and pineal glands. **Metastatic tumors** can be found inside and/or outside the brain substance.

Cranial tumors cause local and generalized clinical manifestations. The local effects are due to the destructive action of a particular site in the brain and to compression that reduces cerebral blood flow. The effects are varied and include seizures, visual disturbances, unstable gait, and cranial nerve dysfunction. The generalized effects result from increased intracranial pressure.

119

Classification of Common Primary Brain Tumors

Tumor Type	Frequency	Age Group	Feature
Astrocytoma (astrocytes)	50% (brain/spinal cord)	Adults	Slow growing, invasive
Oligodendroglioma, (oligodendrocytes)	10% to 15% (brain)	Adults	Slow growing, encapsulated
Ependymoma (ependymal cells)	6% to 10% (brain ventricles)	All ages	Variable growth rate, invasive
Meningioma (arachnoid cells, possibly from fibroblasts)	15% to 20% (brain)	All ages	Slow growing, encapsulated, compressive

Intracranial brain tumors do not metastasize as readily as tumors in other organs because there are no lymphatic channels within the brain substance. If metastasis does occur, it is usually through seeding of cerebral blood or CSF, during cranial surgery, or through artificial shunts.

An estimated 25% of people with cancer develop metastasis to the brain. One third of metastatic brain tumors arise from the lung, approximately one sixth arise from the breast, and a lesser number arises from the gastrointestinal tract and kidney. Other tumors metastasize less frequently. Carcinomas are disseminated to the brain by the circulation. Metastatic brain tumors carry a poor prognosis. If a solitary tumor is found, surgery and/or radiation therapy is used; however, if multiple tumors exist, symptomatic relief only is pursued.

The principal treatment for cerebral neoplasms is surgical or radiosurgical excision or surgical decompression if total excision is not possible. Chemotherapy and radiotherapy also may be used. Supportive treatment is directed at reducing edema.

Spinal cord tumors are relatively rare and are classified as **intramedullary tumors** if they originate within the neural tissues and as **extramedullary tumors** if they originate in tissues outside the spinal cord. Intramedullary tumors have the same cellular origins as brain tumors. Extramedullary tumors arise from the meninges, epidural tissue, or vertebral structure. The most common primary extramedullary spinal cord tumors are neurofibromas and meningiomas. Metastatic spinal cord tumors are usually carcinomas, lymphomas, or myelomas. Their location is often extradural.

The acute onset of clinical manifestations suggests a vascular insult caused by thrombosis of the vessels that supply the spinal cord. Clinical manifestations fall into three major categories: a compressive syndrome, an irritative syndrome, or, rarely, a syringomyelic syndrome. In the **compressive syndrome,** the motor dysfunction is paresis and spasticity, depending on the level of involvement. The sensory manifestations of tingling paresthesias have a similar pattern to that of the motor signs. Pain and temperature dysfunctions are more commonly found than are touch, vibration, and proprioceptive changes. Bladder and bowel deficits usually appear when paresis develops in the legs.

The **irritative syndrome** combines the clinical manifestations of a cord compression with radicular pain. This pain is in the sensory root distribution and indicates root irritation. Sensory changes include paresthesia and impaired pain and touch perception; motor disturbances include cramps, atrophy, fasciculation, and decreased or absent deep tendon reflexes.

Intradural-extramedullary tumors are surgically removed or decompressed by excision of the posterior vertebral arch or laminectomy. Laminectomy with decompression and excision is used for gliomas and is followed by radiotherapy. Extradural metastatic tumors are often managed by radiotherapy, chemotherapy, hormonal therapy, or pain management protocols.

8. **Compare meningitis with encephalitis.**
   Study text pages 620 and 622 through 626; refer to Figures 17-32, 17-35 and Tables 17-10 and 17-11. See the table on page 121.

9. **Characterize CNS abscesses.**
   Study text pages 624 and 625. Refer to Figure 17-36.

   Abscesses are localized collections of pus within the parenchyma or functioning cells of the brain and spinal cord. Abscesses occur following open trauma and during neurosurgery. The foci of infection include the middle ear, mastoid cells, nasal cavity, and nasal sinuses; the abscesses can spread through metastatic or hematogenous means from distant foci. Streptococci, staphylococci, and *Bacteroides* in combination with anaerobes are the most common bacteria that cause abscesses. However, yeast and fungi have also been found in CNS abscess.

   Initially, a localized inflammatory process leads to edema, hyperemia, softening, and petechial hemorrhage. After a few days, fibroblasts from capillaries deposit collagen fibers that contain and encapsulate the purulent focus. The infection becomes limited, with a center of pus and a wall of granular tissue.

   Clinical manifestations of **brain abscesses** include fever, headache, nausea, vomiting, decreasing cognitive abilities, paresis, and seizures. These signs and symptoms develop because of the infection and expanding mass. Clinical manifestations **of spinal cord abscesses** are spinal discomfort, root pain accompanied by spasms of the back muscles and limited vertebral movement due to pain and spasm, weakness due to progressive cord compression, and paralysis.

120

Meningitis and Encephalitis

	Bacterial Meningitis	Aseptic Meningitis	Encephalitis
Site	Pia mater, arachnoid, subarachnoid space, CSF, ventricles	Meninges	Meninges, white and gray matter
Infectious agents	*Neisseria meningitidis, Streptococcus pneumoniae, Haemophilus influenzae*	Enteroviral viruses, herpes simplex 1, mumps, adenoviruses	Arthropod-borne viruses, herpes simplex 1, complications of systemic viral infection
Lesion	Meningeal vessels become hyperemic and permeable	Similar to bacterial meningitis	Nerve cell degeneration
Manifestations	Throbbing headache, flexion of legs and thighs, stiff neck, projectile vomiting, confusion	Mild but similar symptoms compared with bacterial meningitis	Fever, delirium, confusion, coma, seizure, cranial nerve palsies, paresis and paralysis
CSF	Increased pressure, bacteria, elevated protein levels, decreased glucose levels, neutrophils and monocytes	Increased pressure, normal glucose levels, lymphocytes	Same as aseptic meningitis
Treatment	Antibiotics	Antiviral agents and steroids	Herpes infections—antiviral agents, control of intracranial pressure

NOTE: Fungal meningitis is a chronic, much less common infection than bacterial or viral meningitis. Tubercular (TB) meningitis is on the rise in the United States because of AIDS.

Aspiration or excision accompanied by antibiotic therapy is the recommended treatment for brain abscesses. Intracranial pressure must be managed. Spinal cord abscesses are treated with surgical excision or aspiration, because decompression is necessary. Antibiotic and supportive therapies are also required.

10. Identify the neurologic complications of AIDS.

Study text pages 626 through 629; refer to Box 17-6 and Table 17-12.

Approximately 40% to 60% of all people with AIDS develop neurologic complications. The most common neurologic disorder is HIV-associated cognitive dysfunction. Other common neurologic disorders are peripheral neuropathies, vacuolar myelopathy, opportunistic infection of the CNS, and neoplasms.

HIV-associated dementia is characterized by insidious onset and unpredictable but progressive cognitive dysfunction in conjunction with motor and behavioral alterations. Later dysfunction is accompanied by psychomotor slowing, loss of balance, ataxia, spastic paralysis or paraparesis, and generalized hyperreflexia. HIV cognitive dysfunction is likely the result of direct brain tissue infection by the virus. HIV is mostly found in white matter subcortical areas.

Vacuolar myelopathy and multinucleated giant cell encephalitis involving diffuse degeneration of the spinal cord may occur in people with AIDS. A progressive spastic paraparesis with ataxia is the predominant clinical manifestation. Leg weakness, upper motor neuron signs, incontinence, and posterior column sensory loss may be present.

Peripheral neuropathy, which is an HIV neuropathy, is a sensory neuropathy. Individuals experience painful dysthesias and paresthesias in the extremities. Weakness and decreased or absent distal reflexes may be present.

Some individuals develop an acute **aseptic meningitis** at approximately the time of positive seroconversion. Headache, fever, and meningismus with cranial nerve involvement, especially of cranial nerves V and VII, may appear.

Opportunistic viral infections may cause nervous system disease. Papovavirus may produce a demyelinating disorder called progressive multifocal leukoencephalopathy, which causes sensory and motor deficits, aphasia, and apraxia. People with cytomegalovirus encephalitis experience nystagmus and cranial nerve deficits.

Opportunistic nonviral infections are the most common CNS disorders associated with AIDS. Clinical manifestations of CNS toxoplasmosis, which is a common AIDS disorder, are highly variable and include clumsiness, hemiplegia, aphasia, seizures, ataxia, and cognitive changes.

CNS neoplasms associated with AIDS include CNS lymphoma, systemic non-Hodgkin lymphoma, and metastatic Kaposi sarcoma.

11. Describe demyelinating and degenerative CNS disorders.

Study text pages 630 through 638; refer to Boxes 17-7 through 17-9, Figures 17-38 and 17-39, and Tables 17-13 and 17-14. See table on page 122.

12. Distinguish between the classes of neuropathies.

Study text pages 635 and 636.

121

Multiple Sclerosis, Guillain-Barré Syndrome, and Amyotrophic Lateral Sclerosis

	Multiple Sclerosis	Guillain-Barré Syndrome	Amyotrophic Lateral Sclerosis (ALS)
Lesion site	CNS demyelination	Peripheral nerve demyelination	Scarring of corticospinal tract in lateral column of spinal cord, upper and lower motor neurons degenerate
Etiology	Immunogenetic-viral, genetic/environmental, T cells become autoreactive to myelin protein, B cells produce autoantibodies and inflammatory cytokines	Humoral and cell-mediated immunity, influx of macrophages destroys myelin and denudes axons	Genetics, defective superoxide dismutase gene
Onset	Between 20 and 40 years	All age groups	40s, peaks in early 50s
Manifestations	Remissions and exacerbations but progressive paresthesia, diplopia, cerebellar incoordination, urinary and bowel dysfunction	Motor paralysis, usually ascending, respiratory insufficiency, dysphagia, dysarthria, cardiovascular autonomic dysfunction	Muscle weakness, atrophy, paralysis, normal intellectual and sensory function until death
Treatment	Steroids to shorten exacerbations, drugs to reduce relapses, supportive and rehabilitative management	Ventilatory support, autonomic nervous system management	Antiglutamates may reduce excitotoxicity and lengthen survival, support and rehabilitation

Neuropathies can be classified as (1) generalized symmetric polyneuropathies, (2) generalized neuropathies, and (3) focal or multifocal neuropathies. **Generalized symmetrical polyneuropathies** are characterized by symmetric involvement of sensory, motor, or autonomic fibers although, with clinical signs, one type of fiber may predominate. Generalized symmetric polyneuropathies further subdivide into **distal axonal polyneuropathy** and **demyelinating polyneuropathy.** Distal axonal polyneuropathy affects peripheral axons and is the generalized peripheral neuropathy commonly seen. The clinical feature of distal axonal polyneuropathy is involvement of the longest nerve of the body, those going to the feet, first. Sensory impairment is greater than motor impairment. Symptoms are burning pain, tingling, and numbness of the feet. The myelin or Schwann cells are affected in demyelinating polyneuropathy, which occurs far less frequently. Guillain-Barré syndrome is the most recognized example of the demyelinating neuropathies.

Generalized neuropathies affect the cell body of only one type of peripheral neuron. The dorsal root ganglion cell is affected in sensory neuropathies, producing numbness that may begin in a focal or asymmetric distribution or in a distal symmetric pattern. **Sensory neuropathies** are seen in leprosy, some industrial solvent poisonings, some hereditary disorders, and chloramphenicol toxicity. The anterior horn in motor neuropathy is affected, causing weakness that may be symmetric or asymmetric. Motor neuropathies are caused by anterior horn cell disease, such as amyotrophic lateral sclerosis (ALS) or paralytic poliomyelitis.

Focal or **multifocal neuropathies** affect sensory and motor fibers in one or more nerves as is seen in common compression neuropathies such as carpal tunnel syndrome (median nerve compression), ulnar nerve compression (at the elbow), peroneal nerve compression, or sciatic nerve compression. Focal neuropathies can involve one or more cranial nerves. Plexus injuries and radiculopathies also fall into this category.

13. **Describe myasthenia gravis.**
    Study text pages 6387 through 640; refer to Figure 17-40 and Table 17-15.

Myasthenia gravis is a disorder of voluntary or striated muscles that is characterized by muscle weakness and fatigability because of a defect in nerve impulse transmission at the neuromuscular junction. Between 70% and 80% of people with myasthenia gravis have pathologic changes in the thymus; this disorder is an autoimmune disease. Different types of myasthenia gravis exist. In **neonatal myasthenia,** immune globulin is transferred from mother to neonate via the placenta. Symptoms of **congenital** and **juvenile myasthenia** are present in infancy and childhood. **Ocular myasthenia,** which is more common in males, involves muscle weakness confined to the eye muscles. **Generalized myasthenia** involves the proximal musculature throughout the body and exhibits varying rates of progression with possible remissions.

In myasthenia gravis, postsynaptic acetylcholine receptors on the muscle cell's plasma membrane are no longer recognized as "self"; therefore IgG antibody is secreted against the acetylcholine receptors. These antibodies fix onto the receptor sites and block the binding of acetylcholine. Eventually, the antibody action causes the destruction

122

of receptor sites and the diminished transmission of the nerve impulse across the neuromuscular junction.

The muscles of the eyes, face, mouth, throat, and neck are usually affected first. Manifestations include diplopia, ptosis, and ocular palsies; facial droop and an expressionless face; difficulty in chewing and swallowing; drooling, episodes of choking, and aspirations; and a nasal, low-volume, high-pitched, monotonous speech pattern. The muscles of the neck, shoulder girdle, and hip flexor are less frequently affected.

Myasthenic crisis occurs when severe muscle weakness causes extreme quadriparesis or quadriplegia, respiratory insufficiency that can lead to respiratory arrest, and extreme difficulty swallowing. **Cholinergic crisis** is caused by the muscle hyperactivity that occurs secondary to excessive accumulation of acetylcholine at the neuromuscular junctions and excessive parasympathetic activity. As in myasthenic crisis, the individual is in danger of respiratory arrest.

Anticholinesterase drugs, steroids, and immunosuppressant drugs are used to treat myasthenia gravis and myasthenic crisis. Treatment of individuals with cholinergic crisis involves withholding anticholinergic drugs until blood levels fall out of the toxic range while providing ventilatory support.

14. Identify tests of nervous system function.

Review text pages 474 through 476; refer to Table 14-9.

Tests of nervous system function include x-rays (localize bony defects), computed tomography (demonstrates tissue density), magnetic resonance imaging and angiography (orient physiologic atomic particles, visualizes blood vessels), positron emission tomography (visualizes radioactive substance activity of metabolic processes), brain scan (visualizes vascular tissue uptake of radioactive agents), cerebral angiography (demonstrates cerebrovascular blood flow), myelogram (demonstrates radioactive dye activity within the spine), echoencephalography or ultrasound (detects structural characteristics of mass lesions), electroencephalography (records cortical brain electrical patterns), evoked potentials (detects electrical brain activity from sensory stimulation), and cerebrospinal fluid analysis (measures CSF pressure and constituent characteristics).

PRACTICE EXAMINATION

Multiple Choice

Circle the correct answer for each question.

1. In blunt head trauma:
   a. brain tissues are exposed.
   b. only focal injury occurs.
   c. the dura is severed.
   d. the dura remains intact.
2. In an automobile accident, an individual's forehead struck the windshield. The coup/contrecoup would be in the:
   a. frontal/parietal region.
   b. frontal/occipital region.
   c. parietal/occipital region.
   d. occipital/frontal region.

3. In severe diffuse axonal injury:
   a. coma lasts less than 24 hours.
   b. coma lasts longer than 24 hours.
   c. disruption of axons occurs in cerebral hemispheres and in those that extend into the diencephalon and brainstem.
   d. an increase in ICP appears in 4 to 6 days after injury.
4. The regions where most spinal cord injuries occur are the:
   a. cervical and thoracic regions.
   b. cervical and lumbar regions.
   c. thoracic and lumbar regions.
   d. lumbar and sacral regions.
5. Injury of the cervical cord may be life threatening because of:
   a. increased intracranial pressure.
   b. disrupted reflexes.
   c. spinal shock.
   d. loss of bladder and rectal control.
   e. diaphragmatic impairment.
6. Autonomic hyperreflexia is characterized by:
   a. hypotension.
   b. rapid heart rate.
   c. stimulation of sensory receptors below the level of the cord lesion.
   d. hyporeflexia.
7. Intervertebral disk herniation:
   a. usually occurs at the thoracic level.
   b. in the lumbosacral area causes pain over the gluteal region and into the calf or ankle.
   c. is infrequent in the lumbosacral disks.
   d. affects females more often than males.
8. Transient ischemic attacks are:
   a. unilateral neurologic deficits that slowly resolve.
   b. generalized neurologic deficits that occur for a few seconds every hour.
   c. focal neurologic defects of the brain or retina that usually clear within 1 hour without an infarct.
   d. neurologic deficits that slowly evolve or develop.
9. Which of the following is a risk factor for the development of a CVA?
   a. Viral infections
   b. Hypertension
   c. Diabetes insipidus
   d. Hypohomocysteinemia
   e. b and d are correct
10. Which of the following most typically characterizes the victims of a cerebral embolic stroke?
    a. Individuals older than 65 years of age with a history of hypertension
    b. Individuals with a long history of transient ischemic attacks
    c. Middle-age individuals with a history of heart disease
    d. Individuals with gradually occurring symptoms that then rapidly disappear

123

11. Blood in the CSF of an individual is most likely in _____ cerebrovascular accidents.
    a. lacunar
    b. thrombotic
    c. embolic
    d. hemorrhagic
12. Which of the following is a primary intracerebral neoplasm?
    a. Astrocytoma
    b. Meningioma
    c. Pituitary adenoma
    d. Acoustic neuroma
13. In bacterial meningitis, the CSF has:
    a. normal glucose levels.
    b. an elevated number of lymphocytes.
    c. neutrophilic infiltration.
    d. lower protein levels.
14. HIV-associated dementia is:
    a. static.
    b. regressive.
    c. believed to be due to an opportunistic infection.
    d. insidious and unpredictably progressive.
15. Saccular aneurysms occur:
    a. as a result of arteriosclerotic changes.
    b. as a result of arteritis.
    c. in terminal portions of the internal carotid arteries.
    d. as a result of congenital weakness in an arterial wall.
16. Migraine headaches likely involve:
    a. neuroimmunologic dysregulation of parasympathetic ganglia.
    b. serotonergic and other neurotransmitter alterations.
    c. sympathetic deficit.
    d. hypersensitivity of pain fibers from the trigeminal nerve.
17. Slow-growing, well-encapsulated, and relatively easy-to-remove CNS tumors are:
    a. neurofibrosarcomas.
    b. meningiomas.
    c. ependymomas.
    d. astrocytomas.

18. Encephalitis manifests with:
    a. decreased glucose levels in the CSF.
    b. nerve cell degeneration.
    c. projectile vomiting.
    d. ventricular infection.
19. The type of hematoma involving rupture of veins, not arteries, is:
    a. extradural.
    b. subdural.
    c. intracerebral.
    d. subarachnoid.
20. The manifestations of ALS include:
    a. remissions and exacerbations with progression.
    b. ascending motor paralysis.
    c. onset between 20 and 40 years of age.
    d. normal intellectual and sensory function until death.

Fill in the Blanks

Supply the correct response for each statement.

21. The _____ sign exhibits pain and increased rigidity of the neck.

22. A(n) _____ is the violent displacement of brain tissue due to acceleration or deceleration.

23. A(n) _____ is the site of dysfunction in myasthenia gravis

24. _____ involve(s) an influx of macrophages to destroy peripheral nerve myelin.

25. The disorder exhibiting remissions and exacerbations but progressively destroying CNS myelin is _____.

Mrs. B. is an overweight 71-year-old white woman who slurred to daughter, "My right hand hurts. Can you understand me?" Upon hospital admission, she had a severe right-sided headache, slurred speech, and some severe right-handed numbness with a weak left hand grip. Her smile was asymmetric. Mrs. B. has a history of smoking moderately for 50 years and use of estrogen replacement for 20 years. Her mother had adult-onset diabetes and died of breast cancer at age 62; her father died of a gunshot accident at 29; one sister died of a subarachnoid hemorrhage at age 63, and another sister is hemiparetic because of a CVA. One brother is hypertensive, and three other younger siblings are apparently healthy.

Vital signs showed a normal temperature, elevated heart rate, and normal respirations, but Mrs. B. had a severely elevated blood pressure. Blood chemistry was normal except for elevated glucose. A lumbar puncture was negative for blood with normal protein and glucose levels. A normal electrocardiogram was found. EEG showed localized activity in the left hemisphere. A CT showed increased density on the left.

Question

How do you interpret Mrs. B.'s history, her family history, and her symptoms and signs.

Chapter **17** **Disorders of the Central and Peripheral Nervous Systems**

18 Neurobiology of Schizophrenia, Mood Disorders, and Anxiety Disorders

FOUNDATIONAL KNOWLEDGE OBJECTIVE

a. **See this study guide's Foundational Knowledge Objective "a" in Chapter 17.**

LEARNING OBJECTIVES

After studying this chapter, the learner will be able to do the following:

1. **Describe the pathophysiology, manifestations, and treatment of schizophrenia.**

   Study text pages 647 through 652; refer to Figures 18-1 through 18-4.

   Schizophrenia is a common and potentially devastating psychiatric illness that strikes 1% of the world's population across all socioeconomic levels. Schizophrenia is the term used to describe a collection of illnesses that are characterized by **thought disorders.** Thought disorders reflect a break in reality or a splitting of the cognitive from the emotional side of one's personality. A schizophrenic individual may exhibit feelings of happiness when recollecting a terrible event or emotional indifference when describing a joyful occasion. Thought disorders are also manifested by incoherent speech, delusions, abnormal beliefs, and hallucinations, which are imaginary perceptions. During a psychotic episode, the individual loses touch with reality. These psychotic episodes are characterized as **positive symptoms.** Schizophrenic individuals may exhibit blunted affect, apathy, poverty of speech, and lack of social interactions; these latter characteristics are considered **negative symptoms.** Negative symptoms of schizophrenia result from decreased dopamine. The hypersecretion of mesolimbic dopamine may contribute to the manifestation of positive symptoms.

   Studies point to the importance of genetic and neurodevelopmental abnormalities in schizophrenia. Schizophrenia likely results from neurodevelopmental defects that occur during fetal life. Within the neurodevelopmental framework, viral infection during pregnancy, prenatal nutritional deficiencies, and perinatal complications such as birth defects and neonatal hypoxia may lead to schizophrenia.

   Among the most prominent structural brain abnormalities in some schizophrenic individuals is the enlargement of the lateral and third ventricles and the widening of fissures and sulci in the frontal cortex. Increased ventricular volume is associated with a reduction in cortical matter. The dorsolateral prefrontal cortex (DLPFC) appears to play an important role in both the origin and course of schizophrenia. The DLPFC is hypoactive with decreased blood flow, and glutamic acid decarboxylase is reduced and thus lowers gamma-aminobutyric acid (GABA), the inhibitory neurotransmitter in schizophrenia, and likely alters cognition and behavior. In schizophrenics, smaller neurons are found in the hippocampus. The smaller neuron size may lead to cognitive impairments and inability to engage in goal-directed behavior.

   An abnormal elevation in dopaminergic transmission contributes to the onset of the disease. Drugs that increase dopaminergic transmission produce schizophrenic-like psychosis, and these drug-induced psychotic states are reversed by dopamine blockers, drugs having an affinity for dopamine D_2 receptors.

   In the treatment of schizophrenia, the first generation of drugs blocked the dopamine receptor. The second generation are called atypical antipsychotic drugs, which block not only dopamine receptors but also a combination of dopamine, serotonin, and other neurotransmitter receptors. In addition to drug medications, psychosocial therapy is used to increase compliance and encourage coping strategies.

2. **Describe the pathophysiology, manifestations, and treatment of depression and mania.**

   Study text pages 652 through 658; refer to Figures 18-5 through 18-8.

   Mood refers to a sustained emotional state as opposed to brief emotional feelings, which are called affective states. When emotional states such as euphoria (mania) and depression are maintained and become predominant, the individual may be diagnosed with a mood disorder. The two major classifications of mood disorder are **unipolar** or major depressive disorder, also known as major depression or clinical depression, which consists of episodes of depression; and **bipolar** disorder, also known as **manic-depression,** which is classified into bipolar I and bipolar II disorder.

   Major (unipolar) depression is the most common mood disorder. The lifetime prevalence rate for depression is about 16% of the population. Individuals with major depression are unable to experience pleasure and display no outside interests. Females have a twofold greater risk of experiencing a major depression during their lifetime than do males. Approximately 25% of individuals with major depression eventually experience a

127

manic episode A strong genetic basis exists for the development of mood disorders. There is a strong tendency for mood disorders to run in families. Nongenetic environmental factors such as psychosocial stressors play an important role in depression. Depression occurs with a deficit in brain monoamines, norepinephrine, or serotonin. Individuals with major depression commonly have elevated levels of cortisol. Increased cortisol secretion appears to be a reflection of the elevated secretion of corticotropin-releasing hormone (CRH), which is hypothesized to produce some of the symptoms associated with depression. Neuroendocrine abnormalities that involve thyroid and growth hormones also are found in depression. Individuals with hypothyroidism have depressed mood and cognitive impairments.

Structurally, frontal lobe and limbic system volumes are reduced in depression. Functionally, the blood flow to these two brain areas are altered—decreased to the prefrontal regions and increased in frontal regions with interconnections to the amygdala of the limbic system.

Depression is characterized by unremitting feelings of sadness and despair. The dysphoric or intensely painful mood is accompanied frequently by insomnia, loss of appetite and body weight, and reduced interest in sex. Interest or pleasure in activities decreases dramatically. Feelings of worthlessness and guilt are common in depression. The ability to function and concentrate is greatly diminished. Thoughts of suicide and the risk of suicide are elevated in depressed individuals.

Individuals experiencing recurrent patterns of depression and mania have a condition called **bipolar disorder**; this is in contrast with unipolar disorder, which involves only depression. **Manic** individuals experience elevated euphoria. Self-esteem is elevated as are feelings of grandiosity. Restlessness and irritability occur frequently in mania and these individuals are easily distracted both when speaking and when performing tasks. Hallucinations and delusions may occur during both depression and mania. Bipolar individuals have deficits in Reelin expression linked to genetic loci located on chromosome 22. Genetic studies suggest regions on chromosomes 18 and 22 are linked to both bipolar disorder and schizophrenia. Mania also may result from elevated levels of brain monoamines.

Pharmacotherapy is effective in the treatment of mood disorders. Unipolar depressed individuals generally respond when treated with monoamine oxidase inhibitors (MAOIs), tricyclic antidepressants (TCAs), and selective serotonin reuptake inhibitors (SSRIs).

Manic and bipolar individuals can be treated with lithium or a mood stabilizer. Severely depressed and manic people not responding to pharmacotherapy are administered electroconvulsive therapy (ECT) and then treated with drugs.

3. **Describe the pathophysiology, manifestations, and treatment of panic disorders, generalized anxiety disorder, posttraumatic stress disorder, and obsessive-compulsive disorder.**
   Study text pages 658 through 662; refer to Figures 18-9 and 18-10.

In anxiety disorders, fear and anxiety normally arise in threatening or harmful situations. An anxiety disorder develops when these situations become intrusive and uncontrollable.

Panic disorder is characterized by intense autonomic arousal that involves a wide variety of symptoms. Lightheadedness, a racing heart, difficulty breathing, chest discomfort, generalized sweating, general weakness, trembling, abdominal distress, and chills or hot flashes can be experienced. **Agoraphobia**, or phobic avoidance of places or situations from which escape is not possible, can lead to house-bound individuals.

Genetic factors appear to play a large role in panic disorder, although other factors may be acting on vulnerable brainstem regions to provoke a panic attack. Panic disorder may be caused by an oversensitive brain system regulating autonomic functions. Potential brain regions involved are the locus ceruleus, hippocampus, and amygdala. Pathophysiology in the brain GABA-benzodiazepine receptor system may also contribute to the production of panic attacks. Psychosocial stressors may facilitate the occurrence of panic in vulnerable individuals.

Behavioral therapy and antidepressant medication are used to treat panic disorder. The individual learns to control the intensity of anxiety and panic through breathing exercises and biofeedback techniques. Medication includes the use of TCAs and SSRIs. Benzodiazepines also are prescribed as an adjunct or augmentation for individuals nonresponsive to SSRIs or TCAs.

Excessive and persistent worries are the hallmarks of **generalized anxiety disorder (GAD)**. The individual with GAD worries extensively about life events such as marital relationships, job performance, health, money, or social status. Symptoms include restlessness, motor tension, irritability, fatigue, difficulty in concentrating, and sleep disturbances. Abnormalities in norepinephrine, serotonin, and GABA-benzodiazepine systems may contribute to the disorder.

Serotonin/norepinephrine reuptake inhibitors are first-line therapeutics for managing GAD. GAD treatment also includes behavioral therapy that incorporates relaxation techniques.

Exposure to terrifying or life-threatening events may produce **posttraumatic stress disorder (PTSD)**. Individuals with a history of psychiatric illness, major depression, or panic disorder or those who lack strong social support are more likely to develop PTSD. These individuals may be more sensitive to the effects of the stressor. The traumatic event is reexperienced persistently by the individual through thoughts or dreams. Exposure to cues associated with the traumatic event will trigger psychological distress and intense autonomic arousal. Consequently, the individual attempts to avoid stimuli associated with the trauma.

A flashback involving images, odors, sounds, and emotions may make the person reenact the event. The duration of the flashback varies from only a few seconds or hours to, in rare cases, several days. Persistent symptoms of PTSD may include difficulty in sleeping, irritability, lack of concentration, hypervigilance, and exaggerated startle response.

Pathology of brain regions, including the prefrontal cortex, hippocampus, and amygdala, may underlie the development of PTSD. These brain regions play important roles in how fearful memories are stored, retrieved, and forgotten. Neurotransmitter systems such as norepinephrine, dopamine, opiate, and corticotropin-releasing factor (CRF) may mediate the occurrence of PTSD.

Treatment of PTSD involves a combination of psychotherapy and SSRI medication. In psychotherapy, the individual learns to control the feelings of anxiety. Antidepressants decrease the incidence of recurrent nightmares and flashbacks.

Repetitive, intrusive thoughts and/or compulsions are the hallmarks of **obsessive-compulsive disorder (OCD)**. These thoughts and acts are irrational, impair normal functioning, and may cause marked distress. Obsessions may involve a preoccupation with contamination, doubting, religious or sexual themes, or the belief that a negative outcome will occur if a specific act is not performed.

Compulsions are physical and mental ritualized acts such as washing, cleaning, checking, counting, organizing, hoarding, and repeating specific thoughts or prayers.

Orbitofrontal and anterior cortical hyperactivity may be responsible for intrusive thoughts, obsessions, and anxiety, which drives the basal ganglia to engage in compulsive ritualized acts as a means to alleviate the anxious obsessions. Studies further suggest that when provoked, OCD individuals consistently show increased activity in orbitofrontal, anterior cingulate, and caudate nucleus. Serotonin agonists exacerbate the symptoms of OCD, and serotonin synthesis is decreased in the prefrontal cortex and caudate nucleus. Stimulation of the dopamine system increases repetitive acts, which may be blocked by dopamine antagonists.

OCD is a chronic illness that requires long-term treatment consisting of cognitive-behavioral therapy and drug medication, such as SSRIs. Severe OCD may require neurosurgery to disconnect the basal ganglia from the frontal cortex.

PRACTICE EXAMINATION

Matching
Match the descriptor with mental illness(es).

_____ 1. Thought disorder

_____ 2. Hypoactive DLPFC

_____ 3. Unremitting feelings of sadness and despair

_____ 4. Feelings of grandiosity

_____ 5. Task distraction

_____ 6. Triggering cues

_____ 7. Excessive worry

_____ 8. Exhibit happiness when recalling a terrible event

_____ 9. Unable to express pleasure

_____ 10. Elevated levels of brain serotonin

_____ 11. Deficit in brain norepinephrine

_____ 12. Intense autonomic arousal

_____ 13. Neurodevelopmental defects

_____ 14. Elevated dopaminergic transmission

_____ 15. Deficit in brain serotonin

a. depression

b. generalized anxiety disorder

c. mania

d. panic disorder

e. posttraumatic stress disorder

f. schizophrenia

g. obsessive-compulsive disorder

Chapter **18** **Neurobiology of Schizophrenia, Mood Disorders, and Anxiety Disorders**

_____ 16. Ventricular enlargement

_____ 17. Decreased serotonin synthesis in prefrontal cortex

_____ 18. Elevated levels of cortisol

_____ 19. Difficult breathing

_____ 20. Stimuli avoidance

_____ 21. Racing heart

_____ 22. GABA-benzodiazepine receptor disorder

_____ 23. Flashbacks

_____ 24. Biofeedback therapy

_____ 25. Psychotic episode

CASE STUDY

Ms. B. is a 28-year-old woman who is a computer specialist for a major corporation. She is living at home with her biologic mother, who has a long history of mood disorder. She tells her mother, "I feel worthless, useless, and lonely all the time." Two months ago, Ms. B.'s best friend was killed in a car accident, and she is still crying every day. She cannot concentrate at work, and she feels overwhelmed and sad all of the time. She has no appetite and only sleeps for a few hours during the night. Her clothes are not fitting because she has lost 20 pounds. Ms. B. often feels guilty about the death of her friend because she did not stop her friend from driving while under the influence of alcohol. Last year, Ms. B. had an episode of extreme lethargy and sadness. She even attempted suicide, but her mother intervened. In fact, this is the third time since she turned 25 years old that Ms. B. has felt worthless and that life does not seem worth living.

Questions
What mental disorder do you suspect?

What may be causing the disorder to be expressed at this time?

Identify the usual signs and symptoms of the disorder that Ms. B. exhibits.

Chapter **18   Neurobiology of Schizophrenia, Mood Disorders, and Anxiety Disorders**

19 Alterations of Neurologic Function in Children

FOUNDATIONAL KNOWLEDGE OBJECTIVES

a. **Identify the six embryologic stages of neurologic development.**
Review text pages 665 through 667; refer to Figures 19-1 through 19-3

MEMORY CHECK!

- Embryonic development of the nervous system occurs in six stages: (1) dorsal or posterior induction, (2) ventral or anterior induction, (3) proliferation, (4) migration, (5) organization, and (6) myelination.

b. **Identify the infant neurologic reflexes.**
Refer to Table 19-1.
c. **Identify the major differences between adult and infant neurologic functioning.**
Review text page 668.

MEMORY CHECK!

- Several differences between adults and children are notable. First, the head of a normal infant accounts for approximately one fourth of the total height, whereas an adult's head is one eighth of the total body height. Second, the bones of the infant's skull are separated at the suture line to form anterior and posterior fontanels or "soft spots." The posterior fontanel may be open until 2 to 3 months of age, whereas the anterior fontanel normally closes by 18 months. The adult's cranium is a closed cavity with sutures that firmly hold the cranial bones together; the infant's cranium has room for expansion through the fontanels and increases in circumference during the first 5 years of life. An adult's head size cannot expand, regardless of trauma or increased production of cerebrospinal fluid. The infant's head circumference, on the other hand, increases in size as a result of normal growth up to the age of 5 years. The head is the fastest growing body part during infancy. In children, abnormal intracranial conditions characterized by increased intracranial pressure may also increase head circumference in excess of that expected with normal growth. Healthcare providers carefully monitor head growth during the first 5 years of life by measuring head circumference and comparing the results with a standardized growth chart.

LEARNING OBJECTIVES

After studying this chapter, the learner will be able to do the following:

1. **Describe the major forms of central nervous system malformation.**
Study text pages 668 through 675; refer to Figures 19-5 through 19-11 and Table 19-2.
Neural tube defects are caused by an arrest in development of the brain and spinal cord. A strong association with fetal death obscures the actual incidence somewhat. These defects can be subdivided into posterior defects (anencephaly), the myelodysplasias (defects of the vertebral column and spinal cord), and the less frequent

anterior midline defects. Ingestion of the daily allowance of folic acid before conception or early in pregnancy reduces the risks for neural tube defects.

Anencephaly is the absence of the skull and parts of the brain that results from early closure of the anterior neural tube. It is a relatively common disorder that is fatal.

Encephalocele is the herniation of the brain and meninges through a midline defect in the skull. An encephalocele may be located in the nasopharynx, in which case no obvious deformity is noted, but the defect may cause nasal congestion. Central nervous system tissue may be seen on nasal examination. This type of defect has a good prognosis for surgical repair. Size, location, and timing of

133

the development of encephalocele determine the potential outcome for the child's development and cognition.

Meningocele is the protrusion of meninges through a vertebral defect. The spinal cord is not involved. The meningocele is present at birth as a protruding sac at the level of the defect. Abnormal neurologic function may be present, and hydrocephaly is a common complication. Damage and infection may result from manipulation of the sac. Surgical closure is optimal during the first 72 hours of life. The size and level of the defect determine the eventual outcome.

Myelomeningocele (spina bifida) is a herniation of the meninges, spinal fluid, spinal cord, and nerves through a vertebral defect; 80% of these defects are located in the lumbosacral region. Myelomeningocele is observed as a "sac on back." The covering membrane may leak cerebrospinal fluid (CSF). Function is dependent on the degree of spinal cord involvement. Deficits will be distal to the defect and include weakness, paralysis, spasticity, and either bowel or bladder dysfunction; these deficits may worsen with age because of tethering of the cord with development. Hydrocephalus occurs in 85% of cases. Myelomeningocele is detectable through prenatal ultrasound and alpha-fetoprotein sampling. Treatment includes early surgical correction of the defect and its complicating hydrocephaly and multidisciplinary therapy for related problems.

Spina bifida occulta is a less serious form of myelomeningocele, with the defect occurring in the lumbar or sacral area of the spine because of incomplete fusion of the vertebral laminae. Spina bifida occulta is more common than myelomeningocele and usually causes no neurologic deficits; it may occur in 10% to 25% of infants to some degree. Physical findings may include abnormal hair growth along the spine, a midline sacral dimple with or without a sinus tract, angioma over the defect, or an overlying subcutaneous mass. Spina bifida occulta may cause dysfunctions during periods of rapid growth. These abnormalities can be observed in the gait, as positional feet deformities because of muscle weakness, or sphincter disturbances of bladder and bowel. Surgical closure is usually completed in the neonatal period.

Craniosynostosis is the premature closure of cranial sutures during the first 20 months of life. Asymmetry of the skull or interference with brain growth may result if multiple sutures are involved. Diagnosis is made by physical examination, head circumference measurements, and radiologic studies. Surgical treatment is indicated for cases that restrict brain growth.

Microcephaly is a defect in brain growth as a whole. The brain may be only 25% of normal weight, with growth of the frontal lobes severely stunted. Primary microcephaly may be caused by chromosomal abnormality, toxin exposure, radiation, or chemical exposure during periods of induction and major cell migration. Secondary microcephaly may be caused by various insults during the third trimester. Manifestations range from decerebrate posturing and profound retardation to motor impairment and mild retardation.

Congenital hydrocephalus is characterized by an increase in the volume of CSF that may be due to overproduction, a defect in reabsorption, or a blockage of the ventricular drainage system. The incidence rate is approximately 3 of every 1000 live births. The most frequent cause is congenital aqueduct stenosis; but other causes include brain tumors, cysts, trauma, arteriovenous malformations, infections, and blood clots. The resultant pathology is because of increased intracranial pressure (pressure on the brain) that eventually causes tissue damage. At first, sutures and fontanels of the skull are able to accommodate the increased fluid by separating, which allows the head to grow in diameter; this enlargement in utero may require cesarean delivery. After birth, the increasing pressure causes neurologic symptoms including irritability, high-pitched crying, vomiting, and lethargy; serious, irreversible brain damage; and, eventually, death. Diagnosis is made by physical examination, radiologic imaging (computed tomography [CT] or magnetic resonance imaging [MRI]), and head circumference measurement. Treatment includes surgical placement of a shunt from the affected ventricle to another cavity of the body, usually the peritoneal cavity. In the event of shunt malfunction, acute, life-threatening increases in intracranial pressure may result and require emergency surgery.

2. **Compare and contrast the pathophysiology of the static encephalopathies of cerebral palsy, phenylketonuria, Tay-Sachs disease, and seizure disorders**
   Study text pages 675 through 681; refer to Figure 19-12 and Tables 19-3 and 19-4.

   Cerebral palsy (CP) is a static encephalopathy, which means that the resulting damage does not change over time. Several factors can produce the brain damage leading to cerebral palsy. Prenatal cerebral hypoxia, congenital malformations, and placental pathology can contribute to the systemic degeneration of immature areas of the brain white matter and interfere with cell maturation. The severity of the damage depends on the gestational age at the time of injury and the degree of injury sustained. Low birth weight and birth asphyxia are risk factors for CP. Hypoxia and asphyxia cause edema in the brain; lack of oxygen and incorporation of amino acids during protein synthesis lead to acidosis. Carbon dioxide and lactic acid accumulation leads to more acidosis and osmotic pressure changes. This contributes to generalized cerebral swelling and CNS damage. Children with CP manifest spasticity, seizures, mild to severe intellectual impairment, and visual impairment. Although the brain injury is static, the clinical picture changes with growth and development. Therefore, ongoing treatment plans must change. Intrathecal baclofen pumps, botulinum toxin, and selective dorsal rhizotomy for spasticity have shown improvement in selected children with cerebral palsy.

   Phenylketonuria (PKU) is an encephalopathy caused by an inherited metabolic disorder, and it is progressive in nature. The disorder involves an inability to metabolize the amino acid phenylalanine and occurs once in every 14,000 births worldwide. A high level of phenylalanine causes insufficient amounts of other amino acids entering the brain that results in malformation, defective myelination, or cystic degeneration of the white and gray matter. Diagnosis is usually made by nonselective newborn screening. Treatment is to restrict phenylalanine in the diet, which generally results in normal growth and development.

Tay-Sachs disease is a fatal autosomal recessive disorder caused by impairment of the lysosomal enzyme hexosaminidase A. Approximately 80% of the individuals affected are of Jewish ancestry. In Tay-Sachs disease, the pathologic changes predominate in the CNS, but neurons throughout the body contain characteristic cytoplasmic changes. With time, neurons become distorted and balloon; and microglial cells, which also are swollen and filled with large granules, proliferate. Cystic degeneration of the cerebral white matter and atrophy of the cerebellar hemispheres often occur. Changes in the spinal cord, particularly in the motor cells, result in hypotonia, hyporeflexia, and overall weakness. Onset of the disease occurs when the infant is 3 to 6 months old, and death usually occurs by 2 to 5 years of age.

Seizure disorders change in pattern and frequency over time during childhood because of the maturation of neurons and their patterns of connection. The nervous system in children has a decreased capability for generating well-organized seizures, because the immature neuron is unable to generate long bursts of high-frequency signals and has relatively underdeveloped intracortical connections. Seizures during infancy and childhood may be the result of asphyxia, intracranial bleeding, CNS infection, electrolyte imbalance, or inborn errors of metabolism. Many seizure disorders are idiopathic, which means that they have no known cause. Frequently occurring seizure disorders in infancy and childhood include **infantile spasms, Lennox-Gastaut syndrome, juvenile myoclonic epilepsy,** and **febrile seizures.**

3. **Describe the pathophysiology of the acute encephalopathies of Reye syndrome, CNS intoxications, meningitis, and HIV.**
   Study text pages 681, 682, and 684; refer to Figure 19-13.

   Reye syndrome is an acute encephalopathy that is believed to be caused by an interaction of salicylate, viruses, and liver dysfunction. The pathophysiology includes the induction of hypoglycemia, hyperammonemia, and an increase in short-chain fatty acids, all of which lead to an encephalopathy frequently referred to as a hepatic encephalopathy. The brain eventually becomes severely edematous, which leads to tissue damage and transtentorial herniation. Clinical manifestations begin with vomiting and lethargy (stage 1) and progress to disorientation, delirium, central neurologic hyperventilation, and stupor (stage 2). Obtundation, coma, and decorticate rigidity (stage 3) are followed by rapidly developing seizures, flaccidity, and respiratory arrest (stages 4 and 5). Avoiding aspirin during viral illnesses in children is the accepted preventive measure. Treatment ranges from rapid diagnosis and supportive therapy in the early stages to highly complicated neurointensive care in later stages.

Drug-induced encephalopathies must be considered in a child with unexplained neurologic changes. Such encephalopathies may result from accidental ingestion, therapeutic or intentional overdose, or ingestion of environmental toxins. High blood levels of lead, if not treated, lead to encephalopathy that causes serious and irreversible neurologic damage. **Pica** is the habitual, purposeful, and compulsive ingestion of nonfood substances, such as clay, dirt, and paint chips.

Bacterial meningitis refers to inflammation of the meningeal coverings of the brain and spinal cord. The origin of the inflammation and acute encephalopathy also can be viral in nature. **Aseptic meningitis** has no evidence of viral infection but may be associated with systemic disease or drugs. *Escherichia coli* and group B beta-hemolytic streptococci are the most common causes of meningitis in the newborn. *Streptococcus pneumoniae* is the most common microorganism in children 1 to 23 months of age. The second most common microorganism causing bacterial meningitis in children under 4 years of age is *Neisseria meningitidis*. Bacterial toxins increase cerebral vascular permeability causing edema. Thrombosis and increased intracranial pressure can cause neurologic damage and obstruction to CSF circulation, resulting in communicating hydrocephalus. Herniation of the brainstem causes death.

The hallmark of **viral meningitis** is a mononuclear response in the CSF instead of a neutrophilic response as in bacterial meningitis and normal sugar levels instead of decreased sugar levels as in bacterial meningitis. The symptoms are similar but milder than those seen in bacterial meningitis. Malaise, fever, headache, nuchal and spinal rigidity, nausea, and vomiting are common.

The site in infants and children that is most vulnerable and most commonly affected by **HIV** is the CNS. Transmission of HIV to infants and children occurs perinatally through the placenta by exposure to infected maternal blood, vaginal secretions, and by postpartum ingestion of milk. HIV affects all body systems. Manifestations include progressive encephalopathy, deterioration of gross and fine motor skills, developmental and language delays, behavioral impairment, and onset of seizures. Progressive encephalopathy indicates a poor prognosis. Monitoring CD8 and CD4 lymphocytes and monocytes can predict the risk for progressive encephalopathy. Decreases in CD8 T lymphocytes diminish defense against viral infection. In general, treatment is focused on maintenance of immunity, response to opportunistic infections, and antiretroviral therapy.

4. **Describe cerebrovascular disease in children.**
   Study text pages 684 and 685.

   Occlusive cerebrovascular disease in children is rare but may result from embolism, sinovenous thrombosis, or congenital or iatrogenic narrowing of vessels, which decreases blood flow and oxygen to the brain. **Moyamoya disease** is a rare, chronic, progressive vascular stenosis of the circle of Willis that obstructs arterial flow

135

to the brain. The vascularity may be a congenital anomaly or it can develop as a result of cranial radiation therapy. Treatment is surgical bypass of the occluded region. **Hemorrhagic cerebrovascular disease** results from congenital cerebral arteriovenous malformations that can lead to intracranial bleeding and hemorrhagic stroke in children. Treatment options include surgery, radiation therapy, and embolic occlusion of the malformation.

5. **Describe the types of childhood brain tumor and characterize their presentation.**

Study text pages 685 through 691; refer to Figures 19-14 through 19-17 and Tables 19-5 and 19-6.

Brain tumors are the most common solid tumor in childhood and the second most common neoplasm in children; leukemia is the most common neoplasm. Genetic, environmental, and immune factors are all implicated in causation. Maternal employment with exposure to teratogens also is a possible etiologic factor. Most childhood brain tumors arise from glial tissue, with two thirds of tumors found in the posterior fossa (the infratentorial area). In contrast, two thirds of adult tumors are found in the anterior fossa (the supratentorial area).

Brain tumors are unique in their presentation by virtue of their locations. **Infratentorial tumors** often cause increased intracranial pressure because of a mass blockage of the fourth ventricle. Signs include early morning vomiting with neither nausea nor headache, lethargy, and somnolence. **Supratentorial tumors** frequently cause localized neurologic symptoms, such as truncal ataxia, impaired coordination, gait anomalies, and loss of balance. Diagnosis is confirmed by radiologic imaging.

The most common brain tumors in childhood are **medulloblastoma, ependymoma, astrocytoma, brainstem glioma,** and **optic nerve glioma. Neuroblastoma** is an embryonal neoplasm of the sympathetic nervous system and can be located anywhere there is nervous tissue. Causes of neuroblastoma have a genetic basis in chromosomal alterations and the presence of the *Myc-N* oncogene. More than 90% of children with neuroblastoma have increased catecholamines in their urine. **Retinoblastoma** is a rare congenital eye neoplasm that has both hereditary and nonhereditary forms. Approximately 40% of retinoblastomas are inherited as an autosomal dominant disorder caused by mutations in the *RB1* gene; the others are acquired. The primary sign of a retinoblastoma is a white pupillary reflex called a cat's eye reflex that is caused by the mass behind the lens.

PRACTICE EXAMINATION

True or False

For each statement, write T (true) or F (false) in the blank provided.

_____ 1. Childhood seizures are not well organized.

_____ 2. The cause of most childhood bacterial meningitis is *H. influenzae* type B.

_____ 3. Progressive encephalopathy in HIV infection can be monitored by the CD8 T-lymphocyte count.

_____ 4. Environmental influences play an important role in neural tube defects.

_____ 5. Approximately 60% of retinoblastomas are caused by mutations in the RB1 gene.

_____ 6. Neurologic function at birth is chiefly at the subcortical level.

_____ 7. The prognosis for an individual with meningocele depends on the level and extent of the defect.

_____ 8. Hydrocephaly may be due to overproduction of CSF, blockage of CSF flow, or inhibition of reabsorption.

_____ 9. In Tay-Sachs disease, the changes in the spinal cord occur in the motor cells.

_____ 10. Seizure disorders in children are usually static and resolve naturally, because the neurons and the neuronal pathways are constantly maturing.

_____ 11. An obvious "sac" on the back of a newborn should be thoroughly probed and examined to determine where it is attached to underlying structures.

Fill in the Blanks

Supply the correct response for each statement.

12. Aspirin administration during a viral illness has been associated with _____ syndrome, which is considered to be a _____ encephalopathy.

13. Early morning vomiting without associated nausea may be indicative of a _____ fossa brain tumor.

14. Focal neurologic findings such as ataxia may be associated with an _____ fossa brain tumor.

15. A child who is becoming significantly more ill with symptoms of headache, lethargy, and stiff neck after several days of treatment for a respiratory infection may be showing findings consistent with _____.

16. _____ is a disease that is associated with premature closure of the sutures of the skull.

Matching

Match the description with the alteration.

_____ 17. Involves the sympathetic nervous system

_____ 18. May result from increased CSF

_____ 19. Protrusion of the meninges through a vertebral defect

_____ 20. May require cesarean section for delivery

_____ 21. Static disease that has changing findings over time

_____ 22. Defect in metabolism of an amino acid with severe neurologic involvement

_____ 23. Exhibits hereditary and nonhereditary forms

_____ 24. Very small head

_____ 25. Infectious process that may cause nuchal and spinal rigidity in children

a. meningitis

b. microcephaly

c. retinoblastoma

d. PKU

e. cerebral palsy

f. hydrocephaly

g. meningocele

h. congenital hydrocephaly

i. neuroblastoma

A.S. is an 11-year-old white boy who presents to the pediatric nurse practitioner's office for a school physical. His past medical history is unremarkable, and the family history also is benign. After the examination has started, Allen's mother requests that the practitioner pay particular attention to her son's lower back. She explains, "He has an area 'down there' that is extremely tender and has been tender as long as can remember. The problem worsened this year when Allen was hit from behind while playing sandlot football, and he was paralyzed and 'numb' from the hips down for approximately 15 minutes." When asked about the findings when he was taken to the emergency department for the injury, his mother stated, "I never sought care for him because his symptoms subsided within a few minutes and he seemed fine." The practitioner gently admonished and advised the mother that failure to seek care might have caused permanent damage in this case.

As the physical examination continues, it is noted that A.S. has an exquisitely tender area over the lower lumbar spine and that palpation causes pain in both of his legs. This area feels and appears to be perfectly normal. Allen is noted to have a very deep, dime-sized, sacral dimple and highly fissured skin over the lower sacral spine. Deep tendon reflexes, strength, and sensation are all within normal limits. Bowel and bladder function are normal as well. Spine radiographs are ordered.

Questions

What do you expect the radiographs to reveal?

What is the likely resolution of this disorder?

20 Mechanisms of Hormonal Regulation

PREREQUISITE KNOWLEDGE OBJECTIVES

After reviewing the primary text where referenced, the learner will be able to do the following:

1. **Identify the functions of the endocrine system, and describe the regulation of hormone secretion.**
   Review text pages 696 through 699; refer to Figures 20-1 and 20-2 and Table 20-2.

2. **Classify the types of hormones, their receptors, and their proposed mechanisms of action.**
   Refer to Figures 20-3 through 20-6 and Tables 20-1, 20-3, and 20-4.

3. **State the relationship between the hypothalamus and the pituitary gland; identify the hormones of the anterior pituitary and posterior pituitary glands, their target organs, and their functions.**
   Refer to Figures 20-7 through 20-10 and Table 20-5.

4. **Identify the thyroid hormones and their functions.**
   Refer to Figures 20-11 and 20-12 and Tables 20-6 and 20-7.

5. **Cite the physiologic effects of parathyroid hormone and the variables that affect its secretion.**
   Refer to Figures 20-13 and 20-14.

6. **Identify the production sites of pancreatic somatostatin, insulin, and glucagon production, and state their roles in metabolism.**
   Review text pages 712 through 715; refer to Figures 20-15 and 20-16 and Table 20-8.

7. **Describe the effects of the adrenal cortical glucocorticoids, mineralocorticoids, and gonadotropins; note the adrenal medullary secretions and their roles.**
   Review text pages 715 through 720; refer to Figures 20-17 through 20-20.

8. **Describe endocrine gland changes that are associated with normal aging.**
   Review text pages 720 through 722.

PRACTICE EXAMINATION

Multiple Choice
Circle the correct answer for each question.

1. Organs that respond to a particular hormone are called the:
   a. target organs.
   b. integrated organs.
   c. responder organs.
   d. hormone attack organs.

2. A major feature of the "plasma membrane receptor" mechanism of hormonal action is:
   a. receptors exist for lipid-soluble hormones.
   b. increased lysosomal activity.
   c. that a "second messenger" is required.
   d. that hormones attach to a receptor in the cytosol.

3. A major feature of the "activation of genes" mechanism of hormonal action is that:
   a. a "second messenger" is used.
   b. a hormone–Golgi complex is used.
   c. the hormone enters the cell.
   d. lysosomal activity increases.

4. A hormone that has an antidiuretic effect similar to antidiuretic hormone (ADH) is:
   a. insulin.
   b. oxytocin.
   c. growth hormone (GH).
   d. aldosterone.
   e. adrenocorticotropic hormone (ACTH).

5. The hypothalamus controls the adenohypophysis by the direct involvement of:
   a. nerve impulses.
   b. prostaglandins.
   c. cerebrocortical controlling factors (CCCFs).
   d. regulating hormones.

139

6. Amylin:
   a. is a lipid hormone.
   b. has an antihyperglycemic effect.
   c. depresses glucagon secretion after meals.
   d. None of the above is correct.
7. If calcium levels in the blood are too high, thyrocalcitonin (calcitonin) concentrations in the blood should:
   a. increase, thereby inhibiting osteoclasts.
   b. increase, thereby stimulating osteoclasts.
   c. increase, but this would not affect osteoclasts.
   d. decrease, thereby inhibiting osteoclasts.
   e. decrease, thereby stimulating osteoclasts.
8. In the negative feedback mechanism that controls thyroid hormone secretion, which of the following is the nontropic hormone?
   a. Thyrotropin-releasing hormone (TRH)
   b. Thyroid-stimulating hormone (TSH)
   c. Thyroxine
   d. All of the above are tropic hormones.
9. The control of parathyroid hormone is most accurately described as:
   a. negative feedback controlled by the hypothalamus.
   b. positive feedback controlled by the pituitary gland.
   c. negative feedback involving the pituitary gland.
   d. negative feedback not involving the pituitary gland.
10. The renin-angiotensin-aldosterone system begins to operate when renin is secreted by the:
    a. adrenal cortex.
    b. adrenal medulla.
    c. pancreas.
    d. kidneys.

11. The effects of adrenal medullary hormones and the effects of sympathetic stimulation can be described as:
    a. opposites in all respects.
    b. overlapping in some respects.
    c. opposites in some respects.
    d. variable depending on the sex of the person involved.
    e. overlapping in most respects.
12. Which of the following best describes the respective effects of insulin and glucagon on blood sugar?
    a. Insulin raises it, glucagon lowers it.
    b. Both raise blood sugar.
    c. Insulin lowers it, glucagon raises it.
    d. Both lower blood sugar.
    e. None of the above is correct.
13. Mediators of the anabolic function of GH include:
    a. insulin growth factor (IGF)-2 receptors.
    b. somatostatin.
    c. melatonin.
    d. IGFs.
14. Which of the following is an anabolic protein hormone?
    a. TSH
    b. Aldosterone
    c. Follicle stimulating hormone (FSH)
    d. Insulin
15. Aldosterone maintains electrolyte balance by:
    a. retaining potassium.
    b. eliminating sodium.
    c. retaining both sodium and potassium.
    d. Both a and b are correct.
    e. None of the above is correct.

Matching

Match the appropriate hormone with the target organ.

_____ 16. ACTH

_____ 17. TSH

_____ 18. Thyrotropin- releasing hormone (TRH)

_____ 19. Prolactin

a. mammary glands

b. adrenal cortex

c. adrenal medulla

d. thyroid gland

e. adenohypophysis

f. kidneys

Match the hormone with its role.

_____ 20. Epinephrine

_____ 21. Glucocorticoids

_____ 22. Mineralocorticoids

_____ 23. Somatostatin

a. immunity

b. growth inhibition

c. fight or flight

d. controls Na^+, H_2O, and K^+ excretion

e. suppresses T helper lymphocytes

f. inhibits insulin and glucagon secretion

Match the categories of hormones with the hormone.

_____ 24. Water soluble hormone

_____ 25. Lipid soluble hormone

a. growth hormone

b. thyroxine

c. epinephrine

d. cortisol

Chapter **20** **Mechanisms of Hormonal Regulation**

21 Alterations of Hormonal Regulation

FOUNDATIONAL KNOWLEDGE OBJECTIVES

a. Diagram the negative-feedback system of hormone secretion.
Review text pages 697 and 698; refer to Figure 20-2.

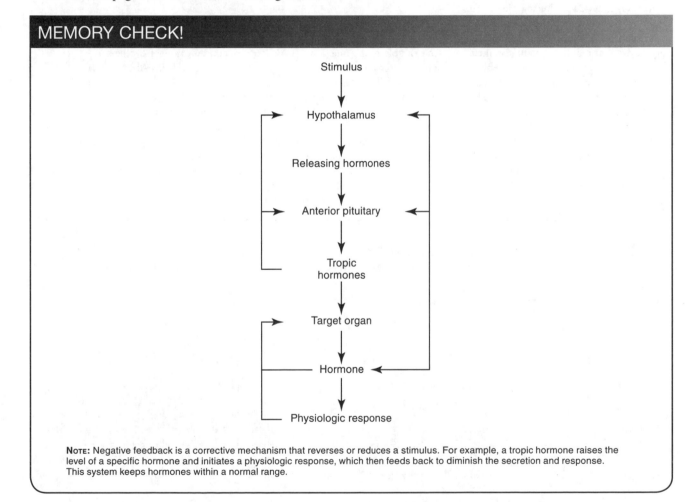

MEMORY CHECK!

NOTE: Negative feedback is a corrective mechanism that reverses or reduces a stimulus. For example, a tropic hormone raises the level of a specific hormone and initiates a physiologic response, which then feeds back to diminish the secretion and response. This system keeps hormones within a normal range.

b. Describe hormone receptors as recognizing and signaling mechanisms for hormonal action.
Review text pages 699 through 703; refer to Figures 20-3 through 20-6 and Tables 20-3 and 20-4.

MEMORY CHECK!

- Hormone receptors are located on the plasma membrane or in the intracellular compartment of a target cell. Water-soluble hormones, which include the protein hormones and epinephrine or norepinephrine, cannot cross the cell membrane and interact or bind with receptors located in or on the cell membrane. Fat-soluble hormones, steroids, vitamin D, and thyroid hormones diffuse freely across the plasma and nuclear membranes to bind primarily with nuclear receptors.
- In the plasma membrane model, the hormones are called "first messengers." The receptors for the water-soluble hormones first recognize the hormone on the plasma membrane and then bind with the hormone. Once recognition and binding have occurred, the hormone-receptor complex initiates the transmission of an intracellular signal by a "second messenger"; the second messenger relays the message inside the cell, where a response can occur. The best-known second messenger is cyclic adenosine monophosphate (cAMP), although other substances are also known as second messengers. Others include cyclic guanosine monophosphate (cGMP); calcium, which associates with inositol triphosphate (ITP); and diacylglycerol (DAG) to produce physiologic effects.
- For cells that have cAMP as a second messenger, the purpose of these interactions is to activate the intracellular cyclic nucleotides such as adenylate cyclase; this enzyme converts adenosine triphosphate (ATP) to cAMP. Elevated levels of cAMP alter cell function in specific ways. An example of the function of cAMP as a second messenger can be seen in the action of epinephrine. The epinephrine-receptor complex interaction increases the synthesis of cAMP. cAMP, in turn, activates an elaborate enzyme cascade in which inactive enzymes are converted in sequence to active enzymes that lead to glycogen breakdown into glucose. For cells that have calcium as their second messenger, a rise in intracellular calcium causes calcium to bind with calmodulin, a regulatory protein. This step then initiates other intracellular processes. Cells that have cCMP as their their second messenger are activated by the enzyme guanylyl cyclase.
- In the lipid-soluble hormonal model, relatively small hydrophobic molecules cross the plasma membrane by simple diffusion. These are the steroid and thyroid hormones. Once inside the cytosol, some hormones bind to receptor molecules in the cytoplasm and then diffuse into the nucleus. Hormones without cytoplasmic receptors diffuse directly into the nucleus and bind with an acceptor molecule. The resulting hormone-receptor complex binds to a specific site on the promoter region of DNA. This binding activates RNA polymerase, which stimulates DNA transcription and increases synthesis of specific proteins.

c. Identify the origins and functions of hormones.
Review the structure and function of endocrine glands in the summary of Chapter 20 on pages 723 and 724

Site of Origin and Effects of Hormones

Site	Hormone	Effect
Hypothalamus	Releasing hormones	Act on anterior pituitary to release specific hormones
Posterior pituitary	Antidiuretic hormone (ADH)	Causes conservation of body water by promoting water reabsorption by renal tubules
	Oxytocin	Stimulates uterine contraction and lactation
Anterior pituitary	Adrenocorticotropic hormone (ACTH)	Stimulates production of glucocorticoids by adrenal cortex
	Melanocyte-stimulating hormone (MSH)	Stimulates pigment production in the skin
	Growth hormone (GH)	Promotes growth/maturation of body tissues
	Thyroid-stimulating hormone (TSH)	Stimulates production and release of thyroid hormones, decreases apoptosis
	Follicle-stimulating hormone (FSH)	Initiates maturation of ovarian follicles; stimulates spermatogenesis
	Prolactin	Stimulates secretion of breast milk
	Luteinizing hormone (LH)	Causes ovulation and stimulates the ovary to produce estrogen and progesterone; stimulates androgen production by interstitial cells of the testes

Site of Origin and Effects of Hormones—cont'd

Site	Hormone	Effect
Thyroid	Thyroxine (T4)	Increases rate of cellular metabolism
	Calcitonin	Osteoblastic; lowers serum cholesterol
Parathyroid	Parathyroid hormone (PTH)	Osteoclastic; raises serum cholesterol
Pancreatic islets of Langerhans	Insulin	Promotes use of glucose; lowers serum glucose
	Glucagon	Promotes use of glycogen; raises serum glucose
	Somatostatin	Inhibits insulin and glucagon secretion
Adrenal cortex	Glucocorticoids, mostly cortisol	Antagonize effects of insulin; inhibit inflammation and fibroblastic activity
	Mineralocorticoids, mostly aldosterone	Promotes retention of sodium by renal tubules
	Androgens and estrogens	Causes development of secondary sex characteristics
Adrenal medulla	Catecholamines (epinephrine and norepinephrine)	Regulates blood pressure by effects on vascular smooth muscle and heart

LEARNING OBJECTIVES

After studying this chapter, the learner will be able to do the following:

1. Identify the causes of hormonal alterations.

Study text pages 727 and 728; refer to Table 21-1.

Any significantly elevated or depressed hormone levels have a variety of causes. Feedback systems may fail to function properly or may respond to inappropriate signals. Inadequate amounts of biologically free or active hormone occur when the secretory cells are unable to produce. A gland also may synthesize or release excessive amounts of hormone. Once in the circulation, hormones may be degraded too fast or too slow, or they may be inactivated by antibodies before reaching their target cell. Hormones produced by nonendocrine tissues also may result in abnormally elevated hormone levels.

The target cell may fail to respond to its hormone. The general types of abnormal target cell responses are receptor-associated disorders and intracellular disorders. **Receptor-associated disorders** may exhibit any of the following: decreased numbers of receptors, defective hormone-receptor binding, impaired receptor function with insensitivity to the hormone, presence of antibodies against specific receptors that either reduce available binding sites or mimic hormone action, or unusual expression by some tumor cells having abnormal receptor activity.

Intracellular disorders may involve inadequate synthesis of the second messenger, such as cAMP, needed to signal intracellular events. The target cell for water-soluble hormones such as insulin may not respond to hormone-receptor binding and thus fail to generate the required second messenger. The cell also may fail to respond to the second messenger if levels of intracellular enzymes or proteins are altered.

The target cell response for lipid-soluble hormones such as TH is thought to occur less frequently than those affecting the water-soluble hormones. For lipid-soluble hormones, the number of intracellular receptors may be decreased or their receptors may have an altered affinity for hormones. Alterations of new messenger RNA or absence of substrates for new protein synthesis also may alter target cell response.

2. Distinguish between SIADH and diabetes insipidus.

Study text pages 728 through 731.

Diseases of the posterior pituitary are usually related to abnormal antidiuretic hormone (ADH/vasopressin) secretion. **Syndrome of inappropriate ADH** (SIADH) secretion is characterized by high levels of ADH without normal physiologic stimuli for its release. Normal adrenal and thyroid function must be present because TH and glucocorticoids are essential for water clearance by the kidneys.

SIADH is associated with several forms of cancer because of the ectopic secretion of ADH by tumor cells. Tumors associated with SIADH include small cell carcinoma of the stomach duodenum and pancreas; cancers of the bladder, prostate, and endometrium; lymphomas; and sarcomas. SIADH may follow pituitary surgery, because stored ADH is released in an unregulated fashion. SIADH may be seen in infectious pulmonary diseases because of the ectopic production of ADH by infected lung tissue or by increased posterior pituitary secretion of ADH in response to hypoxia. SIADH may also occur after treatment with a variety of drugs that stimulate ADH release.

The main features of SIADH are water retention and solute loss, particularly of sodium; this leads to hyponatremia and hypoosmolality. Because ADH is released continually, water retention results from the normal action of ADH on the renal tubules and collecting ducts; this action increases their permeability to water, thereby increasing water reabsorption. Hyponatremia suppresses renin and aldosterone secretion, thereby decreasing proximal tubule reabsorption of sodium.

145

Thirst, impaired taste, anorexia, dyspnea on exertion, fatigue, and dulled consciousness occur when the serum sodium level falls from 140 to 130 mEq/L. Vomiting and abdominal cramps occur with a drop in sodium level from 130 to 120 mEq/L. With a serum sodium level below 115 mEq/L, confusion, lethargy, muscle twitching, and convulsions may occur. Symptoms usually resolve with correction of the hyponatremia. The treatment of SIADH involves the correction of any underlying causal problems, the correction of severe hyponatremia by administration of hypertonic saline, and fluid restriction to 600 to 800 ml/day.

Diabetes insipidus is related to an insufficiency of ADH that leads to polyuria and polydipsia. There are two forms of diabetes insipidus: the neurogenic or central form and the nephrogenic or renal form.

The **neurogenic form** of diabetes insipidus occurs when any organic lesion of the hypothalamus, infundibular stem, or posterior pituitary interferes with ADH synthesis, transport, or release. This results in too little ADH.

Diabetes insipidus in the **nephrogenic form** is an insensitivity of the renal tubules to ADH, particularly of the collecting tubules. This type of diabetes is generally related to disorders and drugs that damage the renal tubules or inhibit the generation of cAMP in the tubules. Genetic causes are related to alterations in aquaporin 2, the signaling protein for ADH in the collecting duct.

The clinical manifestations of diabetes insipidus are due to the absence of ADH. These signs and symptoms include polyuria, nocturia, continuous thirst, polydipsia, low urine osmolality, and high-normal plasma osmolality. Individuals with longstanding diabetes insipidus develop a large bladder capacity and hydronephrosis.

Individuals who have excessive urine output and a low urine osmolality after a dehydration or water restriction test may require ADH replacement with a synthetic vasopressin analog. Drugs that potentiate the action of otherwise insufficient amounts of endogenous ADH may be used to stimulate ADH release from the hypothalamus in less severely affected individuals.

3. **Describe the disorders of the anterior pituitary as either hypofunctions or hyperfunctions of the gland**.
   Study text pages 731 through 736; refer to Figures 21-2 through 21-5.

Anterior pituitary hypofunction may develop from infarction of the gland, removal or destruction of the gland, or space-occupying pituitary adenomas or aneurysms that compress secreting pituitary cells. Spontaneous mutations of pituitary transcription factor (*Prop-1*) gene involved in early embryonic pituitary development leads to combined hormonal deficiencies. **Hyperfunction of the anterior pituitary** generally involves an adenoma that is composed of secretory pituitary cells. An adenoma may lead to hypersecretion of the hormone produced by the adenoma and hyposecretion of another hormone because of the compressive effects of the tumor.

The pituitary gland is extremely vascular and therefore is extremely vulnerable to infarction; it may be susceptible to necrosis because its blood supply through the hypophyseal system is already partially deoxygenated. The likelihood of infarction is increased during pregnancy, because oxygen demands are increased. The primary pathologic mechanism in postpartum pituitary infarction, which is rare, called **Sheehan syndrome**, is a vasospasm of the artery that supplies the anterior pituitary. Following tissue necrosis, edema occurs, which expands the pituitary gland within the fixed confines of the sella turcica; this further impedes blood supply to the pituitary and promotes hypofunction.

The signs and symptoms of **hypofunction** of the anterior pituitary are highly variable and depend on which hormones are affected. If all hormones are absent, a condition called **panhypopituitarism** develops. The individual with this condition suffers from cortisol deficiency from lack of ACTH, thyroid deficiency from lack of TSH, diabetes insipidus from a lack of ADH, and gonadal failure and loss of secondary sex characteristics from an absence of FSH and LH. Gonadotropic hyposecretion frequently results in menstrual irregularity in women. Decreased libido and diminished secondary sex characteristics in both men and women are present.

When there is a GH deficiency in children, **hypopituitary dwarfism** infrequently occurs. A dwarf has a normal face with normal proportions of head, trunk, and limbs; a dwarf also has normal intelligence. In adult GH deficiency, there is social withdrawal, fatigue, loss of motivation, osteoporosis, and reduced lean body mass.

In cases of hypopituitarism, the underlying disorder should be corrected as quickly as possible. Thyroid and cortisol replacement therapy may need to be initiated and maintained. Sex steroid replacement may be required depending on the needs and desires of the individual.

Pituitary adenomas that cause **hyperpituitarism** are usually benign, slow-growing tumors. Effects from an increase in tumor size include nonspecific complaints of headache, fatigue, neck pain or stiffness, and seizures. Visual changes produced by pressure on the optic chiasm include visual field impairments. If the tumor infiltrates other cranial nerves, various neuromuscular functions are affected. Hypersecretion of hormones secreted by the adenoma leads to symptoms associated with the particular hormone that is affected.

Acromegaly occurs in adults who are exposed to continuously excessive levels of GH. Acromegaly is uncommon. The most common cause of acromegaly is a primary autonomous GH-secreting pituitary adenoma. Acromegaly occurs more frequently in women than in men and is a slowly progressive disease. If untreated, this condition is associated with a decreased life expectancy due to an increased occurrence of hypertension, congestive heart failure, and diabetes mellitus. Colon cancer is also more common in individuals with acromegaly.

In the adult with acromegaly, after epiphyseal closure has occurred, increased amounts of GH and somatomedins cannot stimulate further long bone growth. Instead, these elevations cause connective tissue and cytoplasmic increases.

146

Bony proliferation involves periosteal vertebral growth and enlargement of the facial bones and the bones of the hands and feet. The associated growth results in protrusion of the lower jaw and forehead. Because somatomedins stimulate cartilaginous growth, there is elongation of the ribs at the bone-cartilage junction, which causes a barrel-chested appearance and increased proliferation of cartilage in the joints. Because of bony and soft-tissue overgrowth, nerves may be entrapped and damaged; this may be manifested by weakness, muscular atrophy, foot-drop, and sensory changes in the hands. Because of a space-occupying lesion, central nervous system symptoms of headache, seizure activity, and visual disturbances may develop. The metabolic effects of GH hypersecretion include impaired carbohydrate tolerance and increased metabolic rate. Diabetes mellitus type 2 occurs when the pancreas is unable to secrete enough insulin to offset the effects of GH.

In children and adolescents whose epiphyseal plates have not yet closed, the effect of increased GH levels is **giantism.** Giantism is very rare because of early recognition and treatment of the adenoma. It occurs when the epiphyses are not fused and high levels of somatomedins stimulate excessive skeletal growth.

The goal of treatment is to protect the individual from the effects of tumor growth and to control hormone hypersecretion while minimizing damage to appropriately secreting portions of the pituitary. Surgery, long-acting somatostatin analog, and radiation therapy are used, depending on the extent of tumor growth.

Pituitary tumors that secrete prolactin, called **prolactinomas,** are common. Pathologic elevation of prolactin in women results in amenorrhea, galactorrhea, hirsutism, and osteopenia due to estrogen deficiency. Hyperprolactinemia in men causes hypogonadism.

Prolactinomas are best treated with dopaminergic agonists that usually reverse the gonadal effects. If medications fail, surgery and radiotherapy are options.

4. Describe the disorders of hyperthyroidism.

Study text pages 736 through 739; refer to Figures 21-6 through 21-9.

Whenever THs from any source exert greater-than-normal responses, **thyrotoxicosis** exists. **Hyperthyroidism** is a form of thyrotoxicosis in which excess TH is secreted by the thyroid gland. Specific diseases that can cause hyperthyroidism include Graves disease and toxic multinodular goiter. **Thyrotoxicosis** other than hyperthyroidism is seen in subacute thyroiditis, increased TSH secretion, ectopic thyroid tissue, and ingestion of excessive TH. All forms of thyrotoxicosis share some common characteristics because of increased circulating levels of TH. The major types of therapy used to control the elevated levels of TH include drug therapy, radioactive iodine therapy, and surgery.

Graves disease is the most common form of hyperthyroidism and is likely associated with autoimmune abnormalities. Thyroid receptor antibodies of the IgG class bind to the plasma membrane and initiate thyroid growth, vascularity, and hypersecretion of hormone. Ophthalmopathy appears in 50% to 70% of individuals with

Graves disease. This disease is characterized by edema of the orbital contents, exophthalmos, and extraocular muscle weakness that sometimes leads to diplopia and pain, lacrimation, photophobia, and blurred vision.

Diffuse toxic goiter occurs when the thyroid gland enlarges in response to increased demand for TH. The demand for TH increases in puberty, pregnancy, iodine deficiency, and immunologic, viral, or genetic disorders. The increased number of follicles is compensatory in response to increased TSH levels. The thyroid gland returns to its original size when the stimulus for increased TH no longer exists. During the demand status, some follicular cells may be injured and produce less TH than the body requires; the remainder of the gland then functions to supply the body's need. After thyrotoxicosis results, the condition is called toxic multinodular goiter, and the manifestations are similar to those of Graves disease, although infiltrative ophthalmopathy and myxedema do not occur.

Thyrotoxic crisis (thyroid storm) is a rare but dangerous worsening of the thyrotoxic state; death can occur within 48 hours without appropriate treatment. This condition occurs most frequently in individuals who have undiagnosed or partially treated severe hyperthyroidism and who are subjected to excessive stress from other causes. The systemic symptoms of thyrotoxic crisis include hyperthermia, tachycardia, high-output heart failure, agitation or delirium, and nausea, vomiting, or diarrhea contributing to fluid depletion. The symptoms may be attributed to increased beta-adrenergic receptors and catecholamines. The treatment is to reduce circulating TH levels by blocking TH synthesis.

5. Describe the disorders of hypothyroidism.

Study text pages 739, 741, and 742; refer to Figures 21-10 through 21-12.

Deficient production of TH by the thyroid gland results in **hypothyroidism,** which may be either primary or secondary. Primary causes include congenital defects or loss of thyroid tissue following treatment for hyperthyroidism and defective hormone synthesis resulting from antithyroid antibodies or endemic iodine deficiency. Causes of the less common secondary hypothyroidism are insufficient pituitary stimulation of the normal gland and peripheral resistance to TH.

Hypothyroidism can result from several distinct and rare disorders. **Subacute thyroiditis** is a nonbacterial inflammation of the thyroid that is often preceded by a viral infection. **Autoimmune thyroiditis,** which is also called **Hashimoto disease,** results in destruction of thyroid tissue by circulating thyroid antibodies and the infiltration of lymphocytes. Autoimmune thyroiditis may also be caused by an inherited immune defect. **Subclinical hypothyroidism** is defined as elevated TSH with normal levels of circulating TH.

Hypothyroidism generally affects all body systems and has an insidious onset over months or years. The characteristic sign of severe or longstanding adult hypothyroidism is **myxedema.** In myxedema, the connective fibers are separated by an increased amount of protein and mucopolysaccharides. This protein-mucopolysaccharide

147

complex binds water, which develops nonpitting, boggy edema, especially around the eyes.

Myxedema coma is a medical emergency that is associated with severe hypothyroidism. Symptoms include hypothermia without shivering, hypoventilation, hypotension, hypoglycemia, and lactic acidosis. Older patients with severe vascular disease and with moderate or untreated hypothyroidism are particularly at risk for developing myxedema coma; it may also occur after overuse of narcotics or sedatives or after an acute illness in individuals with hypothyroidism.

Hypothyroidism in infants occurs because of absent thyroid tissue and hereditary defects in TH synthesis. Signs may not be evident for at least 4 months after birth and include abdominal protrusion, umbilical hernia, subnormal temperature, lethargy, excessive sleeping, and slow pulse. If not treated, skeletal growth is stunted, and the child will be dwarfed with short limbs if not treated; these signs constitute **cretinism.** Mental retardation in individuals with cretinism is a function of the severity of hypothyroidism and the delay before initiation of thyroxine treatment.

Hypothyroidism is difficult to identify at birth, but high birthweight, hypothermia, delay in passage of the meconium, and neonatal jaundice are suggestive signs. There is a high probability of normal growth and intellectual function if treatment is started before the child is 3 or 4 months old.

Thyroid carcinoma is the most common endocrine malignancy, but it is still relatively rare. The most consistent causal risk factor for the development of thyroid cancer is exposure to ionizing radiation during childhood. Changes in voice and swallowing and difficulty in breathing are related to tumor growth that impinges on the esophagus or trachea. Treatment for this rare entity may include partial or total thyroidectomy, TSH suppressive therapy, radioactive iodine therapy, postoperative radiation therapy, and chemotherapy.

6. **Characterize the manifestations of hypothyroidism and hyperthyroidism**.
   Refer to Tables 21-2 and 21-3.
   See table below.

7. **Distinguish between primary and secondary hyperparathyroidism and hypoparathyroidism**.
   Study text pages 742 through 745; refer to Table 21-4.

Primary hyperparathyroidism disorders result from failed feedback mechanisms that cause an increased secretion of PTH; this causes hypercalcemia and decreased serum phosphate levels. **Secondary hyperparathyroidism** may be a compensatory response of the parathyroid glands to chronic hypocalcemia. Loss of calcium by failing kidneys leads to increased secretion of PTH. Hypersecretion of PTH causes excessive osteoclastic and osteolytic activity that results in bone resorption.

Chronic hypercalcemia may be associated with insulin resistance, kidney stones, gastrointestinal disturbances, muscle weakness and lethargy, dehydration, and confusion. Definitive treatment requires the surgical removal of the hyperplastic parathyroid glands.

Hypoparathyroidism is most commonly caused by damage to the parathyroid glands during thyroid surgery. In the absence of PTH, the ability to resorb calcium from bone and to regulate calcium reabsorption from the renal tubules is impaired. Hypocalcemia lowers the threshold for nerve and muscle excitation. Muscle spasms, hyperreflexia, clonic-tonic convulsions, laryngeal spasms, and, in severe cases, death from asphyxiation are seen with hypocalcemia.

The definitive treatment of primary hyperparathyroidism is surgery. Treatment for secondary hyperparathyroidism in chronic renal disease requires calcium replacement, dietary phosphate restriction, and vitamin D replacement.

8. **Describe the similarities and differences between insulin-dependent (type 1) and non–insulin-dependent (type 2) diabetes mellitus; note the other types of diabetes mellitus**.

Manifestations of Hypothyroid and Hyperthyroid States

Characteristic	Hypothyroidism	Hyperthyroidism
Basal metabolic rate	Decreased	Increased
Sympathetic response	Decreased	Increased
Weight	Gain	Loss
Temperature tolerance	Cold intolerance, decreased sweating	Heat intolerance, increased sweating
Gastrointestinal function	Constipation, decreased appetite	Diarrhea, increased appetite
Cardiovascular function	Decreased cardiac output, bradycardia	Increased cardiac output, tachycardia, and palpitations
Respiratory function	Hypoventilation	Dyspnea
Muscle tone and reflexes	Decreased	Increased
General appearance	Myxedematous, deep voice, impaired growth (child)	Exophthalmos, lid lag, decreased blinking, enlarged thyroid gland
General behavior	Mental retardation (infant), mental and physical sluggishness, somnolence	Restlessness, irritability, anxiety: hyperkinesis; wakefulness

NOTE: Hypothyroidism is more common than hyperthyroidism.

Study text pages 745 through 754; refer to Figures 21-13 through 21-15 and Tables 21-5 through 21-9. See Table below.

The term **diabetes mellitus** encompasses many etiologically unrelated diseases and includes many different causes of disturbed glucose tolerance. Diabetes mellitus is a syndrome that is characterized by chronic hyperglycemia and other disturbances of carbohydrate, fat, and protein metabolism. The major types of diabetes mellitus are primary beta cell defect or failure/absolute insulin deficiency (type 1 diabetes mellitus), non–insulin-dependent diabetes mellitus/insulin resistance and deficit (type 2 diabetes mellitus), insulin resistance with inadequate insulin secretion, and other types of diabetes mellitus. Types 1 and 2 are the most common.

The diagnosis of diabetes is based on three observations: first, more than one fasting plasma glucose level greater than 126 mg/dl; second, elevated plasma glucose levels in response to an oral glucose tolerance test greater than 200 mg/dl confirmed on a subsequent day; and third, random plasma glucose levels above 200 mg/dl without regard to time of last meal combined with classic symptoms of polydipsia, polyphagia, and polyuria. In individuals with poorly controlled diabetes, increases in the quantities of glycosylated hemoglobins are seen. Once a hemoglobin molecule is glycosylated, it remains that way.

Type 1 diabetes mellitus is characterized by a lack of insulin and a relative excess of glucose and is most commonly diagnosed among whites peaking at 12 years of age. In type 1 immune diabetes mellitus, beta cells are destroyed, and islet cell antibodies appear. This disease seems to be caused by a gradual process of autoimmune destruction in genetically susceptible individuals. Macrophages T and B lymphocytes and natural killer cells are often present. Viral infections likely cause autoimmune damage to beta cells. In type 1 nonimmune diabetes mellitus, genetic abnormalities or injury to the beta cells impairs or inhibits insulin secretion. When an individual is heterogeneous for HLA-DR3 and HLA-DR4, the risk is 20 to 40 times greater than the general population's risk for type 1 diabetes mellitus.

Because of the decreased use of glucose, glucose accumulates in the blood and is subsequently released in the urine. This in turn causes polyuria and polydipsia resulting from osmotic diuresis. Ketoacidosis (which is caused by increased levels of circulating ketones without the inhibiting effects of insulin), increased levels of

Classifications of Diabetes and Glucose Intolerance States

Classification	Former Terminology	Characteristics
Type 1 diabetes mellitus	Juvenile-onset diabetes	Few or no islet cells; acute onset at puberty; long preclinical record; insulin-dependent; ketosis-prone; autoimmune and genetic-environment etiology; thin individual (peaks at age 12, rare in those younger than 1 year old and older than 30 years)
Beta cell deficiency/destruction	Insulin-dependent diabetes mellitus (IDDM)	
Type 2 diabetes mellitus (resistant to insulin with an insulin secretory deficiency)	Adult-onset, maturity-onset diabetes	Usually some insulin production; decreased islet cells; not ketosis-prone; frequently obese; strong familial pattern; rapidly increasing in children; related to hypertension and dyslipidemia (age 18 years and older)
	Non–insulin-dependent diabetes mellitus (NIDDM)	
Other forms	Secondary diabetes, maturity-onset diabetes of the young (MODY)	Normal weight to underweight; mutation in gene responsive for insulin secretion or action; mutation in B-cell glucose sensor, glucokinase
Gestational diabetes mellitus (GDM)	Asymptomatic diabetes Subclinical diabetes Latent diabetes	Glucose intolerance develops during pregnancy (third trimester); increased risk of developing within 15 years after parturition

NOTE: *Impaired glucose tolerance (IGT)*
Abnormal response to oral glucose tolerance test:
2 hr PG >140 and <200 mg/dl
10% to 25% will convert to type 2 diabetes within 10 years
Impaired fasting glucose (IFG)
Fasting plasma glucose ≥100 and <126 mg/dl

circulating fatty acids, and weight loss are all manifestations of type 1 diabetes mellitus.

Type 2 diabetes mellitus is more common than type 1 and is probably caused by genetic susceptibility that is triggered by environmental factors. It generally affects those older than 30 years. The greatest risk factor for type 2 diabetes is obesity. In the obese, insulin has a diminished ability to influence glucose uptake and metabolism. In type 2 diabetes, amyloid deposits in the islets, fatty atrophy of the pancreas and liver, and vascular sclerosis are generally present. Some insulin production continues in type 2 diabetes mellitus, but the mass and number of beta cells are decreased. Insulin resistance in glucose and lipid metabolism and decreased insulin secretion are the major abnormalities in type 2 diabetes mellitus.

There is a deficiency of amylin, a hormone co-secreted with insulin by the beta cells, in both type of diabetes. Altered glucagon control on assimilation of nutrients is related to amylin deficit. Amyloid deposition also may be related to amylin loss.

In the management of type 1 diabetes, insulin is most commonly given subcutaneously one to four times daily. Self-monitoring of blood glucose is required. The individual with type 1 diabetes mellitus must consume sufficient calories to achieve and maintain normal weight for height and age. Caloric intake should be regulated with consideration of age, activity, and severity of the diabetes. Exercise by individuals with type 1 diabetes may result in hypoglycemia. Reducing the insulin dosage before exercising will reduce the possibility of hypoglycemia.

Autoimmune type 1 diabetes may be prevented with immunizations using low doses of insulin or oral insulin-like agents.

The treatment of the individual with type 2 diabetes requires appropriate meal planning as in type 1 diabetes; however, only oral medication may be needed for optimal management. Oral hypoglycemic agents need a pancreas that is capable of synthesizing insulin; thus there must be some functioning beta cells. Insulin may also be used in the treatment of some individuals with type 2 diabetes. Exercise or weight loss is an important aspect of treatment for the individual with type 2 diabetes. Exercise reduces after-meal blood glucose levels and diminishes insulin requirements. Increases in the level of good, high-density lipoprotein (HDL) cholesterol are achieved by exercise. Also, exercise increases weight loss in the overweight individual.

9. **Describe the acute complications of diabetes mellitus; describe the features of each**.
   Study text pages 754 through 758; refer to Tables 21-10 through 21-12.

Acute complications of diabetes mellitus include hypoglycemia or insulin shock, diabetic ketoacidosis (DKA), and hyperosmolar hyperglycemic nonketotic syndrome (HHNKS). See table below.

10. **Describe the chronic complications of diabetes mellitus.**
    Study text pages 758 through 765; refer to Figures 21-16 through 21-20 and Tables 21-13 and 21-14. See table below.

Acute Complications of Diabetes Mellitus

Variable	Hypoglycemia Insulin Shock	DKA	HHNKS
Onset	Rapid	Slow	Slowest
Symptoms	Weak, anxious, confused, tachycardia	Nausea, vomiting, polyuria, polyphagia, polydipsia, headache, irritable, comatose, fruity and shortness of breath	Similar to DKA, stuporous, hypotension, dehydration
Skin	Sweating	Hot, flushed, dry	Very dry
Mucous membranes	Normal	Dry	Extremely dry
Respiratory	Normal	Hyperventilation, "fruity" or acetone odor to breath	Normal
Those at risk	Type 1 and 2 diabetes mellitus; fluctuating blood glucose levels; insufficient food intake; excessive exercise; oral medication; excessive insulin	Type 1 diabetes mellitus; stressful situations; omission of insulin	Elderly or young; type 2 diabetes mellitus; high carbohydrate diets; diuresis; hyperosmolar dialysis
Blood sugar/dl	30 mg or less in newborns, 60 mg or less in adults	>250 mg	>600 mg
Treatment	Fast-acting carbohydrate; intravenous glucose; subcutaneous glucagon	Low-dose insulin; electrolyte and fluid replacement	Fluid replacement with crystalloids and colloids

NOTE: The Somogyi effect occurs if an overdose of insulin induces hypoglycemia followed by rebound hyperglycemia because of release of hormones that stimulate lipolysis gluconeogenesis, and glycogenolysis leading to elevated serum glucose. It is most common in individuals with type 1 diabetes mellitus and in children. The dawn phenomenon is an early-morning hyperglycemia caused by nocturnal elevation of growth hormone.

150

Chronic Complications of Diabetes Mellitus

	Chronic hyperglycemia involves		
	*Nonenzymatic glycosylation		
	*Shunting of glucose to polyol and hexosamine pathways		
	*Activation of protein kinase C		
	leading to:		
Diabetic Neuropathies	**Microvascular Disease**	**Macrovascular Disease**	**Infection**
Axonal and Schwann cell degenerations, altered motor nerve conduction, sensory alterations	Retinopathy* Nephropathy* Capillary basement membrane thickening, decreased tissue perfusion or ischemia, hypertension	Coronary heart disease* CVA* Peripheral vascular disease* Proliferation of fibrous plaques, atherosclerosis because of high serum lipids, ischemia	Sensory impairment, atherosclerosis, ischemia, hypoxia, leukocytic impairment

*Major consequences.

NOTE: Microalbuminuria is the first manifestation of renal dysfunction.

11. **Describe the etiology, pathogenesis, and manifestations of hyperfunction and hypofunction of the adrenal cortex.**

Study text pages 765 through 772; refer to Figures 21-21 through 21-24 and Tables 21-15 and 21-16.

Cushing syndrome refers to excessive levels of circulating cortisol regardless of the cause or from autonomous cortisol production by adrenal tissue. Corticotropin-dependent Cushing syndrome is more common, particularly in women and is caused by ACTH-secreting pituitary tumors. Corticotropin-independent Cushing syndrome is less common and is usually caused by an adrenal tumor. **Cushing disease** refers specifically to pituitary-dependent hypercortisolism due to an ACTH-secreting pituitary microadenoma. Individuals with Cushing disease lose diurnal and circadian patterns of ACTH and cortisol secretion and lack the ability to increase secretion of these hormones in response to stressors. Cushing-like syndrome also may develop as a result of the exogenous administration of cortisone.

Most of the clinical signs and symptoms of Cushing syndrome are caused by hypercortisolism. The most common feature is the accumulation of adipose tissue in the trunk, facial, and cervical areas; this has been described as "truncal obesity," "moon face," and "buffalo hump." Protein wasting is commonly observed in hypercortisolism, and this is caused by the catabolic effects of cortisol on peripheral tissues. Muscle wasting is especially obvious in the muscles of the extremities. Loss of the protein matrix in bone leads to osteoporosis and accompanying pathologic fractures, vertebral compression fractures, bone and back pain, kyphosis, and reduced height. Loss of collagen also leads to thin, weakened integumentary tissues through which capillaries are more visible; this accounts for the characteristic purple striae observed in the trunk area. Loss of collagenous support around the small vessels makes them susceptible to rupture and easy bruising. Glucose intolerance occurs because of cortisol-induced insulin resistance. Diabetes mellitus can develop.

With elevated cortisol levels, vascular sensitivity to catecholamines is significantly increased, and this leads to vasoconstriction and hypertension. Chronically elevated cortisol levels also cause suppression of the immune system and increased susceptibility to infections. Hyperpigmentation in Cushing syndrome is likely caused by the melanotropic activity of ACTH. Approximately 50% of individuals with Cushing syndrome experience irritability and depression.

Without treatment, approximately 50% of individuals with Cushing syndrome die within 5 years of onset because of infection, suicide, complications from generalized arteriosclerosis, and hypertensive disease. Treatment is specific for the cause of hypercorticoadrenalism and includes medication, radiation, and surgery.

Hyperaldosteronism is characterized by excessive aldosterone secretion by the adrenal glands. An aldosterone-secreting adenoma or excessive stimulation of the normal adrenal cortex by substances such as angiotensin, ACTH, or elevated potassium may cause hypersecretion.

Conn disease, which is also called **primary aldosteronism,** presents a clinical picture of hypertension, hypokalemia, renal potassium wasting, and neuromuscular manifestations. The most common cause of primary aldosteronism is a benign, single adrenal adenoma followed by multiple tumors or idiopathic hyperplasia of the adrenals. Because aldosterone secretion is normally stimulated by the renin-angiotensin system, **secondary hyperaldosteronism** can result from sustained elevated renin release and the activation of angiotensin. Increased renin-angiotensin secretion occurs with decreased circulating blood volume and decreased delivery of blood to the kidneys.

Hypertension and hypokalemia are the essential manifestations of hyperaldosteronism. Hypertension usually

151

results from increased intravascular volume and from altered serum sodium concentrations. If hypertension is sustained, left ventricular hypertrophy and progressive arteriosclerosis develop.

Aldosterone-stimulated potassium loss can result in the typical manifestations of hypokalemia: hypokalemic alkalosis as potassium moves from the intracellular to the extracellular space in exchange for hydrogen ions and renal loss of hydrogen ions to facilitate sodium reabsorption. Individuals with hypokalemic alkalosis may experience (1) tetany and paresthesia, (2) skeletal muscle weakness, (3) cardiovascular alterations, and (4) loss of urine-concentrating mechanisms, which can cause polyuria or nocturia.

Treatment involves the management of hypertension and hypokalemia and the correction of any underlying causal abnormalities. If an aldosterone-secreting adenoma is present, it must be surgically removed.

Hypersecretion of adrenal androgens and estrogens may be caused by adrenal tumors, Cushing syndrome, or defects in steroid synthesis. The clinical manifestations depend on the hormone secreted, the sex of the individual, and the age at which the hypersecretion occurs. Hypersecretion of estrogens causes **feminization,** which is the development of female sex characteristics. Hypersecretion of androgens causes **virilization,** which is the development of male sex characteristics.

The effects of an estrogen-secreting tumor are most evident in males and cause gynecomastia, testicular atrophy, and decreased libido. In female children, such tumors may lead to the early development of secondary sex characteristics. Androgen-secreting tumor changes are more easily observed in females and include excessive face and body hair growth or hirsutism, clitoral enlargement, deepening of the voice, amenorrhea, acne, and breast atrophy. In children, virilizing tumors promote precocious sexual development and bone aging. Treatment of androgen-secreting tumors usually involves surgical excision.

Hypocortisolism develops either because of inadequate stimulation of the adrenal glands by ACTH or because of an inability of the adrenals to produce and secrete the adrenal cortical hormones. Hypofunction of the adrenal cortex may affect glucocorticoid or mineralocorticoid secretion or a combination of both. Primary adrenal insufficiency is called **Addison disease,** and this is a relatively rare adult disease.

Addison disease is characterized by elevated serum ACTH levels with inadequate corticosteroid synthesis and output. The most common cause is destruction of the adrenal cortex. In idiopathic Addison disease, a combination of cell membrane and cytoplasmic antibodies and cell-mediated immune mechanisms contributes to the pathology of the disease. Apparently, a genetic defect in immune surveillance mechanisms causes a deficiency of immune suppressor cells. The symptoms of Addison disease are primarily a result of hypocortisolism and hypoaldosteronism; these manifestations include weakness, gastrointestinal disturbances, hypoglycemia, hyperpigmentation from increased ACTH secretion, and hypotension.

Secondary hypocortisolism has low or absent ACTH levels, which cause inadequate adrenal stimulation, adrenal atrophy, and decreased corticosteroidogenesis. The exogenous administration of glucocorticoids for nonendocrine disease results in this form of hypocortisolism.

The treatment of Addison disease involves glucocorticoid and possibly mineralocorticoid replacement therapy and dietary modifications to include adequate sodium. Hypocortisolism requires daily chronic glucocorticoid replacement therapy, and additional cortisol must be administered during acute stress.

12. Describe adrenal medulla hyperfunction.

Study text pages 772; refer to Figure 21-25.

The most prominent cause of adrenal medulla hypersecretion is **pheochromocytoma.** Fewer than 10% of these tumors metastasize; if they do, they are usually found in the lungs, liver, bones, or paraaortic lymph glands. Most pheochromocytomas produce norepinephrine, although large tumors of this type secrete both epinephrine and norepinephrine.

Pheochromocytomas cause the excessive production of epinephrine and norepinephrine due to autonomous functioning of the tumor.

The clinical manifestations of a pheochromocytoma include persistent hypertension associated with flushing, diaphoresis, tachycardia, palpitations, and constipation.

Hypermetabolism may develop because of stimulation of the thyroid gland by the catecholamines. Glucose intolerance may occur because of catecholamine-induced inhibition of insulin release by the pancreas.

The usual treatment of pheochromocytoma is surgical excision of the tumor. Medical therapy with adrenergic-blocking agents is used to stabilize blood pressure before surgery.

13. Summarize the effects of endocrine disorders and provide examples.

Study the summary on text pages 773 through 775.

Endocrine disorders affect fluid and electrolyte balance, cardiovascular function, general growth patterns, reproductive function, metabolism of glucose, and metabolic rate.

Endocrine System Disorders

Effect	Examples
Fluid and electrolyte imbalances	Addison disease, hypoaldosteronism, hyperaldosteronism, diabetes insipidus, SIADH, hypoparathyroidism, hyperparathyroidism
Cardiovascular dysfunction	Addison disease, hyperthyroidism, pheochromocytoma, diabetes mellitus
General growth alterations	Dwarfism, giantism, acromegaly, pituitary hyposecretion, hypersecretion
Reproductive irregularities	Precocious puberty, adrenogenital syndrome, gynecomastia
Altered glucose metabolism	Addison disease, Cushing disease, diabetes mellitus
Metabolic rate abnormalities	Hyperthyroidism, hypothyroidism, cretinism, myxedema

PRACTICE EXAMINATION

Multiple Choice

Circle the correct answer(s) for each question.

1. Which of the following laboratory values would be expected in an individual with SIADH?
   a. Serum sodium = 150 mEq/L and urine hypoosmolality
   b. Serum potassium = 5 mEq/L and serum hypoosmolality
   c. Serum sodium = 120 mEq/L and serum hypoosmolality
   d. Serum potassium = 3 mEq/L and serum hyperosmolality

2. Hypopituitarism in an adult male likely includes:
   a. decreased libido.
   b. connective tissue increases.
   c. visual field impairments.
   d. altered neuromuscular function.

3. Excessive secretion of GH in an adult may cause:
   a. diabetes mellitus type 2.
   b. diabetes insipidus.
   c. hypoglycemia.
   d. decreased metabolic rate.

4. A characteristic shared by both diabetes mellitus and diabetes insipidus is:
   a. elevated blood and urine glucose levels.
   b. the inability to produce ADH.
   c. the inability to produce insulin.
   d. polyuria.
   e. elevated blood urine and ketone body levels.

5. The manifestations of hyperthyroidism include all of the following *except:*
   a. diarrhea.
   b. constipation.
   c. heat intolerance.
   d. weight loss.
   e. wakefulness.

6. Hypothyroidism in adults is:
   a. myxedema.
   b. Addison disease.
   c. Cushing disease.
   d. Graves disease.
   e. cretinism.

7. Graves disease is:
   a. hyperthyroidism.
   b. associated with autoimmunity.
   c. manifested by ophthalmopathy.
   d. All of the above are correct.

8. Inadequate levels of thyroid hormones at birth may cause:
   a. mental retardation.
   b. immediate death.
   c. thyroid crisis.
   d. myxedema.
   e. dwarfism.

9. Hyperparathyroidism causes which of the following?
   a. Increased osteoclastic activity
   b. Decreased plasma calcium
   c. Increased phosphorus absorption from the gastrointestinal tract
   d. Hypocalcemia

10. Manifestations of hypocalcemia include:
   a. myopathy.
   b. lethargy.
   c. hypertension.
   d. tetany.
   e. bone cysts.

11. What is the most common cause of acromegaly?
   a. Anterior pituitary adenoma
   b. Overproduction of ACTH
   c. Overproduction of TSH
   d. Pituitary atrophy

12. If a 19-year-old woman had shortness of breath, weight loss, excessive sweating, exophthalmos, and irritability, which hormone would you expect to find elevated in her serum?
   a. Cortisol
   b. Thyroxine
   c. ACTH
   d. 17-Ketosteroid

13. A 24-year-old woman with a history of taking sulfonylurea agents is found in a stuporous state. She is pale and has cold, clammy skin. What is the likely etiology of her condition?
   a. Hyperglycemia
   b. Insulin shock/hypoglycemia
   c. Renal failure
   d. Peripheral neuropathy

14. A 10-year-old boy came into the emergency department dehydrated with metabolic acidosis, hyperkalemia, elevated ketones, and a blood glucose level of 800 mg/dl. The most probable disease in this child is:
    a. cretinism.
    b. type 1 diabetes mellitus.
    c. type 2 diabetes mellitus.
    d. impaired glucose tolerance (IGT).
    e. gestational diabetes mellitus (GDM).
15. Your neighbor has not previously been diabetic but has gained 80 pounds during the past year and is able to produce some insulin. Her fasting blood sugar is always elevated. She is being treated with oral insulin-stimulating drugs. This is likely:
    a. diabetes insipidus.
    b. type 1 diabetes mellitus.
    c. type 2 diabetes mellitus.
    d. IGT.
    e. GDM.
16. Panhypopituitarism in children causes:
    a. excessive ACTH secretion.
    b. increased libido.
    c. dwarfism.
    d. giantism.
17. Hormonal alterations can be caused by:
    a. inadequate synthesis of cAMP.
    b. increased numbers of intracellular receptors for lipid-soluble hormones.
    c. increased substrates for new proteins.
    d. presence of antibodies against specific receptors.
18. Chronic renal failure causes:
    a. dehydration.
    b. hypercalcemia.
    c. secondary hyperparathyroidism.
    d. primary hyperparathyroidism.
19. The end result of hyperthyroidism is:
    a. the production of a goiter.
    b. Graves disease.
    c. overstimulation of the basal metabolic rate.
    d. depression of metabolism.
20. If an individual is heterogeneous for HLA-DR3 and HLA-DR4, the risk is far greater for:
    a. excess insulin
    b. type 1 diabetes mellitus.
    c. type 2 diabetes mellitus.
    d. All of the above are correct, plus diabetes insipidus.
21. Intragenic hyperadrenalism leads to primary adrenal insufficiency if treatment is stopped suddenly because of:
    a. destruction of the adrenal cortex by steroid treatment.
    b. destruction of the adrenal medulla by steroid treatment.
    c. pituitary gland atrophy.
    d. adrenal gland atrophy.
22. Which electrolyte change occurs in Addison disease?
    a. Hypokalemia
    b. Hypernatremia
    c. Hyperkalemia
    d. Hypocalcemia
23. A benign tumor of the adrenal glands that causes the hypersecretion of aldosterone is:
    a. Addison disease.
    b. a pheochromocytoma.
    c. Cushing disease.
    d. Cushing syndrome.
    e. Conn disease.

Matching

Match the hypersecretion with the consequence.

_____ 24. Hypersecretion of aldosterone

_____ 25. Hypersecretion of glucocorticoids

a. decreased cardiac output

b. hyperglycemia and/or osteoporosis

c. basal metabolic rate increases

d. hypernatremia

e. hyponatremia

CASE STUDY 1

Scott, a 17-year-old high school football player, was brought to the hospital emergency department in a coma. According to his mother, he had lost weight during the past month despite eating large amounts of food. Besides losing weight, he was excessively thirsty and voided several times during the night. The family history revealed others with diabetes mellitus. Physical examination was not significant except for tachycardia and hyperpnea.

Laboratory serum studies revealed the following:
Glucose on admission = 1000 mg/dl (high)
pH = 7.25 (low)
P_{CO_2} = 30 mmHg (low)
HCO_3^- = 12 mEq/L (low)
Ketones = 4+ (high)
Glycosylated hemoglobin = high

Question

What do you think Scott's symptoms, signs, and diagnostic studies suggest?

A 49-year-old short, overweight Native American female seeking care at a clinic was diagnosed with type 2 diabetes several years ago. She ignored recommendations for care and is now complaining of weakness in her right foot. The patient said, "My foot has been weak for a long time, it is hard to bend, and it feels numb." She denies any other problems except being thirsty and having to get out of bed at night to urinate; but admits gaining about 20 pounds lately.

Notable findings on physical examination reveal a weight of 198 pounds and a blood pressure of 166/101. Her retina shows mild arteriolar narrowing. The right limb strength is less than half of that of the left limb and sensory perception to light touch on the soles of both feet is diminished.

Questions

What laboratory tests are required (1) now and (2) after fasting?

Interpret the laboratory reports. What treatment would you recommend?

22 Structure and Function of the Reproductive Systems

PREREQUISITE KNOWLEDGE OBJECTIVES

After reviewing the primary text where referenced, the learner will be able to do the following:

1. **Describe the development of the reproductive systems.**
   Review text pages 781 through 784; refer to Figures 22-1 through 22-3.

2. **Identify female external and internal genitalia; identify female sex hormones.**
   Review text pages 784 through 792; refer to Figures 22-4 through 22-9.

3. **Describe the menstrual cycle; note its differential hormonal effects, levels, and cellular events.**
   Review text pages 792 through 796; refer to Figure 22-10 and Table 22-1.

4. **Identify male external and internal genitalia.**
   Review text pages 796 through 800; refer to Figures 22-11 through 22-15.

5. **Describe spermatogenesis and male sex hormones.**
   Review text pages 800 through 802; refer to Figures 22-16 through 22-18.

6. **Describe the progressive and cyclic hormonal changes associated with female breast tissue development; note the lymphatic drainage.**
   Review text pages 802 through 805; refer to Figures 22-19 and 21-20.

7. **List the tests used to evaluate reproductive health and function.**
   Refer to Tables 22-2 through 22-4.

8. **Identify normal changes in the reproductive systems that occur with advancing age; describe perimenopause.**
   Review text pages 807 and 809 through 812; refer to Figure 22-21 and Tables 22-5 through 22-7.

PRACTICE EXAMINATION

Multiple Choice

Circle the correct answer for each question.

1. GnRH reaches the anterior pituitary gland through the hypothalamic hypophyseal-portal system and causes the release of:
   a. growth hormone.
   b. FSH.
   c. ADH.
   d. oxytocin.

2. Which of the following is a structure of the female external genitalia?
   a. Vagina
   b. Clitoris
   c. Cul-de-sac
   d. Cervix

3. During the follicular/proliferative phase, the anterior pituitary gland secretes:
   a. LH.
   b. GH.
   c. estrogen.
   d. progesterone.
   e. FSH.

4. Progesterone:
   a. stimulates lactation.
   b. increases uterine tube motility.
   c. thins the endometrium.
   d. maintains the thickened endometrium.
   e. causes ovulation.

5. The ovaries produce:
   a. ova, estrogen, and oxytocin.
   b. ova only.
   c. ova and estrogen.
   d. testosterone and semen.
   e. None of the above is correct.

6. During which days of the menstrual cycle does the endometrium achieve maximum development?
   a. 2 through 6
   b. 7 through 12
   c. 14
   d. 20 through 24
   e. 26 through 28

7. The hormone(s) necessary for the growth and development of female breasts is (are):
   a. estrogens and progesterone.
   b. oxytocin and ADH.
   c. androgens and steroids.
   d. gonadocorticoids.
   e. relaxin.

8. The structure that releases a mature ovum is the:
   a. corpus albicans.
   b. graafian follicle.
   c. primary follicle.
   d. corpus luteum.
   e. infundibulum.

157

9. A major duct of the female reproductive system is the:
   a. suspensory tube.
   b. uterosacral duct.
   c. broad duct.
   d. mesovarian duct.
   e. uterine tube.
10. Prostate is to accessory gland as ovary is to:
    a. ejaculatory duct.
    b. gonad.
    c. bulbourethral gland.
    d. accessory gland.
    e. urethra.
11. Cells that produce testosterone are called:
    a. interstitial endocrinocytes.
    b. testicular endocrine cells.
    c. sustentacular cells.
    d. spermatogonia.
    e. None of the above is correct.
12. Testosterone:
    a. decreases renal erythropoietin production.
    b. has an anabolic effect on skeletal muscle.
    c. levels depend the activity of Sertoli cells.
    d. production is without diurnal influences.
13. Immediately after the sperm cells leave the ducts epididymis, they enter the:
    a. ejaculatory duct.
    b. ductus deferens.
    c. urethra.
    d. exterior of the body.
14. A substance that is produced in the reproductive system mainly by the bulbourethral glands is:
    a. fructose.
    b. HCl.
    c. mucus.
    d. an alkaline, viscous fluid.
15. Which of the following produces a secretion that helps maintain the motility of spermatozoa?
    a. Prostate
    b. Penis
    c. Greater vestibular glands
    d. Interstitial tissues

16. Semen is:
    a. a vaginal secretion needed to activate sperm.
    b. the product of the testes.
    c. the sperm and secretions of the seminal vesicles, prostate, and bulbourethral gland.
    d. responsible for the engorgement of the erectile tissue in the penis.
    e. the secretion that causes ovulation in the female.
17. The uterus:
    a. increases in size and moves upward and forward during sexual excitement.
    b. is usually backward to rest on the urinary bladder.
    c. has four layers in its wall.
    d. has a functional layer responsive to sex hormones.
18. The major difference between female and male hormone production is that:
    a. LH is without effect in the male.
    b. GnRH does not cause the release of FSH in the male.
    c. daily hormonal levels vary more in females than in males.
    d. FSH is without effect in the male.
19. The primary spermatocyte has:
    a. 46 chromosomes.
    b. the same number of chromosomes as a sperm.
    c. 23 chromosomes.
    d. a haploid number of chromosomes.
20. Which is correct?
    a. Infant gender cannot be predicted based on the timing of intercourse.
    b. Men need to "save up sperm" to enhance their fertility.
    c. Sperm retain their fertility for up to 10 days.
    d. All of the above are correct.
21. Most of the lymphatic drainage of the female breasts occurs through the:
    a. axillary nodes.
    b. internal mammary nodes.
    c. subclavian nodes.
    d. brachial nodes.
    e. anterior pectoral nodes.

Matching

Match the reproductive event with the circumstance.

_____ 22. Primary follicles resist gonadotropin stimulation.

_____ 23. Elevated FSH, decreased inhibin, normal LH, and slightly elevated estradiol

_____ 24. Less effective erection

_____ 25. First menstruation

a. menarche

b. perimenopause

c. menopause

d. vasomotor flush

e. decreased vasocongestion

23 Alterations of the Reproductive Systems

FOUNDATIONAL KNOWLEDGE OBJECTIVES

a. **Describe the relationships of hormones to the normal menstrual cycle.**
   Review text pages 792 through 796; refer to Figure 22-10.

MEMORY CHECK!

- The three phases of the menstrual cycle are the follicular/proliferative phase, the luteal/secretory phase, and menstruation. During menstruation, the functional layer of the endometrium disintegrates and is discharged through the vagina. Menstruation is followed by the follicular/proliferative phase. During this phase, the anterior pituitary gland secretes FSH, which causes an ovarian follicle to develop. While the follicle is developing, it secretes estrogen, which causes cells of the endometrium to proliferate. By the time the ovarian follicle is mature, the endometrial lining is restored. At this point, ovulation occurs.
- Ovulation marks the beginning of the luteal/secretory phase of the menstrual cycle. The ovarian follicle begins its transformation into a corpus luteum. LH from the anterior pituitary stimulates the corpus luteum to secrete progesterone, which initiates the secretory phase of endometrial development. If conception occurs, the nutrient-laden endometrium is ready for implantation. If conception and implantation do not occur, the corpus luteum degenerates and ceases its production of progesterone and estrogen. Without progesterone or estrogen to maintain it, the endometrium enters the ischemic phase and disintegrates; menstruation then occurs, which marks the beginning of another cycle.

b. **Characterize the structure and development of the female breast**.
   Review text pages 802 through 805; refer to Figures 22-19 and 22-20.

MEMORY CHECK!

- The female breast is composed of 15 to 20 pyramid-shaped lobes that are separated and supported by Cooper ligaments. Each lobe contains 20 to 40 lobules that subdivide into many functional units called acini. Each acinus is lined with a layer of epithelial cells that are capable of secreting milk and a layer of subepithelial cells that are capable of contracting to squeeze milk from the acinus. The acini empty into a network of lobular collecting ducts that reach the skin through openings in the nipple. The lobes and lobules are surrounded and separated by muscle strands and fatty connective tissue. An extensive capillary network surrounds the acini. Lymphatic drainage of the breast occurs largely through the axillary nodes.
- The nipple is a pigmented, cylindrical structure that has multiple openings. The areola is the pigmented, circular area around the nipple. A number of sebaceous glands are located within the areola, and these aid in the lubrication of the nipple during lactation. The nipple's smooth muscle is innervated by the sympathetic nervous system.
- During childhood, breast growth is latent, and growth of the nipple and areola keeps pace with the growth of the body surface. At the onset of puberty in the female, estrogen secretion stimulates mammary growth. Full differentiation and development of breast tissue are mediated by a variety of hormones including estrogen, progesterone, prolactin, growth hormone, thyroid hormone, insulin, and cortisol.
- During the reproductive years, the breast undergoes cyclic changes in response to changes in the levels of estrogen and progesterone associated with the menstrual cycle. Because the length of the menstrual cycle does not allow for complete regression of new cell growth, breast growth continues at a slow rate until the woman reaches approximately 35 years of age. The number of acini increase with each cycle, so epithelial tissue proliferation is under the influence of hormones as long as secretion occurs.

c. Identify the circumstances required for normal reproductive function in the male and female.
Review text page 761; refer to Tables 22-3 and 22-4.

MEMORY CHECK!

- The male must have normal numbers, structure, and motility of sperm with no obstruction along the reproductive tract. The female must have the cervix, uterus, and fallopian tubes adequately patent to allow passage of ovum and sperm. She must also have normal ovulation, an endometrium that responds to hormones, and reproductive organs and tissues that are free of tumors or infections.

LEARNING OBJECTIVES

After studying this chapter, the learner will be able to do the following:

1. Distinguish between the causes of delayed and precocious puberty.
Study text pages 817 through 819; refer to Boxes 23-1 through 23-4.

In 95% of cases of **delayed puberty**, hormonal levels are normal, and the hypothalamic-pituitary-gonadal axis is intact, but maturation is happening slowly. The delay tends to be familial and is more common in boys than in girls. It may be related to the consequences of any chronic condition that delays bone development and aging. Exogenous sex steroid administration is used in cases of delayed puberty to reduce the psychological impact of esteem issues or embarrassment.

Precocious puberty can be defined as sexual maturation before age 6 years in black girls or age 7 years in white girls and before age 9 in boys. **Central precocious puberty** is GnRH-dependent and occurs when the hypothalamic-pituitary-gonadal axis is functioning normally but prematurely. Besides the premature development of secondary sex characteristics, there is premature closure of the epiphysis of long bones, which results in short stature. **Peripheral puberty** is GnRH-independent and develops when sex hormones are produced by some mechanisms other than stimulation by the gonadotropins. Gonadal tumors, testotoxicosis, and exposure to exogenous sex steroids are some of the causes.

2. Distinguish among various menstrual disorders; describe premenstrual syndrome.
Study text pages 819 through 828; refer to Figures 23-1 through 23-4 and Tables 23-1 and 23-2.

Premenstrual syndrome (PMS) is the cyclic recurrence in the luteal phase of the menstrual cycle of physical, psychological, or behavioral changes distressing enough to impair interpersonal relationships or usual activities. It has been estimated that 5% to 10% of menstruating women have severe to disabling premenstrual symptoms, and 3% to 8% of these women have exaggerated feelings of depression known as **premenstrual dysphoric disorder (PMDD)** warranting treatment. Currently, it is believed that PMS is the end result of abnormal tissue response of nervous, immunologic, vascular, and gastrointestinal systems to the normal hormone changes of the menstrual cycle. This biologic response may be triggered by fluctuating preovulatory estrogen and postovulatory progesterone levels. Serotonin levels likely play a role in type and severity of symptoms.

A predisposition to PMS runs in families and is likely due to genetics or environmental factors or both. There is some evidence that supports a relationship between the severity and frequency of premenstrual

Menstrual Disorders

Disorder	Alteration
Primary dysmenorrhea	Excessive endometrial prostaglandin production
Secondary dysmenorrhea	Related to pelvic disorders (pelvic adhesions, inflammation, cervical stenosis, or uterine fibrosis)
Painful menstruation	Increases myometrial contractions and constricts blood vessels

Amenorrhea
    Absence of menstruation
	Amenorrhea is divided into compartments that reflect the underlying disorder:
	    Compartment I—disorders of outflow tract or uterine target organ
	    Compartment II—disorders of the ovary
	    Compartment III—disorders of the anterior pituitary
	    Compartment IV—central nervous system disorders or altered hypothalamic factors

Menstrual Disorders—cont'd

Disorder	Alteration
Primary: amenorrhea	No ovulation occurs; no menstruation or secondary sex characteristics by 14 years of age or by 16 years of age if secondary sex characteristics are present
Secondary: amenorrhea	Absence of menstruation for 3 cycles or 6 months after menarche
Dysfunctional uterine bleeding (DUB) Heavy or irregular bleeding caused by disturbance of menstrual cycle	Estrogen proliferates endometrium, and progesterone limits it; large mass of tissue available for heavy, irregular bleeding because of lower levels of progesterone in relation to higher levels of estrogen
Polycystic ovarian syndrome (PCOS)	Related to hyperinsulinemia, and dyslipidemia leading to infertility, hirsutism, acne, endometrial hyperplasia, cardiovascular disease, and diabetes mellitus; a hyperandrogenic state excessive androgens, affect follicular growth while insulin affects follicular decline by suppressing apoptosis thus enabling follicles to survive

symptoms and perfectionism, increased stress, poor nutrition, lack of exercise, low self-esteem, and history of sexual abuse or family conflict. Depression, anger, irritability, and fatigue have been reported as the most prominent and the most distressing symptoms; physical symptoms seem less prevalent and problematic.

Treatment for PMS is symptomatic. Nonpharmacologic therapies tend to be more effective in controlling symptoms than medication alone. For example, dietary changes, such as eating six small meals a day, increasing complex carbohydrate and water intake while decreasing caffeine, alcohol, sugar, and animal fats can be beneficial. Various medications, such as selective serotonin reuptake inhibitors, may be added to the treatment plan even if their efficacy in the treatment of PMS is questionable.

3. Describe pelvic inflammatory disease.

Study text pages 828 through 830; refer to Figures 23-5 through 23-7.

Pelvic inflammatory disease (PID) is an acute inflammatory process caused by infection. PID involves organs of the upper genital tract, the uterus, the fallopian tubes or uterine tubes, or the ovaries.

In its most severe form, the entire peritoneal cavity may be involved. Infection of the fallopian tubes is **salpingitis;** infection of the ovaries is **oophoritis.** Most cases of PID are caused by sexually transmitted microorganisms that ascend from the vagina (bacterial vaginosis) to the uterus, fallopian tubes, and ovaries. PID is considered a polymicrobial infection with the majority of cases being caused by gonorrheal and chlamydial microbes. These organisms may induce a response that causes tubonecrosis with repeated infections, and this may predispose a woman to PID. After one episode of pelvic infection, 15% to 25% of women develop long-term sequelae, such as infertility, ectopic pregnancy, chronic pelvic pain, and pelvic

adhesions. The incidence of complications increases markedly with repeated infections.

The clinical manifestations of PID are variable; 65% to 75% of women with salpingitis have subclinical infections. The first sign of the ascending infection may be the gradual onset of low bilateral abdominal pain often characterized as dull and steady. Symptoms are more likely to develop during or immediately after menstruation. The pain of PID may worsen with walking, jumping, or intercourse. Other manifestations of PID are difficult or painful urination and irregular bleeding. Conditions such as ectopic pregnancy, threatened abortion, or appendicitis, which also cause pelvic pain, must be excluded before treatment.

Treatment involves bed rest, avoidance of intercourse, and combined antibiotic therapy. Intravenous administration of antibiotics and treatment of peritonitis or tuboovarian abscess is required for 25% to 40% of women with this condition.

4. Define and cite causes of vaginitis, cervicitis, vulvovestibulitis, and bartholinitis.

Study text pages 830 and 832 and 833 refer to Figure 23-8.

Vaginitis is an infection of the vagina that is most often caused by sexually transmitted pathogens and *Candida albicans.* Because the acidic nature of vaginal secretions during the reproductive years provides protection against a variety of sexually transmitted pathogens, variables that alter the vaginal pH may predispose a woman to infection. The use of antibiotics may destroy *Lactobacillus acidophilus,* which helps maintain an acidic vaginal pH. With fewer *L. acidophilus* organisms, there may be an overgrowth of *C. albicans,* causing a yeast vaginitis.

Cervicitis is an inflammation of the cervix that is usually caused by one or more sexually transmitted

161

pathogens. A mucopurulent exudate drains from the external os. After diagnosis, oral antibiotics are used to prevent reinfection; sexual partners are treated as well.

Vulvovestibulitis is an inflammation of the skin of the vulva and often of the perianal area. It can be caused by contact with soaps, detergents, lotions, hygienic sprays, menstrual pads, perfumed toilet paper, or nonabsorbent or tight-fitting clothes. The condition also may represent an autoimmune reaction.

Bartholinitis is an inflammation of one or both of the ducts that lead from the vaginal opening to the Bartholin glands. The causes of bartholinitis are microorganisms that infect the lower female reproductive tract; this disorder is usually preceded by cervicitis, vaginitis, or urethritis. Infection or trauma may cause inflammatory changes that narrow the distal portion of the duct, thereby leading to obstruction and stasis of glandular secretions and causing further inflammation. Infection is treated with antibiotics. Pain is relieved with analgesics and warm sitz baths. Abscesses are surgically drained.

5. **Describe pelvic organ prolapse disorders.**

   Study text pages 787 through 790; refer to Figures 23-9 and 23-10 and Table 23-3.

   The bladder, urethra, and rectum are supported by the endopelvic fascia and perineal muscles. This muscular and fascial tissue loses tone and strength with aging and may fail to maintain the pelvic organ in the proper position. Trauma such as childbirth or pelvic surgery damages or weakens the supporting structures.

   Uterine prolapse is the descent of the cervix or entire uterus into the vaginal canal. **Cystocele** is the descent of the bladder and the anterior vaginal wall into the vaginal canal. A cystocele may cause the woman to lose urine when she laughs, sneezes, coughs, or does anything that strains the abdominal muscles. Cystocele is usually accompanied by **urethrocele,** which is the sagging of the urethra. Urethrocele is usually caused by the shearing effect of the fetal head on the urethra during childbirth. A **rectocele** is the bulging of the rectum and posterior vaginal wall into the vaginal canal. An enterocele is the herniation of the rectouterine pouch into the rectovaginal septum.

   Treatment includes isometric exercises to strengthen muscles, estrogens to improve tone and vascularity of fascial support, a pessary device to hold the uterus in position, stool softeners, and rarely surgery.

6. **Characterize the benign growth and proliferative conditions of the female reproductive system.**

   Study text pages 836 through 840; refer to Figures 23-11 through 23-16. See the table below.

7. **Characterize the malignant tumors of the female reproductive system**.

   Study text pages 841 through 848; refer to Figures 23-17 through 23-21 and Tables 23-5 through 23-8. See the table on page 163.

8. **Define the terms used to discuss female sexual dysfunction**.

   Study text pages 848 through 850; refer to Table 23-9.

   Inhibited sexual desire may be a biologic manifestation of depression, alcohol or other substance abuse, prolactin-secretin pituitary tumors, or testosterone deficiency. β-adrenergic blockers used for heart disease may also inhibit sexual desire.

Benign Lesions of the Female Reproductive System

Lesion	Causes	Manifestations
Ovarian cyst		
Follicular cyst	Ovarian follicle does not release ovum, fluid is not reabsorbed from degenerating follicle	Pelvic and abdominal pain, menstrual irregularities
Corpus luteum cyst	An underdeveloped, low-FSH corpus luteum, low progesterone and LH	Pelvic pain, amenorrhea with subsequent heavy bleeding
Endometrial polyps	Estrogen stimulation	Premenstrual or intermenstrual bleeding
Leiomyomas (smooth muscle tumor)	Unknown, estrogen/hormonal fluctuations alter size	Abnormal or increased uterine bleeding, pain, pressure
Adenomyosis (endometrial tissue in the myometrium)	Repeated pregnancies, women taking tamoxifen	Dysmenorrhea, uterine enlargement, tenderness
Endometriosis (ectopic endometrial functioning tissue)	Depressed Tc cells tolerate ectopic tissue, genetics	Ectopic tissues respond to hormonal stimulation, bleeding causes pelvic adhesions and pain

NOTE: Dermoid cysts are ovarian teratomas having malignant potential and should be removed. Ovarian torsion may occur as a complication of ovarian cysts.

Malignant Tumors of the Female Reproductive System

	Causes	Manifestations
Cervical cancer*	STD, human oncogenic papillomavirus (HPV), HIV, immunosuppression, early sexual activity, multiple sex partners, *Chlamydia trachomatis* infection inhibits host cell apoptosis, smoking, diet and vitamin deficiencies, genetic alternations	Asymptomatic vaginal bleeding or discharge, grade of epithelial thickness (Pap test) enables precursor lesion diagnosis
Vaginal cancer	Previous cervical cancer (similar etiology to cervical cancer), nonsteroidal estrogens	Asymptomatic vaginal bleeding or discharge
Vulvar cancer	HPV infection	Pruritus, bloody discharge, hard ulcer
Endometrial cancer	Obesity, no pregnancies, early menarche, late menopause, tamoxifen, unopposed estrogen replacement	Vaginal bleeding
Ovarian cancer†	Unknown, risk factors are similar to those for endometrial cancer, familial and personal history of breast cancer	Pain and abdominal swelling, postmenopausal bleeding, increased carcinoembryonic antigen in serum

*Preceding invasive cervical carcinoma are the progressively serious alterations of cervical intraepithelial neoplasia (cervical dysplasia) and cervical carcinoma in situ.

†CA-125 is a tumor marker for ovarian cancer. When elevated, it is highly suggestive.

NOTE: Treatments for these malignancies depend on the clinical staging, the extent of mestastases, and the age of the individual. Each lesion can be managed by surgery, radiation, or chemotherapy; a combination of all these modalities may be necessary as well as lymphadenectomy.

Vaginismus is an involuntary muscle spasm in response to attempted penetration. Common causes include prior sexual trauma, fear of sex, or organic disorders.

Anorgasmia is the inability of the woman to achieve orgasm. This inability ranges from difficulty in arousal to lack of orgasm. Any chronic illness may affect arousal. Orgasmic dysfunction is linked to organic causes in less than 5% of cases. Drugs such as narcotics, tranquilizers, antidepressants, and antihypertensive medications can inhibit orgasm.

Dyspareunia, which is another name for painful intercourse, is common. Inadequate lubrication may make penetration or intercourse unpleasant. Drugs with a drying effect (e.g., antihistamines, certain tranquilizers, marijuana) and disorders such as diabetes, vaginal infections, and estrogen deficiency can decrease lubrication. Other causes of dyspareunia include infections and anatomic constraints around the introitus or the vulva.

Infertility is the inability to conceive after 1 year of unprotected intercourse and affects approximately 15% of all couples. Important causes of infertility in the female are malfunctions of the fallopian tubes, the ovaries, or the reproductive hormones. Endometriosis also may contribute to infertility.

9. **Define and cite causes of common disorders of the male reproductive system.**
   Study text pages 850 through 860; refer to Figures 23-11 through 23-34 and Tables 23-10 and 23-11.

Urethritis is an inflammatory process that is usually caused by sexually transmitted microorganisms. Nonsexual origins of urethritis are inflammation or infection as a result of urologic procedures, insertion of foreign objects into the urethra, anatomic abnormalities, or trauma.

Urethral stricture is a narrowing of the urethra because of scarring. The scars may be congenital but are more likely to result from trauma or untreated or severe urethral infections.

Phimosis and **paraphimosis** are both disorders in which the penile foreskin, or prepuce, is "too tight" to be moved easily over the glans penis. In phimosis, the foreskin cannot be retracted back over the glans; whereas, in paraphimosis, the foreskin is retracted and cannot be moved forward to cover the glans. Phimosis can occur at any age and is most commonly caused by poor hygiene and chronic infection.

Peyronie disease is a fibrotic condition that causes lateral curvature of the penis during erection. The problem usually affects middle-aged men and is associated with painful erection, painful intercourse for

163

both partners, and poor erection distal to the involved area.

Priapism is a prolonged painful erection not stimulated by sexual arousal. The corpora cavernosa fill with blood that does not drain because of venous obstruction. It is associated with spinal cord trauma, sickle cell disease, leukemia, pelvic tumors, and intracavernous injection therapy for impotence.

Balanitis is an inflammation of the glans penis that usually occurs with an inflammation of the prepuce. It is associated with poor hygiene and phimosis. The accumulation under the foreskin of glandular secretions, sloughed epithelial cells, and *Mycobacterium smegmatis* can irritate the glans directly or lead to infection. Balanitis is most commonly seen in men with poorly controlled diabetes mellitus and candidiasis.

Penile cancer is rare in the United States. Although the exact etiology is unknown, cancer of the penis is likely a result of chronic irritation caused by smegma beneath a phimotic foreskin. A major risk factor is infection with HPV.

Varicocele, hydrocele, and spermatocele are common intrascrotal disorders. **Varicocele** is an abnormal dilation of a vein within the spermatic cord and most often occurs on the left side. Varicoceles may be painful or tender; they occur in 10% to 15% of males, frequently after puberty. The cause of varicoceles is incompetent or congenitally absent valves in the spermatic veins that normally prevent the backflow of blood; thus blood pools in the veins rather than flowing into the venous system. Decreased blood flow through the testis interferes with spermatogenesis and can cause infertility.

A **hydrocele** is a collection of fluid within the tunica vaginalis and is the most common cause of scrotal swelling. Hydroceles in infants are congenital malformations that frequently resolve spontaneously by 1 year of age. Hydroceles in adults may be caused by an imbalance between the secreting and absorptive capacities of scrotal tissues.

The **spermatocele** is a cyst that is located between the head of the epididymis and the testis. It is usually is asymptomatic or produces mild discomfort that is relieved by scrotal support.

Cryptorchidism is a condition in which one or both testes fail to descend into the scrotum. It is the most common congenital condition involving the testes. The cause of cryptorchidism is not clear, but it may result from a developmental delay, a defect of the testis, deficient maternal gonadotropin stimulation, or some mechanical factor that prevents descent through the inguinal canal. Untreated cryptorchidism is associated with lowered sperm count and impaired fertility. Undescended testes are susceptible to neoplastic processes.

Torsion of the testis is a condition in which the testis rotates on its vascular pedicle; this interrupts its blood supply. Onset may be spontaneous or follow physical exertion or trauma. If not corrected within 4 to 6 hours, necrosis and atrophy of testicular tissue occur.

Orchitis is an acute inflammation of the testes and is uncommon except as a complication of systemic infection or as an extension of an associated epididymitis. Mumps is the most common infectious cause of orchitis and usually affects post-pubertal males. The onset is sudden and occurs 3 to 4 days after the onset of parotitis. Irreversible damage to spermatogenesis results in about 30% of affected testes.

Testicular cancers are rare, accounting for approximately 1% of all cancers in males; however, they are the most common solid tumors of young adult men. The cure rate is greater than 95%. The etiology of testicular neoplasms is unknown. Because young men are affected most frequently, it is believed that high levels of androgens may contribute to carcinogenesis. A genetic predisposition also exists. Cryptorchidism also is statistically associated with the development of testicular cancer. Apparently, the undescended testis has a developmental defect or undergoes gradual involution and degeneration over time that may contribute to neoplastic changes.

Painless testicular enlargement usually is the first sign of testicular cancer. Enlargement is gradual and may be accompanied by a sensation of testicular heaviness or dull ache in the lower abdomen. Occasionally, acute pain occurs because of rapid growth; if this happens, there may be hemorrhage and necrosis.

Epididymitis, which is an inflammation of the epididymis, generally occurs in sexually active young males. In men younger than 35, the usual cause is a sexually transmitted microorganism. In men who are older than 35 years, intestinal bacteria and *Pseudomonas aeruginosa* found in urinary tract infections and prostatitis may also cause epididymitis. The pathogenic microorganism reaches the epididymis by ascending the vas deferens from an infected urethra or bladder. Acute and severe scrotal or inguinal pain is caused by inflammation of the epididymis and surrounding tissues. The individual may have pyuria and bacteriuria and a history of urinary symptoms including urethral discharge. Complications of epididymitis include abscess formation, infarction of the testis, recurrent infection, scarring of epididymal endothelium, and infertility.

10. **Distinguish among benign prostatic hyperplasia, prostatitis, and prostatic cancer.**
    Study text pages 860 through 869; refer to Figures 23-35 through 23-42.

Benign prostatic hyperplasia (BPH) is also called benign prostatic hypertrophy and causes problems as enlarged prostatic tissue compresses the prostatic urethra. Approximately 80% of men will have prostatic enlargement before age 80, and there is a 25% to 30% lifetime chance of needing prostatectomy for BPH once a man reaches 50 years of age. During the third decade of life, the prostate reaches adult size. Between 40 and 45 years of age, BPH begins and continues slowly until death. Current etiologic theories of BPH implicate estrogen/androgen synergism or undefined prostatic growth factors with possible additional hormonal involvement.

BPH begins in the periurethral glands, which are the inner glands or layers of the prostate. As nodular hyperplasia

164

and cellular hypertrophy progress, the compressed prostatic urethra usually (but not always) causes bladder outflow obstruction. During the early stages of urethral obstruction, the detrusor muscle hypertrophies to expel urine against increasing urethral resistance. The urge to urinate frequently, some delay in starting urination, and decreased force of the urinary stream develop. Over a period of several years, the bladder is unable to empty all of the urine, and urine retention becomes chronic.

Progressive bladder distention causes sacculations or diverticular outpouchings of the bladder wall. The ureters may be obstructed as they pass through the hypertrophied detrusor muscle; bladder or kidney infection then develops. Hyperplastic tissue may be removed surgically, drugs can be used to relax the smooth muscle of the bladder, and a specific drug may shrink the prostate gland by interrupting the action of hormones.

Prostatitis is an inflammation of the prostate that is usually limited to a few of the gland's excretory ducts. Prostatitis is categorized as acute bacterial prostatitis, chronic bacterial prostatitis, or nonbacterial prostatitis.

Acute bacterial prostatitis is an ascending infection of the urinary tract that tends to occur in men who are between 30 and 50 years of age, but it is also associated with BPH in older men. Coliform bacteria are common causes of bacterial prostatitis.

Symptoms include dysuria, urinary frequency, and lower abdominal and suprapubic discomfort. The individual may also have a slow, small urinary stream, an inability to empty the bladder, and the need to urinate frequently during the night. Systemic signs of infection include the sudden onset of a high fever, fatigue, joint pain, and muscle pain. Long-term, broad-spectrum antibiotics may be required to resolve the infection and control its spread. Pain relievers, antipyretics, bed rest, and adequate hydration are also used therapeutically.

Chronic bacterial prostatitis is characterized by recurrent urinary tract infections and the persistence of pathogenic bacteria. This type of prostatitis is the most common recurrent urinary tract infection in men.

Symptoms are variable and may be similar to those of acute bacterial prostatitis. The prostate may be only slightly enlarged, but fibrosis causes it to be firm and irregular in shape. Treatment of chronic bacterial prostatitis is difficult mainly because fibrosis blocks the passage of antibiotics into prostatic tissues; therefore, therapeutic levels are hard to achieve. The usual treatment is a 12-week course of antibiotics. If chronic bacterial prostatitis is not cured medically, a radical transurethral prostatectomy may be required.

Nonbacterial prostatitis is the most common prostatitis syndrome and consists of prostatic inflammation without evidence of bacterial infection. Its etiology is unclear. Men with nonbacterial prostatitis may complain of continuous or spasmodic pain in the suprapubic, infrapubic, scrotal, penile, or inguinal area. The prostate gland generally feels normal upon palpation. Nonbacterial prostatitis is diagnosed by exclusion. There is no generally accepted treatment for this condition; a course of antibiotics for both affected individuals and their sexual partners may minimize symptoms.

Prostatic cancer accounts for more than 14% of all cancer deaths in men in the United States; only lung cancer accounts for more male deaths. By age 85, the incidence is 1 in 6 for all American men; the incidence increases with advancing age. Prostatic cancer rarely occurs in men who are younger than 40 years. It is believed that both genetic/epigenetic and dietary influences play a role in the etiology of prostate cancer. Androgens act as tumor promoters through receptor mechanisms to enhance endogenous DNA carcinogens, including reactive oxygen species (ROS), reactive estrogen metabolites and estrogen, and environmental carcinogens. Also, there are changes in the balance between autocrine/paracrine growth-promoting and growth-inhibiting factors such as insulin growth factors (IGFs). Vasectomy has been identified as a possible risk factor for prostate cancer, because free testosterone levels elevate after vasectomy. There is no clear evidence of a causal link between BPH and prostate cancer even though they frequently occur together.

More than 95% of prostatic neoplasms are adenocarcinomas, and most occur in the periphery of the prostate. The aggressiveness of the neoplasm appears to be related to the degree of differentiation rather than the size of the tumor. Local extension is usually posterior, although late in the disease the tumor may invade the rectum or encroach on the prostatic urethra and cause bladder outlet obstruction. Sites of distant metastasis occur via lymph and blood vessels and include the lymph nodes, bones, lungs, liver, and adrenals. The pelvis, lumbar spine, femur, thoracic spine, and ribs are the most common sites of bone metastasis.

Prostatic cancer often causes no symptoms until it is far advanced. The first manifestations of disease are slow urinary stream, hesitancy, incomplete emptying, frequency, nocturia, and dysuria. Unlike the symptoms of obstruction caused by BPH, the symptoms of obstruction caused by prostatic cancer are progressive and do not temporarily remit. Symptoms of late disease include bone pain at sites of bone metastasis, edema of the lower extremities, enlarged lymph nodes, liver enlargement, pathologic bone fractures, and mental confusion associated with brain metastases.

Transrectal ultrasound (TRUS), prostatic-specific antigen (PSA) blood tests, and digital examination can validate the symptoms of prostatic cancer. The cutoff point between normal and abnormal PSA is a serum level of 4 ng/ml. Because PSA is organ specific, but not cancer specific, it can increase and overlap with BPH, prostatitis, infarct, manipulation from instrumentation, and ejaculation. Therefore progressions of PSA values have been proposed. These include the ratio between PSA and prostate gland volume, the rate of change in PSA with time, age-specific reference ranges, and total PSA or the ratio of free and bound PSA in the serum. Serial measures of PSA are useful in determining the response to treatment.

Treatment options include hormonal therapy, immunotherapy, chemotherapy, radiation therapy, surgery, or

165

any combination of these. Symptomatic relief of urinary obstruction, bladder outlet obstruction, colon obstruction, and spinal cord compression may be required.

11. Describe sexual dysfunction in the male.

Study text pages 869 through 871.

Male sexual dysfunction is the impairment of erection, emission, and ejaculation. In men who are older than 40 years, organic factors are involved in more than 50% of dysfunction cases.

Some arterial diseases diminish or interrupt circulation to the penis, thereby preventing the engorgement of erectile tissues in the corpora cavernosa and corpus spongiosum; erection is not possible. Inadequate secretion of the pituitary gonadotropins, feminizing tumors, estrogen therapy, and testicular atrophy from any cause decrease testosterone levels and contribute to sexual dysfunction.

Neurologic disorders can interfere with the important sympathetic, parasympathetic, and central nervous system mechanisms of erection, emission, and ejaculation. Upper motor neuron lesions prevent emission and ejaculation. Lesions that affect the lower motor neurons usually prevent erection and often prevent emission and ejaculation.

Diabetes mellitus causes both peripheral vascular and neurologic pathology, which lead to erectile dysfunction. Pelvic surgery can create erectile dysfunction by severing small nerve branches that are essential for erection. Men who are taking antihypertensives, antidepressants, antihistamines, antispasmodics, sedatives, tranquilizers, barbiturates, diuretics, sex hormone preparations, narcotics, or psychoactive drugs or who consume ethyl alcohol experience sexual dysfunction.

Spermatogenesis can be impaired by disruptions of the hypothalamic-pituitary-testicular axis that reduces testosterone secretion, as well as by testicular trauma or atrophy from any cause. Sperm production is also impaired by neoplastic disease, cryptorchidism, or increased testicular temperature from any factor.

12. Describe galactorrhea.

Study text pages 871 and 872; refer to Box 23-14.

Galactorrhea, or inappropriate lactation, is the persistent secretion of a milky substance by one or both breasts in a nonpregnant, nonlactating woman. Its most common cause is a rise in severe prolactin levels unassociated with pregnancy and childbirth. Hyperprolactinemia can be caused by medication, benign pituitary tumors, hypothyroidism, chronic stress, or "persistent and repeated" suckling.

If a pituitary tumor is found, it may be surgically removed. A microadenoma and a macroadenoma may be treated with appropriate medication depending on the size and location.

13. Differentiate between benign and malignant female breast disease.

Study text pages 872 through 875, 877, 880 through 893, and through 909; refer to Figures 23-43 through 23-62 and Tables 23-12 through 23-19.

14. Describe gynecomastia and male breast cancer.

Study text page 909.

Gynecomastia is the overdevelopment of breast tissue in a male. Gynecomastia accounts for approximately 85% of all masses that develop in the male breast, and it affects approximately 35% of the male population. Incidence is greatest among adolescents and men who are older than 50 years.

Gynecomastia usually involves an imbalance of the estrogen-testosterone ratio. The ratio can be altered by tumor- and drug-induced hyperestrogenism that elevates the estrogen levels while the testosterone levels remain normal. Testosterone levels may be extremely low with normal estrogen levels in hypergonadism. Gynecomastia also can be caused by increased breast tissue responsiveness to estrogen or decreased responsiveness to androgen. Estrogen-testosterone imbalances are associated with hypogonadism, Klinefelter syndrome, testicular neoplasms, cirrhosis of the liver, infectious hepatitis, chronic renal failure, chronic obstructive lung disease, hyperthyroidism, tuberculosis, and chronic malnutrition.

Hyperplasia results in a firm, palpable mass at least 2 cm in diameter that is located beneath the areola. Treatment with androgen is likely to resolve the gynecomastia.

Male breast cancer accounts for 1% of all male cancers and is seen most often after age 60 years. Most are estrogen-receptor positive. The lesion is usually a unilateral solid mass located near the nipple and crusting and nipple discharge are typical manifestations. Male breast cancer tends to be advanced at the time of diagnosis and therefore has a poor prognosis. Endocrine therapy is used; however, the mainstay of treatment is modified mastectomy with axillary node removal to assess stage.

PRACTICE EXAMINATION

Multiple Choice

Circle the correct answer for each question.

1. The cause of dysmenorrhea usually involves:
   a. excessive endometrial prostaglandin production.
   b. failure of ovarian follicle maturation.
   c. decreased myometrial contractions.
   d. purulent material draining from the uterine tube.
2. Secondary amenorrhea is:
   a. failure to begin menstruation by age 20.
   b. menarche failure.
   c. increased myometrial vasculature constriction.
   d. the absence of menstruation following menarche.
3. What is the likely pathophysiology of PMS?
   a. Elevated prolactin levels cause salt and water retention.
   b. Elevated aldosterone levels cause salt and water retention.
   c. An abnormal nervous, immunologic, vascular, and gastrointestinal response to the menstrual cycle is causative.
   d. Both a and b are correct.

166

Benign/Malignant Female Breast Disorders

Disorder	Risks	Pathophysiology	Manifestations	Treatment
Proliferative lesions without atypia • Epithelial hyperplasia • Sclerosing adenosis • Complex sclerosing lesions (radial scar)* • Papilloma* • Fibroadenoma *Proliferative lesions with atypia* • Atypical ductal and lobular hyperplasia	Puberty to lifetime; proliferative lesions without atypia generally demonstrate no added risk for cancer; proliferative lesions with atypia hyperplasia have increased risk for cancer development	Increased estrogen levels, alterations in estrogen-to-progesterone ratio; genetic alterations	Fluctuating lesion size; mobile multiple lesions; cysts are evident radiographically; possible nipple discharge; breast tenderness with menstrual cycle	Cyst drainage; surgical excision of mass or duct or breast segment, possible mastectomy (extend of surgery depends on atypia); pain relief by synthetic androgens
Breast cancer	Increases with age: Lifetime risk is 1 in 8 for non-Hispanic white women and less for others No term pregnancies, long reproductive life; ionizing radiation; high-fat diet; physical inactivity; alcohol ingestion; first-degree relatives	Estrogens (endogenous and exogenous) and their receptors have a proliferative effect on mammary gland epithelium; estrogens may increase susceptibility to environmental carcinogens, oxidative catabolism of estrogens generate reactive oxygen species (ROS) that cause genetic damage transforming growth factor (TGF), insulin-like growth factor (IGF), epidermal growth factor (EGF), platelet-derived growth factor (PDGF); mutations of *BRCA1* and *BRCA2*, and other related genes *(p53, Bcl-2, Her2, c-myc)*	Painless or painful mass, skin retraction over lesion; nipple puckering and discharge; hemorrhage *After metastasis:* palpable axillary lymph nodes, bone pain, site-specific signs and symptoms; approximately 50% of breast cancers occur in the upper quadrant because of predominant glandular tissue at site	Surgery to remove lesion; radiation to prevent metastasis; chemotherapy; hormones for hormone-dependent tumors; herceptin (antibody), antiestrogens (tamoxifen) antiestrogens, bone marrow transplantation; treatment depends on stage or extent

NOTE: Breast carcinogenesis involves uncontrolled cellular proliferation, alterations in cell signaling pathways, and aberrant or loss of apoptosis as a consequence of accumulated genetic damage. Germline mutation or acquired somatic mutations as a result of environment carcinogens transform the phenotype. Changes in malignant cells are accompanied or preceded by alterations in the supporting myoepithelial and stromal cells because of genetic and epigenetic events. The final alteration, invasion of the stroma, likely is the result of loss of myoepithelial and stromal cells that maintain the basement membrane.

NOTE: Ductal carcinoma in situ (DCIS) refers to a heterogenous group of lesions. These lesions are presumed to be malignant epithelial cells of the ductal system. The increase in the incidence of DCIS may reflect an increase in cancer or increased detection by mammography.

4. A yeast vaginitis may be caused by:
   a. an overgrowth of *Candida albicans.*
   b. a declining number of lactobacilli.
   c. the chronic use of antibiotics.
   d. a, b, and c are correct.
   e. None of the above is correct.
5. Vulvovestibulitis:
   a. is an inflammation of the cervix.
   b. can be caused by contact with perfumed toilet paper or menstrual pads.
   c. is an inflammation of the Bartholin glands.
   d. is a vaginal infection that has spread to the labia.
   e. Both b and c are correct.
6. Ovarian cancer exhibits:
   a. smooth muscle lesion features.
   b. human papillomavirus infection.
   c. ectopic endometrial functioning tissue.
   d. increased serum levels of CA-125.
   e. Both b and c are correct.
7. Depressed T-cell function is associated with:
   a. follicular cysts.
   b. endometrial polyps.
   c. leiomyomas.
   d. adenomyosis.
   e. endometriosis.
8. It is possible that repeated pregnancies cause:
   a. ovarian cysts.
   b. endometriosis.
   c. leiomyomas.
   d. adenomyosis.
   e. polyps.
9. A 42-year-old retired prostitute who became sexually active at 14 years of age is at risk to develop:
   a. endometriosis.
   b. cervical carcinoma.
   c. breast cancer.
   d. uterine carcinoma.
10. Your neighbor's obese grandmother has breast cancer. Your neighbor's risk factors are greatest for which of the following types of cancer?
   a. cervical
   b. vaginal
   c. endometrial
   d. ovarian
11. Painful intercourse is:
   a. the inability to achieve orgasm.
   b. inhibited sexual desire.
   c. muscle spasm in response to attempted penetration.
   d. dyspareunia.
12. Female breast cancer pathophysiology involves:
   a. *BRCA1* and *BRCA2* mutations.
   b. reactive oxygen species.
   c. endogenous and exogenous estrogens and their receptors.
   d. *Her-2/neu* gene mutations.
   e. All of the above are correct.

13. Phimosis is:
   a. a thickening of the fascia in the erectile tissue of the corpora cavernosa.
   b. a condition in which a retracted foreskin cannot be moved forward.
   c. a condition in which the foreskin cannot be retracted.
   d. caused by poor hygiene and chronic infection.
   e. Both c and d are correct.
14. A varicocele is an intrascrotal disorder that:
   a. results in a collection of fluid within the tunica vaginalis.
   b. occurs because of independent or congenitally absent valves in the spermatic veins.
   c. is located between the head of the epididymis and the testis.
   d. does not interfere with spermatogenesis.
15. Cryptorchidism is:
   a. underdevelopment of the testes.
   b. the absence of scrotal tissue.
   c. relieved by scrotal support.
   d. failure of the testes to descend into the scrotum.
   e. an imbalance between the secreting and absorptive capacities of scrotal tissues.
16. The infectious cause of orchitis is:
   a. streptococci.
   b. gonococci.
   c. chlamydial organisms.
   d. mumps virus.
17. Which of the following organisms can cause epididymitis?
   a. Enterobacteriaceae
   b. *Neisseria gonorrhoeae*
   c. *Pseudomonas aeruginosa*
   d. All of the above are correct.
   e. None of the above is correct.
18. In benign prostatic hyperplasia, enlargement of periurethral tissue of the prostate causes:
   a. obstruction of the urethra.
   b. inflammation of the testis.
   c. decreased urinary outflow from the bladder.
   d. abnormal dilation of a vein within the spermatic cord.
   e. tension of the spermatic cord and testis.
19. A major cause of recurrent urinary tract infections in the male is:
   a. orchitis.
   b. balanitis.
   c. epididymitis.
   d. chronic bacterial prostatitis.
   e. nonbacterial prostatitis.
20. A symptom or sign of late-stage prostatic cancer is:
   a. a slow urinary stream.
   b. frequency of urination.
   c. incomplete emptying of the bladder.
   d. mental confusion.
   e. a, b, and c are correct.

21. Male sexual dysfunction may be caused by:
    a. infection around the introitus.
    b. diabetes mellitus.
    c. infected hymenal remnants.
    d. None of the above is correct.
22. Which of the following is true about acute pelvic inflammatory disease (PID)?
    a. It primarily affects males.
    b. It is usually caused by viruses.
    c. It never causes peritonitis.
    d. It involves the epididymis.
    e. It may cause infertility or tubular pregnancy.
23. Female breast disorders exhibiting proliferative lesions with atypia have:
    a. no added risk for cancer development.
    b. similar risks for fibrocystic disease.
    c. slightly increased risk for cancer development.
    d. increased risk for cancer development.

24. Breast cancer:
    a. exhibits fluctuating lesion size.
    b. pain increases as menstruation approaches.
    c. exhibits painless lumps.
    d. at age 50 years affects 1 in 200 females.
25. After metastasis, female breast cancer manifests as:
    a. nipple puckering.
    b. bone pain.
    c. nipple discharge
    d. skin refraction over the lesion.
    e. a, c, and d are correct.

CASE STUDY 1

B.J. is a 63-year-old retired white female who is physically fit and socially active. She is the mother of two children and has high blood pressure and high cholesterol, both are controlled with medications. On her annual visit to her gynecologist, Dr. F., she reported that she recently had developed a serous, lightly blood-tinged vaginal discharge. Having been postmenopausal since age 52, she expressed concern about this discharge. She also reported that she had been trying to decrease the amount of the hormone replacement therapy (HRT) she had been using since her perimenopausal phase which began at age 49. B.J. asks Dr. F., "What is going on here? I am too old to be having periods again." After the typical gynecological exam including a pap smear, Dr. F. suggested that B.J.'s recent self-regulating of her hormone therapy and a possible irritated vaginal wall could account for the discharge and prescribed a vaginal hormone cream to be used for two weeks, and suggested that B.J. continue low dose HRT. This did not stop the discharge, and so a few weeks later, an endometrial biopsy and culture of the discharge were done. Both came back negative, as had the pap smear, so Dr. F. prescribed additional progesterone for two months. After 4 months of continual serous discharge becoming more blood-tinged, B.J. again contacted Dr. F. and said, "This discharge is continual, getting bloodier, and cannot be normal, what do we need to do right now?"

Questions
What further diagnostic tests are indicated?

169

What additional diagnostic tests are necessary?

After the completed tests and results are available, what is needed?

Mrs. B. is a 46-year-old woman who consults her physician about the nature of a lump in her left breast. About 3 months ago, Mrs. B.'s spouse noticed a small lump in her left breast; however, Mrs. B was unconcerned because she experienced small lumps in her breast around the time of her menses. However, this lump seemed to be growing and did not seem to fluctuate in size, as it had in the past. Three small lumps that fluctuated in size were noticed by Mrs. B. in her right breast. She stated, "I am in excellent health, exercise daily, and neither smoke nor drink alcohol."

Mrs. B. is the mother of two preteen children. After the birth of her last child, she took birth control pills for 8 years and then selected an alternative method of birth control. Her onset of menses occurred at age 10. Her family history reveals that her mother and one of her three aunts died of breast cancer; otherwise, her history is noncontributing.

On examination, a 2- to 3-cm mass was palpated in the upper quadrant of Mrs. B.'s left breast. This mass was firm, affixed to the chest wall, and slightly tender to touch. The skin and nipple appeared normal. Under the left axilla, a node about the size of a pea was palpable. Three 1- to 2-cm soft, movable masses were palpated in Mrs. B.'s right breast.

Mammography confirmed the presence of a 3-cm mass in the left breast and four 1.5-cm masses in the right breast. All other diagnostic procedures were negative.

Question

What thoughts do you have concerning Mrs. B.'s examination and her risk factors?

24 Sexually Transmitted Infections

FOUNDATIONAL KNOWLEDGE OBJECTIVES

a. Identify the female reproductive structures.
Refer to figures 22-4 and 22-5.

MEMORY CHECK!

- The external genitalia collectively are called the vulva and comprise the visible structures: the mons pubis, the labia majora, the labia minora, the clitoris, and the vestibule. The urethral meatus, the vaginal opening, and two sets of glands (the Skene glands and the Bartholin glands) open onto the vestibule. The internal organs of the female reproductive system are two ovaries, two fallopian tubes (uterine tubes), the uterus, and the vagina. The ovaries are the primary female reproductive organs. They are located on both sides of the uterus and are suspended and supported by ligaments.
- The fallopian tubes extend from the ovaries to the uterus and open into the uterine cavity, thereby providing a direct communication from the peritoneal cavity to the uterine cavity. The uterus lies centrally in the pelvis and is divided structurally into the body (the corpus) and the cervix. The inner layer, which is the endometrium, consists of surface epithelium, glands, and connective tissue. The endometrium is shed during menstruation. At the lowest portion of the corpus is the internal os of the cervix. The external os is at the lower end of the cervix. The canal of the cervix provides a direct communication from the cavity of the uterine body through the internal os and the external os to the vagina.
- The vagina extends from the cervix of the uterus to the vaginal opening; thus there is continuous communication from outside the body to the peritoneal cavity through the reproductive system structures.

b. Identify the male reproductive structures.
Refer to figures 22-11, 22-13, 22-14.

MEMORY CHECK!

- The male reproductive structures are the penis, the testes in the scrotal sac, the duct system (including the epididymis), the vas deferens, the ejaculatory ducts, the urethra, and the accessory glands, which include the seminal vesicles, the prostate, and the bulbourethral glands.
- The testes are divided internally into lobules that contain the seminiferous tubules and Leydig cells. Sperm production takes place in the seminiferous tubules; Leydig cells secrete testosterone. On the posterior portion of each testis is a coiled duct, which is the epididymis. The head of the epididymis is connected with the seminiferous tubule of the testis, and its tail is continuous with the vas deferens. The vas deferens is the excretory duct of the testis. It extends to the duct of the seminal vesicle and joins with it to form the ejaculatory duct. The ejaculatory duct joins the urethra, which is the common passageway to the outside of the body for both sperm and urine. The accessory glands communicate with the duct system. The prostate surrounds the neck of the bladder and the upper urethra. Its glandular ducts open into the urethra. The bulbourethral glands, which are also called Cowper glands, are located near the urethral meatus. The penis is composed of three elongated cylindrical masses of erectile tissue, which comprise the shaft of the penis. The inner, ventral mass is the corpus spongiosum, which contains the urethra. The two outer, dorsal, parallel masses are the corpora cavernosa. The distal end of the penis or the glans is covered by the prepuce, also called the foreskin.

173

c. Identify tests used to diagnose sexually transmitted infections (STIs).
Refer to Table 22-2.

MEMORY CHECK!

Diagnostic Tests for Common STIs

Tests for Gonorrhea

Culture	Isolation and detection of *Neisseria gonorrhoeae* in urethral, anal, and/or pharyngeal secretions
Gram stain	Direct smear and staining of cervical or urethral discharge to identify gram-negative intracellular diplococci within polymorphonuclear leukocytes
DNA probe	A sample fragment of DNA hybridizes DNA of microbe

Tests for Syphilis

	Detection of antibodies to *Treponema pallidum*
RPR	Rapid plasma reagin
FTA	Fluorescent treponemal antibody absorption test
Dark-field examination	Direct smear of serous exudate from moist lesions to detect *T. pallidum* with corkscrew appearance

Tests for Chlamydia

Antigen detection	Direct immunofluorescence staining of cervical and/or urethral specimens to detect monoclonal antibodies or genetic probe to detect DNA or probe DNA sequence
Tissue culture	Isolation and detection of *Chlamydia trachomatis* from epithelial cells of endocervix and urethra
Cervical wet mount	Wet mount preparation of endocervical secretions, to rule out gonococci and *C. trachomatis*

Tests for HIV Infection

ELISA (enzyme-linked immunosorbent assay)	Detects the presence of antibodies to HIV
IFA (indirect fluorescent antibody)	A more specific, definitive test for HIV
WB (Western blot)	An even more specific, definitive test for HIV

Tests for Other Viral Infections

TORCH test	Detects elevations of IgA and IgM caused by toxoplasma, rubella, cytomegalovirus, syphilis, and herpes simplex in mother and newborn infant; herpes requires more specific follow-up testing if positive
Cytomegalovirus	Cell culture with samples from urine, cervix, semen, saliva, and blood can reveal cytopathic effects of virus
HPV testing	Detects human papillomavirus (HPV), which is a primary cause of cervical cancer

LEARNING OBJECTIVES

After studying this chapter, the learner will be able to do the following:

1. **State the current status of sexually transmitted infections.**

   Study text pages 923 and 924; refer to Table 24-1.

   The study and categorization of sexually transmitted infections (STIs) have broadened to include bacterial, viral, protozoan, parasitic, and fungal agents as causes of STIs. The virus-induced STIs are generally considered incurable. The incidence and increase in STIs are due to earlier sexual activity and a greater number of lifetime sexual partners, increased premarital sex, nonmonogamy among married

people, and bisexuality. These factors contribute to an increased exposure to STIs. The number of individuals who fail to take protective measures when engaging in sexual activities also contributes to the problem. STIs are prevalent among all individuals in all socioeconomic groups.

2. **Characterize the bacterial STIs; focus on infectious agents, manifestations, and complications.**

   Study text pages 924 through 930 and 932 through 938; refer to Figures 24-1 through 24-10 and Table 24-2. See page 175.

3. **Characterize the viral STIs; focus on infectious agents, manifestations, and complications.**

   Study text pages 938 through 942; refer to Figures 24-11 through 24-15. See page 175.

Bacterial and Bacterial-like STIs

Disease/Infectious Agent	Manifestations	Major Complications
Gonorrhea/*Neisseria gonorrhoeae* (gram-negative diplococcus)	Possibly asymptomatic; urethritis; cervicitis; mucopurulent discharge; anorectal infection; pharyngitis; conjunctivitis	Epididymitis and lymphangitis; salpingitis; infertility; disseminated bloodstream infection; neonatal blindness
Syphilis*/*Treponema pallidum* (anaerobic spirochete)	Primary: nonpainful chancre at site of invasion; secondary: systemic involvement with skin rash and lymphadenopathy; tertiary: gummas	Destructive lesions in cardiovascular and nervous systems; congenital: dental deformations, destructive bone lesions
Chancroid/*Haemophilus ducreyi* (gram-negative bacillus)	Papule erodes into painful ulcer; superficial exudate; painful lymphadenopathy	Phimosis; paraphimosis; ulcers that heal in one area while spreading to another area
Granuloma inguinale/ *Calymmatobacterium granulomatis* (predominant in tropical climates) (gram-negative bacillus)	Painless; indurated, subcutaneous nodules of distal penis and introitus	Possible spread to bones, joints, and liver
Bacterial vaginosis/*Gardnerella vaginitis* and other anaerobes (gram-negative bacilli)	Thin and scant malodorous vaginal discharge	Possible PID; chorioamnionitis; preterm labor; postpartum endometriosis
Urogenital infections (gram-negative intracellular microbe) Lymphogranuloma venereum (LGV)/*Chlamydia trachomatis* (endemic in southern hemisphere)	Commonly associated with other STIs; purulent discharge; cervicitis; urethritis; proctitis; newborn conjunctivitis and pneumonia; tender lymph node and inguinal buboes	Epididymitis; Reiter syndrome; tubule infertility in women; arthritis; in secondary LGV, there may be disrupted lymph node function, meningitis, or pneumonitis

NOTE: Bacterial STIs and bacterial-like STIs are treated with appropriate antibiotics. (Gonorrhea: cephalosporin; syphilis: parenteral penicillin G; chancroid: IM ceftriaxone or multiple doses of ciprofloxacin or erythromycin; vaginosis: 7 days of metronidazole; and LGV: 21 days of doxycycline or erthromycin). Simultaneous treatment of sexual partners and condom use are recommended to prevent reinfection. All genital ulcerative lesions play a role in HIV transmission.

*Latent syphilis exhibits no clinical signs of infection but transmission of infection is possible.

Viral STIs

Disease/Infectious Agent	Manifestations	Major Complications
Genital herpes/Herpes simplex virus (HSV-1 or HSV-2)	Painful blister-like lesions on external genitalia and genital involvement	Spontaneous abortion; neonatal morbidity and mortality from CNS tracts
Condylomata acuminata (warts)/Human papillomavirus (HPV)	Soft, skin-colored single or clustered growths	Cervical dysplasia and cancer; anorectal and penile cancer
Molluscum contagiosum virus (STI and fomites)	Flesh-colored papules with a thick, creamy core	Papules persist months or years because of autoinoculation

NOTE: Treatment for HSV is not curative, but oral and topical antiviral agents (acyclovir) are used to lower recurrence and reduce symptoms; HPV lesions are treated with topical agents and surgery. Molluscum contagiosum can be treated by curettage or cryotherapy.

4. **Characterize the parasitic STIs by infectious agents and manifestations**.

Study text pages 942 through 946; refer to Figures 24-16 through 24-18. See table below.

5. **Identify systemic infections that may be transmitted sexually**.

Study text pages 946 through 948; refer to Figure 24-19. See table below.

Parasitic STIs

Disease/Infectious Agent	Manifestations
Trichomoniasis/*Trichomonas vaginalis* (protozoa)	Vaginal walls are erythematous; vaginal discharge; pruritus; painful intercourse; dysuria
Scabies/*Sarcoptes scabiei* (female itch mite)	Intense pruritus
Pediculosis pubis (crabs)/*Phthirus pubis* (crab louse, STI, and fomites)	Pruritus

NOTE: Treatment of these conditions is with antitrichosmomal agents, scabicides, prescription creams, and effective hygiene practices.

Other Systems Affected by STIs

Disease/Infectious Agent	Transmission Modes	Manifestations
Shigellosis/*Shigella sp.* (gram-negative bacillus) and *Campylobacter enteritis* (gram-negative bacillus)	Contact with infected feces by anal-oral or genital-anal contact	Fever; abdominal distention: diarrhea; dysentery with bloody discharge
Giardiasis/*Giardia lamblia* (protozoa)	Anal-oral or genital-anal contact	Sudden and explosive diarrhea; abdominal distention; flatulence; epigastric pain; nausea and vomiting
Amebiasis/*Entamoeba histolytica* (protozoa)	Anal-oral or genital-anal contact	Mild diarrhea to severe dysentery; may spread to liver
Hepatitis B/Hepatitis B virus	Needle puncture; blood transfusion; cuts in mucous membranes and skin; perinatal transmission	Rash; urticaria; polyarthralgias; arthritis; jaundice; liver enlargement with infected body fluids; neonatal death
AIDS/Human immunodeficiency virus (HIV)	Inoculation with contaminated blood; perinatal transmission	Depressed immune system and opportunistic infections; malignancies
Cytomegalic inclusion disease/ Cytomegalovirus (CMV)	Interpersonal contact or direct transfer of cells or body fluids; perinatal transmission	Mild subclinical illness; life-threatening in the immunocompromised; congenitally infected may have hepatosplenomegaly and neurologic deficits

NOTE: Treatment is as earlier indicated for bacterial, protozoan, and viral diseases.

Matching

Match the STI with the causative agent.

_____ 1. Gonorrhea

_____ 2. Syphilis

_____ 3. Condylomata acuminata

_____ 4. Pediculosis pubis

_____ 5. Amebiasis

a. *Haemophilus ducreyi*

b. *Mycoplasma hominis*

c. *Neisseria gonorrhoeae*

d. *Gardnerella vaginalis*

e. *Treponema pallidum*

f. Human papillomavirus

g. *Sarcoptes scabiei*

h. *Phthirus pubis*

i. *Entamoeba histolytica*

j. *Trichomonas vaginalis*

Fill in the Blanks

Supply the correct response for each statement.

6. Gonococcal infectious transfer to the newborn results in _____.

7. The organism that causes syphilis can be identified by _____.

8. The organism that causes trichomoniasis is a _____.

9. A clinical manifestation associated with HSV-2 infection is _____.

10. *Treponema pallidum* spirochetes infect fetuses by crossing the _____.

11. Chlamydial infections in women may result in _____.

12. Bacterial vaginosis produces a thin, _____ vaginal discharge.

13. The risk of developing gonorrhea with an infected male partner is _____ for females, and with an infected female partner is 20% to 30% for males.

14. Women who have gonorrhea are frequently _____.

15. The secondary stage of syphilis is characterized by a _____.

16. _____ is an _____ bacteria *not* cultured in standard bacterial medium.

17. _____ is a treatment for genital herpes that minimizes recurrent infections.

18. _____ are warts.

19. _____ is a manifestation of scabies.

20. Amebiasis may spread to the _____.

21. Human papillomaviruses may lead to _____ or _____ cancer.

22. A _____ can detect gonorrhea and is helpful since anaerobic incubation is not required.

23. A complication of chlamydial infection in men is _____.

24. Giardiasis may exhibit _____ pain.

25. Neonatal infection with hepatitis B virus may result in neonatal _____.

Ms. C.T., a 23-year-old, recently divorced woman, presented to her physician for her annual gynecologic examination. She states, "I am experiencing a gray-white, creamy vaginal discharge that has a heavy, fishy odor." She admits to having more than one current sex partner, to a history of multiple sex partners, and to not using nonbarrier contraception.

Ms. C.T.'s physical examination reveals lower abdominal and pelvic pain; all other physical signs are normal except that she has a slightly elevated temperature. There are no blisters on the vulva. Her pelvic examination shows cervical edematous congestion and a mucopurulent discharge. A Gram stain of the mucopurulent discharge revealed no intracellular gram-negative diplococci within the polymorphonuclear leukocytes.

Questions

What do you consider to be the most likely cause of Ms. C.T.'s signs and symptoms?

What tests might be ordered to validate any presumptive diagnosis?

25 Structure and Function of the Hematologic System

PREREQUISITE KNOWLEDGE OBJECTIVES

After reviewing the primary text where referenced, the learner will be able to do the following:
1. **Identify the constituents of blood plasma.**
   Review text pages 952 through 954; refer to Table 25-1.
2. **Identify the structural characteristics, normal values, and functions of the cellular elements of blood.**
   Review text pages 954 through 957; refer to Figures 25-1 through 25-4 and Tables 25-2 and 25-3.
3. **Describe the lymphoid organs.**
   Review pages 957 through 960; refer to Figures 25-5 through 25-7.
4. **Define hematopoiesis and describe erythropoiesis; identify the CSFs and nutritional requirements necessary for these processes.**
   Review text pages 960 through 963, 965 through 969, 971; refer to Figures 25-8 through 25-16 and Tables 25-4 through 25-6.
5. **Describe the development of leukocytes and platelets.**
   Review text pages 971 and 972; refer to Figures 25-9.
6. **Describe the sequence of events in hemostasis.**
   Review text pages 972, 973 and 976 through 979; refer to Figures 25-16, 25-17 through 25-24 and Tables 25-7 and 25-8.
7. **Diagram the fibrinolytic system.**
   Refer to Figure 25-28.
8. **Describe information that can be obtained from bone marrow biopsy and various blood tests.**
   Refer to Tables 25-9 and 28-10.
9. **Identify various hematologic values during infancy and childhood.**
   Refer to Table 25-11.

PRACTICE EXAMINATION

Multiple Choice

Circle the correct answer for each question.
1. Which is *not* a plasma component?
   a. Colloids
   b. Electrolytes
   c. Gases
   d. Glucose
   e. Platelets

2. Which is the most abundant protein in blood plasma?
   a. Fibrinogen
   b. Albumins
   c. Globulins
   d. Immunoglobulins
   e. Hormones
3. A fragment of megakaryocytic cytoplasm is the:
   a. reticulocyte.
   b. normoblast.
   c. promyelocyte.
   d. proerythroblast.
   e. platelet.
4. Mast cell mediators are available to:
   a. vascular endothelial cells.
   b. nerves.
   c. immune cells.
   d. a and c are correct.
   e. a, b, and c are correct.
5. Identify the differentiation pathway in the development of erythrocytes.
   a. Uncommitted pluripotential stem cell—normoblast—reticulocyte
   b. Normoblast—reticulocyte—basophilic erythroblast
   c. Normoblast—committed proerythroblast—reticulocyte
   d. Normoblast—basophilic erythroblast—reticulocyte
6. A differential count of WBCs includes all of the following *except*:
   a. granulocytes.
   b. agranulocytes.
   c. reticulocytes.
   d. monocytes.
   e. lymphocytes.
7. The main regulator of platelet circulating mass is:
   a. GP IIb/IIIa complex.
   b. ADP.
   c. thrombopoietin.
   d. thromboxane.
8. The normal platelet count/mm^3 of blood is about:
   a. 4 to 10 $\times$ 10^3.
   b. 50 to 100 $\times$ 10^3.
   c. 140 to 340 $\times$ 10^3.
   d. 5 $\times$ 10^6.
   e. 150 to 300 $\times$ 10^6.

179

9. The hematocrit is the:
   a. number of RBCs in plasma.
   b. aqueous portion of blood.
   c. criterion of blood flow.
   d. percentage of RBCs in a given volume of blood.
   e. amount of hemoglobin by weight in blood.
10. If the total leukocytic count of an individual was 7000/mm^3, about how many neutrophils would normally be present in a mm^3 of blood?
    a. 400
    b. 700
    c. 2100
    d. 3000
    e. 4200
11. Which granulocyte functions in antibody-mediated defense against parasites?
    a. Lymphocyte
    b. Monocyte
    c. Neutrophil
    d. Eosinophil
    e. Basophil
12. About how many times more RBCs than WBCs are there in a mm^3 of blood?
    a. 15
    b. 90
    c. 100
    d. 1000
    e. None of the above is correct.
13. Which is an agranulocyte?
    a. Basophil
    b. Lymphocyte
    c. Neutrophil
    d. Polymorph
14. Which are the most effective phagocytes?
    a. Neutrophils and basophils
    b. Lymphocytes and eosinophils
    c. Basophils and monocytes
    d. Neutrophils and monocytes
    e. None of the above is correct.

15. Erythropoiesis requires vitamins:
    a. C and E.
    b. B$_2$ and B$_{12}$.
    c. A and D.
    d. Both a and b are correct.
    e. a, b, and c are correct.
16. Nitric oxide and prostacyclin:
    a. inhibit platelet adhesion and aggregation.
    b. are vasoconstrictors.
    c. are produced by erythrocytes.
    d. are sporadically produced.
17. Which test reflects bone marrow activity?
    a. Reticulocyte count
    b. Mean corpuscular hemoglobin (MCH)
    c. Mean corpuscular volume (MCV)
    d. Hematrocit (HCT)
18. As an individual ages:
    a. the erythrocyte life span is shortened.
    b. lymphocytic function decreases.
    c. platelet numbers decrease.
    d. All of the above are correct.

Fill in the Blanks

Supply the correct response for each statement.

In the coagulation cascade, (19) _____ is the primary cellular initiator of blood coagulation at the injury/wound site. After vessel injury, the (20) _____ complex leads to platelet activation and fibrin deposition. In the fibrinolytic system, (21) _____ is released from perturbed endothelial cells near the site of vascular injury and converts plasminogen to plasmin. Both t-PA and plasminogen bind to (22) _____, causing plasmin generation and localized (23) _____.

Matching

Match the colony-stimulating factor with the cells that are stimulated.

_____ 24. IL-3

_____ 25. G-CSF

a. erythrocyte

b. pluripotent stem cell

c. macrophage, fibroblast, neutrophil

d. normoblast

e. erythroblast

26 Alterations of Erythrocyte Function

FOUNDATIONAL KNOWLEDGE OBJECTIVES

MEMORY CHECK!

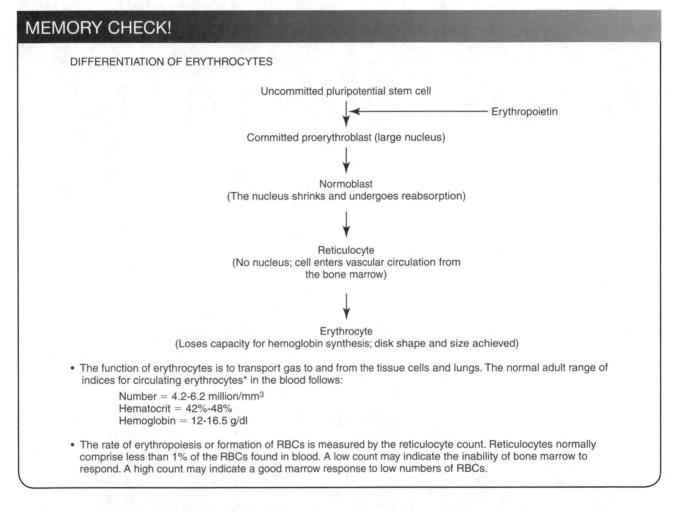

DIFFERENTIATION OF ERYTHROCYTES

Uncommitted pluripotential stem cell

← Erythropoietin

Committed proerythroblast (large nucleus)

Normoblast
(The nucleus shrinks and undergoes reabsorption)

Reticulocyte
(No nucleus; cell enters vascular circulation from
the bone marrow)

Erythrocyte
(Loses capacity for hemoglobin synthesis; disk shape and size achieved)

- The function of erythrocytes is to transport gas to and from the tissue cells and lungs. The normal adult range of indices for circulating erythrocytes* in the blood follows:

  Number = 4.2-6.2 million/mm^3
  Hematocrit = 42%-48%
  Hemoglobin = 12-16.5 g/dl

- The rate of erythropoiesis or formation of RBCs is measured by the reticulocyte count. Reticulocytes normally comprise less than 1% of the RBCs found in blood. A low count may indicate the inability of bone marrow to respond. A high count may indicate a good marrow response to low numbers of RBCs.

a. Identify the differentiation sequence, function, and normal values for erythrocytes.

Review text pages 965 through 969 and 971; refer to Figures 25-1 and 25-12 through 25-16 and Tables 25-2 and 25-4 though 25-6.

LEARNING OBJECTIVES

After studying this chapter, the learner will be able to do the following:

1. Define anemia.

Study text page 989.

Anemia is a reduction in the total number of circulating erythrocytes or a decrease in the quality or quantity of hemoglobin.

2. Classify the anemias.

Study text page 989; refer to Figure 26-1 and Tables 26-1 and 26-2.

Whether there is decreased/defective production or destruction of erythrocytes, anemias are classified according to their **etiologic basis** (see Box 26-1 in the text) **or morphologic appearance.**

181

Anemias

Anemia	Etiology	High-Risk Groups	Symptoms
Macrocytic-Normochromic			
Pernicious (PA)	Insufficient influence of vitamin B_{12} on developing cells because of deficient intrinsic factor (IF); antibodies develop against parietal cells; gastrectomy or ilectomy therapies; chronic gastritis	Northern European populations, blacks and Hispanics, females, >60 years of age	Typical*: digestive symptoms from lack of HCl and enzymes; glossitis; peripheral neuropathy; tingling numbness, loss of vibratory sense
Folate (folic acid)	Dietary deficiency inhibits DNA synthesis	Alcoholics, chronically malnourished individuals	
Microcytic-Hypochromic			
Iron deficiency (IDA)	Excessive bleeding that depletes iron; poor diet; possible *H. pylori* infection	Pregnant women, adolescents, children, elderly, individuals with chronic blood loss	Typical*
Sideroblastic (SA)	Dysfunctional iron uptake by erythroblasts; decreased heme synthesis; enzymes; genetic	Acquired from drugs, ingestion of ethanol, lead, chloramphenicol, antituberculosis agents	Typical*; mild hepatomegaly and splenomegaly; erythropoietic hemochromatosis
Thalassemia	Inherited genetic defect of hemoglobin synthesis; phagocytosis of abnormal erythroblasts in bone marrow	Greeks, Jews, Italians, Asians, blacks	Typical*; hepatomegaly and splenomegaly; fetal intrauterine congestive heart failure
Normocytic-Normochromic			
Aplastic (AA)	Radiation; viruses; drugs; lesions within red bone marrow; immune response that halts erythropoiesis; genetic (Fanconi anemia)	Anyone	Typical*; petechiae; ecchymosis; bleeding; infection; pancytopenia
Posthemorrhagic	Sudden and acute blood loss; depletion of body iron	Surgery, trauma	Shock; acidosis
Hemolytic	Premature dysfunction of mature erythrocytes in circulation; genetics result in fragile cells; acquired from infections, drugs, autoimmunity, warm IgG, or cold IgM antibodies	Anyone	Splenomegaly; jaundice; childhood skeletal abnormalities
Anemia of chronic disease (ACD)	Bacterial toxins; cytokines from activated macrophages and lymphocytes suppress progenitor cells; reduced iron in blood via lactoferrin	AIDS, autoimmunity; neoplasms, inflammatory disorders, chronic hepatitis, chronic renal failure	Mild because of disability caused by chronic condition

*Typical signs and symptoms include: fatigue, weakness, dyspnea, and pallor.
Treatment: Remove cause, if possible, and replace the deficient element; marrow transplants; or immunosuppression.
NOTE: Thalessemia presents in early childhood and has no cure; anemia and cardiovascular compromise lead to early death. See objective 6 in chapter 28.

Etiologic classification is based on either (1) decreased or defective production of erythrocytes or (2) increased erythrocyte destruction. Fewer erythrocytes are caused by altered hemoglobin synthesis, altered DNA synthesis because of deficient nutrients, stem cell dysfunction, bone marrow infiltration, or RBC aplasia. Destruction of erythrocytes is due to blood loss or hemolysis. Descriptions of anemias based on erythrocyte cellular structure refer to the cell size and hemoglobin content. The morphologic classification is widely used. Terms that refer to cellular size end with "-cytic." Terms that describe hemoglobin content end with "-chromic." An erythrocyte can be **macrocytic**, which means that it is abnormally large; **microcytic**, which means that it is abnormally small; **hyperchromic**, which means that it contains an unusually high concentration of hemoglobin within its cytoplasm; or **hypochromic**, which means that it contains an abnormally low concentration of hemoglobin. For comparison, cells of normal size are termed **normocytic**, and cells with normal amounts of hemoglobin are termed **normochromic**. In some anemias, the erythrocytes take on various sizes or they have various shapes; these characteristics are **anisocytosis** and **poikilocytosis**, respectively.

3. **Describe the pathophysiology of the clinical manifestations of anemias.**

   Study text pages 989 and 990; refer to Figure 26-2.

   Compensation for reduced oxygen-carrying capacity of the blood requires the cardiovascular, respiratory, and hematologic systems to respond. A reduction in the number of circulating erythrocytes after hemorrhage affects the consistency and volume of the blood. To compensate for reduced blood volume, fluids from the interstitium move into the blood vessels, and plasma volume expands. The thinner, less viscous blood flows faster and more turbulently than normal blood.

   Hypoxemia, reduced oxygen in the blood, resulting from anemia causes arterial dilation leading to less vascular resistance, thus reducing heart afterload and increasing heart preload. The heart must pump harder and faster to meet normal oxygen demand and to prevent cardiopulmonary congestion. Congestive heart failure can develop.

   Tissue **hypoxia**, inadequate cellular oxygen, causes the rate and depth of breathing to increase in an attempt to make more oxygen available to the remaining erythrocytes. If compensation mechanisms are inadequate, shortness of breath, a rapid pounding heartbeat, dizziness, and fatigue occur.

   A number of systemic symptoms occur subsequent to this shunting of blood. The skin, mucous membranes, lips, nail beds, and conjunctivae become pale because of reduced hemoglobin concentration or yellowish due to accumulation in the skin of products of RBC breakdown or hemolysis. Decreased oxygen delivery to the skin results in impaired healing and loss of elasticity. Thinning and early graying of the hair can occur.

Decreased blood flow is sensed by the kidneys, and in an effort to improve kidney perfusion, the renal renin-angiotensin response is activated. This results in salt and water retention, which causes an increased workload for the heart.

If the anemia is due to vitamin B_{12} deficiency, the nervous system is affected. Myelin degeneration may occur with a loss of nerve fibers in the spinal cord. Paresthesias, gait disturbances, extreme weakness, spasticity, and reflex abnormalities may then result.

Decreased oxygen supply to the gastrointestinal tract often produces abdominal pain, nausea, vomiting, and anorexia. Low-grade fever of less than 101° F occurs in some anemic individuals, and it may be the result of leukocytic pyrogens being released from ischemic tissues.

Therapeutic intervention for any anemic condition requires treatment of the underlying disorder and palliation of symptoms. Therapies for anemia include transfusions, dietary corrections, and administration of supplemental vitamins or iron.

4. **Develop a comparative, morphologic chart of the macrocytic-normochromic, microcytic-hypochromic, and normocytic-normochromic anemias.**

   Study text pages 990, 991, and 993 through 1008; refer to Figures 26-3 through 26-9 and Table 26-3.

5. **Describe the types, causes, manifestations, and treatment of polycythemia.**

   Study text pages 1008 through 1011.

   Polycythemia is an increase in red cell production, and it exists in two forms: relative and absolute. **Relative polycythemia** results from any cause of dehydration, such as decreased water intake, diarrhea, excessive vomiting, or increased use of diuretics. Its development is temporary, and it resolves with appropriate fluid administration or treatment of the underlying condition.

   Absolute polycythemia is primary when it results from an abnormality of the bone marrow stem cells. Secondary polycythemia, the most common type, is caused by an increase in erythropoietin as a normal physiologic response to chronic hypoxia or an inappropriate response to erythropoietin-secreting tumors. Individuals who live at higher altitudes, smokers who have increased levels of CO_2 in their blood, individuals with chronic obstructive pulmonary disease (COPD), and individuals who have congestive heart failure develop secondary polycythemia. Secondary polycythemia also develops in individuals who have abnormal hemoglobin because of genetic mutations in the hemoglobin chains.

   Primary polycythemia is known as polycythemia vera. Most primary absolute polycythemias are acquired and occur at various ages; however, there are some that are hereditary, present at birth, and identified as familial and congenital polycythemias. **Polycythemia vera (PV)** is a neoplastic, nonmalignant condition characterized by splenomegaly and increases in red cells, white cells, and platelets. Erythrocytosis is the most serious complication and the essential manifestation for diagnosis. Clonal proliferation of erythroid progenitors occurs in the bone marrow.

183

independent of erythropoietin, although the cells express a normal erythropoietin receptor. PV-affected individuals have an acquired mutation in Janus kinase (JAK2). This kinase increases the activity of the erythropoietin receptor and is also self-regulating, so JAK2 activity diminishes over time. Thus, the erythropoietin receptors are active regardless of the level of erythropoietin.

Clinical manifestations of absolute PV result from marrow erythropoiesis causing increased cellularity of the blood, which increases blood volume and viscosity. Circulatory alterations prevalent in PV, caused by thick, sticky blood, give rise to specific manifestations, such as plethora (ruddy, red color of the face, hands, feet, ears, and mucous membranes) and engorgement of the retinal and cerebral vessels. Individuals also experience headache, drowsiness, delirium, mania, psychotic depression, chorea, and visual disturbances. Death from cerebral thrombosis is approximately five times greater in individuals with PV. A unique feature of PV and potentially instrumental in diagnosis is extreme, painful itching upon exposure to water (aquagenic pruritus).

Treatment of PV is guided by two objectives: minimize the risk of thrombosis and prevent the progression to myelofibrosis and acute leukemia. **Phlebotomy** remains the primary treatment modality. Hydroxyurea, which blocks DNA synthesis and reduces vascular cellularity, reduces thrombotic complications. Aspirin is also antithrombotic. Radioactive phosphorus (^{32}P) is also used to suppress erythropoieses. It is generally effective for an extended time and as many as 18 months may elapse between treatments. Side effects of ^{32}P treatment include suppression of hematopoiesis, resulting in anemia, leukopenia, or thrombocytopenia. Development of acute leukemia is also a major side effect of ^{32}P, occurring after 7 or more years of treatment, making this therapy more useful in elderly individuals. Interferon alpha (IFN-α) inhibits the growth of the abnormal clone, which leads to the reduction of the clinical and laboratory signs of myeloproliferation.

Without proper treatment, 50% of individuals with PV die within 18 months of the onset of initial symptoms. The primary cause of death is thrombosis, which is more prevalent in older individuals and those with prior vascular complications.

PRACTICE EXAMINATION

Multiple Choice

Circle the correct answer for each question.

1. Anemia refers to a deficiency of:
   a. blood plasma.
   b. erythrocytes.
   c. platelets.
   d. hemoglobin.
   e. Both b and d are correct.

2. Etiologic classification of anemia is based on:
   a. size.
   b. color.
   c. shape.
   d. decreased or defective erythrocytes.

3. Tissue hypoxia causes:
   a. arterioles, capillaries, and venules to constrict.
   b. the heart to contract less forcefully.
   c. the rate and depth of breathing to increase.
   d. increased afterload.

4. Which of the following symptoms are consistent with aplastic anemia but not with pernicious anemia?
   a. Petechiae and purpura
   b. Pallor
   c. Fatigue
   d. Hypoxia
   e. Neuropathy

5. If a reticulocyte count were done on an individual with iron deficiency anemia because of chronic bleeding, it would be:
   a. high.
   b. low.
   c. normal.
   d. meaningless.

6. A 40-year-old white, pregnant woman with four children experienced weakness, loss of appetite, and pallor. Her CBC revealed the following:
   Macrocytic RBCs 2.5 × 10^6/mm^3
   Hematocrit level of 32%
   Hemoglobin level of 8.7 g/dl
   She most likely has:
   a. sickle cell anemia.
   b. folic acid anemia.
   c. iron deficiency anemia.
   d. pernicious anemia.

7. A cause of macrocytic-normochromic anemia is:
   a. iron deficiency.
   b. deficiency of vitamin B$_{12}$ and folic acid.
   c. an enzyme deficiency.
   d. inheritance of abnormal hemoglobin structure.

8. Hemolytic anemia may result in:
   a. jaundice.
   b. loss of vibratory sense.
   c. acidosis.
   d. petechiae.

9. The end result of anemia is:
   a. anoxia.
   b. hypoxia.
   c. infection.
   d. bleeding.
   e. hypoxemia.

10. An individual who has chronic gastritis and tingling in his or her fingers requires which of the following for treatment?
    a. Oral vitamin B_{12}
    b. Vitamin B_{12} by intramuscular injection
    c. Ferrous fumarate by intramuscular injection
    d. Oral folate
    e. Transfusions

11. Individuals at risk for iron deficiency anemia include those:
    a. who have undergone a gastrectomy.
    b. who are Italian.
    c. with neoplastic disease.
    d. with warm antibodies.
    e. with minor, chronic blood loss.

12. The symptoms of sideroblastic anemia may include:
    a. glossitis.
    b. hepatomegaly and splenomegaly.
    c. bleeding and recurrent infections.
    d. neuropathy
    e. jaundice.

13. Primary (absolute) polycythemia exists when there is:
    a. an increase in circulating RBCs, WBCs, and platelets.
    b. a decrease of circulating plasma.
    c. a physiologic response to hypoxia.
    d. chronic obstructive pulmonary disease in an individual.

14. Secondary (absolute) polycythemia may be caused by:
    a. dehydration.
    b. chronic obstructive pulmonary disease.
    c. excessive use of diuretics.
    d. an abnormality of bone marrow stem cells.
    e. diarrhea.

15. The pathophysiology of polycythemia vera is essentially caused by:
    a. fewer erythrocytes than normal.
    b. decreased blood volume.
    c. an acquired mutation in Janus kinase 2.
    d. increased rate of blood flow.

Matching

Match the etiology of the anemia disorder with its morphologic appearance.

_____ 16. Vitamin B_{12} deficiency

_____ 17. Iron deficiency

_____ 18. Folic acid deficiency

_____ 19. Bone marrow depression

_____ 20. Chronic infection

_____ 21. Hemolysis

_____ 22. Posthemorrhagic

_____ 23. Decreased heme synthesis

_____ 24. Chloramphenicol therapy

_____ 25. Malignancy

a. macrocytic-normochromic

b. microcytic-hypochromic

c. normocytic-normochromic

A. is an apparently healthy 26-year-old white woman. Since the beginning of the current golf season, A. has noted increased shortness of breath and low levels of energy and enthusiasm. These symptoms seem worse during her menses. Today, while playing poorly in a golf tournament at a high, mountainous course, she became light-headed and was taken by her golfing partner to the emergency clinic of a multi-specialty medical group. The attending physician's notes indicated a temperature of 98° F, an elevated heart rate and respiratory rate, and low blood pressure. A. states, "Menorrhagia and dysmenorrhea have been a problem for 10 to 12 years, and I take 1000 mg of aspirin every 3 to 4 hours for 6 days during menstruation." During the summer months, while playing golf, she also takes aspirin to avoid "stiffness in my joints." Laboratory values are as follows:

Hemoglobin = 8 g/dl

Hematocrit = 32%

Erythrocyte count = $3.1 \times 10^6/mm^3$

RBC smear showed microcytic and hypochromic cells

Reticulocyte count = 1.5%

Other laboratory values were within normal limits.

Questions

Considering the circumstances and the preliminary workup, what type of anemia does A. most likely have?

Which clinical sign demonstrates that her body is attempting to compensate for the anemia?

27 Alterations of Leukocyte, Lymphoid, and Hemostatic Function

FOUNDATIONAL KNOWLEDGE OBJECTIVES

a. Identify the differentiation sequence for granulocytes, agranulocytes, and platelets.
Refer to Figure 25-9

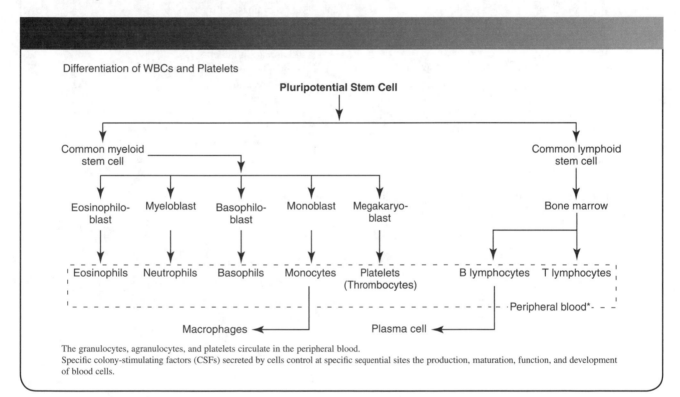

Differentiation of WBCs and Platelets

The granulocytes, agranulocytes, and platelets circulate in the peripheral blood.
Specific colony-stimulating factors (CSFs) secreted by cells control at specific sequential sites the production, maturation, function, and development of blood cells.

b. Identify the normal numbers in circulating blood, the function, and the life span of leukocytes and platelets.
   Refer to Table 25-2.

MEMORY CHECK!

Cell	Normal Amounts	Function	Life Span
Leukocyte	5,000 to 10,000/mm³	Bodily defense mechanisms	
Lymphocyte	25% to 33% of leukocytes	Immunity	Days or years
Monocyte and macrophage	3% to 7% of leukocytes	Phagocytosis, mononuclear phagocyte system	Months or years
Eosinophil	1% to 4% of leukocytes	Phagocytosis, antibody-mediated defense against parasites, allergic reactions, recovery phase of infection	Unknown
Neutrophil	57% to 67% of leukocytes	Phagocytosis, particularly during early phase of inflammation/infection	4 days
Basophil	0% of 0.75% of leukocytes	Unknown but associated with allergic reactions and mechanical irritation	Unknown
Platelet	140,000 to 340,000/mm³	Hemostasis following vascular injury, normal coagulation, and clot formation/reactions	8 to 11 days

c. Summarize the coagulation cascade and the fibrinolytic systems.
   Refer to Figures 25-22 and 25-25. See the following page.

Coagulation Cascade

Extrinsic Pathway
Activated by damaged tissue (TF)

Intrinsic Pathway
Activated by contact with damaged vessel surfaces

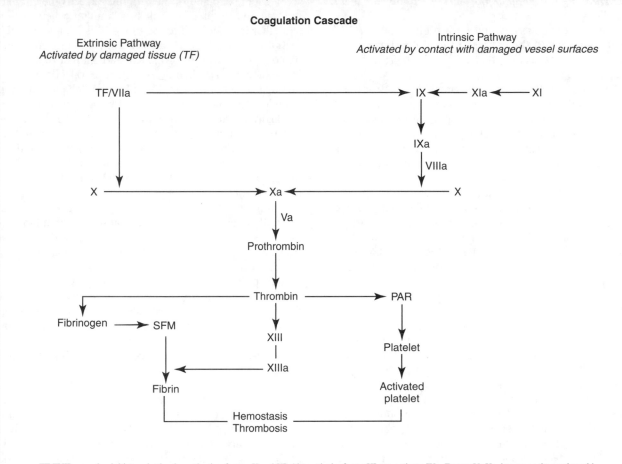

TF:FVIIa complex initiates clotting by activating factors X and XI. Alternatively, factor XI can activate IXa. Factors Va:Xa, known as the prothrombinase complex, activate prothrombin. Thrombin activates several proteases and cofactors. Clot formation finally occurs when thrombin cleaves fibrinogen to soluble fibrinogen monomers (SFMs), which are cross-linked by factor XIIIa, and with activation of protease-activated receptors (PARs) on platelets. Tissue factor (TF) is different depending on tissue type.

Fibrinolytic System

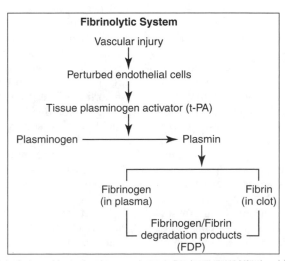

Note: Although t-PA initiates intravascular fibrinolysis, urokinase plasminogen activator (u-PA) is the major activator of fibrinolysis in tissue (extravascular).

189

LEARNING OBJECTIVES

After studying this chapter, the learner will be able to do the following:

1. Describe terms associated with high or low leukocyte counts and the causes of the alterations.

Study text pages 1014, 1015, and 1017; refer to Table 27-1.

Quantitative leukocyte disorders result from decreased production in the bone marrow or accelerated destruction of cells in the circulation. **Qualitative leukocyte disorders** consist of leukocytic dysfunction.

Leukocytosis exists when the leukocyte count is higher than normal; **leukopenia** is a condition in which the leukocyte count is lower than normal. Leukocytosis is a normal, protective response to invading microorganisms, strenuous exercise, emotional changes, temperature changes, anesthesia, surgery, pregnancy, some drugs, hormones, and toxins. Malignancies and hematologic disorders also cause leukocytosis. Increased levels of circulating neutrophils, eosinophils, basophils, and monocytes are chiefly a physiologic response to infection. Elevations can also occur as a result of polycythemia vera and chronic myelocytic leukemia, which increase stem cell proliferation in the bone marrow.

Leukopenia is never beneficial. As the leukocyte count falls below 1000/μL, the individual is at risk for infection. The risk for very serious life-threatening infections develops with counts below 500/μL. Leukopenia can be caused by radiation, anaphylactic shock, systemic lupus erythematosus, and certain chemotherapeutic agents. Decreased leukocytic counts occur when infectious processes delete the circulating granulocytes and monocytes. Infectious agents draw them out of the circulation and into infected tissues faster than they can be replaced. Decreases can also be caused by disorders that suppress marrow function.

Granulocytosis or **neutrophilia** is prevalent in the early stages of infection or inflammation, when stored neutrophils from the venous sinuses are released into the circulating blood. Emptying of the venous sinuses stimulates granulopoiesis to replenish normal stores of granulocytes in the marrow.

Neutropenia, which is a low neutrophilic count, may be caused by decreased or ineffective neutrophil production, because the marrow is producing other formed elements. Also, autoimmunity, reduced neutrophil survival, and abnormal neutrophil distribution and sequestration in tissues lead to neutropenia. Neutropenia exists when the neutrophil count is less than 2000/μL. If the entire granulocyte count is extremely low, less than 500/μL, a very serious condition called **agranulocytosis** or **granulocytopenia** results. The usual cause of agranulocytosis is interference with hematopoiesis in the bone marrow or increased cell destruction in the circulation. Chemotherapeutic agents used in the treatment of hematologic and other malignancies and some drugs cause bone marrow suppression. Clinical manifestations of agranulocytosis include respiratory infection, general malaise, septicemia, fever, tachycardia, and ulcers in the mouth and colon. If untreated, sepsis caused by agranulocytosis can result in death within 3 to 6 days.

When the demand for neutrophils exceeds the circulatory supply, the marrow releases immature neutrophils and other leukocytes into the blood; this is called a **shift to the left,** or a **leukemoid reaction,** because the morphologic findings in blood smears are similar to those of individuals with leukemia. As infection or inflammation diminishes, granulopoiesis replenishes the circulating granulocytes, and the levels return back to normal.

Eosinophilia is an absolute increase in the total numbers of circulating eosinophils. Allergic disorders associated with asthma, hay fever, parasitic invasion, and drug reactions are frequently the cause of eosinophilia. Chemotactic factor of anaphylaxis (CTF-A) and histamine released from mast cells attract eosinophils to the area. **Eosinopenia** is a decrease in circulating eosinophils generally due to migration of eosinophils into inflammatory sites. It may also be seen in Cushing syndrome as a result of stress due to surgery, shock, trauma, burns, or mental distress.

Basophilia is quite rare and is generally seen as a response to inflammation and hypersensitivity reactions of the immediate type. An increase in basophils is also seen in chronic myeloid leukemia and myeloid metaplasia. **Basopenia** is seen in hyperthyroidism, acute infection, and long-term therapy with steroids and during ovulation and pregnancy.

Monocytosis, which is an increase in monocytes, is often transient and correlates poorly with disease states. When present, it is most commonly associated with bacterial infections during the late stages of recovery, when monocytes are needed to phagocytize any surviving microorganisms and debris. Monocytosis is seen in chronic infections such as tuberculosis and subacute bacterial endocarditis. **Monocytopenia,** which is a decrease in monocytes, is rare but has been identified with hairy cell leukemia and prednisone therapy.

A **lymphocytosis** is rare in acute bacterial infections and occurs most often in acute viral infections, especially in those caused by the Epstein-Barr virus (EBV). Lymphocytopenia may be associated with neoplasias, immune deficiencies, and destruction by drugs. It may be that the lymphocytopenia associated with heart failure and other acute illnesses is caused by elevated levels of cortisol. **Lymphocytopenia** is a major problem in people with AIDS. The lymphocytopenia seen with this condition is caused by the HIV, which is cytopathic for helper T lymphocytes.

2. Describe the pathogenesis of infectious mononucleosis.

Study text pages 1017 through 1019; refer to Figure 27-1.

Infectious mononucleosis (IM) is an acute infection of B lymphocytes. The most common etiologic virus is the EBV; however, cytomegalovirus (CMV), other viruses, and several bacteria have been identified as causative agents for this disease.

Approximately 50% to 85% of children by age 4 years and more than 90% of adults are infected with EBV, but

190

are asymptomatic. Symptomatic IM usually affects young adults between the ages of 15 and 35.

Transmission of EBV is usually through saliva, hence the term "kissing disease." The virus also may be present in other mucosal secretions, as well as blood. Aerosol transmission through sneezing or coughing does not occur. The infection begins with the invasion of B lymphocytes that possess an EBV receptor site. The virus infects the oropharynx, nasopharynx, and salivary epithelial cells. Infection of B cells permits the virus to enter the blood which spreads the infection systemically. The proliferation of clones of B and T cells and the removal of dead and damaged leukocytes are largely responsible for the swelling of cervical lymphoid tissues. The proliferation of B and T cells is responsible for the rise in absolute lymphocyte count and the presence of **atypical lymphocytes,** which are actually CD8 cytotoxic T cells.

Flulike symptoms, such as headache, malaise, fatigue, arthralgia, fever, and chills, may appear in 3 to 5 days and vary in severity for the next 7 to 20 days. The individual will develop the classic triad of symptoms; fever, pharyngitits, and lymphadenopathy of the cervical lymph nodes. Splenomegaly is clinically evident 50% of the time and demonstrated radiologically 100% of the time. IM is usually self-limiting, and recovery occurs in a few weeks.

Diagnosis of IM is based on at least 50% lymphocytes and at least 10% atypical lymphocytes in the blood in the presence of classic symptoms confirmed by a positive serologic test. **Heterophile antibodies** are a heterogeneous group of IgM antibodies that are agglutinins against nonhuman (sheep or horse) and are detected by the Monospot test. Treatment consists of rest and alleviation of symptoms with analgesics and antipyretics.

3. Characterize the general features of leukemia.
Study text pages 1019 through 1021.

Leukemia is a malignant disorder of the blood and blood-forming organs, and it exhibits an uncontrolled proliferation of dysfunctional leukocytes. Leukemias are considered clonal disorders in that a single progenitor cell undergoes malignant transformation. The excessive proliferation of leukemic cells crowds the bone marrow and causes decreased production and function of other normal hematopoietic cells. This results in **pancytopenia** or a reduction in all cellular components of the blood. Leukemia is a primary disruption of the bone marrow.

The current classification of leukemia is based on (1) the predominant cell of origin, whether myeloid or lymphoid; and (2) the rate of progression, which usually reflects the degree at which cell differentiation was arrested when the cell became malignant, whether acute or chronic. There are four types of leukemia: acute lymphocytic leukemia (ALL), acute myelogenous leukemia (AML), chronic lymphocytic leukemia (CLL), and chronic myelogenous leukemia (CML).

Acute leukemia is characterized by undifferentiated immature or blastic cells. The onset of disease is abrupt and rapid, and the affected individual can experience a short survival time. In **chronic leukemia**, the predominant cell appears to be mature, but it does not function

normally. The onset of disease is gradual, and the prolonged clinical course results in a relatively longer survival time. Leukemia occurs with varying frequencies at different ages and is more frequent in adults than in children in the United States.

Although the exact cause of leukemia is unknown, several risk factors and related genetic aberrations are associated with the onset of malignancy. There is a tendency for leukemia to occur in families. There is also an increased incidence of leukemia associated with hereditary abnormalities such as Down syndrome, Fanconi aplastic anemia, Bloom syndrome, and some immune deficiencies. The most common genetic abnormality is the reciprocal translocation between chromosomes 9 and 22, the **Philadelphia chromosome.** It is present in 95% of individuals with CML. Large doses of ionizing radiation particularly result in myelogenous leukemia. Infection with HIV or hepatitis C virus increases the risk for leukemia, as well as, by infection with the human T-cell leukemia/lymphoma virus 1. Drugs such as chloramphenicol and certain alkylating agents cause bone marrow depression, and they can also predispose an individual to leukemia.

4. Contrast and describe the four types of leukemia.
Study text pages 1021 through 1029; refer to Figures 27-2 through 27-7.

Acute leukemias consist of two types: **acute lymphocytic leukemia (ALL)** and **acute myelogenous leukemia (AML)**. They are seen in both genders and in all ages and the incidence increases dramatically in individuals older than 50 years. **ALL** is a progressive neoplasm defined by the presence of more than 30% lymphoblasts in the marrow or blood. Most cases of ALL occur in children, and it is the most common leukemia in children. Approximately 75% of ALL in children originates from transformed precursor B cells; whereas adult ALL is a mixture of cancers of precursor B-cell or precursor T-cell origin. Risk factors for childhood ALL include prenatal or postnatal exposure to x-rays. Individuals with Down syndrome have an increased risks for ALL and AML. Genetic conditions, including neurofibromatosis, Shwachman syndrome, and Bloom syndrome increase the risk for ALL.

AML is the most common adult leukemia. It results from a proliferation of myeloid precursor cells, a decreased rate of apoptosis, and an arrest in cellular differentiation. The bone marrow and peripheral blood are characterized by leukocytosis and a predominance of blast cells. As the immature blast cells increase, they replace normal myelocytic cells, megakaryoctes, and erythrocytes. This displacement eventually leads to complications of bleeding, anemia, and infection. AML increases with age, peaking in the sixth decade of life.

All acute leukemias exhibit similar signs and symptoms related to bone marrow depression, including fatigue caused by anemia, bleeding resulting from thrombocytopenia, and fever caused by infection. Liver, spleen, and lymph node enlargement are more common in ALL than in AML. Splenomegaly and hepatomegaly usually occur together.

191

The two main types of chronic leukemia are **chronic myelogenous leukemia (CML)** and **chronic lymphocytic leukemia (CLL).** Unlike cells in acute leukemia, cells in chronic leukemic are well differentiated and can be readily identified. Individuals with chronic leukemia have a longer life expectancy, usually extending several years from the time of diagnosis. The chronic leukemias account for the majority of leukemic cases in adults. The incidences of CLL and CML increase significantly in individuals over 40 years of age, with prevalence in the sixth through eight decades.

CLL is derived from transformation of partially mature B cells that have not yet encountered antigen. CLL cells that accumulate in the marrow do not interfere with normal blood cell production to the extent that occurs in acute leukemias. Because the major deficit in CLL is the failure of B cells to mature into plasma cells that synthesize immunoglobulin, hypogammaglobulinemia is found in 60% of patients. The most significant effect of CLL is suppression of humoral immunity and increased infection with encapsulated bacteria. Invasion of most organs is uncommon, but infiltration does occur in lymph nodes, liver, spleen, and salivary glands

CML is a member of myeloproliferative disorders that includes polycythemia vera, essential thrombocythemia, chronic idiopathic myelofibrosis, chronic neutrophilic leukemia, and chronic eosinophilic leukemia. CML is clonal and believed to arise from a hematopoietic stem cell. The Philadelphia chromosome is present in more than 95% of cases of CML. Chronic leukemia advances slowly and insidiously. Individuals with CML may progress through three phases of the disease: a chronic phase lasting 2 to 5 years, during which symptoms may not be present; an accelerated phase of 6 to 18 months, during which primary symptoms develop; and a terminal "blastic crisis" phase with a survival of only 3 to 6 months. Splenomegaly is the most common finding, which is prominent and painful, but lymphadenopathy generally is not present. Liver enlargement also occurs, but liver function is rarely altered. Hyperuricemia is common and produces gouty arthritis.

Diagnosis of chronic leukemia depends on laboratory analyses of peripheral blood and bone marrow; diagnosis of CLL is based on detection of a monoclonal B-cell lymphocytosis in the blood. Combination chemotherapy is the treatment of choice for all leukemias; however, there is no cure nor increased survival for the chronic leukemias. Stem cell transplantation has increased during the past two decades. Five-year survival rates for adults is 65% and for children 85%, The presence of the Philadelphia chromosome is a poor prognostic indicator.

5. **Compare Hodgkin lymphoma (HL) to non-Hodgkin lymphoma (NHL), and describe Burkitt and lymphoblastic lymphomas.**
Study text pages 1030 through 1037; refer to Figures 27-8 through 27-13 and Tables 27-5 through 27-8.

Lymphomas are a diverse group of neoplasms that develop from the proliferation of malignant lymphocytes in the lymphoid system. Their classification is based on the cell type from which the lymphoma originated. In general, lymphomas are the result of genetic mutations or viral infection.

Malignant Lymphomas

	Hodgkin lymphoma	Non-Hodgkin lymphoma
Cause	No apoptosis of B cell nor immunoglobulin gene rearrangement; EBV; Reed-Sternberg cells* release cytokines	Translocations on proto-oncogenes and tumor suppression genes, cancer causing suppressor genes, cancer causing viruses, immunodeficiency, *H. pylori* infection
Cellular deviation	B cells	B cells (85%), T cells and NK cells (15%)
Nodes involved	Painless node in neck; single node or chain: cervical, inguinal, axillary, retroperitoneal	Noncontinuous nodes: cervical, axillary, inguinal, femoral
Symptoms	Mostly localized manifestations of systemic fever, night sweats, weakness, weight loss, pericardial involvement from mediastinal nodes	Similar to Hodgkin plus pleural effusion, abdominal pain, splenomegaly, and hepatomegaly (generalized manifestations more likely)
Treatment	Radiotherapy or surgery for localized, chemotherapy for generalized; bone marrow or stem cell transplants	Chemotherapy, immunotherapy, and radiotherapy; autologous stem cell transplantation
Curability	More than 75%	Long term, nodular lymphoma has better (15-year) prognosis than diffuse disease (42% for 10 years)

*Reed-Sternberg cells are malignant tissue macrophages that are scattered among normal cells.

Burkitt lymphoma is a B-cell tumor involving the jaw and facial bones of children that occurs in east central Africa and New Guinea. It is rare in the United States and usually involves the abdomen and exhibits extensive bone marrow invasion and replacement.

Lymphoblastic lymphoma is a rare variant of NHL (2% to 4 %) but accounts for a third of cases of NHL in children; it is predominant in males. The vast majority, 85%, has a T-cell origin.

6. **Describe malignant myeloma and differentiate it from the leukemias; note Waldenström macroglobulinemia features.**

Study text pages 1037, 1038, and 1040 through 1042; refer to Figures 27-15 through 27-18.

Malignant myeloma (MM) arises from chromosomal translocations. The primary translocation involves the immunoglobulin heavy chain on chromosome 14 that relocates to multiple other chromosomes. Malignant plasma cells arise from one clone of B cells that produce abnormally large amounts of IgG, occasionally IgA, but rarely IgD or IgE. The malignant transformation may begin before the B cell encounters antigen in secondary lymphoid organs. This disorder originates in the bone marrow and moves through the circulation to and from lymph nodes.

Myeloma cells in the bone marrow directly secrete growth factors that induce the production of several cytokines. All of these cytokines, especially IL-6, act to stimulate osteoclasts to reabsorb bone. This process results in bone lesions and and hypercalcemia. The antibody produced by the transformed plasma cell is usually defective. The abnormal antibody, called **M-protein**, becomes the protein with the highest level in the blood. The myeloma produces free immunoglobulin light chain, **Bence-Jones protein,** that is present in both blood and urine and contributes to renal tubular cell damage.

The most common initial symptom of myeloma is pain felt in a single bone or the entire skeleton. Renal failure and recurrent bacterial infections also are common. The individual also may complain of weakness, fatigue, weight loss, and anorexia in addition to pain. Suppression of humoral immunity occurs as a result of Bence-Jones proteinuria.

Chemotherapy, stem cell transplantation, and drugs to inhibit bone resorption, reduce the incidence of skeletal damage and hypercalcemia, decrease pain, and treat recurring infections. The prognosis for individuals with MM is poor, with survival rarely more than 3 years. Individuals with multiple bone lesions, if untreated, only survive 6 to 12 months.

Waldenström macroglobulinemia is a rare type of slow-growing plasma cell tumor that secretes a monoclonal IgM molecule. Excessive production of IgM leads to abnormally high blood viscosity that interferes with circulation to the eyes, brain, kidneys, and extremities.

7. **Describe thrombocytopenia and thrombocythemia.**

Study text pages 1044 through 1048; refer to Figure 27-19.

Thrombocytopenia exists when platelet count is below 100,000 platelets/mm^3 of blood. It results from decreased platelet production, increased consumption, or both. The condition may be congenital or acquired and may be primary or secondary. Hemorrhage from minor trauma can occur with counts of 50,000 platelets/mm^3 or less. Spontaneous bleeding can occur with counts between 15,000 and 10,000 platelets/mm^3. Severe bleeding results if the count is below 10,000 platelets/mm^3; such bleeding can be fatal if it occurs in the gastrointestinal tract, respiratory system, or central nervous system.

Acquired thrombocytopenia is more common and may occur because of decreased production secondary to viral infections, drugs, nutritional deficiencies, chronic renal failure, aplastic anemia, radiation therapy, or bone marrow infiltration by cancer. Most common deficiencies are the result of increased platelet consumption. One example is **heparin-induced thrombocytopenia**, which is an adverse drug reaction caused by IgG against heparin–platelet factor 4 complex.

Multiple Myeloma/Common Leukemias

Characteristic	Multiple Myeloma	Common Leukemias
Malignant proliferation of WBCs in the bone marrow	Yes	Yes
Anemia	Yes	Yes
Bleeding	Yes	Yes
Recurrent infections	Yes	Yes
Plasma cells	Yes	No
Ineffective immunoglobulins	Yes	Possible
Bence-Jones protein in urine	Yes	No
Pathologic bone fractures	Yes	No
WBC blood elevation	No	Yes
Osteolytic lesions	Yes	Possible
Elevated calcium serum	Yes	Possible
Bone pain	Yes	Possible
Renal disease	Yes	Possible

Chapter **27** **Alterations of Leukocyte, Lymphoid, and Hemostatic Function**

Immune thrombocytopenia purpura (ITP) may be either acute or chronic. ITP is an autoimmune disorder in which an IgG autoantibody (IgM and IgA have also been involved) is formed and binds to and destroys the platelets. The acute form is most common in children and young adults and is usually preceded by a viral infection.

Chronic ITP is more common in females between 20 and 40 years of age. The individual most commonly presents with mucosal or skin bleeding that is often manifested as menorrhagia, purpura, petechiae, and bleeding gums. The antibody-coated platelets are removed from the circulation by mononuclear phagocytes in the spleen.

Treatment is palliative, not curative, focusing on prevention of platelet destruction. Initial therapy for ITP is infusion of glucocorticoids, which suppresses the production of antiplatelet antibodies and prevents sequestering and further destruction of platelets. Intravenous Ig (IVIG) is used to prevent major bleeding. If these therapies are ineffective, splenectomy is considered to remove the primary site of platelet destruction.

In **thrombotic thrombocytopenia purpura (TTP),** platelets aggregate and occlude the microcirculation. The aggregation occurs without activation of the intravascular coagulation cascade. Platelet aggregation and microthrombi formation are found throughout the entire vascular system causing damage to multiple organs. Organs most susceptible to damage are the kidney, brain, and heart. Defects in a cleaving protease result in expression of high molecular weight particles of von Willebrand factor, because this enzyme is responsible for digesting these particles. Subsequently, large aggregates of platelets form and may break off and occlude smaller vessels.

Untreated TTP has a mortality rate of 90%; however, mortality is markedly reduced with treatment. Plasma exchange with fresh frozen plasma to replenish the functional cleaving protease is highly effective; glucocorticoids are also used.

Thrombocythemia has a platelet count of more than 600,000/mm^3 of blood. Transient thrombocytosis is a normal, physiologic response to stress, infection, trauma, exercise, and ovulation. It is usually asymptomatic until the count exceeds 1 million/mm^3, when intravascular clot formation (thrombosis), hemorrhage, or other abnormalities can occur. **Secondary thrombocythemia** may occur after splenectomy because platelets that normally would be stored in the spleen remain in circulating blood.

Essential (primary) thrombocythemia (ET) is a chronic myeloproliferative disorder in which megakaryocytes in the marrow are produced in excess. Microvasculature thrombosis, **erythromyalgia**, is manifested as thrombosis of peripheral blood vessels or, less frequently, thrombosis of hepatic, mesenteric, cardiac, or pulmonary vessels. Arterial thrombosis involves the coronary and renal arteries. Venous thrombosis involves the lower extremities, lungs, and portal and hepatic vessels. Splenomegaly and easy bruising also occur. Other manifestations include headaches, dizziness, paresthesias, TIAs,

strokes, visual disturbances, and seizures. In individuals with thrombotic and hemorrhagic complications, the platelet count is lowered with nonalkylating myelosuppressive agents, interferon, and anagrelide which interferes with platelet maturation and does not affect RBC and WBC growth and development.

8. Describe alterations of platelet function.

Study pages 1048 through 1049.

Qualitative alterations in platelet function occur with increased bleeding time in the presence of normal platelet counts. They may be congenital or acquired. Congenital alterations (thrombocytopathies) are quite rare and may be categorized into five types: disorders of platelet-vessel adhesion, platelet-platelet interactions, platelet granules and secretion, arachidonic acid pathways, and coagulation protein-platelet interactions

Disorders of **platelet-vessel adhesion** result from a deficiency of platelet membrane glycoproteins. The lack of these proteins prevents platelets from adhering to collagen, and this results in impaired hemostasis and clinical hemorrhage.

Disorders of **platelet-platelet interaction** are manifested by the failure of platelets to aggregate with adenosine diphosphate (ADP), collagen, epinephrine, or thrombin because of a deficiency in the glycoprotein that acts as a fibrinogen receptor. The lack of this protein results in a failure to build "fibrinogen bridges" between platelets.

Disorders of **platelet granules and secretion** are characterized by initial normal platelet aggregation with collagen or ADP; however, there is failure of subsequent processes, specifically the secretion of prostaglandins and the release of granule-bound ADP.

Acquired disorders of platelet function are more common than the congenital disorders and may be categorized into three principal causes: drugs, systemic conditions, and hematologic alterations. Clinical manifestations of platelet alterations include petechiae and purpura, mild to moderate mucosal bleeding (bilateral epistaxis, gastrointestinal, genitourinary, and pulmonary), gingival bleeding, and spontaneous bruising.

Multiple drugs are known to affect platelet function. Of this vast array of drugs, aspirin is the only known drug specifically used for its antithrombotic activity. It irreversibly inhibits cyclooxygenase function for several days after administration. Drugs interfere with platelet function in three ways: inhibition of platelet membrane receptors, inhibition of prostaglandin pathways, and inhibition of phosphodiesterase activity.

9. Identify the causes of coagulation disorders.

Study text pages 1049 and 1050.

Disorders of **coagulation** are usually caused by defects or deficiencies of one or more of the clotting factors. Abnormalities of clotting factors prevent the enzymatic reactions by which these factors are normally transformed from circulating plasma proteins to a stable fibrin clot resulting in impaired hemostasis. Two common inherited disorders are the hemophilias and von Willebrand disease; these are caused by deficiencies of specific clotting factors.

194

Other coagulation defects are acquired and usually result from deficient synthesis of clotting factors by an impaired liver. A **deficiency of vitamin K**, which is necessary for normal synthesis of the clotting factors by the liver, is an acquired coagulation defect. The most common cause of vitamin K deficiency is parenteral nutrition in combination with broad-spectrum antibiotics that destroy normal gut flora. Rarely is a deficiency caused by lack of dietary intake; however, bulemia can suppress vitamin K–dependent activity. Clinical manifestations of vitamin K deficiency are caused by a reduction of vitamin K–dependent proteins. The severity of manifestations are related to the degree of deficiency and range from laboratory abnormalities to significant hemorrhage. Parenteral administration of vitamin K is the choice of treatment for this deficiency and usually results in improvement within 8 to 12 hours.

Individuals with **liver disease** have a broad range of hemostasis derangements that may be characterized by defects in the clotting or fibrinolytic systems and by platelet function. The usual sequence of events is an initial reduction in clotting factors, which parallels the degree of hepatic parenchymal cell damage or destruction. Factor VII is the first to decline because of its rapid turnover, followed by declines in prothrombin and factor X. Factor IX levels are less affected and do not decline until liver destruction is well advanced. Fresh frozen plasma administration is the treatment of choice.

10. Characterize disseminated intravascular coagulation.

Study pages 1050 through 1055; refer to Figure 27-20.

Disseminated intravascular coagulation (DIC) is an acquired coagulation disorder that has a variety of predisposing conditions. DIC is a paradoxical condition in which clotting and hemorrhage simultaneously occur within the vascular system. The development of DIC is generally associated with three pathologic processes: endothelial damage; exposure to tissue factor (TF), which complexes with factor VII; and direct activation of factor X. Gram-negative sepsis, septic shock, hypoxia, and low-flow states associated with cardiopulmonary arrest can damage the endothelium and precipitate DIC by activating the intrinsic clotting pathway. Endotoxins of gram-negatives activate both intrinsic and extrinsic clotting pathways.

Release of TF is associated with burns, brain injury, myocardial infarctions, surgeries, obstetric accidents, and malignancies. Excessive amounts of TF in the circulation activate the clotting pathways.

Activation of factor X is stimulated by various substances that enter the bloodstream. Pancreatic and hepatic enzymes and venom from snakebites act in this manner. DIC also can be precipitated by blood transfusion. Transfused blood dilutes the clotting factors and the circulating, naturally occurring antithrombins.

In DIC, the extrinsic system is most often involved. When either the intrinsic or the extrinsic system is activated, widespread, unrestricted coagulation occurs throughout the body and leads to thrombic events within the vasculature. The clotting factors are consumed as widespread clotting develops. Thrombosis in the presence of hemorrhage comprises this paradoxical alteration.

The amount of thrombin that enters the systemic circulation during DIC greatly exceeds the ability of the body's naturally occurring antithrombins. The obstruction that results from the circulatory deposition of thrombin interferes with blood flow and causes widespread organ hypoperfusion that can lead to ischemia, infarction, and necrosis with manifestations of multisystem organ dysfunction.

Plasmin, which is present because of the overstimulation of the clotting cascade, begins to degrade fibrin before a stable clot can develop. As fibrin is broken down by plasmin, fibrin degradation products (FDPs) are released into the circulation; these are potent anticoagulants. The macrophage system likely is unable to clear the blood of FDPs because of a lack of fibronectin. The clearance of particulate matter or fibrin clumps is mediated by the adhesive properties of fibronectin.

The **D-dimer test** is the most reliable and specific test for the diagnosis of DIC. D-dimer is a neoantigen produced by plasmin lysis of cross-linked fibrin clots. Monoclonal antibodies are formed against D-dimer antigen and identified. This documents the activity of thrombin (cross-linking) and plasmin (fibrinolysis).

Treatment of DIC attempts to remove the underlying pathology, restore an appropriate balance between coagulation and fibrinolysis, and maintain organ viability. Interventions based on restoring or replacing coagulation factors, platelets, and other coagulation elements is an effective treatment modality. Heparin is only indicated in certain instances. It seems to be effective in DIC caused by a retained dead fetus or in promeylocytic leukemia. Organ function is compromised by microthrombi, and there is a risk of losing an extremity because of vascular occlusion; thus, heparin is indicated in these conditions. Organ viability is treated primarily by adequate fluid replacement to ensure adequate circulating blood volume so that optimal tissue perfusion can be maintained.

11. Characterize thromboembolic diseases.

Study text pages 1055 through 1057; refer to Figure 27-21 and 27-22.

Thromboembolic diseases occur from a fixed clot (**thrombus**) or a moving clot (**embolus**) that obstructs blood flow. Death is possible whenever clots are lodged in the heart, brain, or lungs.

Hypercoagulability results from a deficiency of anticoagulation proteins. Secondary causes are conditions that promote venous status. The term **triad of Virchow** refers to three factors that can cause spontaneous thrombus formation: (1) loss of vessel wall integrity, (2) blood flow abnormalities, and (3) blood constituent alteration. Anticoagulant and fibrinolytic therapies are used depending on the severity of threat of the disorder. Parenteral heparin is used for inpatients and oral Coumadin is widely used for outpatients.

A large number of inherited conditions increase the risk of thrombosis. Most are autosomal dominant. These

195

include mutations in coagulation proteins, fibrinolytic proteins, and platelet receptors. An acquired hypercoagulable state is antiphospholipid syndrome, which is an autoimmune syndrome characterized by autoantibodies against plasma membrane phospholipids and phospholipid-binding proteins. Individuals that are at risk include those with arterial and venous thrombosis and those with obstetrical complications of miscarriage and preeclampsia/eclampsia. Unfractionated or low-molecular-weight heparin with low-dose aspirin can prevent obstetrical complications.

PRACTICE EXAMINATION

Multiple Choice

Circle the correct answer for each question.

1. Leukocytosis is found in all of the following *except*:
   a. inflammatory responses.
   b. allergic responses.
   c. bacterial infections.
   d. bone marrow depression.
2. What is a notable characteristic of infectious mononucleosis?
   a. Short incubation period of less than 1 week
   b. Affects preteens
   c. Presence of atypical lymphocytes
   d. Widespread invasion of T cells
3. Which of the following likely is not associated with leukemia?
   a. Radiation
   b. Hereditary abnormalities
   c. Polycythemia vera
   d. Chloramphenicol
   e. Increased production of other hematopoietic cells
4. The cell from which ALL most often arises is a:
   a. stem cell.
   b. T cell.
   c. B cell.
   d. monoblast.
5. Signs and symptoms of acute leukemia include all of the following *except*:
   a. splenomegaly.
   b. petechiae.
   c. lymphadenopathy.
   d. polycythemia.
   e. pallor.
6. CML is characterized by its:
   a. high blastocyst numbers.
   b. high incidence in children.
   c. association with the presence of hyperuricemia.
   d. survival time of weeks to months.
7. A bone marrow analysis reveals an abnormally high number of lymphoblasts. The likely diagnosis is:
   a. multiple myeloma.
   b. ALL.
   c. CML.
   d. CLL.

8. Clinical manifestations of multiple myeloma include all of the following except:
   a. bone pain.
   b. decreased serum calcium.
   c. M protein.
   d. renal damage.
   e. pathologic fractures.
9. Thrombocytopenia may be caused by all of the following except:
   a. an IgG autoantibody.
   b. drug hypersensitivities.
   c. viruses that stimulate platelet production.
   d. bacterial infections that consume platelets.
   e. viruses that destroy circulating platelets.
10. A thrombocytopenia with a platelet count of $40,000/mm^3$ likely will cause:
    a. hemorrhage from minor trauma.
    b. spontaneous bleeding.
    c. death.
    d. polycythemia.
11. Thromboembolic disorders can be caused by all of the following except:
    a. injured vessel walls.
    b. tissue damage that releases excessive TF.
    c. obstructed blood flow.
    d. deficient dietary intake of vitamin K.
    e. polycythemia.
12. Essential thrombocythemia exhibits:
    a. fewer megakaryocytes than normal in the marrow.
    b. thrombosis.
    c. erythromyalgia.
    d. Both b and c are correct.
    e. a, b, and c are correct.
13. DIC is associated with:
    a. endothelial damage.
    b. the activation of factor X.
    c. the release of tissue factor.
    d. gram-positive sepsis.
    e. a, b, and c are correct.
14. In DIC, plasmin:
    a. begins to degrade fibrin before a stable clot develops.
    b. complexes with factor VII.
    c. activates factor V.
    d. All of the above are correct.
15. The manifestations of leukemia include:
    a. petechial hemorrhage.
    b. hyperuricemia.
    c. weight loss.
    d. night sweats.
    e. All of above are correct.

Matching

Match the leukocytic alteration with the cause.

_____ 16. Eosinophilia

_____ 17. Granulocytosis

a. immune deficiencies

b. allergic disorders

c. radiation

d. early stages of infection

e. AIDS

f. surgical stress

g. acute viral infections

Match the characteristic with the malignant lymphoma.

_____ 18. Localized nodal involvement

_____ 19. Reed-Sternberg cells

_____ 20. Pleural effusion

a. Hodgkin lymphoma

b. non-Hodgkin lymphoma

Multiple Choice

Circle the correct answer for each question.

21. Philadelphia chromosome is observed in:
    a. AML/CML.
    b. AML/CLL.
    c. ALL/CLL.
    d. ALL/CML.
22. B cells fail to mature into plasma cells in:
    a. AML.
    b. ALL.
    c. CML.
    d. CLL.
23. Death in MM is most commonly due to:
    a. infection.
    b. hypercalcemia.
    c. anemia.
    d. pathologic fractures.

24. Acute ITP is:
    a. more common in individuals older than 40 years of age.
    b. usually preceded by a viral infection.
    c. often manifested by menorrhagia.
    d. more common in females.
    e. c and d are correct.
25. A deficiency of vitamin K is caused by:
    a. lack of clotting factor VII.
    b. impaired platelet function.
    c. altered gut flora.
    d. a and b are correct.

197

L.L., a 9-year-old boy, was taken to his dentist for a regular checkup. Previous dental visits had been routine except for 2 years ago, when L.L. missed one appointment because of chickenpox. The dentist and the boy's mother were having a chatty conversation when L.L.'s mother stated that her son had recently stopped showing interest in sports and complained of fatigue. During the dental examination, the dentist noted gingival bleeding whenever the tissue was lightly probed. Three nontender lymph nodes were palpable in the submandibular nodes; no other abnormalities were noted. The dentist advised the mother to take L.L. to the medical clinic next door.

The physical examination by a nurse practitioner showed L.L.'s skin to be pale with ecchymoses and petechiae of the trunk. The spleen and liver were not palpable, and the remaining examination was unremarkable. A sample of blood was withdrawn. The CBC revealed the following:

Hemoglobin = 9.2 g/dl
Hematocrit = 30%
RBCs = $3 \times 10^6/mm^3$
WBCs = $16 \times 10^3/mm^3$
Neutrophils = $8 \times 10^3/mm^3$
Basophils = $250/mm^3$
Eosinophils = $445/mm^3$
Monocytes = $1900/mm^3$
Lymphocytes = $4500/mm^3$
Blastocysts = much higher than normal
Platelets = $30 \times 10^3/mm^3$

Question

Considering the examinations and the CBC results, what would the nurse practitioner likely suspect and do?

28 Alterations of Hematologic Function in Children

FOUNDATIONAL KNOWLEDGE OBJECTIVES

a. Describe fetal and neonatal hematopoiesis.
Review text pages 1062 and 1063; refer to Figure 28-1.

MEMORY CHECK!

- When the developing embryo becomes too large for the oxygenation of tissues by simple diffusion, the production of erythrocytes begins within the vessels of the yolk sac. At approximately the eighth week of gestation, erythrocyte production shifts from the vessels to the liver sinusoids, the spleen, and the lymph nodes. Erythropoiesis in these sites reaches a peak at approximately 4 months. Hepatic blood cellular formation declines steadily thereafter, but it does not disappear entirely during the remainder of gestation. By the fifth month of gestation, hematopoiesis begins to occur in the marrow and increases rapidly until marrow fills the entire bone marrow space. By the time of delivery, the marrow is the only significant site of hematopoiesis. During childhood, hematopoietic tissue retreats to the vertebrae, ribs, sternum, pelvis, scapulae, skull, and proximal ends of the femur and humerus. A biochemically distinct type of hemoglobin is synthesized during fetal life and is composed of two alpha and two gamma chains of polypeptides, whereas the adult hemoglobins are composed of two alpha and two beta chains.

b. Identify the postnatal changes that occur in the blood throughout childhood.
Review text pages 1063 and 1064; refer to Table 28-1.

MEMORY CHECK!

- Blood cell counts tend to rise above adult levels at birth and then decline gradually throughout childhood. The immediate rise in values is the result of accelerated hematopoiesis during fetal life, the trauma of birth, and the cutting of the umbilical cord. These events that surround birth also are accompanied by a "shift to the left," which is the presence of large numbers of immature erythrocytes and leukocytes in peripheral blood. The shift to the left usually disappears within the first 2 to 3 months of life.

Learning Objectives

After studying this chapter, the learner will be able to do the following:

1. **Describe the etiology of childhood iron deficiency anemia and identify appropriate preventive, diagnostic, and treatment measures.**
Study text pages 1065 and 1066; refer to Table 28-2.
Iron deficiency anemia is the most common childhood anemia and is caused by poor dietary iron intake, occult blood, or both. Early exposure to cow's milk protein often causes hemorrhagic bowel inflammation and occult blood loss in the infant. The onset of menstruation in females also is a contributor. Poor socioeconomic

status can be a significant causal factor. The highest incidence of iron deficiency anemia occurs at 6 months to 2 years of age and peaks again in adolescence during rapid growth periods.

There are few symptoms in infants and young children until moderate anemia develops. General irritability, activity intolerance, and weakness are indicators of anemia. When the hemoglobin level falls below 5 g/dl, specific indicators may occur. Iron stores are best measured by serum ferritin and total iron-binding capacity. Treatment for iron-deficiency anemia is iron supplements; oral supplements are preferred.

199

2. **Compare and contrast the two major causes of hemolytic disease of the newborn.**

Study text pages 1066 through 1068; refer to Figures 28-2 and 28-3 and Table 28-2.

The two major causes of hemolytic disease of the newborn are **blood type incompatibility (ABO)** and **Rh factor incompatibility**. Blood type incompatibility of hemolytic disease of the newborn (HDN) is a mild form of hemolytic disease; Rh incompatibility is potentially much more severe.

Blood type incompatibility in the mother occurs when maternal antibodies to fetal erythrocytes are formed because of a prior incompatible pregnancy, other antigenetic factors, or exposure of the mother to fetal erythrocytes during pregnancy. Incompatibility in the infant occurs when sufficient antibody, usually IgG, crosses the placenta from the mother to the infant or when maternal antibodies attach to and damage fetal erythrocytes. ABO incompatibility occurs in 20% to 25% of pregnancies, with only 1 in 10 cases producing HDN. Usual causes are a type O mother with a type A or B infant, a type A mother with a type B infant, or a type B mother with a type A infant. Hemolysis in the newborn is usually limited and requires no treatment; however, mild hemolysis may contribute to hyperbilirubinemia.

Rh incompatibility occurs in less than 10% of pregnancies and rarely is a problem during the first pregnancy; the first pregnancy initiates sensitization. Anti-Rh antibodies are formed only in response to the presence of incompatible (RH-positive) red blood cells (RBCs) to the blood of an Rh-negative mother. Usually this exposure occurs as fetal blood is mixed with the mother's blood at the time of delivery. A problem develops if the baby is Rh positive, having inherited the Rh antigens from the father. The mother's immune system responds by making anti-Rh antibodies to the baby's Rh-positive status. Rh incompatibility becomes a greater problem with subsequent pregnancies when maternal antibodies cross the placenta into fetal blood. It should be noted that HDN caused by Rh incompatibility occurs in only 5% of pregnancies after five or more pregnancies. In the most severe form, Rh incompatibility can lead to **hydrops fetalis** with severe anemia, edema, central nervous system damage, and fetal death. Because the maternal antibodies remain in the neonate's circulatory system after birth, erythrocyte destruction can continue. This causes hyperbilirubinemia **icterus neonatorum (neonatal jaundice)** shortly after birth. Without replacement transfusions, in which the child receives Rh-negative erythrocytes, the bilirubin is deposited in the brain, a condition termed kernicterus. Kernicterus produces cerebral damage and usually causes death (**icterus gravis neonatorum**). Infants who do not die may have mental retardation, cerebral palsy, or high-frequency deafness.

Blood typing in mothers and infants reveals those who are at risk. Indirect Coombs test reveals antibodies in mothers, and direct Coombs test reveals antibodies bound to fetal erythrocytes. In utero testing through the umbilical vein is now available. Immunoprophylaxis with Rh immunoglobulin (RhoGAM) for at-risk mothers has been very successful.

3. **Identify the etiology, pathophysiology, and ethnic groups at risk for glucose-6-phosphate dehydrogenase deficiency.**

Study text pages 1068 and 1069.

Glucose-6-phosphate dehydrogenase deficiency (G6PD) is an X-linked recessive disorder that is fully expressed in homozygous males. G6PD is primarily a problem in blacks, in whom the incidence may be 10%; a frequency range of 5% to 40% exists in Sephardic Jews, Greeks, Iranians, Chinese, Filipinos, and Indonesians. G6PD is caused by a defect of an enzyme that enables erythrocytes to maintain normal function in the presence of certain substances, such as sulfa drugs, salicylates, quinolones, antimalarials, and fava beans, which are a dietary staple in the Mediterranean area. Exposure to these substances causes hemolysis, often very severe, that resolves when the offending substance is removed. Episodes may result in shock or death. Males at risk for G6PD should be tested before they are exposed to certain oxidant drugs.

4. **Describe hereditary spherocytosis.**

Study text page 1070 and 1071; refer to Figure 28-4.

Hereditary spherocytosis, transmitted as an autosomal dominant tract, is the most common of the hemolytic disorders in which there is no abnormality of hemoglobin. Affected cells are unduly permeable to sodium and acquire a particular characteristic structure due to an abnormality of proteins in the RBC membrane.

Circulation of blood to the spleen creates a metabolic environment that is stressful to spherocyte cells, and repeated passages through this stressful environment result in their sequestration and destruction. During infancy and childhood, severity of the anemia varies widely but tends to be similar within families. Slight jaundice usually is present. After infancy, the spleen almost always is enlarged. Although gallstones have been reported to occur; they usually do not develop until late childhood or early adolescence. Aplastic crises are the most serious complications during childhood.

Surgical removal of the spleen should be performed when the child is 5 years of age or older or in those who develop symptomatic gallstones. Partial splenectomy is an alternative procedure that appears to control hemolysis while retaining splenic function.

5. **Describe childhood sickle cell disease, and identify its most common forms of presentation.**

Study text pages 1071 and 1073 through 1076; refer to Figures 28-5 through 28-9 and Table 28-3.

Sickle cell disease (SCD) is an inherited, autosomal recessive disorder most common in the United States among blacks. The disease is characterized by the presence of **hemoglobin S (HbS)** within the erythrocytes. This hemoglobin becomes elongated and sickle shaped whenever it is deoxygenated or dehydrated. Polymerization stiffens the sickled erythrocyte and changes the cell to an inflexible obstacle that starves tissues.

The parents' medical history and clinical findings may generate an index of suspicion about the child. The sickle solubility test and hemoglobin electrophoresis are used to assist diagnosis. Prenatal chorionic villus sampling is now available.

Acute complications or crises occur in sickle cell disease and may be provoked by infection, exposure to cold, low Po$_2$, acidosis, or localized hypoxemia. Infections are frequent in childhood and may generate various degrees of other triggers.

Vaso-occlusive crises result from a "log-jam" effect produced by stiff, sickled erythrocytes in the microcirculation. Symptoms include symmetric swelling of the hands and feet, which may be the first clinical manifestation in infancy. In older children, swollen painful joints, priapism, severe abdominal pain from infarctions of abdominal organs, and strokes may occur. Other complications include sickle cell retinopathy, renal necrosis, and necrosis of the femoral head.

Sequestration crises occur only in the young child. Large amounts of blood may pool in the liver and spleen; these pools can contain as much as one fifth of the blood volume, and thus, precipitate shock. Up to a 50% mortality rate has been reported with these crises.

Aplastic crisis, a transient cessation in red blood cell production resulting in acute anemia, occurs as a result of viral infection, almost always infection with parvovirus B19, which is the virus responsible for the common childhood infection known as fifth disease. The virus causes temporary shutdown of red blood cell production in the bone marrow, or reticulocytosis. However, hemolysis, a component of SCD, continues. The outcome is a severe drop in hemoglobin with an extremely low reticulocyte count. Treatment of SCD consists of supportive care to prevent consequences of anemia and avoiding crisis. Crisis can be avoided by preventing fever, infection, acidosis, dehydration, and exposure to cold. Hydroxyurea increases fetal hemoglobin synthesis in individuals with sickle cell anemia and increases hemoglobin and mean corpuscular volume while decreasing reticulocytes and bilirubin. Splenectomy may be performed if sequestration crises recur. Definitive treatment can be accomplished through stem cell transplantation.

6. Describe the thalassemias.

Study text pages 1076 through 1078.

The alpha- and beta-thalassemias are inherited autosomal recessive disorders that cause an impaired rate of synthesis or decrease of one of the two chains—alpha or beta—of adult hemoglobin. Beta-thalassemia is more common than alpha-thalassemia.

Beta-thalassemia has slowed or defective synthesis of the beta globin chain and is prevalent among Greeks, Italians, some Arabs, and Sephardic Jews. Alpha-thalassemia, wherein the alpha chain is affected, is most common among Chinese, Vietnamese, Cambodians, and Laotians. Both thalassemias are common among blacks. The effects range from mild microcytosis to death in utero, and the pathophysiology depends on the number of defective genes and the mode of inheritance.

The fundamental defect in **beta-thalassemia** is the uncoupling of alpha and beta chain synthesis. The free alpha chains are unstable and easily precipitated in the cell. Most erythroblasts that contain precipitates are destroyed by mononuclear phagocytes in the marrow, and this results in ineffective erythropoiesis and anemia. Individuals with beta-thalassemia minor, which is the mild form, are usually asymptomatic. People with beta-thalassemia major, which is the severe form, may become quite ill; anemia is severe and results in significant cardiovascular overload with high-output congestive heart failure. Today, blood transfusion can increase life span by a decade or two. Death is usually caused by hemochromatosis.

There are differing forms of **alpha-thalassemia**, and the type depends on the number of defective genes. The severity is variable. Individuals who inherit the mildest form of alpha-thalassemia, caused by the alpha trait, usually are symptom free or have mild microcytosis. Alpha-thalassemia major causes hydrops fetalis and fulminant intrauterine congestive heart failure. The fetus has a grossly enlarged heart and liver. Diagnosis usually is made postmortem. In children with thalassemia major, cardiovascular compromise causes death by 5 to 6 years of age if untreated.

Individuals who are carriers or who have thalassemia minor generally have few symptoms and require no specific treatment. For thalassemia major, therapies to support and prolong life are necessary. There is no cure for either condition. Presently, thalassemia major is treated by blood transfusions, iron chelation therapy combined with transfusion, and splenectomy.

7. Describe hemophilias and coagulation disorders; identify their complications.

Study text pages 1078 through 1081; refer to Table 28-4.

Hemophilia, which is spontaneous bleeding, is rare in the first year of life; although recurrent bleeding, both spontaneous and following minor trauma, is a lifelong problem. **Hemophilia A,** the most common of the hemophilias, is caused by factor VIII deficiency. **Hemophilia B** is caused by factor IX deficiency. Both hemophilia A and B are X-linked and limited to males, being transmitted through the female to the second generation. **Hemophilia C** occurs as an autosomal recessive disease and occurs equally in males and females. Bleeding is less severe than in hemophilia A and B. **von Willebrand disease** is an autosomal dominant inherited disease that produces prolonged bleeding because of decreased levels of clotting factor VIII, and platelets that have decreased adhesiveness, because the plasma factor is absent.

Hematoma formation is a more common problem during the first year of life and may be due to injections, firm holding, or the many accidents that occur in the development of movement in children. These accidents may also precipitate bleeding in the joints. Spontaneous hematuria and epistaxis are bothersome but rarely serious. Life-threatening intracranial, cervical, and abdominal bleeding may result from childhood injury. Inherited **thrombophilic** and **hypercoagulability** conditions are caused by defects in clotting inhibitors, so clotting dominates the aspect of hemostasis. These hypercoagulability disorders include C deficiency, protein S deficiency, neonatal purpura fulminans, and antithrombin III deficiency.

The administration of recombinant blood products to replace deficient or absent factors has enhanced the physical capabilities of individuals that have hemophilic

201

defects. Thrombophilic conditions are treated with plasma, antiplatelet, warfarin (Coumadin), or heparinization.

8. Describe the pathophysiology of idiopathic thrombocytopenic purpura, and identify its etiology; note other purpura conditions.

Study text pages 1081 through 1083.

Idiopathic thrombocytopenic purpura (ITP) is the most common thrombocytopenic purpura of childhood. Antiplatelet antibodies attach to platelets that are then sequestered in the spleen, where they are destroyed by mononuclear phagocytes. Destruction far exceeds production, and thrombocytopenia occurs.

Classic symptoms of bruising and petechiae are usually preceded 1 to 4 weeks earlier by a viral illness that may cause sensitization of the platelets and trigger an antibody response. High levels of IgG have been found on the platelets of affected children.

The prognosis is excellent. The acute phase lasts 1 to 2 weeks, although thrombocytopenia may persist longer. Complete recovery is approximately 75% at 3 months after onset, with 90% of individuals recovering by 9 to 12 months. Although serious complications are few, severe intracranial bleeding does occur in less than 1% of cases, and this can be devastating.

Intravenous IgG can increase the platelet count in some children with ITP. Corticosteroids are indicated in some cases to suppress the body's immune response system to platelets. Monoclonal antibody therapy is being used. Splenectomy is reserved for severe, chronic cases.

Autoimmune neonatal thrombocytopenia is an antibody-mediated disorder observed in newborns who were transiently thrombocytopenic and whose mothers exhibited ITP. **Neonatal alloimmune thrombocytopenic purpura** is the production of a maternal antibody against a fetal platelet–specific antigen inherited from the father but not shared by the mother. **Autoimmune vascular purpuras** are caused by the body's responses to allergens in the blood.

9. Describe proposed causative factors and common manifestations of childhood leukemias.

Study text pages 1083 through 1086; refer to Figures 28-10 and 28-11 and Table 28-5.

Leukemia, in its various forms, is the most common childhood cancer; it comprises 40% of the neoplasms of children. Acute lymphoblastic leukemia (ALL) represents 80% to 85% of all childhood leukemias. The remaining leukemias are acute nonlymphocytic leukemias (ANLL). Peak incidence of ALL occurs between 2 and 6 years of age and is twice as common in white children as in non-white children. The etiology of leukemia is probably multifactorial, with genetic predisposition (abnormal morphological and numerical alterations in chromosomes), environment, and viruses playing a role. Inherited diseases that predispose a child to leukemia include Down syndrome, Fanconi anemia, and congenital agammaglobulinemia. Exposure to high levels of radiation also is an established etiologic factor.

The appearance of symptoms may be rapid or slow, but it generally reflects the effects of bone marrow failure. Findings include decreased RBCs and platelets and changes in WBCs. Pallor, fatigue, petechiae, purpura, and fever are generally present. Fever may be due to a hypermetabolic state brought on by the rapid production and destruction of leukemic cells or because of a secondary infection due to neutropenia.

Although WBC counts are generally less than $50,000/mm^3$ in most forms of leukemia, they may exceed $100,000/mm^3$. Renal failure may ensue because of high uric acid levels that produce precipitates of urates in the renal tubules. This phenomenon is the result of rapid cellular breakdown, which liberates high levels of purines that are then metabolized into uric acid. Other symptoms, such as bone and joint pain, may be due to infiltration of leukemic cells into other organs. The central nervous system is a common site of extramedullary infiltration, although few children have this problem at diagnosis.

Combination chemotherapy, with or without radiation to local sites, is the choice for acute leukemia. Prognosis for the childhood leukemias is variable; however, 70% to 80% of children with ALL can be cured.

10. Distinguish between non-Hodgkin lymphoma and Hodgkin lymphoma.

Study text pages 1086 through 1088; refer to Figure 28-12.

Non-Hodgkin lymphoma (NHL) and Hodgkin disease comprise approximately 15% of all childhood cancer; NHL is the most common. Both groups of disease are rare before 5 years of age, and the relative incidence increases throughout childhood. Males are affected more often than females; at particular risk are children with inherited or acquired immunodeficiency syndromes. Etiologic factors likely include defective host immunity, a viral agent, chronic immunostimulation, and genetics.

Childhood **non-Hodgkin lymphoma** is a diffuse rather than a nodular disease. Disease sites commonly involve extranodal sites such as brain, lung, bone, and skin. Rapidly enlarging lymphoid tissue and painless lymphadenopathy are common with abdominal sites. Symptoms often include abdominal pain and vomiting, but a palpable mass is not always present. An anterior mediastinal mass, with or without pleural effusion, may be present. If the mass is large, respiratory compromise, tracheal compression, and superior vena cava syndrome may arise. Central nervous system involvement is common.

Seventy percent to 80% of children with localized NHL can be cured. Optimal treatment is evolving, but combinations of radiation therapy that destroys lymphoma cells and chemotherapy are successful.

Besides a possible viral etiology (an EBV) for **Hodgkin lymphoma** in children, genetic susceptibility and immune deficits have been suggested as causes. Hodgkin disease incidence gradually rises until 11 years of age, with a marked increase through adolescence that continues into the 30s.

Painless lymphadenopathy in the lower cervical chain is the most common symptom. Mediastinal involvement can lead to airway obstruction. Extranodal primary involvement is rare in Hodgkin disease.

Treatment for Hodgkin disease includes chemotherapy and low-dose radiation therapy. The survival rate for children with Hodgkin disease is high; 90% to 95% is common.

PRACTICE EXAMINATION

True or False

For each statement, write T (true) or F (false) in the blank provided.

_____ 1. During fetal life, the synthesized hemoglobin is composed of two alpha and two beta chains.

_____ 2. Although a frequent problem, ABO incompatibility seldom results in significant disease.

_____ 3. Sequestration crisis is a serious complication of sickle cell disease seen only in the young child.

_____ 4. Rh incompatibility is a problem only of Rh-positive women bearing an Rh-negative fetus during a second pregnancy.

_____ 5. Because hemostasis in the newborn is chiefly attained through the extrinsic pathway, serious bleeding in the newborn period is usually not a problem in hemophiliacs.

_____ 6. Idiopathic thrombocytopenic purpura is a genetically transmitted disease.

_____ 7. Leukemias are multifactorial diseases with genetic disposition, environment, and bacterial infections playing a role in their etiology.

Multiple Choice

Circle the correct answer for each question.

8. The blood disorder of infancy and childhood caused by poor dietary iron intake is:
   a. a microcytic-hypochromic anemia.
   b. pernicious anemia.
   c. folate deficiency anemia.
   d. sideroblastic anemia.

9. A first-time pregnancy may initiate Rh sensitization in which conditions?
   a. Rh-positive mother, Rh-negative fetus
   b. Rh-negative mother, Rh-positive fetus
   c. Rh-negative father, Rh-positive mother
   d. Rh-negative father, Rh-negative mother

10. Beta-thalassemia is:
    a. common among Italians.
    b. an X-linked recessive disorder.
    c. an autosomal dominant disorder.
    d. common in the Chinese.
    e. Both a and c are correct.

11. Sickle cell disease is an:
    a. autosomal dominant disorder.
    b. X-linked recessive disorder.
    c. X-linked dominant disorder.
    d. autosomal recessive disorder.

12. Idiopathic thrombocytopenic purpura (ITP) involves:
    a. neutrophilic destruction.
    b. eosinophilic destruction.
    c. a platelet/antibody complex.
    d. thrombocytosis.

13. Which are associated with inherited thrombophilic conditions?
    a. Antithrombin III deficiency
    b. Factor III deficiency.
    c. Decreased platelet adhesiveness.
    d. Both a and c are correct.

14. Which is the most likely cause of idiopathic thrombocytopenic purpura?
    a. Stress and fatigue
    b. High levels of IgG on platelets
    c. Prolonged occult bleeding
    d. Viral sensitization

15. Hodgkin disease has:
    a. extensive extranodal involvement.
    b. rare extranodal involvement.
    c. painful cervical lymphadenopathy.
    d. a mediastinal mass.

16. In sickle cell disease, vaso-occlusive crisis is the result of:
    a. damage to platelets due to IgG.
    b. the "plugging" of peripheral blood vessels by "stiff" sickled erythrocytes.
    c. the ingestion of sulfa drugs.
    d. sequestration of large numbers of erythrocytes in the spleen.

17. Which factor/s may play a part in the development of childhood leukemia?
    a. Genetic predisposition
    b. Environmental factors
    c. Viral infections
    d. Radiation
    e. All of the above are correct.

18. Which characteristic is true about acute lymphocytic leukemia?
    a. It is the most common childhood leukemia.
    b. It usually occurs in nonwhite children.
    c. It is uniformly fatal.
    d. It is easily predicted through genetic testing.

Matching

Match the alteration/circumstance with the disorder (may use answer more than once).

_____ 19. Urate precipitates in renal tubules   a. leukemia

_____ 20. Antibody/cell complexes sequester in the spleen   b. ITP

_____ 21. Sensitization is usually required before problems develop   c. sickle cell disease

_____ 22. May present early as symmetric, painful swelling of the hands and feet   d. Rh incompatibility

_____ 23. May cause severe hemolysis during the newborn period   e. hemophilia

_____ 24. May result in aplastic crises

_____ 25. May result in hydrops fetalis or fetal death

CASE STUDY

S.C. is a 10-year-old white boy seeking physician attention because of possible physical abuse observed by his gym teacher. The teacher noticed severe bruising over much of the boy's upper body when his shirt "rode up" during an exercise. S.C. emphatically states, "I have never been abused by anyone and have had this bruising for 2 to 3 days." He denies any accidents and did not tell anyone about his bruises because he thought they might "get me into trouble." He also denies any systemic symptoms, but he acknowledges that he had a "bad cold" nearly a month ago. His mother is very confused and concerned. She cannot explain the bruises either, and she did not see them before today, because her son performs all of his own hygiene and is quite modest about revealing his body even to family members. S.C.'s physical examination is benign except for multiple, irregular, dark purple bruises over most of his torso and lower extremities. He also has a "shower" of light petechiae over his shoulders and neck. His complete blood count is well within normal limits, except for a low platelet count of 18,000/mm³, exhibiting large cells.

Questions

What is S.C.'s diagnosis?

What is the treatment?

29 Structure and Function of the Cardiovascular and Lymphatic Systems

PREREQUISITE KNOWLEDGE OBJECTIVES

After reviewing the primary text where referenced, the learner will be able to do the following:

1. Describe the function of the circulatory system; distinguish between the pulmonary and systemic circulation.
   Review text pages 1091 and 1093; refer to Figure 29-1.
2. Describe the heart including its wall, chambers, fibrous skeleton, valves, and great vessels; trace the blood flow through the heart.
   Review text pages 1093 through 1096; refer to Figures 29-2 through 29-8 and Table 29-1.
3. Describe the coronary arteries, collateral arteries, capillaries, veins, and lymphatic vessels.
   Review text pages 1096 through 1099; refer to Figure 29-9.
4. Describe the initiation of and the conduction sequence of electrical impulses through the heart; identify the autonomic innervation and its effects on the heart.
   Review text pages 1099 through 1106; refer to Figures 29-10 through 29-13 and Table 29-2.
5. Identify the structure, function, and characteristics of myocardial cells.
   Review text pages 1105 through 1109; refer to Figures 29-14 through 29-18.
6. Describe the factors that affect cardiac performances, use the Frank-Starling and Laplace laws to demonstrate interrelationships that affect cardiac function.
   Review text pages 1109 through 1113; refer to Figures 29-19 and 29-21.
7. Contrast the structure and function of systemic circulatory arteries, capillaries, and veins.
   Review text pages 1113, 1114, 1116, and 1117; refer to Figures 29-22 through 29-31.
8. Describe the determinants of blood flow.
   Review text pages 1117 through 1122; refer to Figures 29-32 through 29-35.
9. Identify the factors that regulate arterial and venous blood pressure; note regulators of coronary circulation.
   Review text pages 1122 through 1128, 1130, and 1131; refer to Figures 29-36 through 29-39 and Table 29-3.

10. Describe the normal structure and function of the lymphatic system.
    Review text pages 1131 through 1133; refer to Figures 29-40 through 29-42.
11. Describe tests of cardiovascular function.
    Review text pages 1133 through 1136; refer to Figure 29-43 and Table 29-4.
12. Note the changes that aging causes in the cardiovascular system.
    Review text pages 1136 and 1137; refer to Table 29-5.

PRACTICE EXAMINATION

Multiple Choice

Circle the correct answer(s) for each question.

1. Oxygenated blood flows through the:
   a. superior vena cava.
   b. pulmonary veins.
   c. pulmonary arteries.
   d. coronary veins.
2. The hepatic vein:
   a. carries blood from the vena cava to the liver.
   b. carries blood from the liver to the vena cava.
   c. carries blood from the aorta to the liver.
   d. carries blood from the liver to the aorta.
3. Insulin protects vascular tissue by:
   a. increasing growth of vascular smooth muscle cells.
   b. increasing endothelial cell production of nitric oxide.
   c. increasing the effect of platelet-derived growth factor.
   d. increasing the binding of monocytes/macrophages to the vessel wall.
4. The pericardial space is found between the:
   a. myocardium and the parietal pericardium.
   b. endocardium and the visceral pericardium.
   c. visceral and the parietal pericardia.
   d. visceral and the epicardial pericardia.
5. The QRS complex of the ECG represents:
   a. atrial depolarization.
   b. ventricular depolarization.
   c. atrial contraction.
   d. ventricular repolarization.
   e. atrial repolarization.

205

6. A person who has a heart rate of 100 beats per minute, a systolic blood pressure of 200 mmHg, and a stroke volume of 40 ml would have an average cardiac output of:
   a. 0.5 ml.
   b. 5 L.
   c. 4 ml.
   d. 8000 ml.
   e. None of the above is correct.
7. During atrial systole, the:
   a. AV valves are open.
   b. atria are filling.
   c. ventricles are emptying.
   d. semilunar valves are open.
8. Which of the following does *not* significantly affect heart rate?
   a. Temperature
   b. Age
   c. Presence of heart murmur
   d. Na^+ and K^+ ions
9. One cardiac cycle:
   a. has a duration that changes if the heart rate changes.
   b. usually requires less than 1 second to complete.
   c. is equal to stroke volume times heart rate.
   d. pumps approximately 5 liters of blood.
   e. Both a and b are correct.
10. Compared with arteries, veins:
    a. have a larger diameter.
    b. are thickly coated.
    c. recoil quickly after distention.
    d. Both a and b are correct.
11. When the intraventricular pressure becomes greater than the pressure in the pulmonary arteries, the:
    a. semilunar valves will open.
    b. semilunar valves will close.
    c. AV valves will open.
    d. AV valves will close.
12. The two distinct heart sounds, *lubb* and *dupp,* are most directly related to:
    a. pulse pressure in the aorta.
    b. the contraction of the ventricles.
    c. turbulence from the closing of valves.
    d. contraction of the atria.
13. Normal end-diastolic pressure within the left ventricle is in the range of:
    a. 100 to 140 mmHg.
    b. 15 to 28 mmHg.
    c. 0 to 8 mmHg.
    d. 4 to 12 mmHg.
14. The Frank-Starling "law of the heart" involves the relationship between:
    a. the length of the cardiac muscle fiber and the strength of contraction.
    b. stroke volume and arterial resistance.
    c. rapidity of nerve conduction and stroke volume.
    d. systolic rate and cardiac output.

15. Blood pressure is measured by the:
    a. pressure exerted on the ventricular walls during systole.
    b. pressure exerted by the blood on the wall of any blood vessel.
    c. pressure exerted on arteries by the blood.
    d. product of the stroke volume times heart rate.
16. The heartbeat is initiated by the:
    a. coronary sinus.
    b. atrioventricular bundle.
    c. right ventricle.
    d. SA node.
    e. AV node.
17. If the sympathetic nervous system stimulation of the heart predominates over parasympathetic nervous stimulation, the heart will:
    a. increase its rate.
    b. contract with greater force and at a slower rate.
    c. decrease its rate and force of contraction.
    d. contract with less force and at a higher rate.
18. Adrenomedullin (ADM):
    a. exhibits powerful vasoconstriction activity.
    b. is present only in cardiovascular tissue.
    c. mediates sodium reabsorption.
    d. exhibits powerful vasodilation activity.
19. Which factor might increase resistance to the flow of blood through the blood vessels?
    a. An increased inner radius or diameter of the blood vessels
    b. A decreased number of capillaries
    c. A decreased blood viscosity
    d. A decreased number of red blood cells
20. Nitric oxide is:
    a. a potent vasodilator.
    b. a potent vasoconstrictor.
    c. endothelium-derived relaxing factor (EDRF).
    d. an inhibitor of platelet adherence to the endothelium.
    e. Both a and c are correct.
21. Which of the following is *true?*
    a. Lymphatic walls consist of multiple layers of flattened endothelial cells.
    b. Lymph from the entire body, except the upper right quadrant, eventually drains into the thoracic duct.
    c. The thoracic duct has approximately the same diameter as the great veins.
    d. Lymph contains more proteins than does blood plasma.
    e. The lymphatic system, like the circulatory system, is a closed circuit.

206

22. Which event(s) is/are part of the normal cardiac cycle?
    a. The right atrium and right ventricles contract simultaneously.
    b. The two atria contract simultaneously while the two ventricles relax.
    c. The two ventricles contract simultaneously while the two atria relax.
    d. Both the ventricles and the atria contract simultaneously to increase cardiac output.
23. What factors assist the return of venous blood to the heart?
    a. Peripheral pooling
    b. Venous valves
    c. Increased intra-abdominal pressure
    d. Respiratory movements
    e. Contraction of skeletal muscles
24. Alphabetize the correct sequence as blood travels through the following structures.
    a. Pulmonary veins
    b. Pulmonary arteries
    c. Lungs
    d. Right ventricle
    e. Left atrium
25. Alphabetize the normal sequence of an electrical impulse through the heart's conduction system.
    a. Atrioventricular bundle
    b. AV node
    c. Purkinje fibers
    d. SA node
    e. Right and left bundle branches

30 Alterations of Cardiovascular Function

FOUNDATIONAL KNOWLEDGE OBJECTIVES

a. Describe the flow of blood through the heart, and identify the coronary vessels.
   Refer to Figures 29-3 and 29-29

MEMORY CHECK!

- The pumping action of the heart consists of the contraction and relaxation of the myocardial layer of the heart wall. During relaxation, which is called diastole, blood fills the chambers. The contraction that follows, called systole, forces the blood out of the chamber and into the pulmonary or systemic circulation. During diastole, veins from the systemic circulation enter the thin-walled right atrium from the superior vena cava and the inferior vena cava. Venous blood from the coronary circulation enters the right atrium through the coronary sinus. The right atrium fills, and its fluid pressure pushes open the right atrioventricular or tricuspid valve; blood fills the right ventricle. The same sequence of events occurs a fraction of a second earlier in the left heart. The four pulmonary veins (two from the right lung and two from the left lung) carry oxygenated blood from the pulmonary circulation to the left atrium. As the left atrium fills, its fluid pressure pushes the cusps of the mitral valve open, and blood flows into the left ventricle. Left atrial contraction, also called "atrial kick," provides a significant increase of blood to the left ventricle. Blood circulates from the left ventricle and returns to the right atrium because of a progressive fall in pressure from the left ventricle to the right atrium of approximately 120 mmHg. Blood always flows from a higher pressure area to a lower pressure area.
- The blood within the heart chambers does not supply oxygen and other nutrients to the cells of the heart. Like all other organs, heart structures are nourished by vessels of the systemic circulation. The coronary circulation consists of coronary arteries and the cardiac veins. The right and left coronary arteries traverse the epicardium and branch several times. The left coronary artery arises from a single opening behind the left cusp of the aortic semilunar valve. It divides into two branches: the left anterior descending artery and the circumflex artery. The left anterior descending artery delivers blood to portions of the left and right ventricles and much of the interventricular septum. The circumflex artery supplies blood to the left atrium and the lateral wall of the left ventricle. The circumflex artery often branches to the posterior surfaces of the left atrium and left ventricle. The right coronary artery originates from an opening behind the right aortic cusp. Three major branches of the right coronary artery supply blood to the right atrium, the upper right ventricle, and both ventricles.
- Collateral arteries are connections or anastomoses between two branches of the same coronary artery or connections of branches of the right coronary artery with branches of the left. They are particularly common within the interventricular and interatrial septa, at the apex of the heart, over the anterior surface of the right ventricle, and around the sinus node. The heart has an extensive capillary network with about one capillary per muscle cell. Blood travels from the arteries to the arterioles and then into the capillaries, where exchange of oxygen and other nutrients takes place.
- Blood from the coronary arteries drains into the cardiac veins that travel alongside the arteries. The cardiac veins feed into the great cardiac vein and then into the coronary sinus, which is located between the atria and ventricles. The coronary sinus empties into the right atrium.

b. Describe the conduction system of the heart.
   Review text pages 1099 through 1106; refer to Figures 29-10 through 29-13 and Table 29-2.

MEMORY CHECK!

- Continuous, rhythmic repetition of the cardiac cycle (systole and diastole) depends on the continuous, rhythmic transmission of electrical impulses. As an electrical impulse passes from cell to cell in the myocardium, it stimulates the fibers to shorten; shortening causes muscular contraction (systole). After the action potential passes, the fibers relax and return to their resting length; this relaxation is diastole.
- The myocardium differs from other muscle tissues; it contains its own intrinsic conduction system. It can generate and transmit action potentials without stimulation from the nervous system. These cells are concentrated at certain sites in the myocardium called nodes. Although the heart is innervated by both sympathetic and parasympathetic fibers, neural impulses are not needed to maintain the cardiac cycle.
- Electrical impulses normally arise in the sinoatrial node (SA node), which is often called the pacemaker of the heart. The SA node lies only a millimeter or less beneath the visceral pericardium, and this makes it vulnerable to injury and disease, especially pericardial inflammation. There are numerous autonomic nerve endings within the node that enable it to respond to the nervous system. In the resting adult, the SA node generates about 75 action potentials per minute. Each action potential travels rapidly from cell to cell and through special pathways in the atrial myocardium, which causes both atria to contract. Atrial contraction initiates systole. Transmission of the action potential from the atrial to the ventricular myocardium occurs through muscle fibers of the conduction system. The action potential travels first to the atrioventricular node (AV node), then to the atrioventricular bundle, then to the common bundle, and finally through the bundle branches of the interventricular septum to Purkinje fibers in the heart wall.
- The extensive network of Purkinje fibers enables the rapid spread of the impulse to the ventricular apices.
- Electrical activation of the muscle cells (depolarization) is caused by the movement of electrically charged solutes (primarily sodium and potassium) across cardiac cell membranes. Deactivation, which is also called repolarization, occurs by ion movement in the opposite direction. Movement of ions into and out of the cell creates an electrical or voltage difference across the cell membrane. This difference or potential of charged ions causes the impulse to flow within cells and from cell to cell.
- Sympathetic neural stimulation of the myocardium and coronary vessels depends on the presence of adrenergic receptors that are able to bind specifically with neurotransmitters of the sympathetic nervous system. The effects of sympathetic stimulation depend on which adrenergic receptors are most plentiful on the cells of the effector tissue and whether the neurotransmitter is norepinephrine or epinephrine. β_1 Receptors are found mostly in the AV and SA nodes, the Purkinje fibers, and the atrial and ventricular myocardia. Norepinephrine binding with β_1 receptors increases the rate of impulse generation and conduction and also the strength of myocardial contraction during systole; these effects enable the heart to pump more blood. At the same time, epinephrine binds with β_2 receptors, which are most plentiful in the coronary arterioles; this causes the coronary arterioles to dilate and supplies the hard-working myocardium with more oxygen and nutrients.

c. Describe the interrelationships between myocardial stretch and chamber wall dimensions and the contractible force of the heart.
   Review text pages 1109 through 1113; refer to Figures 29-20 and 29-21.

MEMORY CHECK!

- Cardiac muscle, like other muscle, increases its strength of contraction within certain limits when it is stretched. The Frank-Starling law of the heart states that there is a direct relationship between the volume of blood in the heart and the stretch or length of cardiac fibers at the end of diastole and the force of contraction during the next systole. The greater the stretch from preload blood volume, the stronger is the contraction. The failing or dilated heart may not be able to respond to increased filling, because its fibers are already lengthened maximally.
- Laplace law states the relationships between wall thickness, pressure, and wall tension. Wall tension is related directly to the product of intraventricular pressure and internal radius and inversely related to the wall thickness. Stated another way, wall tension equals intraventricular pressure times radius of space divided by wall thickness. If solved for pressure, the pressure or contractible force is directly related to wall thickness and wall tension and indirectly related to the radius. The thicker the wall and the greater the wall tension and the smaller the radius, the greater is the force of contraction. With a dilated chamber or vessel, the myocardial fibers in the wall must develop greater tension to produce a given pressure within the chamber or vessel.

d. Establish the determinants of blood flow.

Review text pages 1117 through 1122; refer to Figures 29-32 through 29-35

MEMORY CHECK!

- Blood flow is determined primarily by two factors: pressure and resistance. Pressure in a liquid system is the force exerted on the liquid per unit area. Fluid moves from the arterial "side" of the capillaries, which is a region of greater pressure, to the venous side, which is a region of lesser pressure. Resistance opposes force. In the cardiovascular system, most opposition to blood flow is because of the diameter and length of the blood vessels themselves.
- The relationship between blood flow, pressure, and resistance can be stated as Q equals P divided by R, where Q is blood flow, P is the pressure difference, and R is resistance.
- Resistance to fluid flow considers the length of the tube or vessel, the viscosity of the fluid, and the radius of the lumen. According to Poiseuille's formula, the resistance equals viscosity of blood times length of vessel divided by the fourth power of the lumen's radius.
- Because this equation was derived using straight, rigid tubes with steady, streamlined flow, it cannot be applied exactly to the vascular system. Nevertheless, it is a useful model for vascular resistance assessment. Small changes in the lumen's radius lead to large changes in vascular resistance. Because vessel length is relatively constant, length is not as important as lumen size in determining flow through a single vessel. However, blood flowing through the distributing arteries encounters more resistance than blood flowing through the capillary bed. In the capillary bed, flow is distributed among many short, tiny branches.
- If R equals viscosity times length divided by the fourth power of radius is substituted into the formula Q equals P divided by R, a helpful summary of likely factors affecting blood flow rate can be expressed. Now, blood flow equals pressure times radius to the fourth power divided by the viscosity times the length. The higher the pressure and the greater the vessel radius and the less the viscosity of blood and length of vessel, the greater is the flow of blood.

---

e. Establish the determinants of blood pressure.

Review text pages 1122 through 1128, 1130, and 1131; refer to Figures 29-36 through 29-39 and Table 29-3.

MEMORY CHECK!

- The mean arterial pressure, which is the average pressure in the arteries throughout the cardiac cycle, depends on the elastic properties of the arterial walls and the mean volume of blood in the arterial system. The main determinants of venous blood pressure are the volume of fluid within the veins and the compliance or distensibility of their vessel walls. Veins have much thinner walls than arteries and are more distensible than arteries. The venous system accommodates approximately 60% of the total blood volume at any given moment, with a venous pressure averaging less than 10 mmHg. Conversely, the arteries accommodate about 15% of the total blood volume, with a pressure of about 100 mmHg. Some important relationships include the following:
- Mean blood pressure equals cardiac output times peripheral resistance.
- Cardiac output equals heart rate times stroke volume.
- Peripheral resistance equals blood viscosity times vessel length divided by vessel radius raised to the fourth power.
- Blood pressure equals heart rate times stroke volume times viscosity times length divided by the radius to the fourth power. The higher the heart rate, stroke volume, blood viscosity, and vessel length and the less the vessel radius to the fourth power, the greater is the blood pressure.

LEARNING OBJECTIVES

After studying this chapter, the learner will be able to do the following:

1. Distinguish among venous occlusive diseases.

Study text pages 1142 through 1144; refer to Figures 30-1 and 30-2.

A **varicose vein** is a vein in which blood has pooled. Varicose veins are distended, tortuous, and palpable. Varicose veins in the legs are caused by trauma to the saphenous veins that damages one or more valves or by venous distention from a combination of standing for long periods and the action of gravity on blood within the legs. If a valve is damaged and permits backflow, a section of the vein is subjected to the pressure exerted by a larger volume of blood under the influence of gravity. The vein swells as it becomes engorged, and surrounding tissue becomes edematous, because increased hydrostatic pressure pushes plasma through the stretched vessel wall.

Varicose veins and valvular incompetence can progress to **chronic venous insufficiency (CVI).** This condition is characterized by chronic pooling of blood in the

211

veins of the lower extremities and leads to hyperpigmentation of the skin over the feet and ankles. Edema of the feet and ankles may progress proximally to the knees. Any trauma or pressure lowers the oxygen supply by further reducing blood flow into the area. Cell death occurs, and necrotic tissue develops into **venous stasis ulcers.** Persistent ulceration develops because the high metabolic demands of healing tissue cannot be met by the existing compromised circulation.

Deep venous thrombosis occurs in individuals who have venous stasis (immobility, age, left heart failure), vein wall damage (trauma, intravenous medications), or hypercoagulable states (pregnancy, oral contraceptives, malignancy, genetic coagulopathies).

Deep venous thrombosis is often asymptomatic but may lead to potentially fatal pulmonary emboli. The inflammatory response triggered by the clotting cascade causes extreme tenderness, swelling, and redness in the area of thrombus formation. With venous occlusion, the skin is discolored rather than pale, edema is prominent, and pain is most marked at the site of occlusion.

Treatment of varicose veins begins with thrombolytics and having the individual wear antiembolism stockings and avoid standing and the use of constrictive clothing. If conservative treatment is ineffective, various grafts and intravascular stents may be possible.

Superior vena cava syndrome (SVCS) is a progressive occlusion of the superior vena cava (SVC) that leads to venous distention in the upper extremities and head. The leading cause of SVCS is bronchogenic cancer, and this is followed by lymphomas and metastasis of other cancers. The SVC is a relatively low-pressure vessel that lies in the closed thoracic compartment; therefore, tissue expansion within the thoracic compartment can easily compress the SVC.

Clinical manifestations of SVCS include edema and venous distention in the upper extremities and face, including the ocular beds. Cerebral and central nervous system edema may cause headache, visual disturbance, or impaired consciousness. Respiratory distress may be present because of edema of the bronchial structures or compression of the bronchus by a carcinoma. SVCS is generally not a vascular emergency but rather an oncologic problem.

Treatment consists of radiotherapy for the neoplasm. The administration of diuretics, steroids, and anticoagulants is used for occlusion.

2. Define aneurysm and list the types.

Study text pages 1144 through 1147; refer to Figures 30-3 through 30-5.

An **aneurysm** is a localized dilation or outpouching of a vessel wall or cardiac chamber. The tension on the wall increases as the vessel becomes thinner, so the possibility of rupture increases. This is an example of the law of Laplace. The stretching produces infarct expansion, a weak and thin layer of necrotic muscle, and fibrous tissue that bulges with each systole. With time, the aneurysm can leak, cause pressure on surrounding organs, impair blood flow, or rupture. The aorta is particularly susceptible to aneurysm formation because of the constant stress on its vessel wall and the absence of penetrating vasa

vasorum in its adventitial layer. Most aneurysms occur in the thoracic and abdominal aorta.

True aneurysms are fusiform and circumferential in nature and involve all three layers of the arterial wall; there is weakening of the vessel wall. **False aneurysms** are extravascular hematomas that communicate with the intravascular space as a leak between a vascular graft and a natural artery. **Saccular aneurysms** occur when blood enters the wall of an artery, creating an opening in the vessel wall.

Clinical manifestations of an aneurysm depend on its location. They can create pressure on surrounding organs, impair flow, and cause ischemia or signs of a stroke.

Medical treatment of aneurysms involves reducing blood pressure and volume to prevent further dilation. Surgical treatment is frequently necessary.

3. Distinguish between a thrombus and an embolus.

Study text pages 1147 and 1148.

A **thrombus** is a blood clot that remains attached to a vessel wall. Thrombi tend to develop wherever intravascular conditions promote activation of the coagulation cascade. In the arteries, activation of the coagulation cascade is usually caused by roughening of the tunica intima by atherosclerosis. Thrombi also form on heart valves if there is inflammation of the endocardium or rheumatic heart disease.

An arterial thrombus poses two threats to the circulation. First, the thrombus may be large enough to occlude the artery and cause ischemia in the tissue that is supplied by the artery. Alternatively, the thrombus may dislodge and travel through the vascular system until it occludes flow into a distal systemic or pulmonic vascular bed.

Pharmacologic treatment includes the administration of heparin and warfarin, thrombin inhibitors, or thrombolytics, which interfere with the clotting cascade, thereby slowing or stopping thrombus growth. Also, the intravenous or intra-arterial administration of streptokinase can dissolve the thrombus. A balloon-tipped catheter can be used to remove or compress a thrombus. Drug and catheter therapies are sometimes used concurrently.

Embolism is the obstruction of a vessel by an **embolus** or a bolus of matter that is circulating in the bloodstream. The embolus may be a dislodged thrombus, an air bubble, or an aggregate of fat, bacteria, or foreign matter. An embolus travels in the bloodstream until it reaches a vessel through which it cannot pass; an embolus will eventually lodge in a systemic or pulmonary vessel.

Pulmonary emboli originate mostly from the deep veins of the legs or in the heart. Systemic emboli most commonly originate in the left heart and are associated with thrombi after myocardial infarction, valvular disease, left heart failure, endocarditis, and dysrhythmias.

Pulmonary artery embolism from the right heart causes chest pain and dyspnea. The systemic emboli that pass through the left heart have varied effects. Renal artery embolism causes abdominal pain and oliguria. Mesenteric artery embolism causes abdominal pain and a paralytic, ischemic bowel.

Embolism of a coronary or cerebral artery is an immediate threat to life if the embolus severely obstructs these important major vessels. Occlusion of a coronary artery will cause a myocardial infarction, whereas occlusion of a cerebral artery will cause a stroke or cerebral vascular accident.

4. Distinguish between thromboangiitis obliterans and Raynaud phenomenon and Raynaud disease.

Study text pages 1148 and 1149.

Peripheral artery disease (PAD) refers to atherosclerotic disease that decreases perfusion to the limbs, especially the lower extremities. **Thromboangiitis obliterans,** which is also called Buerger disease, tends to occur in young men who are heavy cigarette smokers. It is an inflammatory disease of the peripheral arteries. Inflammation, thrombus formation, and vasospasm can eventually occlude and obliterate portions of small and medium-sized arteries in the feet and sometimes in the hands. The pathogenesis of thromboangiitis obliterans is unknown, although T-cell activation and autoimmunity are possible causes.

The chief symptom of thromboangiitis obliterans is pain and tenderness of the affected part. Clinical manifestations are caused by sluggish blood flow and include rubor caused by dilated capillaries under the skin and cyanosis caused by blood that remains in the capillaries after its oxygen has diffused into the interstitium.

The most important part of treatment is the cessation of cigarette smoking. Vasodilators may alleviate vasospasm. If vasospasm persists, sympathectomy may be performed, and gangrene necessitates amputation.

Raynaud phenomenon and **Raynaud disease** are characterized by attacks of vasospasm in the small arteries and arterioles of the fingers and, less commonly, the toes. Raynaud phenomenon is secondary to systemic diseases such as collagen vascular disease, pulmonary hypertension, thoracic outlet syndrome, myxedema trauma, serum sickness, or long-term exposure to environmental conditions like cold or vibrating machinery in the workplace. Raynaud disease is a primary vasospastic disorder of unknown origin that tends to affect young women. It consists of vasospastic attacks triggered by brief exposure to cold or by emotional stress. Genetic predisposition may play a role in its development.

The vasospastic attacks of either disorder cause changes in skin color and sensation because of ischemia. Vasospasm occurs with varying frequency and severity and causes pallor, numbness, and the sensation of cold in the digits. Also, sluggish blood flow resulting from ischemia may cause the skin to appear cyanotic. Rubor follows as vasospasm ends and the capillaries become engorged with oxygenated blood.

Treatment of Raynaud disease is limited to prevention or alleviation of vasospasm itself. Cold, emotional stress, and cigarette smoking are avoided. Exercises that build centrifugal force in the extremities are also helpful in the early stages of vasospasm for either entity.

5. Distinguish among primary, secondary, complicated, and malignant hypertension.

Study text pages 1149 through 1152 and 1154 through 1156; refer to Figures 30-6 through 30-10 and Tables 30-2 through 30-4.

Individuals are diagnosed as having hypertension when (1) the average of two or more diastolic blood pressure measurements made on two or more consecutive clinical visits is 90 mmHg or higher, or (2) when the average of systolic blood pressure measurements made on two or more consecutive visits is greater than 140 mmHg. Systolic hypertension, even when unaccompanied by an increase in diastolic pressure, is the most significant factor causing target organ damage. Optimal systolic blood pressure should be less than 120 mmHg, and diastolic blood pressure should be less than 80 mmHg. Adult hypertension can be categorized as follows: prehypertension when the systolic pressure is 120 to 139 and the diastolic pressure is 80 to 89. Stage 1 exists when systolic pressure is 140 to 159 mmHg and diastolic pressure is 90 to 99 mmHg; stage 2 is when systolic pressure is greater than 160 mmHg and diastolic pressure is greater than 100 mmHg.

Hypertension is caused by increases in cardiac output, total peripheral resistance, or both. Cardiac output is increased by any condition that increases heart rate or stroke volume, whereas peripheral resistance is increased by any factor that increases blood viscosity or reduces vessel diameter.

A specific cause for **primary hypertension,** which is also called essential or idiopathic hypertension, has not been identified; a combination of genetic and environmental factors mediated by a host of neurohumoral effects is likely responsible for its development. Primary hypertension affects 90% to 95% of hypertensive individuals. The likely pathogenesis of primary hypertension includes (1) overactivity of the sympathetic nervous system; (2) overactivity of the renin-angiotensin-aldosterone system; (3) a mutated gene for adducin, resulting in a significant increase in renal salt retention; (4) alterations in other neurohumoral mediators of blood volume and vasomotor tone such as atrial natriuretic peptide, brain natriuretic peptide, and C-type natriuretic peptide; and (5) a complex interaction involving insulin resistance and endothelial dysfunction. This dysfunction is characterized by decreased production of vasodilators, such as nitric oxide, and increased production of vasoconstrictors, such as endothelin.

Secondary hypertension is caused by any systemic disease process that raises peripheral vascular resistance or cardiac output (see the box on page 214). Fortunately, if the cause is identified and removed before permanent structural changes occur, blood pressure can return to normal.

Complicated hypertension damages the walls of systemic blood vessels. Smooth muscle cells of the tunica media undergo hypertrophy and hyperplasia with associated fibrosis in both tunicas, intima and media, known as vascular "remodeling."

Complicated hypertension compromises the structure and function of the vessels, heart, kidneys, eyes, and brain. Vascular complications include the formation, dissection, and rupture of aneurysms or outpouchings in vessel walls as well as gangrene resulting from vessel occlusion. Possible renal complications include parenchymal damage, renal arteriosclerosis, and renal insufficiency or failure. Cardiovascular complications include

213

left ventricular hypertrophy, angina pectoris, congestive heart failure or left heart failure, coronary artery disease, myocardial infarction, and sudden death. Complications specific to the retina include retinal vascular sclerosis, exudation, and hemorrhage. Cerebrovascular complications are similar to those of other arterial beds and include transient ischemia, stroke, cerebral thrombosis, aneurysm, and hemorrhage.

Malignant hypertension is a rapidly progressive hypertension in which diastolic pressure is usually above 140 mmHg. It can cause profound cerebral edema that disrupts cerebral function and causes loss of consciousness. High hydrostatic pressures in the capillaries cause vascular fluid to move into the interstitial space. Organ damage is extensive, including encephalopathy, cardiac failure, uremia, retinopathy, and cerebrovascular accident. If blood pressure is not reduced, cerebral edema and organ dysfunction increase until death occurs.

The early stages of hypertension have no clinical manifestations; thus, hypertension is called a silent disease. Some hypertensive individuals never have signs, symptoms, or complications, whereas others become very ill, and their hypertension can cause death. Others have anatomic and physiologic damage caused by past hypertensive disease even if current blood pressure is within normal ranges. The chance of developing primary hypertension increases with aging, but it occurs in children with increasing frequency. Most of the clinical manifestations of hypertensive disease are caused by complications that damage organs and tissues other than the vascular system. Besides elevated blood pressure, the signs and symptoms are specific for the organs or tissues affected. Heart disease, renal insufficiency, central nervous system dysfunction, impaired vision, impaired mobility, vascular occlusion, or edema can be caused by sustained hypertension.

Hypertension is usually managed with both pharmacologic and nonpharmacologic methods. Treatment begins with reducing or eliminating risk factors. The usual dietary recommendations are to restrict sodium intake, increase potassium intake, restrict saturated fat intake, and adjust caloric intake to maintain optimum weight. Physical training increases stroke volume, which lowers heart rate and thus systolic blood pressure. Relaxation reduces levels of circulating catecholamines, which then reduce vascular tone and blood pressure. Discontinuance of cigarettes eliminates the vasoconstrictor effects of nicotine.

When lifestyle modifications fail to manage hypertension, it can be managed pharmacologically. Thiazide diuretics have been shown to be safe and effective for most stage 1 hypertension. If the individual requires two drugs, beta-blockers or angiotensin-converting enzyme (ACE) inhibitors can be added to the thiazide diuretics. Individuals with heart failure or chronic kidney disease or who are post–myocardial infarction or recurrent stroke should begin treatment with an ACE inhibitor, angiotensin receptor blocker, or aldosterone antagonist.

6. Define and identify the causes of orthostatic or postural hypotension.
 Study text pages 1156 and 1157.

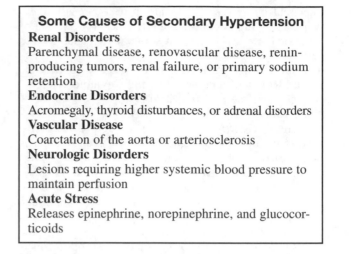

Some Causes of Secondary Hypertension
Renal Disorders
Parenchymal disease, renovascular disease, renin-producing tumors, renal failure, or primary sodium retention
Endocrine Disorders
Acromegaly, thyroid disturbances, or adrenal disorders
Vascular Disease
Coarctation of the aorta or arteriosclerosis
Neurologic Disorders
Lesions requiring higher systemic blood pressure to maintain perfusion
Acute Stress
Releases epinephrine, norepinephrine, and glucocorticoids

Orthostatic or **postural hypotension** is a decrease in both systolic and diastolic arterial blood pressure on standing from a reclining position. The normal or compensatory vasoconstrictor response to standing is replaced by a marked vasodilation and blood pooling in the muscle vasculature and in the splanchnic and renal beds.

Acute orthostatic hypotension may be the result of (1) anatomic variation, (2) altered body chemistry, (3) antihypertensive and antidepressant therapy, (4) prolonged immobility caused by illness, (5) starvation, (6) physical exhaustion, (7) fluid volume depletion, and (8) venous pooling.

Chronic orthostatic hypotension also may be secondary to a specific disease or idiopathic. The diseases that may cause secondary orthostatic hypotension are adrenal insufficiency, diabetes mellitus, intracranial tumors, cerebral infarcts, and peripheral neuropathies.

7. Distinguish between arteriosclerosis and atherosclerosis; describe the development and its consequences of atheromatous plaque.
 Study text pages 1157, 1159, and 1160; refer to Figures 30-11 through 30-13. See the flow chart on page 215.

Arteriosclerosis is a chronic disease of the arterial system that is characterized by abnormal thickening and hardening of the vessel walls. Smooth muscle cells and collagen fibers migrate into the tunica intima, causing it to stiffen and thicken; this decreases the artery's ability to change lumen size as well as narrowing the lumen.

Atherosclerosis is a form of arteriosclerosis in which the thickening of vessel walls is caused by hardening of soft deposits of intra-arterial fat and fibrin that reduce lumen size. Atherosclerosis is an inflammatory disease. Atherosclerosis can take several forms depending on the anatomic vessel location, the individual's age and genetic and physiologic status, and the risk factors to which each individual may have been exposed. It is the leading contributor to coronary artery and cerebrovascular disease.

Atherogenesis begins with injury to the endothelial cells of arteries. Possible injuries to endothelial cells include smoking, hypertension, diabetes, increased low-density lipoprotein (LDL) and decreased high-density lipoprotein, and hyperhomocystinemia. So-called novel

214

risk factors include elevated C-reactive protein, increased serum fibrinogen, oxidative stress, infection, and periodontal disease. Injured endothelial cells are unable to produce normal amounts of antithrombin and vasodilating cytokines. Inflammatory cytokines are released. The release of growth factors stimulates smooth muscle proliferation in the tunica media. Macrophages adhere to injured endothelial cells and release oxygen radicals that result in oxidation of LDL further injuring the vessel wall. The oxidized LDL is engulfed by macrophages; lipid-laden macrophages are called **foam cells,** which accumulate to form the fatty streak. The lesions of atherosclerosis occur primarily within the tunica intima, or the innermost layer. These lesions include the fatty streak, fibrous plaque, and the complicated lesion. The early **fatty streak** is a flat, yellow, lipid-filled smooth muscle cell that causes no obstruction of the affected vessel.

Fibrous plaque is the characteristic lesion of advancing atherosclerosis and consists of lipid-laden smooth muscle cells surrounded by collagen, elastic fibers, and a mucoprotein matrix. The lesion is elevated and protrudes into the lumen of the artery. The growing mass affixes to the inner wall of the tunica intima and may invade the muscular tunica media. Fibrous plaques likely develop from fatty streaks. The core of the fibrous plaque consists of lipids and debris from cellular necrosis caused by insufficient blood supply. If the lesion progresses sufficiently, it occludes the arterial lumen at arterial bifurcations, curves, or regions where the arteries taper.

Complicated lesions occur as the fibrous plaques are altered by hemorrhage, calcification, cellular necrosis, and blood clots throughout the intimal layer. As the altered complex structure becomes rigid, it causes extensive vascular occlusion.

The signs and symptoms of atherosclerosis result from inadequate tissue perfusion because of obstruction of vessels that supply the tissues. Atherosclerosis may have many different manifestations. High blood pressure develops if atherosclerosis elevates systemic vascular resistance. Cerebral or myocardial ischemia is a life-threatening manifestation of atherosclerosis that occurs in the vessels of the brain or heart, respectively.

Management focuses on removing the initial causes of vessel injury and preventing further lesion progression with drugs before plaques rupture. This includes exercise, smoking cessation, and the control of hypertension and diabetes and dyslipidemia.

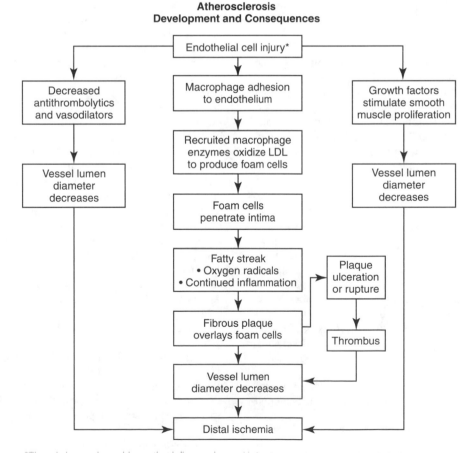

Atherosclerosis Development and Consequences

*There is increasing evidence that inflammation and infection may be causes of endothelial injury.

8. **Characterize coronary artery disease; distinguish between myocardial ischemia and myocardial infarction, and the consequences/complications of each.**

Study text pages 1160 through 1176; refer to Figures 30-14 through 30-24 and Tables 30-5 through 30-7.

Coronary artery disease (CAD), myocardial ischemia, and **myocardial infarction** all impair the pumping ability of the heart by depriving the heart muscle of oxygen and nutrients. CAD diminishes the myocardial blood supply until deprivation impairs myocardial metabolism. The myocardial cells remain alive, but they are unable to function normally. Persistent ischemia or the complete occlusion of a coronary artery causes infarction or death of the deprived myocardial cells and tissues.

In the United States, CAD is the single largest killer of individuals. The risk factors for CAD are classified as either modifiable or nonmodifiable. The nonmodifiable risk factors for CAD are variables that cannot be altered by people who wish to decrease their risk of cardiovascular disease. These include advanced age, male gender or women after menopause, and family history. The modifiable risk factors include dyslipidemia, hyperhomocysteinemia, hypertension, cigarette smoking, diabetes and insulin resistance, obesity, sedentary lifestyle, and atherogenic diet. High levels of low density lipoprotein (LDL) and lipoprotein(a) [Lp(a)], which are genetically determined, and low levels of high density lipoprotein (HDL) have been shown to be high-risk factors for CAD. High levels of HDL may be more protective for the development of atherosclerosis than low levels of LDL. The postmenopausal state is characterized by an increase in LDL and total cholesterol. Newly identified risk factors for atherogenesis and CAD include fibrinogen, serum amyloid, C-reactive protein, uric acid, and infectious agents, notably, *Chlamydia pneumoniae* and *Helicobacter pylori*. C-reactive protein is an acute phase reactant that is a measure of atherosclerotic-related inflammation. Adipokines are hormones released from adipose cells. **Adiponectin** is normally antiatherogenic and is decreased in obesity. It protects vascular endothelium and is anti-inflammatory. Decreased adiponectin is linked to a significant increase in cardiovascular risk.

The most common cause of **myocardial ischemia** is atherosclerosis. The growing mass of plaque, platelets, fibrin, and cellular debris can eventually narrow the coronary artery lumen sufficiently to impede blood flow. Imbalances between blood supply and myocardial demand cause myocardial ischemia. Supply is reduced by increased resistance in coronary vessels, hypotension, arrhythmia, valvular incompetence, shock, or anemia. Demand is increased by high systolic blood pressure, increased ventricular volume, left ventricular hypertrophy, increased heart rate, and valvular disease. Ischemia occurs whether demand exceeds supply.

Myocardial cells become ischemic within 10 seconds of coronary occlusion. After several minutes, the heart cells lose their ability to contract. Anaerobic processes take over, and lactic acid accumulates. Cardiac cells remain viable for approximately 20 minutes under ischemic conditions.

If blood flow is restored, aerobic metabolism resumes, and contractility is restored. If the coronary arteries cannot compensate for a lack of oxygen, **myocardial infarction** occurs. Pathologically, there are two major types of myocardial infarction: **subendocardial infarction** and **transmural infarction.** Clinically, myocardial infarction is categorized as non–ST-segment elevation myocardial infarction **(non-STEMI)** or ST-segment elevation **(STEMI).** Non-STEMI is usually subendocardial and presents with ST depression and T-wave inversion without Q waves. Transmural MI results in marked elevation in the ST segments on ECG and are categorized as STEMI.

Ischemia can be asymptomatic; if so, it is referred to as **silent ischemia.** The absence of angina may be caused by an abnormality in left ventricular symptomatic afferent innervation. Myocardial ischemia induced by mental stress can exist without angina and is thus considered silent. (See page 217) for a comparison of myocardial ischemia and myocardial infarction; the flow chart also on page 217 illustrates the consequences of ischemia.

The number and severity of postinfarction complications depend on the location and extent of necrosis, the individual's physiologic condition before the infarction, and the therapeutic intervention. Arrhythmias, which are disturbances of cardiac rhythm, are the most common complication of acute myocardial infarction and affect more than 90% of individuals. Sudden death resulting from cardiac arrest is often caused by arrhythmias, particularly ventricular fibrillation.

Acute **myocardial infarction** is usually accompanied by left ventricular failure characterized by pulmonary congestion, reduced myocardial contractility, and abnormal heart wall motion. Inflammation of the pericardium, which is called pericarditis, is a frequent complication of acute myocardial infarction. Dressler's postinfarction pericarditis syndrome is thought to be an antigen-antibody response to the necrotic myocardium. Pain, fever, friction rub, pleural effusion, and arthralgias may accompany this syndrome. Transient ischemic attacks or an outright cerebrovascular accident may result from thromboemboli that have broken loose from coronary arteries or cardiac valves to occlude cerebral vessels. Pulmonary emboli are especially common. Rupture of the wall of the infarcted ventricle may be a consequence of aneurysm formation because of decreased muscle mass at the infarcted site.

9. **Characterize the conditions associated with pericardial disease.**

Review text pages 1176 through 1178; refer to Figures 30-25 and 30-26.

Pericardial disease is often a localized manifestation of another disorder. Infection, trauma, surgery, neoplasms, or metabolic, immunologic, or vascular disorders can elicit a pericardial response. Pericarditis, pericardial effusion, or constrictive pericarditis is the consequence of the response.

Acute pericarditis, although idiopathic, is commonly caused by infection, connective tissue disease, or radiation therapy. The pericardial membranes become inflamed and roughened, and an exudate may develop.

Myocardial Ischemia/Infarction

Stable Angina	Prinzmetal Angina	Unstable Angina	Infarction
Cause			
Temporary ischemia, exertion, vessels cannot dilate in response to increased demand	Vasospasm, with or without atherosclerosis; occurs at night and at rest, may be asymptomatic	Advanced reversible ischemia; occurs at rest	Prolonged and irreversible ischemia, cellular necrosis with repair or scarring
Electrocardiography			
Normal, transient ST depression and T-wave inversion	Transient ST elevation	Normal transient ST depression and T-wave inversion	Irreversible, abnormal and pronounced Q waves, ST elevation later
Plasma Enzyme Levels			
Negative	Negative	Negative	CPK-MB fraction, LDH, SGOT, troponins I and T indicate severity
Pain Relief and Treatment*			
Rest and nitrogylcerin, beta-blockers, calcium antagonist	Nitroglycerin, beta-blockers, calcium antagonists	Rest and nitroglycerin ineffective, beta-blockers, calcium antagonist, anticoagulant therapy	Narcotics, anticoagulant therapy (aspirin), thrombolytic agents, ACE inhibitors, beta-blockers, statins, stents, surgery

*When medical therapy fails to relieve angina, percutaneous transluminal intervention (PTCI) or coronary artery bypass grafting (CABG) may be required.

NOTE: The first symptom of myocardial ischemia or infarction is usually sudden, severe chest pain. Infarction is more severe and persistent than ischemia pain; it may be heavy, crushing, and radiating to neck, jaw, back, shoulder, or left arm.

Consequences/Complications of Myocardial Ischemia

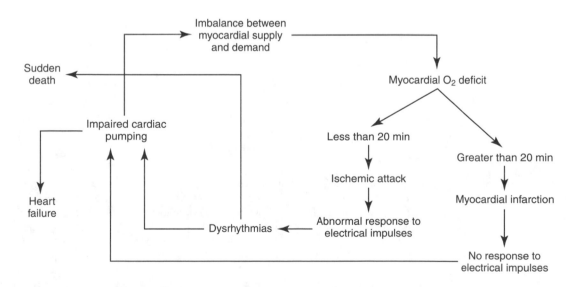

Symptoms include the sudden onset of severe chest pain that worsens with respiratory movements. Individuals with acute pericarditis may also report dysphagia, restlessness, irritability, anxiety, weakness, and malaise. Friction rub, or a short, scratchy, grating sensation similar to the sound of sandpaper, may be heard at the cardiac apex and left sternal border and is pathognomonic for pericarditis.

Treatment for uncomplicated acute pericarditis consists of relieving symptoms. Analgesics are given to relieve pain, and salicylates and nonsteroidal anti-inflammatory drugs are used to reduce inflammation.

Pericardial effusion is the accumulation of fluid in the pericardial cavity and is possible with all forms of pericarditis. The fluid may be a transudate or an exudate.

217

Pericardial effusion indicates an underlying disorder. If the fluid creates sufficient pressure to cause cardiac compression, it becomes a serious condition known as **tamponade.** The danger of tamponade is that the pressure exerted by the pericardial fluid will eventually equal the diastolic pressure within the heart chambers. The first structures to be affected by tamponade are the right atrium and ventricle, where diastolic pressures are normally lowest. Subsequent decreased atrial filling leads to decreased ventricular filling, decreased stroke volume, and reduced cardiac output. Life-threatening circulatory collapse may develop.

The most significant clinical finding in tamponade is pulsus paradoxus. In this circumstance, arterial blood pressure during expiration exceeds arterial pressure during inspiration by more than 10 mmHg. There is impairment of diastolic filling of the left ventricle plus reduction of blood volume within all cardiac chambers.

Treatment of pericardial effusion or tamponade generally consists of aspiration of the excessive pericardial fluid. The fluid may be analyzed to identify the cause of the effusion so that the underlying cause of tamponade may be corrected. If the underlying cause of tamponade is trauma or an aneurysm, surgery may be required.

Constrictive pericarditis is either idiopathic or associated with radiation exposure, rheumatoid arthritis, uremia, or coronary artery bypass grafting. In constrictive pericarditis, fibrous scarring with occasional calcification of the pericardium causes the visceral and parietal pericardial layers to adhere; thus, there is obliteration of the pericardial cavity. Like tamponade, constrictive pericarditis compresses the heart and eventually reduces cardiac output. Unlike tamponade, however, constrictive pericarditis always develops gradually.

Symptoms are exercise intolerance, dyspnea on exertion, fatigue, anorexia, weight loss, edema, distention of the jugular vein, and hepatic congestion. Chest radiographs frequently show prominent pulmonary vessels and calcification of the pericardium.

Initial treatment for constrictive pericarditis involves digitalis, glycosides, diuretics, and sodium restriction. Surgical removal of the pericardium may be indicated, because its removal does not compromise cardiac function.

10. Compare the cardiomyopathies.

Study text pages 1176 through 1180; refer to Figures 30-27 through 30-29 and Tables 30-8.

The **cardiomyopathies** are a diverse group of diseases that primarily affect the myocardium itself and are the result of underlying cardiovascular disorders, such as ischemia heart disease, hypertension, or valvular dysfunction. They may be secondary to infectious disease, exposure to toxins, systemic connective tissue disease, infiltrative and proliferative disorders, or nutritional deficiencies; most cases of cardiomyopathy are idiopathic.

Three categories of cardiomyopathies can be identified: dilated, hypertrophic, and restricted. See the table that follows.

11. Identify the causes and manifestations of valvular dysfunction.

Study text pages 1181, 1183, and 1184; refer to Figures 30-30 through 30-33 and Table 30-9.

In **valvular stenosis,** the valve orifice is constricted or narrowed. This impedes the forward flow of blood and increases the workload of the cardiac chamber "behind" or before the diseased valve. Increased volume and pressure

Characteristics of Cardiomyopathies

	Dilated	Hypertrophic	Restrictive
Associated Conditions	Alcoholism, pregnancy, infection, nutritional deficiency, toxin exposure	Possible inherited defect of muscle growth and development	Infiltrative disease
Structural Changes	Chamber volume increased, mitral valve incompetence	Hypertrophy of left ventricle and interventricular septum, chamber volume normal or decreased, mitral valve incompetence	Reduced ventricular compliance, infiltration of myocardium with amyloid or hemosiderin or glycogen deposits, chamber volume normal or decreased, atrioventricular valve incompetence
Manifestations	Weakness, fatigue, palpitations, eventual left heart failure	Dyspnea, fatigue, dizziness, angina, syncope, palpitations, eventual left heart failure	Dyspnea, fatigue, eventual right heart failure

cause the myocardium to work harder, and myocardial hypertrophy develops.

In **valvular regurgitation,** also known as insufficiency or incompetence, the valve leaflets or cusps fail to close completely; this permits blood flow to continue even when the valve should be closed. During systole, some blood leaks back into the "upstream" chamber; this increases the workload of both atrium and ventricle. Increased volume leads to chamber dilation; increased workload leads to hypertrophy. Although all four heart valves may be affected, those of the left heart are more commonly affected than those of the right heart. See the following table for a comparison of valvular stenosis and regurgitation.

Valvular Stenosis and Regurgitation

Valvular Disorders	Causes	Manifestations
Aortic stenosis	Rheumatic heart disease, congenital malformation, calcification degeneration	Decreased stroke volume, left ventricular failure, dyspnea, angina, systolic murmur
Mitral stenosis	Acute rheumatic heart fever, bacterial endocarditis	Decreased stroke volume, right ventricular failure, chest pain, orthopnea, pulmonary hypertension, dysrhythmia, palpitations, induced thrombi, ascites, diastolic murmurs
Aortic regurgitation	Bacterial endocarditis, hypertension, connective disease disorders	Congestive left heart failure, dyspnea, throbbing peripheral pulse, palpitations, chest pain, decrescendo murmurs in 2nd, 3rd, and 4th intercostal spaces
Mitral regurgitation	Rheumatic heart disease, mitral valve prolapse, CAD, infective endocarditis, connective tissue disorders	Left heart failure, pulmonary hypertension, dyspnea, hemoptysis, palpitations, murmur throughout systole
Tricuspid regurgitation	Congenital, high blood pressure in pulmonary circulation or right ventricle	Right heart failure, peripheral edema, ascites, hepatomegaly, murmur throughout systole
Mitral valve prolapse	Autosomal dominant pattern, hyperthyroidism-related, angiotensin II receptor polymorphism	Regurgitant murmur, fatigue and lethargy, greater risk for infective endocarditis

NOTE: Diuretics and vasodilators can manage valvular disease temporarily. Most disorders eventually require surgical repair or valve replacement.

Rheumatic Heart Disease and Infective Endocarditis

Cause	Pathophysiology	Manifestations	Treatment
Rheumatic Heart Disease Sequel to pharyngeal infection with group A beta-hemolytic streptococci, immune response to streptococcal cell membrane antigens (M proteins)	Carditis of all three layers of heart wall, endocardial inflammation and vegetative growth on valves, valvular stenosis, Aschoff bodies	Fever, lymphadenopathy, acute migratory polyarthritis, chorea, erythema marginatum or truncal rash, history of streptococcal pharyngeal infection, high anti–streptolysin O titer, ECG abnormalities	10 days of oral penicillin or erythromycin, salicylates or NSAIDS, surgical repair of damaged valves for chronic disease; to prevent recurrence: continuous prophylactic antibiotic therapy for as long as 5 years
Infective Endocarditis *Staphylococcus aureus* followed by viridans streptococci, viruses, fungi, rickettsiae	Prior endothelial damage to valves leads to thrombotic endocarditis; blood-borne microbes colonize damaged valve; adhered microbes multiply and form endocardial vegetations	Fever, cardiac murmur, petechial lesions of skin and mucosa, bacteremia, Osler nodes, Janeway lesions	Long-term (4 to 6 weeks) antimicrobial therapy: penicillin and streptomycin, prophylactic antibiotics for procedures increasing risk of transient bacteremia

11. **Distinguish between rheumatic heart disease and infective endocarditis.**

Study text pages 1185 through 1189; refer to Figures 30-34 through 30-37 and Table 30-10. See the table on page 219.

13. **Compare the pathophysiology, manifestations, and treatment of left side and right side heart failure.**

Study text pages 1189, 1190, and 1192 through 1195; refer to Figures 30-38 through 30-42 and Table 30-11.

In addition to the hemodynamic interactions, congestive heart failure (CHF) is characterized by complex neurohumoral and inflammatory processes. These include actions of catecholamines, angiotensin II, arginine vasopressin, natriuretic peptides, endothelial hormones, endotoxin, and tumor necrosis factor alpha.

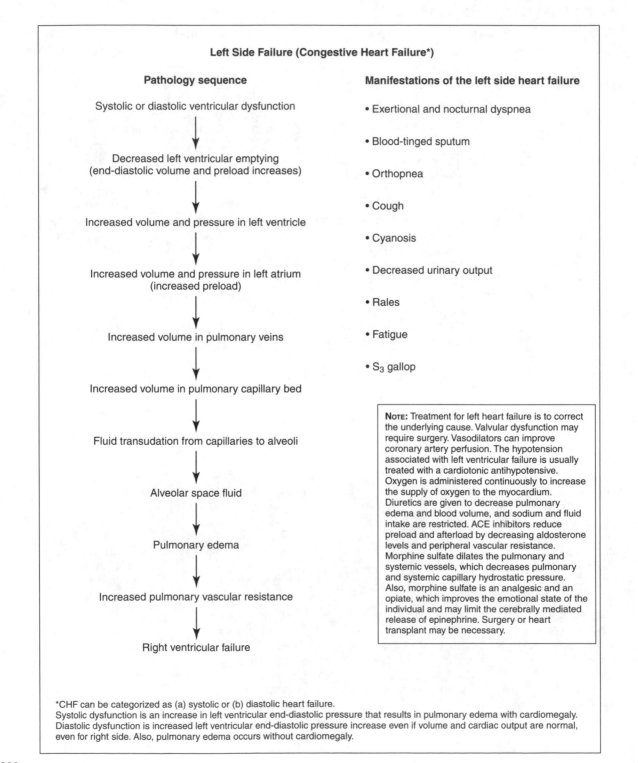

Left Side Failure (Congestive Heart Failure*)

Pathology sequence

Systolic or diastolic ventricular dysfunction

↓

Decreased left ventricular emptying
(end-diastolic volume and preload increases)

↓

Increased volume and pressure in left ventricle

↓

Increased volume and pressure in left atrium
(increased preload)

↓

Increased volume in pulmonary veins

↓

Increased volume in pulmonary capillary bed

↓

Fluid transudation from capillaries to alveoli

↓

Alveolar space fluid

↓

Pulmonary edema

↓

Increased pulmonary vascular resistance

↓

Right ventricular failure

Manifestations of the left side heart failure

• Exertional and nocturnal dyspnea

• Blood-tinged sputum

• Orthopnea

• Cough

• Cyanosis

• Decreased urinary output

• Rales

• Fatigue

• S₃ gallop

> **NOTE:** Treatment for left heart failure is to correct the underlying cause. Valvular dysfunction may require surgery. Vasodilators can improve coronary artery perfusion. The hypotension associated with left ventricular failure is usually treated with a cardiotonic antihypotensive. Oxygen is administered continuously to increase the supply of oxygen to the myocardium. Diuretics are given to decrease pulmonary edema and blood volume, and sodium and fluid intake are restricted. ACE inhibitors reduce preload and afterload by decreasing aldosterone levels and peripheral vascular resistance. Morphine sulfate dilates the pulmonary and systemic vessels, which decreases pulmonary and systemic capillary hydrostatic pressure. Also, morphine sulfate is an analgesic and an opiate, which improves the emotional state of the individual and may limit the cerebrally mediated release of epinephrine. Surgery or heart transplant may be necessary.

*CHF can be categorized as (a) systolic or (b) diastolic heart failure.
Systolic dysfunction is an increase in left ventricular end-diastolic pressure that results in pulmonary edema with cardiomegaly.
Diastolic dysfunction is increased left ventricular end-diastolic pressure increase even if volume and cardiac output are normal, even for right side. Also, pulmonary edema occurs without cardiomegaly.

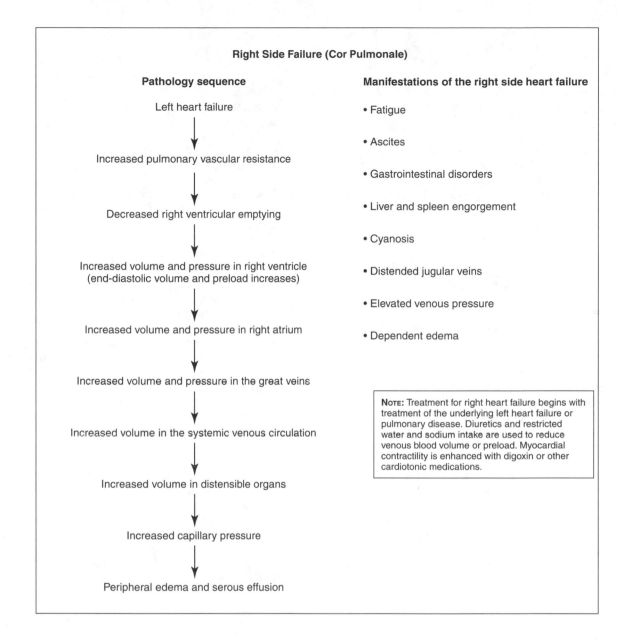

Right Side Failure (Cor Pulmonale)

Pathology sequence

Left heart failure

↓

Increased pulmonary vascular resistance

↓

Decreased right ventricular emptying

↓

Increased volume and pressure in right ventricle
(end-diastolic volume and preload increases)

↓

Increased volume and pressure in right atrium

↓

Increased volume and pressure in the great veins

↓

Increased volume in the systemic venous circulation

↓

Increased volume in distensible organs

↓

Increased capillary pressure

↓

Peripheral edema and serous effusion

Manifestations of the right side heart failure

• Fatigue

• Ascites

• Gastrointestinal disorders

• Liver and spleen engorgement

• Cyanosis

• Distended jugular veins

• Elevated venous pressure

• Dependent edema

NOTE: Treatment for right heart failure begins with treatment of the underlying left heart failure or pulmonary disease. Diuretics and restricted water and sodium intake are used to reduce venous blood volume or preload. Myocardial contractility is enhanced with digoxin or other cardiotonic medications.

14. Describe high-output heart failure.

Study pages 1195 and 1196; refer to Figure 30-43.

High-output failure is the inability of the heart to adequately supply the body with blood-borne nutrients, despite adequate blood volume and normal or elevated myocardial contractility. In high-output failure, the heart increases its output but the body's metabolic needs are still not met. Common causes of high-output failure are anemia, septicemia, hyperthyroidism, and beriberi.

Anemia decreases the oxygen-carrying capacity of the blood. Metabolic acidosis occurs as the body's cells switch to anaerobic metabolism. In response to metabolic acidosis, heart rate and stroke volume increase in an attempt to circulate blood faster.

In **septicemia,** disturbed metabolism, bacterial toxins, and the inflammatory process cause systemic vasodilation and fever. Faced with a lowered systemic vascular resistance (SVR) and an elevated metabolic rate, cardiac output increases to maintain blood pressure and prevent metabolic acidosis. In overwhelming septicemia, however, the heart may not be able to raise its output enough to compensate for vasodilation. Body tissues show signs of inadequate blood supply despite a very high cardiac output.

Hyperthyroidism accelerates cellular metabolism through the actions of elevated levels of thyroxine from the thyroid gland. This may occur chronically (thyrotoxicosis) or acutely (thyroid storm). Because the body's demand for oxygen threatens to cause metabolic acidosis, cardiac output increases.

In the United States, **beriberi** (thiamine deficiency) usually is caused by malnutrition secondary to chronic alcoholism. Beriberi actually causes a mixed type of heart failure. Thiamine deficiency impairs cellular metabolism in all tissues, including the myocardium. In the heart, impaired cardiac metabolism leads to insufficient

221

contractile strength. In blood vessels, thiamine deficiency leads mainly to peripheral vasodilation, which decreases SVR. Heart failure ensues as decreased SVR triggers increased cardiac output, which the impaired myocardium is unable to deliver.

15. Characterize dysrhythmias of the heart.

Study text page 1196; refer to Tables 30-12 and 30-13.

Arrhythmias can be caused by either an abnormal rate of impulse generation by the SA node or an abnormal conduction of impulses. A number of circumstances may lead to dysrhythmias including hypoxia, trauma, electrolyte imbalances, inflammation, and drugs. Arrhythmias can impair the pumping of the heart and cause heart failure.

PRACTICE EXAMINATION

Multiple Choice

Circle the correct answer for each question.

1. Atherosclerosis raises the systolic blood pressure by:
   a. increasing arterial distensibility and vessel lumen radius or diameter.
   b. increasing arterial distensibility and decreasing vessel lumen radius or diameter.
   c. decreasing arterial distensibility and increasing vessel lumen radius or diameter.
   d. decreasing arterial distensibility and lumen radius or diameter.

2. Events in the development of atherosclerotic plaque include all of the following *except:*
   a. oxidation of LDL.
   b. smooth muscle proliferation.
   c. decreased antithrombolytics.
   d. fibrous plaque overlies foam cells.
   e. complement activation.

3. G.P. is a 50-year-old man who was referred for evaluation of blood pressure. If he had a high diastolic blood pressure, which of the following readings would reflect that?
   a. 140/82 mmHg
   b. 160/72 mmHg
   c. 130/95 mmHg
   d. 95/68 mmHg
   e. 140/72 mmHg

4. The complications of uncontrolled hypertension include all of the following *except:*
   a. cerebrovascular accidents.
   b. anemia.
   c. renal injury.
   d. cardiac hypertrophy.

5. Primary hypertension:
   a. is essentially idiopathic mediated by a host of neurohumoral effects.
   b. can be caused by renal disease.
   c. can be caused by hormone imbalance.
   d. results from arterial coarctation.

6. Orthostatic hypotension is caused by all *except:*
   a. increased age.
   b. increased blood volume.
   c. autonomic nervous system dysfunction.
   d. bed rest.
   e. severe varicose veins.

7. Adiponectin is:
   a. an enzyme.
   b. increased in obesity.
   c. antiatherogenic.
   d. inflammatory.

8. Transmural myocardial infarction:
   a. displays non-STEMI.
   b. occurs when infarction is limited to part of the heart wall.
   c. is categorized as STEMI.
   d. displays T-wave inversion.

9. A 76-year-old man came to the emergency department after experiencing chest pain while shoveling snow. Laboratory tests revealed essentially normal blood levels of SGOT or AST, CPK, and LDH enzymes. The chest pain was relieved following bed rest and nitroglycerin therapy. The most probable diagnosis is:
   a. myocardial infarction.
   b. emphysema.
   c. stable angina.
   d. hepatic cirrhosis.
   e. acute pancreatitis.

10. In pericardial effusion:
    a. fibrotic lesions obliterate the pericardial cavity.
    b. there is associated rheumatoid arthritis.
    c. tamponade compresses the right heart before affecting other structures.
    d. arterial blood pressure during inspiration exceeds that during expiration.

11. Increased chamber size is observed in _____ cardiomyopathy.
    a. dilated
    b. hypertrophic
    c. restrictive
    d. constrictive

12. Which of the following is *not* an expected finding in acute rheumatic fever?
    a. history of a pharyngeal infection
    b. elevated ASO titer (anti–streptolysin O)
    c. leukopenia
    d. fever

13. In unstable angina:
    a. pronounced Q waves are evident.
    b. transient ST elevation occurs.
    c. vasospasm occurs.
    d. T-wave inversion occurs.

14. Secondary hypertension is caused by:
    a. sodium retention.
    b. renovascular disease.
    c. genetics.
    d. decreased cardiac contractibility.
    e. increased ventricular preload.

15. Which of the following statements about hypertension is *incorrect?*
    a. Malignant hypertension is characterized by a diastolic pressure of more than 140 mmHg.
    b. Approximately 90% of hypertension cases are of the essential or primary type.
    c. Headache is the most reliable symptom.
    d. When left untreated, the major risks include CVAs and cardiac hypertrophy.
16. A 53-year-old man was admitted to the emergency department after experiencing shortness of breath, weakness, cardiac dysrhythmias, and chest pain that did not subside following nitroglycerin therapy. Laboratory tests revealed the patient had an elevated serum CPK and SGOT or AST level and troponin I monoclonal antibodies. ECG tracings revealed a prominent Q wave and an elevated ST segment. The most probable diagnosis is:
    a. a transient ischemic attack.
    b. an acute myocardial infarct.
    c. an attack of unstable angina pectoris.
    d. Prinzmetal angina.
    e. coronary artery vasospasm.
17. Life-threatening consequences of coronary artery disease include:
    a. angina.
    b. cardiomegaly.
    c. endocarditis.
    d. heart failure.
18. Which accompanies an infarcted myocardium?
    a. unconsciousness
    b. transient ST elevation
    c. left ventricular hypertrophy
    d. arrhythmias
19. The most serious complication of infective endocarditis is:
    a. valvular deformity.
    b. septic emboli.
    c. regurgitated blood by mitral valve.
    d. myocardial hypertrophy.
20. Patients with only left side heart failure would exhibit:
    a. hepatomegaly.
    b. ankle swelling.
    c. pulmonary edema.
    d. peripheral edema.
21. In congestive heart failure, there is:
    a. gastrointestinal disturbances.
    b. elevated venous pressure.
    c. decreased urinary output.
    d. ascites.
22. In right-side heart failure, there is:
    a. nocturnal dyspnea.
    b. dependent edema.
    c. blood-tinged sputum.
    d. rales.

Matching

Match the valvular dysfunction with the appropriate initial consequence.

_____ 23. Tricuspid regurgitation

_____ 24. Mitral stenosis

_____ 25. Mitral regurgitation

a. right ventricular hypertrophy

b. left ventricular hypertrophy

c. right atrial hypertrophy

d. left atrial hypertrophy

e. left atrial/right ventricular hypertrophy

f. right and left ventricular/left atrial hypertrophy

g. hypertrophy of all chambers

Mr. T. is a 45-year-old black male employed as a midlevel corporate manager seeking a physical examination. He appeared somewhat overweight. He denied taking any medications or smoking but admitted drinking alcohol. His father and older brother have hypertension and his paternal grandfather experienced an MI and a CVA at a young age. Mr. T. stated, "A year ago at a health fair, I was told later by mail that my cholesterol was 250."

Questions

What presumptive diagnosis seems likely?

What other questions should be asked of this patient?

What laboratory tests are indicated?

224

W.S., a 51-year-old white man, was assisting in the launching of his best friend's water ski boat from a faulty boat trailer when he began to experience chest discomfort. At first, he believed his discomfort was because of the extreme July heat. Gradually, the discomfort became a crushing pain in his sternal area that radiated into his left arm and lower jaw. His friend suspected an ensuing heart attack and convinced W.S. to check into an emergency department. During the drive down a canyon with steep, winding curves, W.S. collapsed.

On arrival at the emergency department, W.S. was unconscious. His skin was cool, clammy, and very pale. His blood pressure was so low that it had to be palpated, and his pulse was weak and irregular. Established resuscitation procedures were followed. After his return to consciousness, an electrocardiogram showed evidence of anterior myocardial injury, and blood was drawn to check enzyme and electrolyte levels. When history could be obtained, W.S. stated that, "I am a harassed advertising executive and have no significant illnesses but am being treated for high blood pressure." He later acknowledged smoking three packs of cigarettes a day for 30 years and that his father died of a heart attack at the age of 47.

W.S.'s subsequent electrocardiograms and serum levels of myocardium infarction indicators confirmed myocardial infarction. Also, the area of infarction was in the anterior myocardium.

Question

Knowing the diagnosis, identify W.S.'s risk factors, the early causes and precipitating events of his infarction, and the justification for using anticoagulant therapy.

31 Alterations of Cardiovascular Function in Children

FOUNDATIONAL KNOWLEDGE OBJECTIVES

a. Describe the embryologic development of the cardiovascular system.
Review text pages 1209 through 1211; refer to Figures 31-1 through 31-3.

MEMORY CHECK!

- The heart arises from the mesenchyme and begins its development as an enlarged blood vessel with a large lumen and muscular wall. The midsection of this tube begins to grow faster than its ends, so the tube bulges and twists until both ends of the tube come together and fuse. The superior part of the tube is the truncus arteriosus, which divides longitudinally into the pulmonary artery and aorta; the lower part of the tube becomes the superior and inferior venae cavae. The development of the cardiac septa eventually divides the heart into the four chambers. If development of the septa proceeds normally, the four-chambered heart will be present by the sixth or seventh week of gestation.

b. Describe the flow of blood through the fetal circulation.
Review Figure 31-4.

MEMORY CHECK!

- Blood for the fetus is oxygenated in the placenta and returns to the fetus through the umbilical vein. Part of this blood passes through the liver, but about half the flow is diverted from the liver through the ductus venosus (a connection between the hepatic vessels and the inferior vena cava) and into the inferior vena cava. This blood flows into the heart and passes through the foramen ovale (an opening between the right and left atria), through the left ventricle, and into the aorta. From there, it flows to the head and upper extremities. Blood returning from the upper body collects in the superior vena cava. A small portion of this blood enters the lungs; the largest amount, however, flows through the ductus arteriosus (a connection between the pulmonary artery and the aorta), into the descending aorta, to the body, and then back to the placental vein through two umbilical arteries.

c. **Describe the events involved in the change from fetal to independent circulation that take place immediately after birth.**
   Review text page 1213.

MEMORY CHECK!

- After birth, systemic resistance rises, and pulmonary resistance falls. Pulmonary vascular resistance drops suddenly at birth, because the lungs expand and the pulmonary vessels dilate; it continues to decrease gradually over the first 6 to 8 weeks after birth. Decreased resistance causes the right myocardium to thin. Systemic vascular resistance increases markedly at birth, because severance of the umbilical cord removes the low-resistance placenta from the systemic circulation. Increased systemic resistance causes the right myocardium to thicken. Changes in resistance cause the fetal connections between the pulmonary and systemic circulatory systems to disappear. The foramen ovale closes functionally at birth and anatomically several months later. The ductus arteriosus closes functionally 15 to 18 hours after birth and anatomically within 10 to 21 days. The ductus venosus closes within 1 week after birth.

LEARNING OBJECTIVES

After studying this chapter, the learner will be able to do the following:

1. **Describe the defects that occur with increased pulmonary blood flow, their pathophysiology, and their treatment.**

   Study text pages 1218 through 1223; refer to Figures 31-5 through 31-8 and Table 31-5.

   Patent ductus arteriosus (PDA) results from the failure of the ductus arteriosus to close within the first weeks of life. Continued patency permits blood to flow from the higher-pressure aorta to the lower-pressure pulmonary artery, and this causes a left-to-right shunt to develop. Clinical manifestations are usually without cyanosis and include a "machinery" murmur and pulmonary vascular obstructive disease in later life. Treatment is usually by surgical ligation. Other options include coil embolization during catheterization and video-assisted thoracoscopic surgery to place a clip around the vessel to occlude it.

   Atrial septal defects (ASDs) are abnormal communications across the interatrial septum. The size of the ASD determines the direction of flow. If small, the shunt is from left to right; if large, the pressures in the atria are equal, and shunt direction is determined by resistance of the ventricles. At birth, atrial size and resistance are generally equal; as the infant grows, the left ventricle thickens, and systemic pressure rises and causes a left-to-right shunt. These defects may be so mild that they go undetected until preschool age. A soft murmur is often heard at the second intercostal space, and a fixed splitting of the second heart sound also may be heard; this finding is indicative of right ventricular overload. Radiography may demonstrate cardiomegaly and pulmonary vascular congestion. ECG may demonstrate ventricular stress. Echocardiography or cardiac catheterization will demonstrate the defect. Treatment is generally surgical correction.

   Ventricular septal defect (VSD) is essentially a defect in the intraventricular septum that leads to blood flow between the ventricles of the heart. Small defects have very little associated pathology and often close on their own, with the shunt usually flowing from left to right.

   Large defects are a different matter. In a large VSD, pressures may become equal in both chambers, with blood flow again being left to right due to higher systemic pressures. In this case, large amounts of blood flow into the lungs through the pulmonary artery and back to the left heart and cause a great deal of left ventricular stress; heart failure may eventually result. A related physiologic event is a constriction of the pulmonary blood vessels in an effort to limit pulmonary blood flow.

   Radiography and ECG are usually normal unless left ventricular stress is present. Echocardiography illustrates flow across the defect. Surgical correction involves a pericardial patch or sutures to close the defect.

   Atrioventricular caval defect consists of a low atrial septal defect that is continuous with a high ventricular septal defect and clefts of the mitral and tricuspid valves. A large central atrioventricular defect allows blood to flow among all four chambers of the heart. The directions of flow are determined by pulmonary and systemic resistance, left and right ventricular pressures, and the compliance of each chamber. Flow is generally from left to right.

   There is usually moderate to severe left heart failure and a characteristic loud, harsh holosystolic murmur. There may be mild cyanosis. Surgical repair, between 3 and 6 months of age, is performed through a midsternotomy using a one- or two-patch repair to close the septal defects and repair the involved AV valves.

2. **Describe the defects that occur with decreased pulmonary blood flow, their pathophysiology, and their treatment.**

   Study pages 1223 through 1226; refer to Figures 31-9 and 31-10 and Table 31-5.

   The pathophysiology associated with **tetralogy of Fallot** may be varied and depends on the degree of pulmonary stenosis, the size of the VSD, and pulmonary and systemic pressures. Because the VSD is usually large, the shunt may be either left to right or right to left. In any event, these defects result in hypoxia in the systemic circulation while the body attempts to compensate by increasing red cell production and blood flow to the lungs through collateral bronchial vessels. Cyanotic episodes may also be accompanied by syncope or seizures due to

228

hypoxia. Corrective repair involves patch closure of the VSD, resection of infundibular or valvular stenosis, and augmentation of the right ventricle outflow tract through a median sternotomy on cardiopulmonary bypass.

Tricuspid atresia is the failure of the tricuspid valve to develop; thus, there is no communication from right atrium to right ventricle. Blood flows through an atrial septal defect or a patent foramen ovale to the left heart and through a ventricular septal defect to the right ventricle and then to the lungs. This condition is often associated with pulmonic stenosis and transposition of the great arteries; there is mixing of unoxygenated and oxygenated blood in the left heart.

Cyanosis is usually seen during the newborn period. There may be tachycardia, dyspnea, and hypoxemia. Older children exhibit chronic hypoxemia, polycythemia, and clubbing. Individuals are at risk for bacterial endocarditis, brain abscess, and stroke. Corrective repair involves closing the septal defects, removal of previous shunts or bands, and connecting the superior and inferior venae cavae to the pulmonary artery to separated the pulmonary systemic circulation.

3. **Identify the most common congenital defects that obstruct outflow, and describe their pathophysiology.**

    Study text pages 1226, and 1228 through 1230; refer to Figures 31-11 through 31-16 and Table 30-5.

    Coarctation of the aorta (COA) is caused by a narrowing of the aorta anywhere between the origin of the aortic arch and the abdominal bifurcation. This defect may be considered in terms of its proximity to the ductus arteriosus. A narrowing near the ductus arteriosus results in increased blood flow to the head and upper extremities and decreased blood flow to the lower extremities. There are signs of left heart failure in infants. Surgical repair of those younger than 1 year consists of either a subclavian flap aortoplasty to enlarge the constricted area, or resection with end-to-end anastomosis of the arch segments. In children older than 1 year, resection with end-to-end anastomosis is done.

    Aortic stenosis is a narrowing or stricture of the aortic valve that causes resistance to blood flow from the left ventricle, decreased cardiac output, left ventricular hypertrophy, and pulmonary vascular congestion. Children with this condition show signs of exercise intolerance, chest pain, and dizziness when standing for long periods, and there is a characteristic murmur. Individuals are at risk for bacterial endocarditis, coronary insufficiency, and ventricular dysfunction. Aortic valvotomy may be used as an initial procedure. A valve replacement may be required as a subsequent surgical intervention.

    Pulmonic stenosis is caused by the restriction or thickening of the leaflets of the pulmonary valve. Outflow is restricted from the right ventricle; this results in increased afterload and, if severe, may cause right ventricular hypertrophy and dilation. If pressures are high enough, the foramen ovale may reopen, and this results in a right-to-left shunt and cyanosis. Surgical correction involves a pulmonary valvotomy incising the fused commissures.

Hypoplastic left heart syndrome is the underdevelopment of the left heart that results in a hypoplastic left ventricle, aortic arch, and either mitral atresia or stenosis. Most blood from the left atrium flows across the patent foramen ovale to the right atrium, to the right ventricle, and out the pulmonary artery.

Mild cyanosis and signs of left heart failure are present until the patent ductus arteriosus closes, and then there is progressive deterioration with cyanosis and decreased cardiac output that leads to cardiovascular collapse.

A several-stage surgical repair approach is used for correction of this condition. Some believe that heart transplantation in the newborn period may be the best option for these infants.

4. **Describe defects that permit the mixing of pulmonary and systemic blood.**

    Study text pages 1230 through 1234; refer to Figures 31-17 through 31-19 and Table 30-5.

    Complete transposition of the great vessels (TGA) results in the effective switching of the aorta and pulmonary arteries so that the pulmonary artery leaves the left ventricle and the aorta leaves the right ventricle; this creates two separate circulatory systems with no communication between them. Children with minimum communication are severely cyanotic. If large septal defects exist, cyanosis may be less, but symptoms of left heart failure will occur. Cardiomegaly develops a few weeks after birth in individuals with this condition. Switching procedures to make the left ventricle the systemic pump may be the best alternative of the various surgical corrections.

    Total anomalous pulmonary venous connection (TAPVC) is a disorder in which the pulmonary circulation enters the right atrium instead of the left. TAPVC has four different variations with the same resultant pathophysiology, all of which are associated with ASDs. The most common forms of this anomaly are (1) drainage of the pulmonary veins into the superior vena cava and right atrium, (2) drainage into the right atrium through the coronary sinus, and (3) drainage into the right atrium through the inferior vena cava. TAPVC in any form results in a mixture of oxygenated and unoxygenated blood being pumped through the systemic circulation; the shunt is usually right to left. The amount of cyanosis generated by this anomaly depends on the mixture of unoxygenated and oxygenated blood; thus, the greater the pulmonary blood flow, the less is the cyanosis. Congestive heart failure is a frequent complication. Obstructed lesions are repaired at the time of diagnosis; whereas, the unobstructed type generally is repaired during infancy. The procedure is performed on cardiopulmonary bypass and involves anastomosis of the common pulmonary vein to the left atrium, ligating the common pulmonary vein, and closing the ASD, as in the supracardiac and infracardiac types.

    Truncus arteriosus is the failure of normal septation and division of the embryonic vessel trunk into the pulmonary artery and the aorta; the resulting single vessel overrides both ventricles. Blood from both ventricles mixes in the common great artery and causes desaturation

229

and hypoxemia. Blood ejected from the heart flows to the lower-pressure pulmonary arteries and causes increased pulmonary blood flow and reduced systemic blood flow.

Most infants have moderate to severe left heart failure and variable cyanosis, poor growth, and activity intolerance. There is a characteristic murmur, and children are at risk for brain abscess and bacterial endocarditis.

Corrective surgery involves closing the defect so that the truncus arteriosus receives the outflow from the left ventricle, excising the pulmonary arteries from the aorta, and attaching them to the right ventricle by a homograft.

5. **Summarize the preceding four objectives by diagramming the causes and consequences of blood flow defects in congenital hearts defects.**

6. **Describe the pathophysiology related to Kawasaki disease.**

Study text pages 1234 and 1235.

Kawasaki disease is an acute, self-limiting vasculitis that may result in cardiac sequelae. Eighty percent of cases occur in children younger than 5 years of age; peak incidence is during toddlerhood. Currently, Kawasaki disease is the leading cause of pediatric acquired heart disorders in the United States. This disease tends to cluster in miniepidemics and may be related to an infectious process with an autoimmune component. The disease process progresses through four clinical stages:

Stage 1: onset to 12 days: Small venules, arterioles, and the heart become inflamed.

Stage 2: 12 to 25 days: Inflammation of larger vessels occurs, and coronary artery aneurysms appear.

Stage 3: 26 to 40 days: Medium-sized arteries begin granulation, and inflammation subsides in the microcirculation.

Stage 4: day 40 and beyond: The vessels develop scarring, thickening of the intima, calcification, and formation of thrombi; arteritis is most frequent in the coronaries, but it may occur in a variety of arteries; 10% to 20% of children develop aneurysms in this process.

Diagnosis is made by evaluating six major findings, five of which must be present for diagnosis. These findings are as follows: (1) fever greater than 104° F, (2) bilateral conjunctivitis, (3) erythema of the oral mucosa, (4) erythema with desquamation of the palms and soles, (5) polymorphous erythematous rash, and (6) cervical lymphadenopathy. These may be accompanied by arthritis and abdominal pain. Later complications include coronary thrombosis. Echocardiography can be used to monitor the disease in the coronary arteries. Treatment is nonspecific and supportive; high-dose aspirin and intravenous immunoglobulin during the acute phase decrease mortality.

7. **Describe susceptibility and manifestations of hypertension (HTN) in children; note the cardiovascular risks for obese children.**

Study text pages 1235 through 1238; refer to Figure 31-20 and Tables 31-6 through 31-9.

Most **secondary HTN** in children is a result of an underlying disease, such as renal disease or coarctation of the aorta. **Primary HTN** is now known to exist in children and is related to complex interaction of strong predisposing genetic components. Ultimately, these factors impede the ability of the peripheral vascular bed to adjust its own resistance to meet perfusion needs.

Children who are overweight are often hypertensive. Obesity in children is an epidemic in the United States and other countries. Obese children are at risk for HTN, cardiovascular disease, type 2 diabetes, sleep apnea, and asthma. Smoking increases the risk for HTN, and the

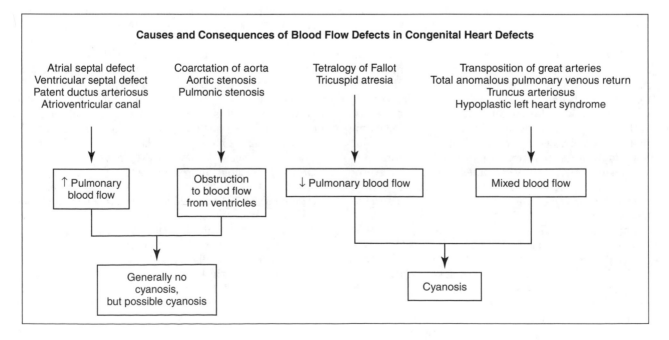

Causes and Consequences of Blood Flow Defects in Congenital Heart Defects

Atrial septal defect
Ventricular septal defect
Patent ductus arteriosus
Atrioventricular canal

Coarctation of aorta
Aortic stenosis
Pulmonic stenosis

Tetralogy of Fallot
Tricuspid atresia

Transposition of great arteries
Total anomalous pulmonary venous return
Truncus arteriosus
Hypoplastic left heart syndrome

↑ Pulmonary blood flow

Obstruction to blood flow from ventricles

↓ Pulmonary blood flow

Mixed blood flow

Generally no cyanosis, but possible cyanosis

Cyanosis

gender or race of the child has not been associated with primary HTN. Recent data suggest that elevated serum uric acid is related to the onset of essential HTN in children.

HTN in children may be asymptomatic, and blood pressures vary from child to child and change as the child grows. The preventive efficacy of antihypertensive therapy during childhood is debatable, and some clinicians prefer to control or eliminate risk factors.

PRACTICE EXAMINATION

True or False

For each statement, write T (true) or F (false) in the blank provided.

_____ 1. Shunts are usually independent of systemic or pulmonary pressures and are due solely to defects within the heart.

_____ 2. A patent ductus arteriosus or VSD is sometimes helpful when it is associated with other cardiac defects.

_____ 3. VSDs always require surgical closure.

_____ 4. In ASDs or VSDs, murmurs indicate defects.

_____ 5. Cyanosis is not a major finding in transposition of the great vessels because the blood is free to travel normally to the lungs.

Matching

Match the description with the association.

_____ 16. Associated with dyspnea when feeding

_____ 17. Likely associated with an infectious etiology and an autoimmune response

_____ 18. Vasculitis associated with aneurysm

_____ 19. If mild, often self-correcting

_____ 20. "Blue spells"

_____ 21. VSD, overriding aorta, pulmonic stenosis, right ventricular hypertrophy

_____ 22. Common complication of congenital heart defects

_____ 23. Immediate cyanosis and distress at birth

_____ 24. Two separate circulatory systems

_____ 25. May be associated with coronary thrombosis

Fill in the Blanks

Supply the correct response for each statement.

6. Abnormal blood flow direction within the heart is usually referred to as a _____.

7. In VSDs, the shunt is generally _____ to ____.

8. Cyanotic defects usually shunt _____ to _____.

9. Cyanosis due to cardiac defects is usually due to a mixture of _____ and _____ blood.

10. Some cardiac defects are not obvious at birth because systemic and pulmonary pressures are nearly _____ at that point.

11. The patent ductus arteriosus has a _____ to _____ shunt.

12. The ductus arteriosus should be totally closed within the _____ of life.

13. Thickening or restriction of the valve from the right ventricle is known as _____ _____.

14. Defects that obstruct outflow from the ventricles tend to cause increased _____, which may lead to _____ _____ _____.

15. Narrowing of the great vessel that leads to the systemic circulation is known as _____ _____ _____.

a. Kawasaki disease

b. VSD

c. tetralogy of Fallot

d. transposition of the great vessels

e. left heart failure

231

D.M. is a 7-year-old boy who presents for a routine physical examination at a practitioner's office. D.M.'s past medical and family history is not unusual. His activity level is normal, and his mother states, "He is quite healthy." D.M's physical examination is normal until the cardiovascular system is evaluated; then, he is noted to have a systolic murmur. There are also bounding pulses in the arms and severely decreased pulses in the legs. A pediatric cardiology consultation is requested.

Question

What cardiac defect causes such a striking discrepancy in blood flow to the upper and lower extremities?

32 Structure and Function of the Pulmonary System

PREREQUISITE KNOWLEDGE OBJECTIVES

After reviewing the primary text where referenced, the learner will be able to do the following:

1. **Identify the sequence of structures of the pulmonary system as air moves into and out of the lungs.**
   Review text pages 1242 through 1244, 1247, and 1249; refer to Figures 32-1 through 32-9.
2. **Identify the defense mechanisms of the pulmonary systems.**
   Refer to Table 32-1.
3. **Describe the neural and chemical control of ventilation.**
   Review text pages 1249 through 1251; refer to Figures 32-10 and 32-11.
4. **Relate changes in the thoracic volume to contractions, alveolar surface tension, elastic properties of the lungs and chest wall, and conducting airway resistance.**
   Review text pages 1251 through 1254; refer to Figures 32-12 and 32-13.
5. **Describe the alveolocapillary membrane and the diffusion of oxygen and carbon dioxide across it.**
   Review text pages 1257 and 1258; refer to Figures 32-8 and 32-17.
6. **Identify the factors in the transport of oxygen to the cells of the body, and describe oxyhemoglobin association and dissociation; identify the factors in the transport of carbon dioxide from the cells.**
   Review text pages 1258 through 1260; refer to Figure 32-18.
7. **Identify the normal values for arterial and venous blood gases and their significance.**
   Refer to Table 32-4.
8. **Note the pulmonary changes that occur with normal aging.**
   Review text page 1263; refer to Figure 32-20.

PRACTICE EXAMINATION

Multiple Choice
Circle the correct answer for each question.

1. Considering the sequence of structures through which air enters the pulmonary system, the pharynx is to the trachea as the:
   a. bronchioles are to the segmental bronchi.
   b. alveoli are to the alveolar ducts.
   c. alveolar ducts are to the respiratory bronchioles.
   d. respiratory bronchioles are to the alveolar ducts.
2. The cilia of the bronchial wall:
   a. ingest bacteria.
   b. trigger the sneeze reflex.
   c. trap and remove bacteria.
   d. propel mucus and trapped bacteria toward the oropharynx.
3. As the terminal bronchioles are approached:
   a. the epithelium becomes thicker.
   b. mucus-producing glands increase.
   c. the epithelium becomes thinner.
   d. cartilaginous support increases.
   e. the smooth muscle layer thickens.
4. The left bronchus:
   a. is shorter and wider than the right.
   b. is symmetrical to the right.
   c. has a course that is more vertical than that of the right.
   d. is more angled than the right.
   e. has more bronchial wall layers than the right.
5. The respiratory unit consists of:
   a. cilia.
   b. bronchiolar arteries and veins.
   c. goblet cells and alveoli.
   d. respiratory bronchioles and alveoli.

6. An increase of carbon dioxide in arterial blood causes chemoreceptors to stimulate the respiratory centers to:
   a. decrease respiratory rate.
   b. increase respiratory rate.
   c. cause hypocapnia.
   d. cause hypercapnia.
7. Surfactant:
   a. facilitates O_2 exchange.
   b. produces nutrients for the alveoli.
   c. permits air exchange between alveolar ducts.
   d. facilitates alveolar expansion during inspiration.
   e. All of the above are correct.
8. During expiration, which of the following relationships is *true*?
   a. As the lung volume decreases, the number of molecules of the gas increases.
   b. As the lung pressure increases, the number of molecules of the gas increases.
   c. As the lung volume decreases, the pressure increases.
   d. As the partial pressure increases, less gas will dissolve in a liquid.
9. When the diaphragm and external intercostal contract:
   a. the intrathoracic volume increases.
   b. the intrathoracic pressure increases.
   c. the intrathoracic volume decreases.
   d. None of the above is correct.
10. Oxygen diffusion from the alveolus to the alveolar capillary occurs because:
    a. the Po_2 is less in the capillary than in the alveolus.
    b. the Po_2 is greater in the atmosphere than in the arterial blood.
    c. oxygen diffuses faster than CO_2.
    d. the Po_2 is higher in the capillary than in the alveolus.
11. A shift to the right in the oxyhemoglobin dissociation curve:
    a. prevents oxygen release at the cellular level.
    b. causes oxygen to bind tighter to hemoglobin.
    c. improves oxygen release at the cellular level.
    d. causes alkalosis.
12. In which sequence does Po_2 progressively decrease?
    a. Blood in aorta, atmospheric air, body tissues
    b. Body tissues, arterial blood, alveolar air
    c. Body tissues, alveolar air, arterial blood
    d. Atmospheric air, blood in aorta, body tissues
13. Most O_2 is carried in the blood _____; most CO_2 is carried _____.
    a. dissolved in plasma, associated with salt or an acid
    b. bound to hemoglobin, associated with bicarbonate or carbonic acid
    c. combined with albumin, associated with carbonic acid and hemoglobin
    d. bound to hemoglobin, bound to albumin

14. Alveoli are well suited for diffusion of respiratory gases because:
    a. they are small and thus have a small total surface area.
    b. vascularization is minimal, thereby allowing greater air circulation.
    c. they contain four thick layers, which prevent air leakage.
    d. they contain surfactant, which helps prevent alveolar collapse.
15. Which ordinarily brings about the greatest increase in the rate of respiration?
    a. Hypercapnia (excess carbon dioxide)
    b. Increased O_2
    c. Increased arterial pH
    d. Sudden rise in blood pressure
16. Given that the oxygen content of blood equals 1.34 ml of O_2 per gram of hemoglobin arterial oxygen saturation percent, if hemoglobin concentration is 15 g/dl and arterial saturation is 98%, what is the arterial oxygen content?
    a. 13.2 ml/dl of blood
    b. 19.7 ml/dl of blood
    c. 14.7 ml/dl of blood
    d. None of the above are correct.
17. Given that an individual has a respiratory rate of 15 breaths per minute and a tidal volume of 500 ml of air, the respiratory minute volume is:
    a. 7.5 L/min.
    b. 75 L/min.
    c. 750 L/min.
    d. 7500 L/min.
18. Stretch receptors:
    a. are sensitive to volume changes in the lung.
    b. are located near capillaries in the alveolar septa.
    c. increase ventilatory rate when stimulated.
    d. prevent lung underinflation when stimulated.
19. Which of the following increases the respiratory rate?
    a. Increased Pco_2, decreased arterial pressure, decreased pH, decreased Po_2
    b. Increased Pco_2, decreased arterial pressure, increased pH, decreased Po_2
    c. Decreased Pco_2, decreased arterial pressure, decreased pH, increased Po_2
    d. Decreased Pco_2, decreased arterial pressure, decreased pH, decreased Po_2
20. The dorsal respiratory group of neurons:
    a. sets the automatic rhythm of respiration.
    b. modifies the rhythm of respiration.
    c. is active when increased ventilation is required.
    d. None of the above is correct.

21. Which of the following does *not* provide chemoreceptor input to the medulla oblongata respiratory centers?
    a. Medullary centers
    b. Olfactory epithelium
    c. Carotid body
    d. Aortic body
22. Parasympathetic stimulation to bronchiolar smooth muscle causes:
    a. muscle relaxation.
    b. increased tidal volume.
    c. bronchodilation.
    d. bronchoconstriction.
23. The pons apneustic center:
    a. inhibits inspiration.
    b. stimulates/prolongs inspiration.
    c. controls respiratory rhythm.
    d. monitors blood gas tensions.
24. During inhalation, the intrapleural pressure approximates:
    a. 1 mmHg.
    b. 1 mmHg.
    c. 6 mmHg.
    d. 6 mmHg.
25. Control of airflow resistance and air distribution in the lungs is controlled by the:
    a. trachea.
    b. alveoli.
    c. bronchioles.
    d. diaphragm.

235

33 Alterations of Pulmonary Function

FOUNDATIONAL KNOWLEDGE OBJECTIVES

a. Compare the structures of the lower airway as the generations of division move toward the alveoli.
Refer to Figures 32-3 through 32-5.

MEMORY CHECK!

- The trachea and mainstem bronchi are composed mainly of cartilage, with a lining of mucous membrane. When the bronchi enter the lungs, they branch further. Instead of cartilaginous rings, smooth muscle encircles the bronchi, with cartilage interspersed among the muscle bundles. By the time the bronchioles are reached, supportive cartilage is no longer present. The bronchioles are capable of constriction because of their layer of smooth muscle. Smooth muscle becomes thinner in the terminal bronchioles. The epithelium changes from pseudostratified and ciliated columnar in the bronchi to nonciliated cuboidal in the terminal bronchioles and finally to squamous in the alveoli. Macrophages must remove any debris that reaches the respiratory bronchioles and alveoli because of the absence of cilia.

b. Describe the diaphragmatic movement in inspiration and expiration; indicate other factors that are involved in the mechanism of breathing.
Review text pages 1251 through 1254; refer to Figure 32-13.

MEMORY CHECK!

- Other factors involved in the mechanics of breathing include alveolar surface tension, elasticity of the lungs and chest wall, and resistance to air flow through the conducting airways. Surface tension occurs at any gas-liquid interface and is the tendency for liquid molecules exposed to air to adhere to one another. This phenomenon decreases the surface area exposed to the air. According to the law of Laplace, the pressure (P) required to inflate a sphere is equal to two times the surface tension (t) divided by the radius (r) of the sphere, or $P = 2T/r$. As the radius of the sphere or alveolus becomes smaller and the surface tension increases, more pressure is required to inflate the alveolus.
- Surfactant in the alveoli has a detergent-like effect that separates the liquid molecules, thereby decreasing alveolar surface tension. Surfactant reverses the law of Laplace. The alveoli are much easier to inflate at low lung volumes after expiration than at high volumes after inspiration. The decrease in the surface tension caused by surfactant also is responsible for keeping the alveoli free of fluid. In the absence of surfactant, the surface tension tends to attract fluid into the alveoli.
- The lung and chest wall have elastic properties that permit expansion during inspiration and relaxation to original dimension during expiration. During inspiration, the diaphragm and intercostal muscles contract, air flows into the lungs, and the chest wall expands. Muscular effort is needed to overcome the resistance of the lungs to expansion. During expiration, the muscles relax, and the elastic recoil of the lungs causes the thorax to decrease in volume until balance between the chest wall and lung recoil forces is reached.
- Compliance is the measure of lung and chest wall distensibility; it represents the relative ease with which these structures can be stretched. Compliance is, therefore, the reciprocal of elasticity. An increase in compliance indicates that the lungs and/or chest wall are abnormally easy to inflate and have lost some elastic recoil. A decrease indicates that the lungs and/or chest wall is abnormally stiff or difficult to inflate.
- Airway resistance is determined by the length, radius, and cross-sectional area of the airways and the density, viscosity, and velocity of the gas. Resistance is inversely proportional to the fourth power of the radius; thus, anything that decreases the radius of the airways increases airway resistance.

237

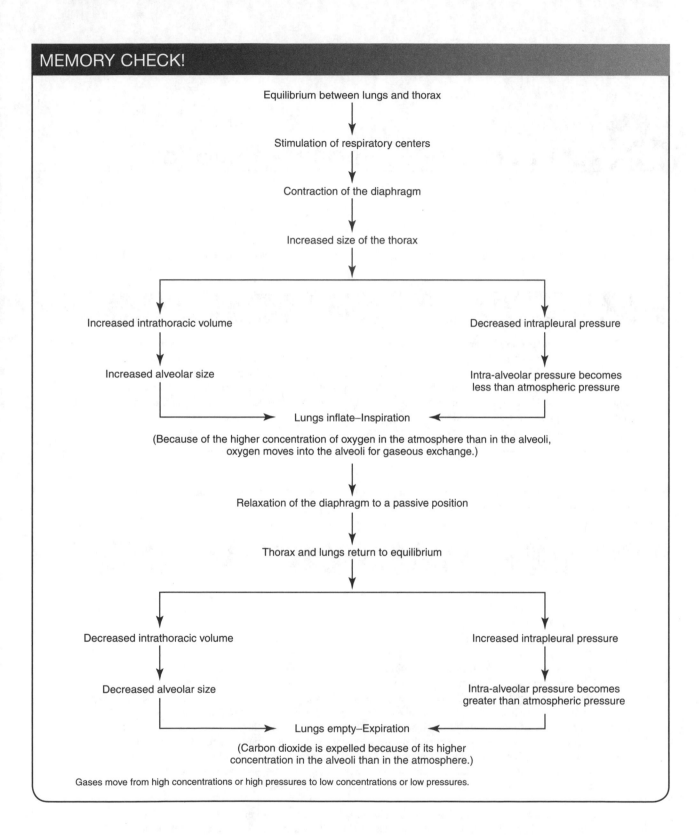

Equilibrium between lungs and thorax

Stimulation of respiratory centers

Contraction of the diaphragm

Increased size of the thorax

Increased intrathoracic volume

Decreased intrapleural pressure

Increased alveolar size

Intra-alveolar pressure becomes less than atmospheric pressure

Lungs inflate–Inspiration

(Because of the higher concentration of oxygen in the atmosphere than in the alveoli, oxygen moves into the alveoli for gaseous exchange.)

Relaxation of the diaphragm to a passive position

Thorax and lungs return to equilibrium

Decreased intrathoracic volume

Increased intrapleural pressure

Decreased alveolar size

Intra-alveolar pressure becomes greater than atmospheric pressure

Lungs empty–Expiration

(Carbon dioxide is expelled because of its higher concentration in the alveoli than in the atmosphere.)

Gases move from high concentrations or high pressures to low concentrations or low pressures.

After studying this chapter, the learner will be able to do the following:

1. **Define the terms used in describing the signs and symptoms of pulmonary disease.**

   Study text pages 1266 through 1269; refer to Figure 33-1.

   Dyspnea is the subjective sensation of uncomfortable breathing; it is often described as breathlessness, air hunger, shortness of breath, or labored breathing. Dyspnea occurs if increased airway resistance or decreased compliance causes respiratory effort that is greater than what is appropriate for the ventilation achieved. The signs of dyspnea include flaring of the nostrils, use of accessory muscles of respiration, and retraction of the intercostal spaces.

   Orthopnea is experienced when an individual is in the horizontal position. This position redistributes body water and causes the abdominal contents to exert pressure on the diaphragm, which decreases its efficiency of contraction and causes dyspnea.

   Paroxysmal nocturnal dyspnea is seen in individuals with left ventricular failure who wake up at night gasping for air and have to sit up or stand to relieve the dyspnea. This dyspnea results from the redistribution of body water into the lungs while the individual is recumbent.

   Strenuous exercise or metabolic acidosis induces **Kussmaul respiration** or **hyperpnea.** Kussmaul respiration is characterized by a slightly increased ventilatory rate, very large tidal volumes, and no expiratory pause.

   Cheyne-Stokes respirations are characterized by alternating periods of deep and shallow breathing. Apnea, which is a cessation of breathing that lasts from 15 to 60 seconds, is followed by increased ventilation after which ventilation decreases again to apnea. Cheyne-Stokes respirations occur in any condition that slows the blood flow to the brainstem or that slows impulses to the respiratory centers of the brainstem.

   Hypoventilation is inadequate alveolar ventilation in relation to metabolic demands. It is caused by alterations in pulmonary mechanics or in the neurologic control of breathing. With hypoventilation, CO_2 removal does not keep up with production and CO_2 rises in the blood, causing **hypercapnia.**

   Hyperventilation is alveolar ventilation that exceeds metabolic demands. The lungs remove CO_2 at a faster rate than it is produced, and this results in **hypocapnia,** which means that there are low levels of CO_2 in the blood.

   Coughing is a protective reflex that cleanses the lower airways by an explosive expiration that removes inhaled particles, accumulated mucus, or foreign bodies. Stimulating the irritant receptors in the airway initiates the cough. Acute cough resolves in 2 to 3 weeks and is most commonly the result of pulmonary infections, allergic rhinitis, acute bronchitis, pneumonia, CHF, pulmonary embolus, or aspiration. Chronic cough persists longer than 3 months. In nonsmokers, it is mostly caused by postnasal drainage, bronchitis, asthma, or gastroesophageal disease.

   Hemoptysis is the coughing up of blood or bloody secretions. Hemoptysis indicates a localized infection or inflammation that has damaged the bronchi or the lung parenchyma.

   Cyanosis is a bluish discoloration of the skin and mucous membranes that is caused by increasing amounts of desaturated or reduced hemoglobin in the blood. Cyanosis can result from decreased arterial oxygenation or decreased cardiac output.

   Pain is caused by pulmonary disorders that originate in the pleurae, airways, or chest wall. Infection and inflammation of the parietal pleura cause pain when the pleura stretches during inspiration. Pain that is pronounced after coughing occurs in individuals with infection and inflammation of the trachea and/or bronchi. Pain in the chest wall occurs with excessive coughing, which makes the muscles sore.

   Clubbing is the selective bulbous enlargement of the end of a finger or toe. Its pathogenesis is unknown, but it is associated with diseases that interfere with oxygenation.

   An **abnormal sputum** is seen with different pulmonary disorders. Changes in the amount and consistency of sputum provide information about the progression of disease and the effectiveness of therapy.

2. **Indicate conditions that are caused by pulmonary disease or injury.**

   Study text pages 1269 through 1279; refer to Figures 33-2 through 33-7 and Tables 33-1 and 33-2. See the table on pages 240 and 241.

3. **Using a flow chart, interrelate the pathogenic factors in acute respiratory distress syndrome (ARDS).**

   Study text pages 1279 through 1282; refer to Figures 33-8 and 33-9. See the flow chart on page 242.

4. **Compare and contrast the obstructive pulmonary diseases.**

   Study text pages 1282 through 1290; refer to Figures 33-10 through 33-14 and Table 33-3. See the table on page 243.

   Obstructive pulmonary disease is characterized by difficult expiration that is not fully reversible. More force or the use of accessory muscles of expiration is required to expire a given volume of air. The most common obstructive diseases are asthma, chronic bronchitis, and emphysema. Because many individuals have both chronic bronchitis and emphysema, these diseases are grouped together and are called chronic obstructive pulmonary disease (COPD). Asthma is more acute and intermittent than COPD, but it can also be chronic.

5. **Define pneumonia and describe its causes, manifestations, and treatment.**

   Study text pages 1290 through 1293; refer to Figure 33-15.

   Pneumonia is an acute infection of the lower respiratory tract that is caused by bacteria, bacteria-like microbes, or viruses. It can be causally grouped as

Conditions Caused by Pulmonary Disease or Injury

Oxygen and Carbon Dioxide Tension

Condition	Pathology	Cause
Hypercapnia	Increased carbon dioxide in arterial blood	Drug depression of respiratory center, infections of CNS or trauma to medulla; spinal cord disruption or poliomyelitis; neuromuscular junction disease as in myasthenia gravis or muscular dystrophy affecting respiratory muscles; thorax cage abnormalities; airway obstruction; emphysema due to physiologic dead space
Hypoxemia	Reduced oxygenation of arterial blood	Decreased oxygen content of inspired gas, hypoventilation diffusion abnormalities in emphysema, abnormal ventilation/perfusion ratios in bronchitis, right-to-left shunts in RDS or atelectasis

Disorders of the Chest Wall and Pleura

Condition	Pathology	Cause
Chest wall restriction	Compromised ventilation, decreased tidal volume	Grossly obese, lateral bending and rotation of spine, arthritis of spine, depression of the sternum, neuromuscular disease
Flail chest	Compromised ventilation	Fracture of ribs or sternum
Pneumothorax	Air or gas in pleural space collapses the lung partially or totally	Rupture of pleura or chest wall or spontaneous rupture of pleura blebs
Pleural effusion	Transudative or exudative fluid in the pleural space collapses the lung partially or totally	Fluid from blood or lymphatic vessels from CHF, hypoproteinemia, infections or malignancies cause mast cell release of capillary permeability mediators, trauma that damages blood vessels
Empyema	Pus in pleural space	Bacterial pneumonia, surgical complications, tumor obstruction

Restrictive Lung Disorders

Condition	Pathology	Cause
Aspiration	Passage of fluid and solids into lungs, obstruction of airway, localized inflammation, noncompliant lungs, disrupted surfactant production, edema, collapse	Decreased levels of consciousness, CNS abnormalities
Atelectasis	Collapse of lung tissue	External pressure from tumor, fluid, or air in pleural space; abdominal distention; bronchi obstruction; inhalation of concentrated oxygen or anesthetics
Bronchiectasis	Persistent abnormal dilation of bronchi	Obstruction of airway, atelectasis, infection, cystic fibrosis, tuberculosis, weakness of bronchial wall
Bronchiolitis	Inflammatory obstruction of bronchioles	Chronic bronchitis, infection, inhalation of toxic gases
Bronchiolitis obliterans	Fibrotic process occludes airways and scars lungs	Same as bronchiolitis; common after lung transplantation
Fibrosis	Fibrous or connective tissue in lung	Scar tissue following ARDS, tuberculosis, or inhalation of dust or asbestos
Toxic gas exposure	Inflammation of airways, alveolar and capillary damage, pulmonary edema	Inhalation of smoke, ammonia, hydrogen chloride, sulfur dioxide, chlorine, phosgene, and nitrogen dioxide; prolonged levels of high concentration of oxygen

240

Conditions Caused by Pulmonary Disease or Injury—cont'd

Condition	Pathology	Cause
Pneumoconiosis	Fibrous tissue or nodules in lungs	Silicosis (inhalation of silica), anthracosis (inhalation of coal dust), asbestosis (inhalation of asbestos)
Allergic alveolitis	Lung inflammation or hypersensitivity pneumonitis	Inhalation of allergens: grains, silage, bird droppings, feathers, cork dust, animal pelts, molds, mushroom compost
Pulmonary edema	Excess water in lungs	Heart disease increases pulmonary capillary hydrostatic pressure, so fluid moves into interstitium; ARDS or inhalation of toxic gases injures capillaries and increases permeability; blockage of lymphatic vessels by congestive heart failure (CHF), edema, or tumors

community-acquired pneumonia, nosocomial pneumonia, and pneumonia of immunocompromised individuals.

Fungi infrequently cause pneumonia, but **fungal pneumonia** can occur in immunosuppressed individuals. The most common cause of **community-acquired pneumonia** is *Streptococcus pneumoniae. Mycoplasma pneumoniae* is the next most common cause of community-acquired pneumonia. The *Legionella* species are widely distributed in water environments and are present in cooling systems, condensers, shower heads, and water reservoirs; infections from these species may occur in outbreaks or sporadically. *Staphylococcus aureus* and *Klebsiella pneumoniae* cause some **nosocomial pneumonia,** usually in individuals with other health problems, such as COPD or alcoholism, or those individuals with a primary viral illness. Most nosocomial or hospital-acquired pneumonias are caused by gram-negative bacteria, such as *Escherichia coli, Klebsiella pneumoniae, Pneumocystis carinii,* and *Pseudomonas aeruginosa.* Viral pneumonia is usually caused by influenza viruses.

Pathogenic microorganisms can reach the lung by inspiration, by aspiration of oropharyngeal secretions, or via the circulation. This last source is usually by systemic infection, sepsis, or contaminated needles of intravenous drug users.

The defense mechanisms of the lungs (the cough reflex, mucociliary clearance, and phagocytosis by alveolar macrophages) normally prevent infection by pathogens. The body's immune system and various components of the inflammatory response further aid healthy individuals in preventing disease. In susceptible individuals, the invading pathogen is not contained. Instead, it multiplies and releases damaging toxins and stimulates full-scale inflammatory and immune responses.

The immune response and the endotoxins released by some microorganisms damage bronchial mucous membranes and alveolocapillary membranes. Inflammation and edema cause the acinus and terminal bronchioles to fill with infectious debris and exudate; ventilation-perfusion abnormalities follow. In pneumococcal pneumonia, the involved lobe has four phases in the inflammatory response: (1) consolidation, (2) red hepatization, (3) gray hepatization, and (4) resolution. If the pneumonia is caused by staphylococci or gram-negative bacteria, necrosis of lung parenchyma may also occur.

The first step in the management of pneumonia is establishing adequate ventilation and oxygenation. Antibiotics are used to treat bacterial and mycoplasmal pneumonia. Viral pneumonia is treated with supportive therapy unless secondary bacterial infection is present.

6. Describe the pathogenesis of tuberculosis.

Study text pages 1293 and 1294.

Tuberculosis (TB) is an infection caused by *Mycobacterium tuberculosis,* which is an acid-fast bacillus that usually affects the lungs but that may invade other body systems. Recently, the number of reported TB cases has increased; a major reason for this trend is the epidemic of acquired immunodeficiency syndrome

Gram-Positive Bacteria	Gram-Negative Bacteria	Nonbacterial Organisms
Streptococcus pneumoniae	*Escherichia coli*	*Pneumocystis carinii*
Staphylococcus aureus	*Pseudomonas aeruginosa*	*Mycoplasma pneumoniae*
Streptococcus pyogenes	*Klebsiella pneumoniae*	Fungi
	Proteus species	Viruses
	Bacteroides species	
	Haemophilus species	
	Legionella species	

ARDS Pathophysiology

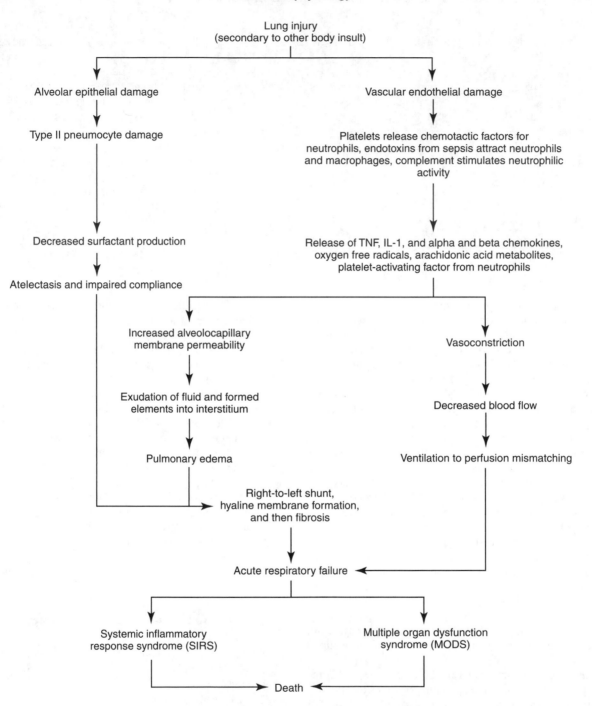

(AIDS). Individuals with AIDS are highly susceptible to respiratory infections, including TB. A second important reason is the growing number of drug-resistant strains of TB bacillus that have evolved because a large number of individuals do not consistently take their medications; this allows resistant strains to develop and spread. Emigration of infected individuals from high-prevalence countries, transmission in crowded institutional settings, substance abuse, and lack of access to medical care have also contributed to the growing problem.

TB is transmitted from person to person in airborne droplets. Once the bacilli are inspired into the lung, they multiply and cause nonspecific lung inflammation. Some bacilli migrate through the lymphatics and become lodged in the lymph nodes, where they encounter lymphocytes and initiate an immune response.

Neutrophils and alveolar macrophages wall off the colonies of bacilli and form a granulomatous lesion called a tubercle. Infected tissues within the tubercle die and form a cheeselike material; this is called **caseation**

Obstructive Pulmonary Diseases

	Asthma	Emphysema	Chronic Bronchitis
Cause of airway obstruction	Bronchial inflammation, smooth muscle spasm, mucosal edema, and increased thick mucus production	Enlargement and destruction of alveoli, loss of elasticity, trapping of air during expiration	Inflammation and thickening of mucous membrane; production of thick, tenacious mucus and pus
Precipitating causes and risk factors	Familial hyperresponsiveness to inflammatory mediators—allergens, histamine, interleukins, IgE prostaglandins, nitric oxide, and leukotrienes—leads to mucus and bronchoconstriction	Alpha-1 antitrypsin deficiency, cigarette smoke	Cigarette smoke, air pollutants, infections
Manifestations	Dyspnea, wheezing, nonproductive cough early but later mucoid, prolonged expiration, tachycardia, pulsus paradoxus, tachypnea, acidosis	Marked dyspnea, no productive cough early but develops later, tachypnea with prolonged expiration, accessory muscles used for ventilation, barrel chest, normal or elevated hematocrit, late cor pulmonale	Exercise intolerance, late dyspnea, wheezing, productive cough, prolonged expiration, polycythemia and cyanosis, early cor pulmonale, CHF
Treatment	Inhaled anti-inflammatory agents, inhaled or oral bronchodilators, immune therapies for allergic individuals	Prophylactic antibiotics for acute infections, bronchodilators, cautious oxygen administration	Bronchodilators, expectorants, postural drainage, percussion, anti-inflammatory agents

NOTE: Acute bronchitis is an acute infection or inflammation of the bronchi following a viral infection and is usually self-limiting.

necrosis. Collagenous scar tissue then grows around the tubercle, which further isolates the bacilli. Once the bacilli are isolated in tubercles and immunity develops, TB may remain dormant for life. However, if the immune system is impaired or if live bacilli escape into the bronchi, active disease occurs and may spread through the blood and lymphatics to other organs. Endogenous reactivation of dormant bacilli in the elderly may be caused by poor nutritional status, insulin-dependent diabetes, long-term corticosteroid therapy, and other debilitating diseases.

In many infected individuals, TB is asymptomatic. In others, symptoms develop so gradually that they are not noticed until the disease is well advanced. Common clinical manifestations include fatigue, weight loss, lethargy, loss of appetite, and a low-grade fever that usually occurs in the afternoon. A cough with purulent sputum develops slowly and becomes more frequent after weeks or months; "night sweats" and general anxiety are often present. Extrapulmonary TB is common in HIV-infected individuals and may cause neurologic deficits, meningitis symptoms, bone pain, and urinary symptoms. A positive tuberculin skin test indicates that an individual has been infected and has sensitized T lymphocytes against the bacillus. Those who have received the TB vaccine

with bacillus Calmette-Guérin (BCG) also will have a positive test. Chest radiographs and culturing the bacillus from the sputum aid in the diagnosis of tuberculosis. Six grades of tuberculosis are possible; the grades aid in evaluation and in the determination of appropriate therapy.

Treatment consists of antibiotic therapy to control active or dormant tuberculosis and to prevent transmission. Today, with the increased numbers of immunosuppressed and susceptible individuals and drug-resistant bacilli, the recommended treatment for those at high risk is a combination of four drugs: isoniazid, rifampin, pyrazinamide, and ethambutol; newer drugs include rifapentine and immune amplifiers. Treatment continues until sputum cultures show that the active bacilli have been eliminated.

7. **Compare and contrast pulmonary embolism, pulmonary hypertension, and cor pulmonale.**
   Study text pages 1294 through 1298; refer to Figures 33-16 through 33-18. See the table on page 244.
   Blood flow through the lungs can be disrupted by a number of disorders that occlude the vessels, increase pulmonary vascular resistance, or destroy the vascular bed. Major disruptive disorders include pulmonary embolism, pulmonary hypertension, and cor pulmonale. See the table on p. 244 for a comparison of these disorders.

243

8. Describe lip and laryngeal cancer.

Study text pages 1298 and 1299 and Figures 33-19 and 33-20.

Lip cancer is more prevalent in men exposed to the sun, wind, and cold over years and results in dryness, chapping, hyperkeratosis, and premalignancy. The cancerous lesion develops in the outer part of the lip along the vermilion border. The most common type is squamous cell, and metastasis is uncommon when lesions are diagnosed and surgically excised early.

The risk for **laryngeal cancer** is increased by and related to the amount of tobacco smoked; the risk is heightened when smoking is combined with alcohol consumption. Carcinoma of the glottis is more common than that of the epiglottis, aryepiglottic folds, arytenoids, and false cords. Squamous cell carcinoma is the most common cell type.

Progressive hoarseness is the most significant symptom, and it can result in voice loss. Dyspnea is rare with supraglottic tumors, but it can be severe in subglottic tumors. Laryngeal pain or a sore throat is likely with supraglottic lesions.

Radiation therapy has shown good results for early carcinoma of the vocal cords. Partial laryngectomies are the preferred treatment for small glottic malignancies. Total laryngectomy is required when lesions are extensive and involve the cartilage.

9. Describe the four major histologic types of lung cancer.

Study text pages 1299 through 1304; refer to Figures 33-21 through 32-23 and Table 33-4. See page 245.

Lung cancers or **bronchogenic carcinomas** arise from the epithelium of the respiratory tract. Lung cancer incidence is rapidly increasing in the United States. The most common cause of lung cancer is cigarette smoking; the chance that a heavy smoker will develop lung cancer is about 25 times greater than that of a nonsmoker. Tobacco smoke carcinogens, along with a probable inherited genetic predisposition, results in chromosomal deletions, the activation of oncogenes, and the inactivation of tumor-suppressor genes (*p53*). Smoke-induced toxic oxygen radical production damages cells. After carcinogen-induced mutations, further carcinogenesis is promoted by epidermal growth factor.

Comparison of Pulmonary Vascular Diseases

	Embolism	Hypertension	Cor Pulmonale
Cause	Blood-borne substances from venous stasis, vessel injury, or hypercoagulation lodge in a branch of pulmonary artery and obstruct blood flow	Pulmonary arterial pressure is elevated by increased left atrial pressure, increased blood flow in pulmonary circulation, obstruction of vascular bed, constriction of the vascular bed produced by hypoxemia or acidosis secondary to lung disease	Right heart failure because of primary pulmonary disease and long-standing pulmonary hypertension
Manifestations	Earlier evidence of deep vein thrombosis of legs or pelvis, tachypnea, dyspnea, chest pain, hypotension, shock, possible radiographic wedge shape bordering the pleura	Fatigue, chest discomfort, tachypnea, dyspnea with exercise, jugular venous distention, accentuated second heart sound, a radiograph or electrocardiogram that shows right ventricle hypertrophy	Chest pain, second heart sound or closure of pulmonic valve is accentuated; tricuspid valve murmur; radiograph and electrocardiagram show right ventricular enlargement
Treatment	Avoid venous stasis; anticoagulant therapy; fibrinolytic agent if life-threatening	Supplemental oxygen, digitalis, and diuretics are palliative; lung transplantation is therapeutic	Same as pulmonary hypertension; success depends on reversal of underlying lung disease

Characteristics of Lung Cancer

Type/Frequency	Growth Rate	Metastasis	Manifestations/Treatment
Adenocarcinoma; 35%-40%	Moderate	Early	Pleural effusion; surgical treatment/ adjunctive chemotherapy
Squamous cell; 30%	Slow	Late	Cough, sputum production, airway obstruction; surgical treatment/ adjunctive chemotherapy
Large cell undifferentiated carcinoma; 10%-15%	Rapid	Early and widespread	Pain, pleural effusion, cough, sputum production, hemoptysis, airway obstruction results in pneumonitis or pleural effusion
Small cell (oat cell) carcinoma; 20%-25%	Very rapid	Very early to mediastinum or distally in lung	Airway obstruction, excessive ACTH secretion with its signs and symptoms; chemotherapy and radiation

NOTE: The current accepted system for the staging of lung cancer is the TNM classification. In this system, *T* denotes the extent of the primary tumor, *N* indicates the nodal involvement, and *M* describes the extent of metastasis.

PRACTICE EXAMINATION

Multiple Choice
Circle the correct answer(s) for each question.

1. High altitudes may produce hypoxemia by:
   a. right-to-left shunts.
   b. atelectasis.
   c. decreased oxygen inspiration.
   d. emphysema.
   e. All of the above are correct.
2. In ARDS, increased alveolocapillary membrane permeability mainly is due to:
   a. alveolar epithelial damage.
   b. decreased surfactant.
   c. vasoconstriction.
   d. ventilation to perfusion mismatching.
   e. inflammatory mediators released.
3. Type II pneumocyte damage causes:
   a. increased alveolocapillary permeability.
   b. chemotaxis for neutrophils.
   c. exudation of fluid from capillaries into the interstitium.
   d. decreased surfactant production.
   e. All of the above are correct.
4. Pulmonary edema may be caused by:
   a. hypoventilation.
   b. CNS abnormalities.
   c. atelectasis.
   d. rupture of pleura.
   e. increased pulmonary hydrostatic pressure.
5. In asthma:
   a. bronchial muscles contract.
   b. bronchial muscles relax.
   c. mucous secretions decrease.
   d. imbalances within the CNS develop.
6. In emphysema:
   a. there is increased area for gaseous exchange.
   b. there are prolonged inspirations.
   c. the bronchioles are primarily involved.
   d. there is increased diaphragm movement.
   e. alveoli are less able to recoil and expel air.
7. In pneumococcal pneumonia, the stage of gray hepatization is characterized by:
   a. solidification of tissue.
   b. fibrin deposition.
   c. alveoli filling with blood cells and pneumococci.
   d. macrophages appearing in alveolar spaces.
8. Pulmonary hypertension:
   a. shows an enlarged pulmonary artery.
   b. involves deep vein thrombosis.
   c. shows right ventricular hypertrophy.
   d. Both a and c are correct.
   e. a, b, and c are correct.
9. Cor pulmonale:
   a. occurs in response to long-standing pulmonary hypertension.
   b. is right heart failure.
   c. is manifested by altered tricuspid and pulmonic valve sounds.
   d. Both b and c are correct.
   e. a, b, and c are correct.
10. A lung cancer characterized by many anaplastic figures and the production of hormones is most likely:
   a. squamous cell carcinoma.
   b. small cell carcinoma.
   c. large cell carcinoma.
   d. adenocarcinoma.
   e. bronchial adenoma.

11. The metastasis of lung squamous cell carcinoma is:
    a. late.
    b. very early and widespread.
    c. early.
    d. early and widespread.
    e. never seen.
12. Which is *true* about tuberculosis?
    a. It is caused by an aerobic bacillus.
    b. It may affect other organs.
    c. It involves a type III hypersensitivity.
    d. Antibodies to it may be detected with a skin test.
13. Pulmonary emboli usually do which of the following?
    a. Obstruct blood supply to lung parenchyma
    b. Have origins from thrombi in the legs
    c. Occlude pulmonary vein branches
    d. Occlude pulmonary artery branches
14. Chronic bronchitis:
    a. is caused by a lack of surfactant.
    b. impairs cilia.
    c. exhibits a nonproductive cough.
    d. causes collapsed alveoli.
15. Emphysema is precipitated by:
    a. histamine.
    b. TNF.
    c. leukotrienes.
    d. alpha-1 antitrypsin deficiency.

Fill in the Blanks

Supply the correct response for each statement.

16. Increased ventilatory rate, very large tidal volume, and no expiratory pause are characteristics of ____.

17. Coughing up blood or bloody secretions is _____.

18. Decreased arterial oxygenation causes _____.

19. Apnea, inward ventilation, then apnea again characterize _____.

20. Alveolar collapse is observed in _____.

21. Abnormal deflation of bronchi is termed _____.

22. Fibrous tissue or nodules in lungs is termed _____.

23. Fractured ribs or sternum cause _____.

24. Pleural space air is termed _____.

25. *Streptococcus pneumoniae* causes _____ _____.

CASE STUDY

Mr. S. is a retired 69-year-old county attorney who was on a buying trip with his wife for old, classic cars in the high, mountainous country of Colorado when he became extremely short of breath. His alarmed wife took him to a multispecialty medical clinic for evaluation. On admission to the clinic, Mr. S. was restless and dyspneic. His chest had an increased anteroposterior dimension.

Mr. S.'s past history revealed a habit of smoking two packs of cigarettes a day for 45 years. During the past few years, Mr. S. had noticed a cough each morning on rising. Recently, while working in his flower garden, he had to stop at times to catch his breath. Even while watching television, he had experienced dyspnea. Also, he indicated a weight loss over the last 2 months.

A chest radiograph was taken, and pulmonary function tests were done. The chest radiograph revealed a flat, low diaphragm with lung hyperinflation but clear fields. Pulmonary function tests showed decreased tidal volume and vital capacity, increased total lung capacity, and prolonged forced expiratory volume.

Question

Which pulmonary disease is exhibited by Mr. S.'s symptoms? Justify your answer.

34 Alterations of Pulmonary Function in Children

FOUNDATIONAL KNOWLEDGE OBJECTIVE

a. **Identify differences between children and adults that affect the pulmonary system**.
   Review text pages 1249 through 1251; refer to Figures 34-1 through 34-3.

MEMORY CHECK!

- Infants and young children have fewer alveoli than adults; their alveoli are much smaller and less complex than those of adults. The small diameter airways of infants and children produce increased resistance to airflow and are easily obstructed by mucosal edema or secretions. The airways and chest walls of the infant are much less rigid than those of the adult. The flexible and compliant infant chest wall may actually flex inward, and the airways collapse somewhat during times of respiratory stress, thereby limiting functional respiratory capacity. Surfactant production begins by 20 to 24 weeks of gestation and is secreted into the fetal airways by 30 weeks. The premature infant, however, may not have attained adequate surfactant production by birth and will be unable to maintain alveolar surface tension. Children have greater metabolic rates and oxygen consumption than adults; respiratory distress, acidosis, and dehydration develop more easily in children than in adults. By virtue of their immature immune systems, children have many more respiratory infections than do adults.

LEARNING OBJECTIVES

After studying this chapter, the learner will be able to do the following:

1. **Compare upper airway infections and obstructions.**
   Study text pages 1313 through 1317; refer to Figures 34-4 through 34-8 and Table 34-1. See the table on page 248.

2. **Describe other causes of upper airway compromise.**
   Study text pages 1317 though 1320; refer to Figures 34-9 and 34-10.

Most children who **aspirate a foreign object** are between 1 and 3 years of age. Often the aspiration is not witnessed nor does not seem significant to the parent, so fewer than one third of children who aspirate an object seek medical care during the first 24 hours. At the time of the aspiration event, the child may cough, choke, gag, or wheeze; occasionally stridor or cyanosis occurs. There may then be a quiescent interval of minutes to even weeks or months before symptoms reappear due to local irritation, granulation, bronchial obstruction, or infection (pneumonia or bronchiectasis).

Foreign bodies lodged in the upper trachea typically produce inspiratory stridor, whereas those located in the lower intrathoracic airways more commonly produce wheezing. About 75% of aspirated foreign bodies lodge in a bronchus. Many objects are not radiopaque; however, if the object has completely occluded a lung segment,

atelectasis will be visible on a chest x-ray examination or air will accumulate distal to the obstruction if the object is causing a ball-valve effect.

Most foreign bodies can be removed by bronchoscopy; rarely is a pulmonary lobectomy required. Food particles, which are soft, must be removed, as well as hard objects, because infection will otherwise occur. Objects lodged in the laryngeal or subglottic regions are particularly dangerous because of their potential for complete or near-complete airway occlusion.

Angioedema is a localized edema involving the deep, subcutaneous layers of skin or mucous membranes. Generally, angioedema causes facial swelling, particularly around the eyes and lips, and may progress to airway swelling. Angioedema is usually secondary to allergic phenomena and standard treatment includes epinephrine, antihistamines, and steroids if airway compromise is apparent. An inherited deficiency of C-1 inhibitor is characterized by recurring attacks of angioedema involving subcutaneous tissue. Laryngeal attacks may be life threatening if not treated.

Traumatic injury to the upper airway with development of **subglottic stenosis** is a well-described complication of endotracheal intubation. Factors that contribute to subglottic stenosis include long-term assisted ventilation, use of an endotracheal tube that is too large, excessive movement of the tube, and individual susceptibility. For significant subglottic stenosis, tracheostomy or tracheal reconstructive surgery may be needed.

247

Upper Airway Infections and Obstruction

Condition	Age	Etiology	Pathology	Symptoms/Treatment
Bacterial tracheitis	1 to 12 yr	S. aureus H. influenzae	Inflammation of upper trachea	High fever, thick harsh cough, purulent secretions/Artificial airway and antibiotics
Retropharyngeal abscess	>6 yr	S. aureus Hemolytic streptococci	Abscess in posterior pharyngeal wall	Sore throat, fever, muffled voice, drools/Artificial airway and antibiotics
Peritonsillar	>9 yr	S. aureus Hemolytic streptococci	Abscess in or around tonsil	Similar to retropharyngeal abscess/Antibiotics, incision and drainage
Acute laryngotracheobronchitis or croup	6 mo to 5 yr	Parainfluenza, influenza A, respiratory syncytial viruses	Inflammation from vocal cords to bronchial lumina	Prodrome of rhinorrhea and sore throat, harsh cough, stridor, fever, nasal discharge, conjunctivitis/Epinephrine and nebulized steroids
Epiglottitis	2 to 6 yr	H. influenzae, Group A streptococci	Inflammation of supraglottic structures	Inflammation of supraglottic structures sore throat, fever, muffled voice, may droll, sits erect and quietly/Artificial airway, antibiotics, and nebulized steroids

Laryngomalacia is the most common cause of chronic stridor in infants, but it is usually mild and improves spontaneously over the first year of life as the supralaryngeal cartilage structures stiffen. In laryngomalacia, the epiglottis or arytenoids or both fold inward with inspiration, partially covering the glottis. Typical signs of laryngomalacia include inspiratory stridor beginning in the first days or weeks of life, accentuated with activity, and sometimes worse with supine or head flexed positions.

In **tracheomalacia**, the tracheal cartilages tend to collapse during the respiratory cycle. Symptoms are more subtle than in laryngomalacia. There may be low-pitched inspiratory stridor for malacia of the upper trachea or centrally located, single-pitch (monophonic) wheeze for malacia of the mid to distal trachea. Both laryngomalacia and tracheomalacia can be confirmed by a laryngoscopy.

Congenital malformations of the trachea and bronchial tree cause airway obstruction. Affected infants develop obvious airway symptoms or feeding difficulties or both. Many children are first thought to have gastroesophageal reflux as the principal problem. Lesions include laryngeal webs, cysts, clefts, subglottic hemangiomas, and abnormalities involving the great vessels that result in tracheal compression (vascular rings). Surgical management is usually required in these conditions.

3. Describe obstructive sleep apnea.

Study text page 1320.

Obstructive sleep apnea syndrome (OSAS) is partial or complete upper airway obstruction (UAO) during sleep with disruption of normal ventilation and normal sleep patterns. OSAS is usually seen in children with adenotonsillar hypertrophy but also may occur in children who are obese or have craniofacial anomalies or neurologic disorders.

There usually is a history of snoring and labored breathing during sleep, which may be continuous or intermittent. There may be episodes of increased respiratory effort but no audible airflow, often terminated by snorting, gasping, repositioning, or arousal. Sleep is often described as restless. Daytime sleepiness is occasionally reported. Children are most often referred for tonsillectomy and adenoidectomy (T&A) on the basis of described symptoms and physical findings, such as enlarged tonsils, adenoidal facies, and mouth breathing.

4. Describe the pathophysiologic processes involved in respiratory distress syndrome of the newborn.

Study pages 1321 through 1323; refer to Figures 34-11 and 34-12.

Respiratory distress syndrome (RDS) of the newborn, which is also known as hyaline membrane disease (HMD), is a lack of adequate surfactant to reduce alveolar surface tension. Although primarily a disease of preterm infants who have inadequate surfactant production, RDS can appear in term infants, particularly those with diabetic mothers or those who have undergone prenatal or birth insults, such as asphyxia or shock. The small, underdeveloped alveoli of preterm infants require very high pressures to inflate. Absence of surfactant compounds this problem, and each breath the infant takes requires as much pressure as the first. Widespread atelectasis occurs, and this causes respiratory distress and increased pulmonary vascular resistance.

248

Increased pulmonary vascular resistance causes shunting of the blood away from the lungs and results in persistent fetal circulation, which further compounds the problem of hypoxia and hypercapnia. Capillary permeability increases, which results in the leakage of plasma proteins. Fibrin deposits in the air spaces create the appearance of the hyaline membranes. Hypoxia and hypercapnia trigger vasoconstriction of the pulmonary vascular bed and exacerbate shunting. Prolonged anaerobic metabolism produces metabolic acidosis.

Tachypnea, expiratory grunting, intercostal and subcostal retractions, nasal flaring, and skin duskiness are clinical manifestations. Treatment is supportive with mechanical ventilation. Exogenous surfactant administration has contributed significantly to the treatment of RDS. Newborns with RDS need oxygen and possible mechanical ventilation. Nitric oxide has been used for persistent pulmonary hypertension of the newborn. Antenatal treatment with glucocorticoids for women in preterm labor (24 to 34 weeks' gestation) induces a significant acceleration of lung maturation and reduces the incidence of RDS.

5. Describe bronchopulmonary dysplasia.

Study text pages 1323 through 1326; refer to Figure 34-13.

Bronchopulmonary dysplasia (BPD) is a severe form of lung damage associated with neonatal chronic lung disease. Risk factors include premature birth, immature lungs, oxygen toxicity, positive pressure ventilation, respiratory infection, antiprotease deficiency, genetic predisposition, and ductus arteriosus. It occurs in infants of 24 to 28 weeks' gestation who have been ventilated.

Clinically, the infants remain oxygen and ventilator dependent and have respiratory symptoms and radiographic abnormalities. Episodes of atelectasis, hyperinflation, pneumothorax, and interstitium air are characteristic.

BPD can cause death because of infection or respiratory factors within a few weeks or can continue for months or years with impaired pulmonary function. Treatment is designed to accelerate lung maturation, maintain normal oxygenation and nutrition, prevent further lung damage, and promote lung repair.

6. Identify the most common etiologic agent in bronchiolitis and bronchiolitis obliterans; describe their pathophysiology.

Study pages 1326 and 1330.

The most common cause of **bronchiolitis** is respiratory syncytial virus, followed by adenoviruses, influenza, parainfluenza, and mycoplasma in older children. Viral infection causes necrosis of the bronchial epithelium and destruction of ciliated epithelial cells. The submucosa of the bronchi becomes edematous and plugged with mucus and cellular debris, and bronchospasm narrows airways. Atelectasis occurs in some areas of the lungs and hyperinflation in others.

The usual manifestation is an infant who develops mild cold symptoms. Symptoms progress to hypoxemia, overexpanded thoracic cage, and diaphragm flattening, causing downward displacement of the liver and spleen. Children younger than 1 year may require assisted ventilation and hydration. Bronchodilators and antiviral agents for respiratory syncytial virus (RSV) may be required.

Bronchiolitis obliterans is fibrotic obstruction of the respiratory bronchioles and alveolar ducts secondary to inflammation. Most cases are associated with pulmonary infections.

7. Describe the most common etiologic agents of pneumonias in children.

Study pages 1327 through 1330; refer to Table 34-2.

Pneumonia involves inflammation and infection in the terminal airways and alveoli. The common etiologic agents are viruses, followed by bacteria and mycoplasma. Widespread childhood vaccination has decreased the incidence of *Haemophilus influenzae* type b and *Streptococcus pneumoniae* infections. The milder viral pneumonias tend to occur in infancy and early childhood and are characterized by an antecedent "cold" followed by cough, fever, rhinorrhea, rales, wheezing, and mild systemic symptoms. RSV causes most viral pneumonia in infants. Mycoplasma and chlamydia cause atypical pneumonia in school-age children and adolescents and exhibit only upper respiratory tract involvement with low grade fever and cough. Bacterial pneumonias, such as those caused by *Streptococcus pneumoniae* (1 to 4 years), *Staphylococcus aureus* (1 week to 2 years), and group A beta-hemolytic streptococci (all ages), tend to have more dramatic systemic features and exhibit high fever, productive cough, shaking, chills, pleuritic pain, and malaise. They are more lobar in nature than those caused by other infectious agents and require antibiotics therapy for resolution. Treatment for viral pneumonia is palliative.

Children at highest risk for **aspiration pneumonitis** are toddlers and children with poor airway reflexes or gastroesophageal reflux. The severity of lung injury after an aspiration incident is determined by the pH of the aspirated material, presence of pathogenic bacteria, and the volatility and viscosity of the substance. Very low or high pH and low viscosity cause significant inflammatory response, whereas high-viscosity substances are less likely to cause a pneumonitis.

8. Describe the pathophysiologic processes, manifestations, and treatment of childhood asthma.

Study pages 1330 through 1334; refer to Figures 34-14 and 34-15.

Asthma is a chronic illness of highly variable severity, which tends to be punctuated with more or less frequent episodes of acute exacerbation. In children, asthma reflects a complex interaction between genetic susceptibility and environmental factors, including early exposure to allergens and infection. In infants and toddlers younger than 2 years, the most common of these is RSV. In older children, the major viral trigger is rhinovirus. The pathophysiologic basis of asthma involves hyperresponsive lower airways responding in an obstructive manner to various triggers. The triggers include allergens, exercise, viruses, and other infectious agents. Responses include spasm of the respiratory smooth muscle that encircles the airways, edema of the airway mucosa, mucus plugging of

249

the airways, and cellular infiltration into the airways. Asthma attacks may have two phases. The early phase of the attack is caused by IgE mediation resulting from mast cell degranulation and histamine, leukotrienes, prostaglandins, platelet activating factor, and certain cytokines released in response to the triggering factors. The late phase follows in 4 to 8 hours and is caused by inflammatory mediators released from cells attracted to the airways. The typical abnormalities in acute asthma are hypoxemia, hypercapnia, and respiratory alkalosis; with severe airway obstruction, respiratory failure with acute CO_2 retention and respiratory acidosis occurs.

Clinical manifestations may include persistent cough, expiratory wheeze, and signs of respiratory distress. On physical examination, there is expiratory wheezing described as high pitched and musical; there is prolongation of the expiratory phase of the respiratory cycle. The child may speak in clipped sentences or not at all because of dyspnea. Sometimes, hyperinflation (barrel chest) is visible.

Treatment involves the administration of adrenergic and bronchodilator aerosols and inhaled and systemic corticosteroids. For allergic asthma, anti-IgE may be appropriate.

9. Describe the pathogenesis of acute respiratory distress syndrome.

Study text pages 1334 through 1336; refer to Figure 34-16.

Acute respiratory distress syndrome (ARDS) is the descriptor for the condition in children that results from a direct pulmonary insult or systemic insult that activates an inflammatory response causing alveolocapillary injury. Its pathogenesis is also detailed in the flow chart of acute respiratory distress syndrome detailed in Chapter 33 learning objective 3.

10. Describe the pulmonary pathophysiology associated with cystic fibrosis and identify general modes of diagnostic testing and therapy.

Study pages 1336 through 1339; refer to Figures 34-17 and 34-18.

Cystic fibrosis (CF) is an autosomal recessive, genetically transmitted, multisystem disease in which exocrine or mucus-producing glands secrete abnormally thick mucus that obstructs the gastrointestinal system and lungs. The CF gene has been located on chromosome 7. Its mutation results in the abnormal expression of the protein, **cystic fibrosis transmembrane conductance regulator (CFTR)**, which is a chloride channel present on the surface of many types of epithelial cells. Although CF is a multiorgan disease, respiratory failure is almost always the cause of death. An obstructed gastrointestinal system leads to malabsorption of nutrients related to pancreatic insufficiency. Thick secretions obstruct the bronchioles in the lung and predispose the lungs to recurrent or chronic infection. Chronic inflammation, subsequent to interleukin-8 actions, neutrophil attraction, and protease activity, leads to destruction of the airway walls and hyperplasia of goblet cells. Bronchiectasis, pneumonia, and widespread pulmonary fibrosis follow in response to bacterial colonization with *Staphylococcus aureus* and *Pseu-*

domonas aeruginosa. End-stage disease is characterized by cor pulmonale, chronic hypoxia, and pulmonary hypertension.

Chronic cough, sputum production, and purulent mucus indicate lung involvement. Labored ventilation results in hypoxia, finger clubbing, and cyanosis. Classic gastrointestinal presentations include meconium ileus at birth, which is pathognomonic for CF. Approximately half of all children present with failure-to-thrive and malabsorptive symptoms, such as frequent, loose, and oily stools. Less frequent manifestations include chronic sinusitis, nasal polyps, and rectal prolapse.

Genetic testing is available to detect carriers. Sweat chloride testing is a definitive diagnostic test because it measures defective epithelial chloride ion transport. Treatment includes aggressive chest physiotherapy, bronchodilators, mucus liquefiers, and judicious use of antibiotics to control infection.

11. Describe sudden infant death syndrome.

Study page 1339.

Sudden infant death syndrome (SIDS) refers to the sudden, unexpected death of any infant or young child in whom a postmortem examination fails to demonstrate a cause for death. The highest incidence is between 3 and 4 months of age; it mostly occurs during sleep and with greater frequency during the winter months.

The cause of SIDS is unknown. There may be a developmental immaturity of ventilatory and arousal responses to hypoxemia or hypercarbia; also, a hyperimmune airway in association with a prior respiratory infection may be causative. However, some risk factors can be avoided, such as prone sleeping, soft bedding surfaces, and maternal smoking.

There is no treatment, because the death is sudden and unexplained.

PRACTICE EXAMINATION

Fill in the Blanks

Supply the correct response for each statement.

1. During times of respiratory distress, the infant's chest wall may flex inward and limit functional respiratory capacity because of chest wall _____ and _____.

2. At birth, the infant has small, immature alveoli that cause _____ to air flow.

3. Surfactant production begins by _____ weeks of gestation.

4. Failure to produce surfactant at birth results in severe _____ and RDS of the newborn.

5. _____ is a disease process primarily caused by hyperresponsive airways that are sensitive to certain environmental triggers.

6. Children have greater _____ and _____ than do adults.

250

Multiple Choice

Circle the correct answer(s) for each question.

7. Epiglottitis is characterized by:
   a. gradual onset.
   b. severe stridor.
   c. harsh cough.
   d. nasal discharge.

8. Laryngotracheobronchitis is characterized by:
   a. drooling.
   b. *H. influenza* infections.
   c. group A streptococcal infections.
   d. inflammation from vocal cords to bronchial lumina.

9. The most common cause of bronchiolitis is:
   a. *H. influenzae.*
   b. exposure to allergens.
   c. parainfluenza virus.
   d. respiratory syncytial virus.

10. Most children who aspirate foreign objects:
    a. exhibit quiescent intervals before symptoms appear.
    b. remove the offending object by coughing.
    c. lodged in the trachea exhibit wheezing.
    d. lodged in airways exhibit stridor.

11. Staphylococcal pneumonia results in:
    a. mild systemic symptoms.
    b. upper respiratory tract involvement.
    c. lobar involvement.
    d. a typical pneumonia.

12. Which is *true* of childhood pneumonias?
    a. All pneumonias are mostly lobar.
    b. Systemic involvement is greater in viral than in bacterial pneumonias.
    c. Viral pneumonias are often preceded by a "cold."
    d. All of the above are correct.

13. Which statement about SIDS is *true?*
    a. It commonly occurs during autumn.
    b. Its etiology is known.
    c. It occurs between 3 and 4 months of age.
    d. It may be effectively treated.

14. Cystic fibrosis is:
    a. a multisystem disease.
    b. a defect that results in the overproduction of viscous mucus.
    c. a disease for which it is difficult to detect carriers through genetic testing.
    d. diagnosed by sweat chloride testing.
    e. a, b, and d are correct.

15. Asthma:
    a. triggers include allergens and viruses.
    b. of affected individuals may be assumed to be cured if they are asymptomatic for a number of years.
    c. is characterized by hyperresponsive airways.
    d. Both a and c are correct.
    e. a, b, and c are correct.

16. Respiratory distress syndrome of the newborn:
    a. exhibits vasodilation of the pulmonary vascular bed.
    b. develops less capillary permeability, which causes fibrin deposits.
    c. can be treated with nitric oxide to alleviate pulmonary hypertension.
    d. can be treated at birth by the administration of glucocorticoids.

Matching

Match the circumstance or cause with the alteration. (More than one answer may be correct.)

_____ 17. Chronic condition

_____ 18. Genetic predisposition

_____ 19. May result in persistent fetal circulation

_____ 20. May be a consequence of prematurity

_____ 21. Acute, life-threatening infection

_____ 22. Parainfluenza virus

_____ 23. Neonatal chronic lung disease

_____ 24. Occurs epidemically in fall and winter

_____ 25. Inflammatory basis with hyperresponsive airways

a. asthma

b. cystic fibrosis

c. laryngotracheobronchitis

d. bronchopulmonary dysplasia

e. epiglottitis

f. respiratory distress syndrome

Chapter **34** **Alterations of Pulmonary Function in Children**

T.C. is a 2-year-old boy who saw his physician 3 days ago with a history of mild nasal congestion without fever, cough, vomiting, or other complaints. His parents stated, "We are just getting over 'terrible winter colds' and hoped they had not given them to T.C."

T.C. is back today because his mother is concerned that he is coughing severely, is not feeding well at all, and "breathes funny." He still has no significant fever but is somewhat lethargic with a respiratory rate consistently high at approximately 90 breaths per minute with moderate intercostal retractions, nasal flaring, and light expiratory wheeze. A chest x-ray shows no specific areas of consolidation but does show hyperinflation and general "haziness." T.C. is admitted to the hospital for further treatment.

Question

What do T.C.'s signs and symptoms suggest?

35 Structure and Function of the Renal and Urologic Systems

PREREQUISITE KNOWLEDGE OBJECTIVES

After reviewing the primary text where referenced, the learner will be able to do the following:

1. **Describe or identify the organs of the urinary system and the gross anatomic features of the kidneys.**
   Review text pages 1344 and 1345; refer to Figures 35-1 and 35-2.
2. **Describe the microscopic structure of the nephron.**
   Review text pages 1345 through 1348 and 1350; refer to Figures 35-3 through 35-7.
3. **Identify the determinants of renal blood flow.**
   Review text pages 1351 and 1352; refer to Figures 35-9 and 35-10 and Table 35-1.
4. **Describe the processes of glomerular filtration and tubular reabsorption and secretion; note major functions of nephron segments.**
   Review text pages 1352 and 1354 through 1357; refer to Figures 35-11 through 35-13 and Table 35-2.
5. **Describe the purposes of the countercurrent exchange system; note the actions of diuretics.**
   Review text pages 1357 and 1358; refer to Figure 35-14 and Table 35-3.
6. **Identify the effects of hormones activated or synthesized by the kidney.**
   Review text pages 1358 through 1360.
7. **Identify the tests of renal functions.**
   Review text pages 1360 through 1362.
8. **Identify the changes that occur in renal functions with advancing age.**
   Review text page 1362.

PRACTICE EXAMINATION

Multiple Choice

Circle the correct answer for each question.

1. Alphabetize the correct sequence of structures through which urine passes as it leaves the body.
   a. Ureter
   b. Renal pelvis
   c. Urinary bladder
   d. Major calyx
   e. Urethra
   f. Minor calyx
2. The functional unit of the human kidney is the:
   a. nephron.
   b. collecting tubule (duct).
   c. major calyx.
   d. minor calyx.
   e. pyramid.
3. One feature of the renal blood circulation that makes it unique is that:
   a. blood flows from arterioles into venules.
   b. blood flows from venules into arterioles.
   c. there is a double set of venules.
   d. there are two sets of capillaries.
4. Which of the following has the opposite effect on urine production from the others?
   a. decreased solutes in blood
   b. decreased blood pressure
   c. increased ambient temperature
   d. dehydration
   e. reduced water consumption
5. A relatively high blood pressure in the glomerulus of the kidney is maintained because:
   a. the afferent arteriole arises from the arcuate artery.
   b. the efferent arteriole is larger than the interlobular artery.
   c. the glomerulus is constricted.
   d. the afferent arteriole is larger than the efferent arteriole.
   e. ADH from the anterior pituitary causes vasoconstriction of the renal arteries.

6. If the following hypothetical conditions exist in the nephron, what would be the net (effective) filtration pressure?
   Glomerular blood hydrostatic = 80 mmHg
   Glomerular blood osmotic = 20 mmHg
   Capsular hydrostatic = 30 mmHg
   a. 40 mmHg
   b. 30 mmHg
   c. 20 mmHg
   d. 10 mmHg
7. The capillaries of the glomerulus differ from other capillary networks in the body because they:
   a. have a larger area of anastomosis.
   b. branch from and drain into arterioles.
   c. lack endothelium.
   d. force filtrate from the blood.
8. Which of the following is not a function of the kidney?
   a. Water volume control
   b. Blood pressure control
   c. Urine storage
   d. Conversion of vitamin D to an active form
9. Potassium is secreted and reabsorbed by:
   a. Bowman's capsule.
   b. the proximal convoluted tubule.
   c. the loop of Henle.
   d. collecting ducts.
10. The primary receptors sensitive to the oncotic pressure of blood are found in the:
    a. kidney cortex.
    b. kidney medulla.
    c. hypothalamus.
    d. juxtaglomerular apparatus.
11. Water reabsorbed from the glomerular filtrate initially enters (the):
    a. afferent arterioles.
    b. efferent arterioles.
    c. Bowman's capsule.
    d. glomerulus.
    e. vasa recta.
12. Plasma contains a much greater concentration of __ _____ than the glomerular filtrate.
    a. sodium
    b. protein
    c. urea
    d. creatinine
13. An increase in water permeability of the distal convoluted tubules and collecting duct is due to:
    a. a decrease in the production of antidiuretic hormone.
    b. an increase in the production of antidiuretic hormone.
    c. a decrease in blood plasma osmolality.
    d. an increase in water content within tubular cells.
    e. None of the above is correct.
14. The descending loop of the nephron allows:
    a. sodium secretion.
    b. potassium secretion.
    c. hydrogen ion secretion.
    d. sodium diffusion inward.

15. Which of the following pressures affect net glomerular filtration?
    a. Blood osmotic pressure opposes capsular hydrostatic and blood hydrostatic pressures.
    b. Blood hydrostatic pressure opposes capsular hydrostatic and blood oncotic pressures.
    c. Capsular hydrostatic pressure opposes blood osmotic and blood hydrostatic pressures.
    d. None of the above is correct.
16. Tubular secretion is accomplished in the:
    a. glomerulus.
    b. urethra.
    c. renal pelvis.
    d. distal convoluted tubule.
    e. None of the above is correct.
17. Tubular reabsorption and tubular secretion differ in that:
    a. secretion adds material to the filtrate; reabsorption removes materials from the filtrate.
    b. secretion is a passive process; reabsorption is an active transport process.
    c. reabsorption tends to increase urine volume; secretion tends to decrease urine volume.
    d. secretion adds materials to the blood; reabsorption removes materials from the blood.
18. The kidneys perform which function?
    a. Conserve H^+, HCO_3^-
    b. Conserve NH_4^+
    c. Eliminate H^+, NH_4^+
    d. Eliminate amino acids
19. If a small person excretes about 1 L of urine during a 24-hour period, estimate the total amount of glomerular filtrate formed.
    a. 4 L
    b. 10 L
    c. 18 L
    d. 100 L
20. Which of the following should *not* appear in the glomerular filtrate (in any significant quantity) just after the process of glomerular filtration has been accomplished?
    a. Protein
    b. Urea
    c. Glucose
    d. Both a and b are correct.
21. Loop of Henle is to vasa recta as convoluted tubules are to:
    a. afferent arterioles.
    b. peritubular capillaries.
    c. efferent arterioles.
    d. renal arteries.
22. The two "currents" used in the countercurrent exchange system are the:
    a. afferent and efferent arterioles.
    b. glomerulus and glomerular (Bowman's) capsule.
    c. ascending and descending limbs.
    d. proximal and distal tubules.
    e. All of the above are correct.

23. The countercurrent exchange system:
    a. prevents water reabsorption from the collecting duct.
    b. concentrates sodium in the renal cortex.
    c. facilitates osmosis.
    d. concentrates chloride in the renal cortex.
    e. None of the above is correct.
24. As ambient temperature increases, what usually happens to the volume of urine production?
    a. No effect at all
    b. Either more or less, depending on other factors
    c. More urine output
    d. Less urine output
25. A waste product of protein metabolism is:
    a. pepsinogen.
    b. trypsin.
    c. amino acid.
    d. urea.
    e. urine.

36 Alterations of Renal and Urinary Tract Function

FOUNDATIONAL KNOWLEDGE OBJECTIVES

a. Define the renal processes of filtration, reabsorption, and secretion.
   Refer to Figures 35-11, 35-12, and 35-14.

MEMORY CHECK!

- Glomerular filtration is the first step in urine formation in which permeable substances from the blood are filtered at the endothelial-capsular membrane and the filtrate enters the proximal convoluted tubule.
- Tubular reabsorption retains substances that are needed by the body, including water, glucose, sodium, potassium, and bicarbonate. This process removes materials from the filtrate and returns them to the blood.
- Tubular secretion excretes chemicals that are not needed by the body, including hydrogen, some amino acids, urea, creatinine, and some drugs. Secretion adds material to the filtrate from the blood.
- In electrolyte movement between body fluids and cells, electrolyte neutrality must be maintained in both extracellular and intracellular compartments. It is necessary that the number of cations equals the number of anions present. This principle is particularly important in renal function.

b. Identify the forces and factors that determine net filtration pressure; explain the cause and effect of decreased filtration pressure.
   Refer to Figure 35-13 and Table 35-2.

MEMORY CHECK!

- Net filtration pressure (NFP) is equal to glomerular blood hydrostatic pressure (GBHP) minus capsular hydrostatic pressure (CHP) plus blood oncotic pressure (BOP). Stated mathematically, the formula is NFP = GBHP − (CHP + BOP). The pressure that promotes filtration into Bowman's space is 47 mmHg due to GBHP, whereas the pressure that resists flow to Bowman's space is 35 mmHg due to 10 mmHg of pressure from Bowman's capsule HP and 25 mmHg from BOP. This provides a small NFP of 12 mmHg. This NFP can be reduced by renal vasoconstriction, hypotension, hypovolemia, or low cardiac output. Any of these circumstances will reduce glomerular filtration rate (GFR). The GFR is directly related to renal blood flow (RBF), which is regulated by intrinsic neural and hormonal autoregulation. The blood flow is determined by arteriovenous pressure differences across the vascular bed divided by the vascular resistance or, stated mathematically, RBF = PA − PV/R. As pressure increases and resistance decreases, renal blood flow increases. Sympathetic nerve activity stimulates renal arteriolar vasoconstriction and decreases both RBF and GFR.

Effects of the Renin-Angiotensin System

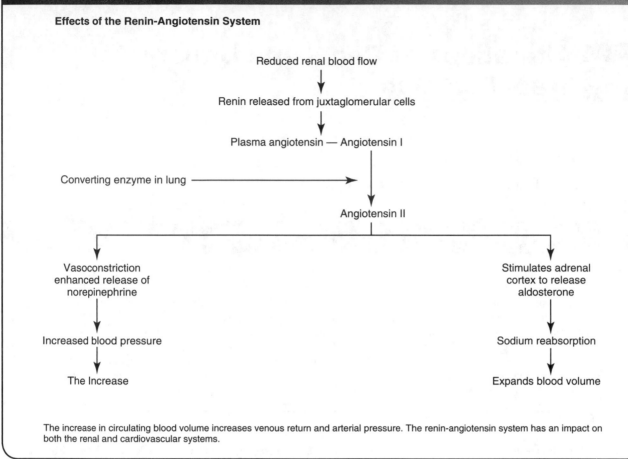

The increase in circulating blood volume increases venous return and arterial pressure. The renin-angiotensin system has an impact on both the renal and cardiovascular systems.

c. **Explain the basis of serum and urinalysis examinations to evaluate renal function.**
   Review text pages 1360 through 1362.

Laboratory Tests for Kidney Function
- **Blood urea nitrogen (BUN)** measures the concentration of urea in the blood. Urea is formed from protein metabolism and is elevated in reduced glomerular filtration. Normal BUN is 10 to 20 mg/dl. The BUN rises in states of dehydration and acute and chronic renal failure, because passage of fluid through the tubules is slowed.
- The **serum creatinine level** should have a stable value, because creatinine is a byproduct of muscle metabolism, and its levels of production are constant and are proportional to muscle mass. Normally, creatinine is not reabsorbed. If serum levels of 0.7 to 1.2 mg/dl exist, it indicates normal renal function. When creatinine rises and accumulates in the plasma, it represents decreasing GFR. If doubled, renal function is probably half of normal. If tripled, about 75% of renal function is lost.
- **Creatinine clearance** is the amount of blood that is theoretically "cleared" of creatinine by the kidney in 1 minute of filtration; 90 to 130 ml/min is normal. Creatinine clearance provides a good measure of renal blood flow and GFR, because serum levels are related to a 24-hour urine volume. Inulin, which is a substance with a stable plasma concentration, can be used to assess clearance. The amount of inulin filtered is equal to the volume of plasma filtered multiplied by the plasma concentration of inulin.
- The **urinalysis** is an essential part of the examination of all patients who may have renal disease, because materials in the urine can be diagnostic for many disorders. It is normal to have inorganic material, such as Na^+, Cl^-, Mg^{2+}, SO_4^2, PO_4^{3-}, and NH_4^+, and organic materials, such as urea, creatinine, and uric acid in the urine. It is abnormal to find RBCs, more than a few WBCs, bacteria protein, glucose, or ketones in the urine.

LEARNING OBJECTIVES

After studying this chapter, the learner will be able to do the following:

1. **Describe the features of upper urinary tract obstruction.**

   Study text pages 1365 through 1368, refer to Figures 36-1 and 36-2.

   Urinary tract obstruction is defined as blockage of urine flow within the urinary tract. Blockage may be caused by an anatomic or a functional defect and is referred to as **obstructive uropathy.** Regardless of its cause, the consequence is an impedance to flow that leads to urinary stasis, dilates the urinary system, increases the risk for infection, and compromises urinary system function.

   Complete obstruction of the upper urinary tract causes dilation of the ureter, or **hydroureter,** and of the renal pelvis and calyces, or **hydronephrosis.** Within days, two deleterious consequences develop: tubulointerstitial fibrosis and apoptosis. Unless the underlying obstruction is relieved, irreversible renal damage occurs. **Tubulointerstitial fibrosis** is the deposition of excessive amount of collagen and proteins within the kidney. **Apoptosis** is a normal process that the body uses to replace damaged or senescent cells with new ones, but the imbalance in growth factors initiated by fibrosis leads to excess cellular destruction of nephrons. Urinary tract obstruction also predisposes an individual to hypertension. Hypertension occurs because the renin-angiotensin-aldosterone cascade is activated.

   Persistent partial obstruction leads to impairment of the ability to concentrate urine, reabsorb bicarbonate, excrete ammonia, or regulate metabolic acid-base balance. Relief of bilateral, partial urinary tract obstruction or complete obstruction of a single kidney causes a transient period of **postobstructive diuresis** that may cause dehydration and dangerous electrolyte imbalances that must be corrected promptly.

   The body is able to partially counteract the negative consequences of unilateral obstruction through the processes of **compensatory hypertrophy** and **hyperfunction.** These processes cause the unobstructed kidney to increase the size of the individual glomeruli and tubules but not the total number of functioning nephrons. These processes diminish with age and are reversible when the obstructed kidney recovers.

2. **Describe the pathophysiology of calculi or urinary stones observed in upper tract obstruction.**

   Study text pages 1368 and 1369.

   Calcium is a common constituent of renal stones; about 70% to 80% of stones or **calculi** or **urinary stones** are composed of calcium oxalate, calcium phosphate, or a combination of both. Another stone, the struvite stone, which is composed of magnesium, ammonium, and phosphate, is caused by the action of some urea-splitting bacteria. Struvite stones are seen more often in women and account for about 15% of all stones. Uric acid stones, which comprise about 7% of stones, may be seen with gout. Rarely, cystine stones are seen in individuals with a genetic defect in transporting cystine. Stones are formed from urine salt supersaturation, precipitation, and crystallization; a stone less than 5 mm in size has about a 50% chance of spontaneous passage, but a 1-cm stone has almost no chance to pass.

   A colicky pain occurs as the rhythmic contractions of the ureter attempt to dislodge and advance the sharp-edged stone. The accumulation of urine behind the stone causes distention or spasm of the ureters. The pain may be in the flank, or it may radiate into the groin if the stone is located in the renal pelvis or proximal ureter. Colic radiating to the flank or lower abdomen indicates the stone is in the mid ureter. Urgency or incontinence indicates obstruction of the lower ureter.

   Treatment involves the dilution of stone-forming substances by a high fluid intake and extraction of larger stones by instrumentation, fragmentation of stones by ultrasonic lithotripsy, or surgical removal by percutaneous nephrolithotomy.

3. **Describe lower urinary tract obstruction, notably, neurogenic bladder.**

   Study text pages 1369 through 1372; refer to Figure 36-3 and Table 36-1.

   Neurogenic bladder is a functional urinary tract dysfunction that disrupts normal bladder filling and emptying, leading to urine retention or urinary incompetence; it is caused by an interruption of the nerve supply to the bladder. The neurologic disruption can occur in the brain or at the level of the spinal cord. Brain lesions produce neurogenic detrusor overactivity and urinary incompetence. Lesions affecting spinal cord segments C4-S1 produce detrusor overactivity called vesicosphincter dyssynergia, meaning "lack of harmonious coordination between detrusor and urethral sphincter muscles." Lesions affecting S2-S4 are associated with loss of the detrusor contraction reflex and denervation of the sphincter mechanism.

   Management involves catheterization, drugs, or surgery to relieve obstructions. Appropriate antibiotics are given to treat infections.

   Overactive bladder syndrome (OAB) is a syndrome of detrusor overactivity characterized by urgency with involuntary detrusor contraction during bladder filling that may be spontaneous or provoked. The detrusor is too weak to empty the bladder, resulting in urinary retention with overflow or stress incontinence. Anatomic causes of resistance to urine flow include **urethral stricture, prostatic enlargement** in men, and **pelvic organ prolapse** in women.

4. **Describe renal and bladder tumors.**

   Study text pages 1372 and 1373; refer to Figures 36-4 and 36-5 and Tables 36-2 and 36-3.

   Renal adenomas are uncommon, but they may become malignant, so they are usually surgically removed. **Renal cell carcinoma** is the most common renal neoplasm, and it usually occurs in men. An association exists between tobacco use, obesity, and long-term analgesic use and renal cell carcinoma. The tumors usually occur unilaterally and spread through the lymph nodes and blood vessels to the lungs, liver, and bones.

The manifestations are hematuria, flank pain, palpable flank or abdomen mass, and weight loss. These signs and symptoms are often silent; when they occur, they indicate an advanced stage of disease.

Treatment is usually surgical removal of the affected kidney in combination with chemotherapy. Radiation therapy and biologic response modifiers are used to treat metastatic disease.

Bladder tumors represent about 3% of all malignant tumors and are the fifth most common malignancy. The development of bladder cancer is most common in men who are older than 60 years. The risk of primary bladder cancer is greater among individuals who smoke or work in the chemical, rubber, or textile industries, and among women who take large amounts of phenacetin. Bladder cancer results from a genetic alteration in normal bladder epithelium associated with mutations in the tumor-suppressor gene *p53* and inactivation of the *pRb* gene. Metastasis is usually to the lymph nodes, liver, bones, and lungs. Secondary bladder cancer develops by the invasion of cancer from bordering organs, such as cervical carcinoma in women and prostatic carcinoma in men.

Bladder tumors may be asymptomatic or accompanied by hematuria. Advanced cancers are associated with pelvic pain and frequent urination. Treatment depends on the type and size of the lesion and involves resection, chemotherapy, or laser therapy.

5. **Compare and contrast the signs, symptoms, and etiology of cystitis and pyelonephritis.**
   Study text pages 1373 through 1378; refer to Figure 36-6 and Table 36-4. See the following table.
6. **Describe the types of glomerulonephritis and its features, manifestations, and treatment.**
   Study text pages 1378 through 1384; refer to Figures 36-7 through 36-10 and Table 36-5 through 36-7. See the table on page 261.

Glomerulonephritis is a group of diseases of the glomerulus that are caused by immune responses, toxins or drugs, vascular disorders, hepatitis, immune deficiency viruses, and other systemic diseases, including diabetes mellitus and lupus erythematosus. Glomerular damage generally occurs from the activation and products of the biochemical mediators of inflammation, namely complement, leukocytes, and fibrin. Damage begins after antibodies against glomerular basement membrane or antigen-antibody complexes have localized in the glomerular capillary wall. Complement is deposited with the antibodies. Complement activation attracts neutrophils and monocytes. The neutrophils and monocytes further the inflammatory reaction by releasing lysosomal enzymes that damage glomerular walls and increase glomerular capillary wall permeability. Membrane damage can lead to platelet aggregation and degranulation wherein platelets release vasoactive amines. Changes in membrane permeability permit the passage of protein molecules and red blood cells into the urine, thereby causing proteinuria and hematuria. The coagulation system also may be activated and lead to fibrin deposition in Bowman's space; this reduces renal blood flow and depresses glomerular filtration.

Depending on the cause, extent, and degree of damage to the glomerulus, increased or decreased filtration results. Mild proteinuria and hematuria occur during the early years of the disease. In later years, after 10 or 20 years, renal insufficiency will develop and be followed by nephrotic syndrome and an accelerated progression to end-stage renal failure.

The diagnosis of glomerular disease is confirmed by a urinalysis that shows (1) hematuria with red blood cell casts and (2) proteinuria that exceeds 3 to 5 g per day. In acute poststreptococcal glomerulonephritis, anti–streptolysin O (ASO) and antistreptokinase (ASK) are elevated, and serum complement is decreased. Creatinine clearance evaluates the extent of glomerular damage.

The basic principles for the treatment of glomerulonephritis are related to treating the primary disease, preventing or minimizing immune responses, and correcting

Cystitis and Pyelonephritis

	Cystitis (Bladder)	Pyelonephritis* (Kidney Tubules, Pelvis, and Interstitium)
	Lower Tract Infection	**Upper Tract Infection**
Signs/symptoms	Low back or suprapubic pain, painful burning on urination, frequent voiding/urgency, hematuria, cloudy urine	Fever, chills, backache, abdominal pain, nausea, vomiting, urinary urgency and frequency, costovertebral tenderness, possible hypertension
Etiology	Urinary obstruction, prostatitis, ascending infection with gram-negative rods ("honeymoon cystitis"), irritable bladder from sphincter dysfunction; interstitial "nonbacterial" cystitis is caused by an inflammatory autoimmune response	Inflammation or scarring of the interstitial tissue and tubules; causative organism is usually an ascending gram-negative rod, but can be fungi or viruses; a risk factor is any urinary obstruction or infection that causes urine reflux or residual urine

*Acute pyelonephritis involves an infection that exhibits inflammation of the pelvis, calyces, and medulla. Chronic pyelonephritis is persistent or recurrent autoimmune infection usually associated with an obstructive pathologic condition. It can lead to renal failure.

Common Types of Glomerulonephritis

Type	Features
Poststreptococcal (group A beta-hemolytic streptococci)	Diffuse; subepithelial deposits of immune IgG and complement complexes; phagocytic infiltration; occlusion of glomerular capillary blood flow; decreased glomerular filtration
Rapidly progressive or crescentic* (nonspecific response to glomerular injury)	Diffuse; accumulation of fibrin or cells proliferate into Bowman's space to form crescents and occlude glomerular filtration; antiglomerular basement membrane antibodies lead to damaged tissue and renal failure
Minimal change disease or lipoid nephrosis (usually idiopathic)	Diffuse fusion of epithelial processes; loss of negative charge in basement membrane and increased permeability lead to proteinuria and nephrotic syndrome
Focal glomerulosclerosis (usually idiopathic)	Similar pathology to minimal change disease
Membranous nephropathy (usually can be associated with systemic disease)	Diffuse thickening of glomerular capillary wall from deposits of antibody and idiopathic complement; increased permeability with proteinuria and nephrotic syndrome
Membranoproliferative (usually idiopathic, associated with activation of complement pathways)	Diffuse; mesangial cell proliferation; thickened basement membrane; subendothelial deposits of immune complex occlude glomerular capillary blood flow and decrease glomerular filtration
IgA nephropathy† (usually idiopathic)	Focal; some diffuse lesions; mesangial cell proliferation with IgA deposits; release of inflammatory mediators with crescent formation; sclerosis; interstitial fibrosis; decreased glomerular filtration rate

*Goodpasture syndrome is a type of crescentic glomerular nephritis associated with antibody formation against both pulmonary capillary and glomerular basement membrane.

†IgA nephropathy is the most common type of glomerulonephritis in developed countries, especially in Asia.

NOTE: Membranous, focal, and minimal change diseases are associated with nephrotic syndrome.

accompanying problems such as edema, hypertension, and hyperlipidemia.

7. Identify and explain the key features of nephrotic syndrome.

Study text pages 1384 and 1385; refer to Figure 36-11 and Table 36-8.

In **nephrotic syndrome**, there is increased glomerular permeability and protein leakage of 3.5 gram or more in the urine per day across an injured glomerular filtration, membrane. Genetic defects that affect the function and structure of the glomerular capillary wall can cause nephrotic syndrome. Systemic diseases implicated in secondary nephrotic syndrome include diabetes mellitus, amyloidosis, systemic lupus erythematosus, and Henoch-Schönlein purpura.

The key features of nephrotic syndrome include proteinuria, edema, hypoalbuminemia, hyperlipidemia, lipiduria, and vitamin D deficiency. Proteinuria occurs with protein leakage from the serum into the urine and excretion of up to 10 g protein in the urine per day.

This process reduces blood oncotic pressure; water leaves the capillaries more easily, and tissue edema follows. The edema is soft, pitting, and generalized. Hypoalbuminemia develops as albumin leaks through the capillaries and depletes its serum level. Hyperlipidemia occurs as the liver responds to the hypoalbuminemia by synthesizing replacement albumin. While synthesizing albumin, the liver also synthesizes lipoproteins in large amounts; therefore, hyperlipidemia develops. As tubular cells that contain fat are sloughed into the urine, lipiduria can be seen. Also, free fat from hyperlipidemia leaks across the glomerulus. Hypocalcemia develops in response to loss of vitamin bound to circulatory globulin. Loss of protein immunoglobulins increases susceptibility to infection in nephrotic syndrome. Treatment is with a normal protein, low-fat diet; salt restriction; diuretics; and steroids.

8. Define and identify the common etiologies of prerenal, intrarenal, and postrenal disease/failures; note the phases.

Study text pages 1386 through 1389; refer to Figure 36-12 and Tables 36-9 through 36-11. See the table on page 262.

Acute kidney injury renal failure is the rapid deterioration of renal function with a decrease in glomerular filtration and an accompanying elevation of BUN and plasma creatinine; oliguria also develops. The cause may be either prerenal (before kidney) because of renal hypoperfusion, intrarenal (within kidney) from renal functional impairment, or postrenal (after kidney) following obstruction of urinary flow.

The clinical progression has three phases: oliguria, diuresis, and recovery of renal function. BUN and plasma creatinine concentrations increase.

The primary goal is to maintain life until renal function returns. Management involves correcting fluid and

261

Causes of Acute Renal Failure

Prerenal	Intrarenal	Postrenal
Hypovolemia	Prolonged renal ischemia	Urethral obstruction
Water and electrolyte losses	Nephrotoxins	Edema, tumors, stones, clots
Hemorrhage	Glomerulopathies	Bladder outlet obstruction
Hypotension	Malignant hypertension	Prostatic hyperplasia, urethral
Septic shock	Coagulation defects	strictures
Cardiac failure		
Pulmonary embolism		
Interruption of renal artery flow		

electrolyte imbalances, treating infections, and providing nutrients. Dialysis is indicated for patients with uncontrollable hyperkalemia, acidosis, or severe fluid overload. Acute renal failure is rapidly progressive within hours, although it may be reversible.

9. **Describe chronic kidney disease; identify the systemic manifestations of uremia.**

Study pages 1389 through 1396; refer to Figure 36-13 and Table 36-12.

Chronic kidney disease symptoms and signs usually do not develop until GFR and renal function decline to 25% of normal. The chronic alteration is primarily because of loss of nephron mass. The disease is associated with hypertension, diabetes mellitus, or intrinsic kidney disease. Two factors, proteinuria and angiotensin II, advance kidney disease. **Proteinuria** contributes to tubulointerstitial injury by accumulating in the interstitial space and activating mediators that promote progressive fibrosis. **Angiotensin II** promotes glomerular hypertension and hyperfiltration caused by efferent arteriolar vasoconstriction, thus systemic hypertension. The **uremic state** is characterized by a decline in renal function and the accumulation of toxins in the blood and associated systems manifestations identified in the following table. If the lesions are tubular, electrolyte imbalances, volume depletions, and metabolic acidosis occur. In glomerular lesions, hematuria and nephrotic syndrome develop.

Uremia Manifestations

Skeletal	Cardiopulmonary	Neurologic	Hematologic
Bone demineralization	Hypertension	Fatigue	Anemia
	Pericarditis	Attention deficit	Bleeding
	Pulmonary edema	Peripheral neuropathy	Infection
		Stupor	Suppressed immunity
		Coma	
Endocrine	**Gastrointestinal**	**Integumentary**	**Reproductive**
Retarded growth in children	Diarrhea	Pruritus	Infertility
Osteomalacia	Nausea	Pigmentation	Decreased libido
Increased goiter	Vomiting		Impotence
	Anorexia		Amenorrhea
	Urinous breath		

NOTE: If chronic renal failure cannot be managed with diet, diuretics, and fluid restriction, then hemofiltration, hemodiafiltration, or transplantation becomes necessary.

Multiple Choice

Circle the correct answer for each question.

1. Renal function tests include:
   a. urinalysis.
   b. BUN and serum creatinine.
   c. SGOT/SGPT.
   d. Both a and b are correct.
2. Which substance is an abnormal constituent of urine?
   a. Urea
   b. Glucose
   c. Sodium chloride
   d. Creatinine
3. The presence of albumin in the urine would indicate probable damage to:
   a. glomeruli.
   b. renal columns.
   c. collecting tubules.
   d. pyramids.
4. Upper urinary tract obstruction:
   a. can cause hydroureter.
   b. increases the force of detrusor contraction.
   c. predisposes an individual to hypotension.
   d. increases postvoid residual volume.
5. Renal calculi may be composed of:
   a. calcium oxalate.
   b. uric acid.
   c. cholesterol.
   d. All of the above are correct.
   e. Both a and b are correct.
6. Which is a characteristic of ureteral stones located in the renal pelvis?
   a. Pain radiating to the lower abdomen
   b. Urgency
   c. Incontinence
   d. Pain radiating to the groin
7. A common cause of both pyelonephritis and cystitis is:
   a. urinary calculi.
   b. invading microorganisms, such as *Escherichia coli*.
   c. allergy reactions.
   d. heavy metals.
8. Uremia exhibits:
   a. polycythemia.
   b. electrolyte disorders.
   c. low plasma calcium levels.
   d. increased erythropoiesis.
9. Which renal condition usually involves a history of recent infection with group A beta-hemolytic streptococci?
   a. Pyelonephritis
   b. Chronic renal failure
   c. Nephrosis
   d. Glomerulonephritis
   e. Calculi
10. The most common pathogenesis of cystitis, an infection, is acquired through/from:
    a. an ascending or exogenous route.
    b. a hematogenous route.
    c. a bladder stone obstruction.
    d. pyelitis.
11. Nephrotic syndrome is associated with _____ to plasma _____.
    a. increased glomerular permeability, urea
    b. decreased glomerular permeability, proteins
    c. decreased glomerular permeability, tubular filtrate
    d. increased glomerular permeability, proteins
12. Causes of acute renal failure include:
    a. cholecystitis.
    b. stones and strictures in kidneys or ureters.
    c. heart failure leading to poor renal perfusion.
    d. Both b and c are correct.
    e. a, b, and c are correct.
13. Hypertension of nephrotic syndrome occurs because:
    a. inflammation of glomeruli stimulates the secretion of renin, which elevates blood pressure.
    b. systemic hypoperfusion stimulates the secretion of renin, which elevates blood pressure.
    c. excessive angiotensin is secreted from the adrenal cortex during kidney disease.
    d. localized hypoperfusion of glomeruli stimulates renin secretion, which elevates blood pressure.
14. Chronic kidney disease:
    a. may result from hypertension.
    b. is usually the result of chronic inflammation of the kidney.
    c. may be treated with dialysis or transplants.
    d. All of the above are correct.
    e. Both a and b are correct.
15. Nephrotoxins such as the antibiotics may be responsible for:
    a. acute tubular necrosis.
    b. acute glomerulonephritis.
    c. pyelonephritis.
    d. cystitis.
16. Uremia, as seen in chronic renal failure, would manifest:
    a. metabolic acidosis.
    b. elevated BUN and creatinine.
    c. cardiovascular disturbances.
    d. All of the above are correct.
17. Hematuria in the absence of proteinuria indicates injury to the:
    a. glomerulus.
    b. renal tubule.
    c. ureter.
    d. renal medulla.

18. In chronic renal failure, tubulointerstitial disease leads to:
    a. sodium retention.
    b. sodium wasting.
    c. no significant changes in sodium levels.
    d. increased phosphate excretion.
19. Frequent small voidings suggest:
    a. CHF.
    b. prostatic hyperplasia.
    c. nephrotic syndrome.
    d. hepatic cirrhosis.
20. Bacterial infection of kidney parenchyma is:
    a. pyelitis.
    b. cystitis.
    c. pyelonephritis.
    d. pyuria.
    e. pyelonephrosis.

21. Which sign describes a patient in acute renal failure?
    a. Elevated serum creatinine
    b. Leukocytosis
    c. Low BUN
    d. Fever
22. Lesions affecting spinal cord segments C2-S1 cause:
    a. loss of detrusor contraction reflex.
    b. denervation of sphincter mechanisms.
    c. inharmonious coordination between detrusor and urethral muscles.
    d. detrusor overactivity and urinary incompetence.

Matching

Match the etiology with the condition.

_____ 23. Epithelial proliferation in capsular space

_____ 24. Hypovolemia

_____ 25. Uremia

a. prerenal failure

b. postrenal failure

c. chronic glomerulonephritis

d. rapidly progressive glomerulonephritis

e. pruritus

CASE STUDY 1

Mr. and Mrs. C. returned from a weekend of downhill skiing to find their 9-year-old son, E.C., eliminating bloody urine. About 6 weeks earlier, they had spent a week skiing during which E.C. had a severe sore throat that was not treated because his teenaged babysitter did not take him to a physician.

E.C. was taken to his pediatrician, where his mother stated, "He has been lethargic and without appetite for the past 10 days and has complained of back pain." His physical examination showed a temperature of 101° F and a blood pressure of 140/102 mmHg. The remainder of the physical was noncontributory. E.C.'s urinalysis showed blood, protein, and red blood cell casts with an elevated specific gravity. BUN, serum creatinine, and ASO titer levels were elevated.

Questions

What do you think is the likely cause of E.C.'s symptoms and signs?

What do you think the pediatrician will do?

CASE STUDY 2

Ms. J. is a 26-year-old woman married for 3 years who has just returned from an outdoor camping trip with her husband. with symptoms of dysuria with a burning sensation, urgency to urinate, and frequent urination. She said, "I have had similar symptoms three times over the last 2 years. Pubic and low back discomfort awoke me two nights ago and that is why I am here." On physical examination, her temperature was 98.6° F, blood pressure was 114/64 mm Hg, pulse was 68 beats per minute, and the respiratory rate was 12 breaths per minute. Other than a tender abdominal pelvic area, the examination was unremarkable.

Questions

Without any laboratory values now available, what are the possible diagnoses?

Given the following laboratory results, what is her final diagnosis and treatment?
Notable laboratory results from a dipstick urinalysis, microscopic examination, and urine culture:
Color was dark yellow; trace blood; no casts; bacteria, especially E. coli, and WBCs were too numerous to count.

37 Alterations of Renal and Urinary Tract Function in Children

FOUNDATIONAL KNOWLEDGE OJECTIVES

a. Briefly describe the embryologic development of the renal system, urinary tract, urine formation, and excretion in children.
Review text pages 1402 through 1404; refer to Figure 37-1 and Table 37-1.

MEMORY CHECK!

- The Wilms tumor I gene plays an important role at all stages of kidney development and maintenance. The kidneys develop from three distinct tissues: the pronephros, the mesonephros, and the metanephros. The tissue is present by the third week of gestation, and excretory function is evident by 6 weeks' gestation. The metanephros, the permanent kidney, develops from two structures: the ureteric bud and the metanephrogenic blastema. The bud subdivides to form the ureter, the renal pelvis, the calyces, and the collecting ducts. The blastema develops into primitive glomeruli and uriniferous tubules. After the primitive glomeruli and uriniferous tubules develop from the metanephrogenic tissue on the top of the collecting ducts, they continue to develop into the ninth month. The other structures of the urinary tract form as the kidneys mature. The cloaca becomes the urogenital sinus and follows a differentiation process that develops into the bladder and the urethra. Urine formation and excretion begin by the third month of gestation and contribute to the amniotic fluid. If at any point during this process an injury or insult occurs to the embryo, congenital anomalies may result that will have a major impact on the structure and function of the system. All of the nephrons are present at birth, and their number does not increase as the kidney grows and matures. Maturation of the tubular system increases the size and weight of the kidney 10-fold from birth.
- Immediately at birth, the renal blood flow and glomerular filtration rate (GFR) increase due to a decrease in vascular resistance and required excretory functions no longer performed by the placenta. The resistance progressively declines during the first year of development, and an increasing fraction of the cardiac output goes to the kidney. The GFR continues to increase but remains at 30% to 50% of adult levels until the end of the first year.

b. Describe fluid and electrolyte balance in children; explain the implications of imbalances of either.
Review text page 1404.

MEMORY CHECK!

- Infants and young children have a larger ratio of body water to body weight than do adults; a large proportion of this water is in the extracellular compartment. Children exchange half of their extracellular water each day. Factors that influence water movement are those that affect osmolality.
- The infant has limited ability to concentrate urine because of decreased renal blood flow, high renal vascular resistance, shorter tubular length, and a limited amount of urea available in the loop of Henle. There also is a lower threshold for bicarbonate reabsorption and limited acid excretion; this increases the child's risk for developing metabolic acidosis. Fluid and electrolyte balance is very sensitive to the slightest changes in any of these factors. Imbalance may occur rapidly and can precipitate life-threatening crises in infants.

After studying this chapter, the learner will be able to do the following:

1. **Describe the common congenital anomalies that occur within the renal and urologic systems.**

   Study text pages 1404 through 1407; refer to Figures 37-2 through 37-4.

   Structural defects range from minor, easily correctable anomalies to those that are incompatible with life. **Horseshoe kidney** is a single U-shaped kidney that develops from fusion of the kidneys as they descend from the midline. The kidney may be asymptomatic or associated with hydronephrosis, stone formation, or infection. **Hypospadias,** with or without chordae and its band of fibrous tissue that deviates or bows the penis ventrally, and **epispadias** result in the placement of the urethral meatus on the dorsal surface of the penis. Hypospadias with the urethral meatus opening ventrally on the penis is the more common penile defect, and it is usually easily corrected with surgery. Epispadias is a more complex problem because it can extend into the bladder. It has a lower incidence in girls than in boys. The urethral meatus is located ventrally in females and often has an accompanying cleft. This can also be surgically corrected, but it requires a more involved intervention.

   Exstrophy of the bladder is a defect wherein the bladder and associated urinary tract structures are exposed to the surface of the body; this defect involves the abdominal wall and the pubic bone. This defect allows urine to leak from the ureters and onto the abdominal wall, which leads to excoriation of the skin and the persistent odor of urine. The exposed bladder mucosa becomes edematous, bleeds easily, and is painful. Surgical repair requires several stages, with the first occurring during the first few days of life. Neoplastic changes have been associated with exstrophy of the bladder.

   Ureteropelvic junction obstruction is blockage where the renal pelvic joins the ureter and is often caused by smooth muscle or urothelial malformation or scarring leading to hydronephrosis. Treatment is surgical pyeloplasty or endopyelotomy.

   Bladder outlet obstruction is usually caused by urethral valves or polyps. They often cause obstructions that can impair renal function via reflux and tract infection. Resection using a small cystoscope is ideally done during the first days of life.

   A **dysplastic kidney** results from abnormal differentiation of renal tissues. The kidney is very small but functional.

   Renal agenesis is failure of growth and development. It may be unilateral or bilateral and occur in association with other disorders.

   Polycystic kidney disease is an autosomal dominant disorder. In this disorder, the renal tubule or epithelium proliferates with excessive fluid transport causing cysts and obstruction.

2. **Note glomerular disorders in children; describe the pathophysiology and clinical manifestations of immunoglobulin A nephropathy and hemolytic uremic syndrome and their treatment.**

   Study pages 1407 through 1411; refer to Figure 37-5 and Tables 37-2 and 37-3.

   It is notable that nephrotic syndrome and glomerulonephritis in children express pathophysiologic mechanisms similar to those observed in adults.

   Immunoglobulin A (IgA) nephropathy is the most common form of glomerulonephritis worldwide. It is characterized by deposition mainly of the IgA in glomerular capillaries and mesangium. No systemic immunologic disease is evident. Deposits of IgA cause immune injury to the glomerulus that is usually reversible.

   Children with the disease have recurrent gross hematuria, often after a respiratory infection. Most continue to have microscopic hematuria between the attacks of gross hematuria and have a mild proteinuria as well. Treatment is supportive because kidney damage is generally insignificant. Approximately 20% of affected children develop the progressive form of the disease with hypertension and decreasing renal function. These children eventually require dialysis and transplantation.

   Hemolytic uremic syndrome is associated with a viral or bacterial illness and is preceded 1 or 2 weeks by an upper respiratory or gastrointestinal infection. The antecedent infection causes endothelial injury to the glomerular arterioles. This event triggers the inflammatory cascade, resulting in platelet aggregation and fibrin clot formation that narrows the arterioles. Anemia results when erythrocytes and platelets are damaged while passing through narrowed and inflamed glomerular arterioles and are later removed by the spleen. This same thrombocyte and fibrin clot mechanism activates the fibrinolytic cascade that prompts the release of damaged platelets from the arterioles. These damaged platelets are also removed by the spleen. Thrombocytosis eventually results.

   Classic symptoms of hemolytic uremic syndrome are pallor, bruising or purpura, and oliguria that may be accompanied by fever, vomiting, bloody diarrhea, abdominal pain, and jaundice. Central nervous system involvement, seizures, and lethargy may be features of severe disease.

   Treatment is supportive to maintain nutrition and fluid and electrolyte balance and to control hypertension and seizures. Therapy includes transfusions of red blood cells and platelets to treat the anemia and thrombocytopenia. Peritoneal dialysis may be required to regulate fluids and electrolytes.

3. **Describe childhood urinary tract infections.**

   Study text pages 1411 and 1412.

   Urinary tract infections (UTIs) can result from general sepsis in the newborn but are caused by bacteria ascending the urethra in older children. When the bladder is infected, it is **cystitis,** causing detrusor hyperactivity and a decrease in bladder capacity. If the infection ascends into the kidneys, it is **pyelonephritis.** Infants and young children, with either infection, may present with fever of undetermined origin, and others may present with frequent or urgent urination; enuresis, or incontinence; abdominal, flank, or back pain; foul-smelling urine; and sometimes hematuria may be present. Urinary tract infections must be treated with antibiotics. Urinary tract anomalies must be surgically corrected to prevent recurrent infections.

4. **Identify the structural cause of vesicoureteral reflux, and explain the potential effects on renal function.**

Study pages 1412 and 1413; refer to Figures 37-6 and 37-7.

Primary vesicoureteral reflux is caused by the congenital malpositioning of a ureter or ureters into the bladder that allows urine to retrograde up the ureters. If the urine contains microorganisms and can reach the renal parenchyma, chronic infections and scarring may result. This reflux of urine returns to the bladder after the child voids; the incomplete emptying of the bladder predisposes the child to infection. This condition is classified by a grading system, with grade I being the most mild and grade V (which requires surgery) being the most severe.

Secondary vesicoureteral reflux occurs because an infection causes mucosal edema and interferes with the antireflux mechanisms of the urinary tract. Antireflux mechanisms are somewhat immature at birth and become efficient as the urinary tract matures.

Symptoms associated with vesicoureteral reflux include fever, recurrent urinary tract infections, and poor feeding. Diagnosis is confirmed by a radiologic procedure that allows for the visualization of reflux during voiding. Treatment goals are to prevent infection and to protect and preserve renal function. Recurrent infection is an indication for surgical repair.

5. **Characterize Wilms tumor.**

Study pages 1413 and 1414; refer to Tables 37-5 and 37-6.

Wilms tumor, also called nephroblastoma, is an embryonic tumor with cellular components that are stromal, epithelial, and blastemal. The peak age of diagnosis is 2 to 3 years of age, with an incidence of approximately 500 cases diagnosed yearly in the United States. Wilms tumor may occur as a sporadic phenomenon, or it may be inherited. The tumor is smooth, firm, and usually encapsulated and separated from the renal parenchyma. Wilms tumor has both sporadic and inherited forms. The inherited form is an autosomal dominant disorder, but it is rare. The occurrence has been found to be caused by the deletion or inactivation of genes on various chromosome, notably, the Wilms tumor-suppressor gene *(WTI).* Other congenital genitourinary anomalies have been associated with Wilms tumor in 10% of children having the tumor.

Children may be asymptomatic or may present with vague abdominal pain, hematuria, fever, or hypertension. Diagnosis is made by locating the tumor and assessing its site by radiologic procedures such as ultrasound, computed tomography (CT) scan, or magnetic resonance imaging (MRI).

Treatment is surgical excision with a heminephrectomy of the less involved kidney or total nephrectomy of the other. Depending on the stage of the tumor, chemotherapy, radiation therapy, or both may be required. Prognosis is affected by tumor weight and histologic category, the age of the child, and the extent of lymph node involvement. The survival rate of Wilms tumor is approximately 95% for those with a histologically favorable tumor, stages I through III.

6. **Define primary and secondary enuresis; discuss likely causes and common approaches to the management.**

Study pages 1414 and 1415; refer to Table 37-7.

Enuresis can be classified into two categories: primary and secondary. **Primary enuresis** occurs when a child has never obtained continence; **secondary enuresis** occurs when a child has had and then loses bladder control. Secondary enuresis is also called acquired enuresis.

The origin of enuresis may be neurologic, anatomic, or functional. Psychologic problems have been related to enuresis in some cases, and they must be considered a legitimate cause in the absence of organic findings. All efforts are initially focused on identifying an organic, underlying problem such as urinary tract infection, a congenital defect of the urinary tract, or neurologic dysfunction. Linkages have been proposed between nocturnal enuresis and chromosomes 8, 12, 13, and 22, indicating the presence of genetic factors. The disorder tends to occur during non–rapid eye movement sleep or greater depths of sleep. The child who exhibits smaller functional bladder capacity or experiences episodes of enuresis during deep sleep will most likely outgrow the problem.

Management depends on cause and may include a combination of interventions such as medication, limited fluid intake, behavior modification, alarms, or periodic awakenings during sleep. Psychologic counseling also may benefit the child and family.

PRACTICE EXAMINATION

Fill in the Blanks

Supply the correct response for each statement.

1. Urine formation and excretion begin by the _____ month of gestation.

2. Genetically, the _____ plays an important role at all stages of kidney development.

3. During the first year of life, infant's GFR is about _____ of adult levels.

4. The primitive glomeruli and uriniferous tubules develop from the _____.

5. An infant has a lower threshold for bicarbonate reabsorption and limited acid excretion, this increases the risk for developing _____.

6. When a child has had and then loses bladder control, it is known as _____.

269

7. A _____ kidney is a small but normal functioning organ.

8. _____ is blockage where the renal pelvis joins the ureter.

9. _____ exhibits a urethral meatus on the ventral surface of the penis.

10. Urine seepage onto the abdominal wall from the ureter can be observed in _____.

11. Polycystic kidney disease is an autosomal _____ disorder.

12. Bilateral renal agenesis is usually _____.

13. Congenital malpositioning of a ureter or ureters into the bladder causes _____.

14. _____ is responsible for most school-age children who require dialysis and kidney transplantation.

15. Common childhood glomerular diseases include glomerulonephritis, hemolytic uremic syndrome, and _____.

Multiple Choice
Circle the correct answer for each question.

16. Poststreptococcal glomerulonephritis in children:
    a. is a postinfectious renal disease.
    b. causes hypotension.
    c. causes dehydration.
    d. Both b and c are correct.

17. Infants *cannot* concentrate urine because of:
    a. shorter tubular length.
    b. increased tubular weight.
    c. increased blood flow to the kidneys.
    d. Both a and c are correct.
    e. a, b, and c are correct.

18. Vesicoureteral reflux causes urine to _____ up the ureters and places the young child at risk for _____.
    a. retrograde, glomerulonephritis
    b. regrade, nephrotic syndrome
    c. retrograde, pyelonephritis
    d. regrade, cystitis

19. IgA nephropathy:
    a. occurs in the presence of other systemic immunologic disease.
    b. has no other immunoglobulin present.
    c. damages the glomerulus irreversibly.
    d. manifests as recurrent gross hematuria.

20. Organic causes of enuresis may include:
    a. congenital abnormalities of the urinary tract.
    b. a neurologic origin.
    c. diabetes insipidus.
    d. All of the above are correct.

21. Which clinical manifestation suggests hemolytic uremic syndrome?
    a. polyuria
    b. pallor and bruising
    c. hypotension.
    d. All of the above are correct.

22. Childhood urinary tract infection results from:
    a. bacteria ascending up the ureter in cystitis.
    b. bacteria ascending up the urethra in pyelonephritis.
    c. detrusor muscle hypoactivity.
    d. a pathogenic strain of *E. coli*.

23. Wilms tumor is characterized by:
    a. hypotension.
    b. diagnosis in the early teens.
    c. loss or inactivation of both copies of the Wilms tumor-suppressor gene.
    d. transmission in an autosomal recessive fashion for inherited cases.

24. Alphabetize the sequence of events in hemolytic uremic syndrome that cause anemia.
    a. The damaged cells are removed from the circulation by the spleen.
    b. The endothelial lining of the glomerular arterioles becomes swollen.
    c. Narrowed vessels damage erythrocytes.

25. Childhood nephrotic syndrome is characterized by:
    a. having a peak incidence during the teen years.
    b. increased glomerular permeability to protein.
    c. hypolipidemia.
    d. injured renal interstitial tissue.

A 3-year-old girl is brought to the emergency department of a local hospital because she has bloody stools. The parents complain that "her eyes are puffy and she looks very pale." Her parents reveal a history of gastrointestinal illness 2 weeks ago after a weekend of camping. The girl has been well since the illness until yesterday, when the bloody stools began. At that time, they noticed how pale she was, and they believe that she has not voided at all today. Her assessment reveals pallor and bruising. A urine collection bag was placed on the child; however, she never voided while in the emergency department. A complete blood count revealed low hemoglobin, hematocrit, and platelets. Serum levels showed that Na^+ and K^+ were elevated and that albumin and protein were low; pH was 7.30.

Questions

From the laboratory values, what diagnosis is likely?

What treatment will this child require?

38 Structure and Function of the Digestive System

PREREQUISITE KNOWLEDGE OBJECTIVES

After reviewing the primary text where referenced, the learner will be able to do the following:

1. **List sequentially the parts of the alimentary canal from the mouth to the anus.**
   Refer to Figure 38-1.
2. **Describe the structural layers of the gastrointestinal tract.**
   Review text page 1421; refer to Figure 38-2.
3. **Describe the mouth and esophagus, and note specific structural functions.**
   Review text pages 1421 through 1423; refer to Figures 38-3 and 38-4.
4. **Describe the stomach, and note specific structural function.**
   Review text pages 1423 through 1428; refer to Figures 38-5 through 38-9 and 38-11 and Table 38-1.
5. **Describe the small intestine, and note specific function and secretions.**
   Review text pages 1428 through 1430 and 1432 through 1435; refer to Figures 38-10 through 38-15 and Table 38-2.
6. **Describe the structure and function of the large intestine, and identify normal intestinal flora and their activities.**
   Review text pages 1435 through 1437; refer to Figure 38-16.
7. **Describe the structure and function of the liver and gallbladder.**
   Review text pages 1437 through 1442; refer to Figures 38-17 through 38-23 and Table 38-3.
8. **Explain the relationships between pancreatic cell types and their functions.**
   Review text pages 1443 and 1444; refer to Figure 38-23.
9. **Identify tests of digestive function.**
   Review text pages 1444, 1446, and 1447; refer to Tables 38-4 through 38-8.
10. **Describe the alterations in the digestive system that are associated with normal aging.**
    Review text pages 1447 and 1448.

PRACTICE EXAMINATION

Multiple Choice

Circle the correct answer for each question.

1. The muscularis of the gastrointestinal tract is:
   a. skeletal muscle throughout the tract, particularly in the esophagus and large intestine.
   b. the layer that contains the blood capillaries for the entire wall of the tract.
   c. composed principally of keratinized epithelium.
   d. composed of circular fibers and longitudinal fibers.
2. The digestive functions performed by the saliva and salivary amylase, respectively, are:
   a. moistening and protein digestion.
   b. deglutition and fat digestion.
   c. peristalsis and polysaccharide digestion.
   d. lubrication and carbohydrate digestion.
3. The nervous pathway involved in salivary secretion requires the stimulation of:
   a. receptors in the taste buds, impulses to the motor cortex, and somatic motor impulses to salivary glands.
   b. receptors in the mouth, sensory impulses to a center in the brainstem, and parasympathetic impulses to salivary glands.
   c. taste receptors, sensory impulses to centers in the brainstem, and somatic motor impulses to salivary glands.
   d. pressoreceptors in blood vessels, motor impulses, and autonomic impulses to salivary glands.
4. Food would pass rapidly from the stomach into the duodenum if it were *not* for the:
   a. fundus.
   b. epiglottis.
   c. rugae.
   d. cardiac sphincter.
   e. pyloric sphincter.
5. The secretion of gastric juice:
   a. occurs only when the stomach comes in contact with swallowed food.
   b. is entirely under the control of the hormone gastrin.
   c. is entirely under the control of the hormone enterogastrone.
   d. is stimulated by the presence of saliva in the stomach.
   e. occurs in three phases: cephalic, gastric, and intestinal.

273

6. During nervous control of gastric secretion, the gastric glands secrete before food enters the stomach. This stimulus to the glands comes from:
   a. gastrin.
   b. impulses over somatic nerves from the hypothalamus.
   c. motor impulses from the cerebral cortex and cerebellum.
   d. parasympathetic impulses over the vagus nerve.
7. Pepsinogen:
   a. must be activated by HCl.
   b. is secreted by the chief cells.
   c. is important in the breakdown of proteins.
   d. All of the above are correct.
8. Beginning at the lumen, the sequence of layers of the gastrointestinal tract is:
   a. mucosa, submucosa, muscularis, serosa.
   b. submucosa, mucosa, serous membrane, muscularis.
   c. submucosa, mucosa, muscularis, skeletal muscle.
   d. serous membranes, muscularis, mucosa, submucosa.
9. Normally, when chyme leaves the stomach:
   a. the nutrients are ready for absorption into the blood.
   b. the amount of inorganic salts has been increased by the action of hydrochloric acid.
   c. its pH is neutral.
   d. the proteins have been partly digested.
   e. All of the above are correct.
10. Which layer of the small intestine includes microvilli?
    a. submucosa
    b. mucosa
    c. muscularis
    d. serosa
11. Which of the following is *not* an example of mechanical digestion?
    a. Chewing
    b. Churning and mixing of food in the stomach
    c. Peristalsis and mastication
    d. Conversion of protein molecules into amino acids
12. Pancreatic juice is to trypsin as gastric juice is to:
    a. salivary amylase.
    b. pepsin.
    c. mucin.
    d. intrinsic factor.
13. Which part of the small intestine is most distal from the pylorus?
    a. Jejunum
    b. Pyloric sphincter
    c. Duodenum
    d. Cardiac sphincter
    e. Common bile duct
14. The pancreas:
    a. lies mostly on the left side of the abdominal cavity, anterior to the stomach and the spleen.
    b. secretes all of its products directly into the bloodstream.
    c. is a slender, flattened gland with its duct ultimately opening into the duodenum.
    d. contains cells with endocrine function for the determination of secondary sex characteristics.
    e. is classified as a digestive exocrine gland that does not have endocrine functions.
15. The chief role played by the pancreas in digestion is to:
    a. secrete insulin and glucagon.
    b. churn the food and bring it into contact with digestive enzymes.
    c. secrete enzymes that digest food in the small intestine.
    d. assist in absorbing the digested food.
16. Among the structural features of the small intestine are villi, microvilli, and circular folds. Their function is to:
    a. liberate hormones.
    b. promote peristalsis.
    c. liberate digestive enzymes.
    d. increase the surface area for absorption.
17. The fate of carbohydrates in the small intestine is:
    a. digestion by amylase, sucrase, maltase, and lactase to monosaccharide.
    b. conversion to simple sugars by the activity of trypsin and lipase.
    c. hydrolysis to amino acids by the activity of amylase, sucrase, maltase, and lactase.
    d. conversion to glycerol and fatty acids by the activity of lipase and amylase.
18. The absorptive fate of the end products of digestion may be summarized as:
    a. most fatty acids are absorbed into the blood; glucose and amino acids are absorbed into the lymphatic system.
    b. amino acids and monosaccharides are absorbed into blood capillaries; most fatty acids are absorbed into lymph.
    c. amino acids and fatty acids are absorbed into the lymph capillaries; glycerol and glucose are absorbed into the blood capillaries.
    d. fatty acids are absorbed into blood capillaries; glycerol, glucose, and amino acids are absorbed into lymph.

19. A lobule of the liver contains a centrally located:
    a. vein, with radiating hepatocytes and sinusoids.
    b. arteriole, with radiating capillaries and Kupffer's cells.
    c. hepatic sinus, with radiating sinusoids.
    d. hepatic duct, with radiating Kupffer's cells and cords of hepatic cells.
20. An obstruction of the common bile duct would cause the blockage of bile coming from:
    a. the gallbladder.
    b. the liver but not the gallbladder.
    c. both the liver and the gallbladder.
    d. the pancreatic duct but not the gallbladder.
21. The human adult liver does *not:*
    a. store glycogen.
    b. produce erythrocytes.
    c. convert ammonia to urea.
    d. produce blood coagulation proteins.
22. The chyme that enters the large intestine is converted to feces by activity of:
    a. specific mucosal enzymes.
    b. gastric and duodenal hormones.
    c. bacteria and water reabsorption.
    d. the microvilli, villi, and circular muscles.

Fill in the Blanks

Supply the correct response for each statement.

23. The pyloric gland mucosa in the stomach antrum synthesizes and releases the hormone _____ from G cells.

24. Total serum bilirubin is normally less than _____.

25. Aging is associated with a greater frequency of ____ infection.

275

39 Alterations of Digestive Function

FOUNDATIONAL KNOWLEDGE OBJECTIVES

a. Describe the structure and function of the gastrointestinal tract and accessory organs of digestion.
Review summary; review pages 1448 and 1449; refer to Figure 38-1.

MEMORY CHECK!

- The gastrointestinal system includes the oral structures (mouth, salivary glands, pharynx), the alimentary tract (esophagus, stomach, small intestine, large intestine, appendix, anus), and the accessory organs of digestion (liver, gallbladder, bile ducts, pancreas). The function of the alimentary tract is to digest masticated food, to absorb digestive products, and to excrete the digestive residue and certain waste products excreted by the liver through the bile duct.
- The esophagus is a straight tube that carries food from the pharynx to the stomach. The stomach is a distensible organ. The stomach's mucosal cells secrete hydrochloric acid and proteolytic enzymes that aid in digestion. The mucosa of the lower part of the stomach is lined by mucous cells. The distal end of the stomach is called the pylorus. The small intestine is divided into the duodenum, jejunum, and ileum. The large intestine or colon consists of the cecum, ascending colon, transverse colon, descending colon, sigmoid colon, and rectum. The vermiform appendix is a nonfunctional vestigial structure attached to the cecum. The colon is a storage reservoir for undigested food and a site for water absorption.
- The alimentary tract has four layers: mucosa, submucosa, muscularis, and serosa. The mucosal layer consists of epithelial cells lining the lumen's surface, supporting connective tissue called the lamina propria, and a unique thin, muscular layer called the muscularis mucosae. The structure of inner mucosal layer varies to provide specialized function at each part of the tract. The esophagus is lined by stratified squamous epithelium, which enables rapid gliding of masticated food from the mouth to the stomach. The stomach has a thick glandular mucosa that provides mucus, acid, and proteolytic enzymes to help digest food. The small intestinal mucosa has a villous structure to provide a large surface of cells for active absorption. The large intestinal mucosa is lined by abundant mucus-secreting cells that facilitate storage and evacuation of the residue. Beneath the mucosa is the submucosa, which gives structural support to the tract because of its abundant collagenous tissue. The muscle layer contracts rhythmically to move materials through the alimentary tract. The serosal layer is a thin, smooth membrane present on the outer surface of the alimentary tract. It keeps the tortuous loops of bowel from becoming tangled and is continuous with the mesentery. The mesentery is a connective tissue attachment of the bowel to the abdominal wall; it contains blood vessels, lymphatics, and nerves.
- A wave of muscle contraction carries a bolus of swallowed food down the esophagus where a sphincter at the lower end of the esophagus prevents regurgitation. Contractions in the stomach mix the food and push the partially digested contents into the duodenum. The muscle of the pylorus only partially closes the outlet to the stomach so intestinal contents can regurgitate into the stomach if the small intestine is not emptying properly. Normally, movement of luminal contents in the small intestine is more rapid in the upper small intestine and slows as chyme moves distally. Contents pass from the ileum into the colon where reverse proximal movement is partially prevented by the ileocecal valve. Water is absorbed in the colon and the contents become solid; the solid residue is moved to the left side of the colon and rectum. When the rectum becomes distended, an urge for defecation develops.
- The liver and the pancreas are glandular organs with excretory ducts emptying into the duodenum at a site called the ampulla of Vater. The excretory ducts of the liver are called bile ducts. The gallbladder is a storage reservoir connected to the bile ducts by the cystic duct.
- Most of the blood from the abdominal organs is carried to the liver via the portal veins. Therefore, blood is filtered by the glandular cells of the liver before it returns to the heart via the hepatic vein and vena cava. Because portal blood has little oxygen left after passing through the abdominal organs, the liver has the hepatic artery to provide oxygenated blood. The bulk of the liver is composed of hepatocytes that are aligned in cords with sinusoids between the cords to diffuse the blood

Continued

from the portal areas to the central vein. Between adjacent hepatocytes are tiny canaliculi that carry bile produced by the hepatocytes to the portal area where they empty into epithelial-lined bile ducts. In the sinusoids, waste products and nutrients are removed and metabolized by the hepatocytes. The metabolites may be returned to the blood, stored in the hepatocytes, or excreted into bile canaliculi. The liver also contains many mononuclear cells or Kupffer's cells that line the sinusoids. They phagocytize particulate material from the blood. Metabolically, the liver (1) produces bile salts, (2) excretes bilirubin, (3) metabolizes nitrogenous substances, (4) produces serum proteins, and (5) detoxifies drugs and poisons.

- The gallbladder is a distention of the common bile duct that becomes a storage reservoir for bile. The gallbladder empties its contents into the duodenum after meals when bile salts are needed for fat absorption. This reservoir function is not essential, as the gallbladder can be removed without loss of digestive function.

- The pancreas is a long, narrow glandular organ lying horizontally and retroperitoneally in the midabdomen region. The bulk of the pancreas is made up of glands that secrete digestive enzymes into the pancreatic duct. When activated by intestinal juices, these enzymes digest carbohydrate, fat, and protein. Pancreatic enzymes are essential for life. Scattered among the pancreatic glands are clusters of endocrine cells known as the islets of Langerhans, which produce insulin and other hormones.

- The digestive process begins in the mouth, where carbohydrate-splitting enzymes or amylases from the salivary glands mix with food during mastication. In the stomach, proteolytic pepsin and hydrochloric acid are added to the digesting mixture of food in the duodenum. These include amylases, proteolytic trypsin, and fat-splitting enzymes or lipases. In addition, bile salts secreted by the liver and stored in the gallbladder are added to emulsify lipids into small water-soluble micelles. The final phase of the digestive process occurs at the surface of small intestinal epithelial cells. Here, carbohydrate-splitting disaccharidases and protein-splitting dipeptidases continue the process. Complex endocrine and nervous mechanisms coordinate the timing of the secretion of digestive enzymes, hydrochloric acid, and bile salts. The sight of food may cause salivation and gastric secretions because of nervous stimulation. Distention of the stomach causes release of gastrin, which stimulates acid production and gastric emptying. Movement of food into the duodenum causes the pancreas to secrete more fluid and enzymes and the gallbladder to release bile. The products of both enter the duodenum.

b. **Describe tests used to evaluate the structure and function of the digestive system.**
   Refer to Tables 38-4 through 38-8.

- The structure and function of the gastrointestinal tract can be assessed by x-ray films using contrast media such as barium- or iodine-containing compounds to outline the gastrointestinal lumen, biliary tree and pancreatic ducts, fistulas, and arteriovenous systems. CT scanning is used for diagnosis of pancreatic or hepatic tumors or cysts. Ultrasonic scanning can detect liver-related jaundice and intra-abdominal masses. Fiberoptic endoscopy with flexible endoscopes permits direct visualization of the upper and lower gastrointestinal tract; a biopsy channel in the endoscope allows tissue sampling. Suction can be used to remove gastrointestinal secretions or blood to assess infection, malabsorption syndromes, ulcerative lesions, and tumor growth.

- Imaging techniques similar to those used for the gastrointestinal tract also are useful to evaluate liver structure and function. Serum enzymes are elevated in many liver diseases; aminotransferase and lactate dehydrogenase are released into the circulation when there is damage to hepatocytes. Obstruction of bile canaliculi or ducts causes regurgitation of bile back into the hepatic sinusoids and into the circulation, which elevates bilirubin levels. Blood coagulation times are often prolonged with both hepatitis and chronic liver disease. Serum albumin and globulins may be lowered because of hepatocyte damage. Liver biopsies may be performed to evaluate the extent of liver involvement or degeneration in either cirrhosis or hepatitis.

- Evaluation of structural alterations in the gallbladder uses imaging techniques. Both conjugated and total serum bilirubin values are elevated, urine urobilinogen is increased, stools are clay-colored, and jaundice develops if bile flow to the gastrointestinal tract is obstructed. During inflammation of the gallbladder, the white cell count is elevated. Inflammation or obstruction of the pancreas results in an increase in serum amylase levels. Increased stool fat indicates pancreatic insufficiency because of decreased lipase secretion.

LEARNING OBJECTIVES

After studying this chapter, the learner will be able to do the following:

1. **Describe the common terms used in identifying the signs and symptoms of gastrointestinal dysfunction.**
   Study text pages 1452 through 1456; refer to Figure 39-1 and Table 39-1.

   Anorexia is the absence of a desire to eat despite physiologic stimuli that would normally produce hunger. Anorexia is a nonspecific symptom often associated with nausea, abdominal pain, and diarrhea. Disorders of other systems besides the digestive system are accompanied by anorexia. These include cancer, heart disease, and renal disease.

   Vomiting is the forceful emptying of stomach and intestinal contents or chyme through the mouth. The vomiting reflex is stimulated by presence of ipecac or copper salts in the duodenum, severe pain, or distention of the stomach or duodenum. Torsion or trauma affecting the ovaries, testes, uterus, bladder, or kidney also elicits vomiting.

   Nausea and retching usually precede vomiting. Nausea is a subjective experience associated with many different conditions. **Retching** is a strong, involuntary effort to vomit. In retching, the lower esophageal sphincter and body of the stomach relax but the duodenum and antrum of the stomach go into spasm. The reverse peristalsis forces chyme from the stomach and duodenum up into the esophagus. Because the upper esophageal sphincter is closed, chyme does not enter the mouth. As the abdominal muscles relax, the contents of the esophagus drop back into the stomach. This process may be repeated several times before vomiting occurs.

   Vomiting occurs when the stomach is full of gastric contents and the diaphragm is forced high into the thoracic cavity by strong abdominal muscle contractions. The higher intrathoracic pressure forces the upper esophageal sphincter to open and chyme is discharged from the mouth. Spontaneous vomiting not preceded by nausea or retching is called **projectile vomiting**. This vomiting is caused by direct stimulation of the vomiting center because of neurologic lesions involving the brainstem. The metabolic consequences of vomiting are fluid, electrolyte, and acid-base disturbances.

   Constipation is difficult or infrequent defecation involving decreased numbers of bowel movements per week, hard stools, and difficult evacuation. Constipation is frequently caused by unhealthy dietary and bowel habits combined with inadequate exercise. It also can occur as a result of intestinal immobility or obstructive disorders. Constipation resulting from lifestyle or bowel habits usually has a long duration. Dysfunctional constipation is more likely to be sudden and can accompany the development of organic lesions.

   Diarrhea is increased frequency of defecation accompanied by changes in fecal fluidity and volume. In osmotic diarrhea, the presence of nonabsorbable substances in the intestine causes water to be drawn into the lumen by osmosis. Lactose deficiency is the most common cause of osmotic diarrhea. The excess water and the nonabsorbable substances increase stool weight and volume. This causes **large-volume diarrhea.**

   Secretory diarrhea is a form of large-volume diarrhea caused by excessive mucosal secretion of fluid and electrolytes. Excessive intestinal secretion is caused mostly by bacterial enterotoxins released by cholera or strains of *Escherichia coli*. Gastrinoma or thyroid carcinoma produces hormones that may stimulate intestinal secretion. A lesion that impairs autonomic control of motility such as diabetic neuropathy can cause large-volume diarrhea.

   Excessive motility decreases transit time, mucosal surface contact, and opportunities for fluid absorption. **Motility diarrhea** can be caused by resection of the small intestine, surgical bypass of an area of the intestine, or fistula formation between loops of the intestine.

   Small-volume diarrhea is usually caused by inflammatory disorders of the intestine or by fecal impaction from severe constipation. In the latter case, the diarrhea consists of mucus and fluid produced by the colon to lubricate the impacted feces and move it toward the anal canal.

   Abdominal pain is observed in a number of gastrointestinal diseases. Abdominal organs are sensitive to stretching and distention, which can activate nerve endings in both hollow and solid structures. Histamine, bradykinin, and serotonin, when released during inflammation, stimulate organic nerve endings and produce abdominal pain. The edema and vascular congestion that accompany inflammation also cause painful stretching. Any obstruction of blood flow because of distention of bowel obstruction or mesenteric vessel thrombosis produces ischemic pain. **Parietal pain** arises from the parietal peritoneum and is more localized and intense than **visceral pain,** which arises from the organs themselves.

   Referred pain is visceral pain felt at some distance from a diseased or affected organ. Referred pain is usually well localized and is felt in the skin or deeper tissues that share a central, common afferent pathway with the affected organ.

   Numerous disorders cause gastrointestinal tract bleeding. Acute **gastrointestinal bleeding** is usually characterized by **hematemesis** or the presence of blood in the vomitus; **hematochezia** or frank bleeding from the rectum or **melena**, which is dark, tarry stools. **Occult bleeding** is slow, chronic blood loss that results in iron-deficiency anemia as iron stores in the bone marrow are slowly depleted.

2. **Compare and contrast the various disorders of digestive motility.**
   Study text pages 1456 through 1463; refer to Figures 39-2 through 39-5 and Tables 39-2 through 39-4. See the table on page 280.

3. **Describe the pathogenesis of acute and chronic gastritis.**
   Study text pages 1463 through 1464; refer to Figure 39-6.

   Gastritis is an inflammatory disorder of the gastric mucosa that may be acute or chronic and that affects the fundus or antrum or both. Aspirin and other antiinflammatory drugs are known to cause **acute gastritis**, which erodes the epithelium, probably because they inhibit prostaglandins that normally stimulate the secretion of protective mucus. Alcohol, histamine,

279

Motility Disorders

Disorder	Causes	Manifestations
Dysphagia (swallowing difficulty)	Esophageal obstruction 　Tumors, strictured, or diverticula Impaired esophageal motility 　Neural dysfunction, muscular disease, CVA Achalasia (decreased ganglion cells in myenteric plexus, muscle cell atrophy)	Distention and spasm of esophagus after swallowing, regurgitation of undigested food
Gastroesophageal reflux (chyme reflux into esophagus)	Increased abdominal pressure, ulcers, pyloric edema and strictures, hiatal hernia	Regurgitation of chyme within 1 hour of eating
Hiatal hernia (protrusion upper stomach through diaphragm into thorax); two types*	Congenitally short esophagus, trauma, weak diaphragmatic muscles at gastroesophageal junction, increased abdominal pressure	Gastroesophageal reflux, dysphagia, epigastric pain
Pyloric obstruction (narrow pylorus)	Peptic ulcer or carcinoma near pylorus	Epigastric fullness, nausea and pain, vomitus without bile
Intestinal obstruction (impaired chyme flow through intestinal lumen)	Hernia, telescoping of one part of intestine into another, twisting, inflamed diverticula, tumor growth, loss of peristaltic activity	Colicky pain to severe and constant pain, vomiting, diarrhea, constipation, dehydration and hypovolemia, and acidosis with its complications

*A sliding hernia (90% of the hiatal hernias) moves into and from the thoracic cavity through the diaphragm. A rolling hernia can pass entirely into the thoracic cavity through a secondary opening in the diaphragm; the protruding stomach (a paraesophageal hernia) lies alongside the esophagus.

digitalis, and metabolic disorders such as uremia are contributing factors for gastritis. The clinical manifestations of acute gastritis can include vague abdominal discomfort, epigastric tenderness, and bleeding. Healing usually occurs spontaneously within a few days. Discontinuing injurious drugs, using antacids, or decreasing acid secretion with drugs facilitate healing.

Chronic gastritis is a progressive disease that tends to occur in elderly individuals. This gastritis causes thinning and degeneration of the stomach wall.

Chronic *fundal* gastritis is the most severe type, because the gastric mucosa degenerates extensively. The loss of chief cells and parietal cells diminishes secretion of pepsinogen, hydrochloric acid, and intrinsic factor. Pernicious anemia develops because intrinsic factor is unavailable to facilitate vitamin B_{12} absorption. Chronic fundal gastritis becomes a risk factor for gastric carcinoma, particularly in individuals who develop pernicious anemia. A significant number of individuals with chronic fundal gastritis have antibodies to parietal cells, intrinsic factor, and gastric cells in their sera thus suggesting an autoimmune mechanism as the pathogenesis of the disease.

Chronic *antral* gastritis is more frequent than fundal gastritis. It is not associated with decreased hydrochloric acid secretion, pernicious anemia, nor the presence of parietal cell antibodies. *Helicobacter pylori* is a major etiologic factor associated with the inflammation seen in this chronic gastritis. The individual's response to the infection is infiltration of neutrophils and release of inflammatory cytokines that damage the gastric epithelium. The long-standing inflammatory process and gastric atrophy may develop without a history of abdominal distress. Individuals may report vague symptoms including anorexia, fullness, nausea, vomiting, and epigastric pain. Gastric bleeding may be the only clinical manifestation of gastritis.

Management of gastritis requires avoidance of alcohol, aspirin, or other inflammatory drugs. Antibiotics and vitamin B_{12} are used to treat infection and pernicious anemia, respectively.

4. **Compare duodenal, gastric, and stress ulcers; identify the complications of surgical management of ulcers.**

Study text pages 1464, 1465, and 1467 through 1470; refer to Figures 39-7 through 39-10 and Table 39-5. See the table on page 281.

A **peptic ulcer** is a break or ulceration in the protective mucosal lining of the lower esophagus, stomach, or duodenum. Such breaks expose submucosal areas to gastric secretions and autodigestion. Normally, the gastric and duodenal mucosa are protected from acid and pepsin by mucus and bicarbonate that are secreted by surface epithelial cells. Also, cellular tight junctions prevent back-diffusion of acid.

Risk factors for peptic ulcer disease are smoking and habitual use of nonsteroidal anti-inflammatory drugs (NSAIDs) or alcohol. Some chronic diseases such as emphysema, rheumatoid arthritis, and cirrhosis are associated with the development of peptic ulcers. Infection of the gastric and duodenal mucosa with *H. pylori* may cause peptic ulcers. Studies of life stress and ulcer disease are inconclusive regarding causation of peptic ulcers.

Postgastrectomy syndromes are a group of signs and symptoms that occur after gastric resection. They are caused by alterations in motor and control functions of the stomach and upper small intestine. **Dumping syndrome** is the rapid emptying of hypertonic chyme from the surgically reduced and smaller stomach into the small intestine 10 to 20 minutes after eating. Rapid gastric emptying and creation of a high osmotic gradient within the small intestine cause a sudden shift of fluid from the vascular compartment to the intestinal lumen. Plasma volume decreases may cause increased pulse rate, hypotension, weakness, pallor, sweating, and dizziness. Rapid distention of the intestine produces a feeling of epigastric fullness, cramping, nausea, vomiting, and diarrhea. After a high-carbohydrate meal, hypoglycemia can develop because of an increase in insulin secretion stimulated by the hyperglycemia that follows eating. The symptoms include weakness, diaphoresis, and confusion.

Alkaline reflux gastritis is stomach inflammation caused by reflux of bile and alkaline pancreatic secretions that contain proteolytic enzymes that disrupt the mucosal barrier. Clinical manifestations include nausea, vomiting in which the vomitus contains bile, and sustained epigastric pain that worsens after eating and is not relieved by antacids.

Afferent loop obstruction is a problem caused by volvulus, hernia, adhesion, or stenosis in the duodenal stump on the proximal side of the surgery. Partial obstruction causes bile and pancreatic secretions to accumulate, distend the loop, and delay emptying. The symptoms of afferent loop obstruction include intermittent severe pain and epigastric fullness after eating.

Diarrhea is one of the most common long-term alterations caused by gastric surgery. Postgastrectomy diarrhea appears to be related to rapid gastric emptying of large amounts of high carbohydrate liquids that increase the **osmotic** gradient and attract water into the intestinal lumen.

Many individuals cannot tolerate carbohydrates or a normal-sized meal. **Weight loss** frequently follows gastric resection.

Anemia after gastrectomy results from iron, vitamin B_{12}, or folate deficiency. Iron malabsorption may be caused by decreased acid secretion, which makes it more difficult to absorb iron. The duodenum may no longer be available to absorb iron after gastrectomy. Vitamin B_{12} deficiency may occur because of fewer parietal cells to secrete intrinsic factor that facilitates absorption of vitamin B_{12}.

5. **Define malabsorption syndrome and maldigestion; characterize pancreatic insufficiency and lactase and bile salt deficiency.**
Study text pages 1470 and 1471.

Malabsorption syndromes interfere with nutrient absorption in the small intestine; the intestinal mucosa fails to absorb or transport the digested nutrients into the blood. **Maldigestion** is the result of mucosal disruption caused by gastric or intestinal resection, vascular disorders, or intestinal disease. **Malabsorption** is failed or faulty digestion because of deficiencies of chemical enzymes.

Pancreatic insufficiency occurs because of deficient production of lipase, amylase, trypsin, or chymotrypsin by the pancreas. Causes of pancreatic insufficiency include chronic pancreatitis, pancreatic carcinoma, pancreatic

Features of Ulcers

Feature	Duodenal	Gastric	Stress
Age incidence	25-40 years	50-70 years	Related to severe stress, trauma, head injuries
Sex prevalence	Men	No sex difference	
Stress factors	Average	Increased	Increased
Acid production	Increased	Normal to low	Increased
Ulcerogenic drugs	Heavy use of alcohol and tobacco, NSAIDS	Moderate use of alcohol and tobacco	
Associated gastritis	Seldom	Common	
*Helicobacter pylori**	Usually present	May be present	
Pain	Pain-food-relief, common nocturnal pain, remission and exacerbations	Pain-food-relief, uncommon nocturnal pain, chronic, uncommon remission and exacerbations	Asymptomatic until hemorrhage or perforation
Hemorrhage	Common	Less common	Very common (most frequent complication)
Malignancy	Almost never	Possible	

H. pylori urease leads to ammonia formation, which is toxic to mucosal cells, and the phospholipases of these organisms damage mucosa. Also, *H. pylori* infection stimulates gastrin production, which increases acid secretion.
NOTE: Medical treatment is directed toward inhibiting or buffering acid secretions to relieve symptoms and promote healing. Antacids, dietary management, anticholinergic histamine blockers, and physical and emotional rest are used to accomplish relief and promote healing. *H. pylori* is treated with a combination of antibiotics and bismuth.

281

resection, and cystic fibrosis. Fat maldigestion is the chief problem because salivary amylase and enzymes secreted by the intestinal brush border assist in carbohydrate and protein digestion but do not digest fats. A large amount of fat in the stool is the most common sign of pancreatic insufficiency. Lipase supplementation is usually successful.

Lactase deficiency inhibits the breakdown of lactose or milk sugar into monosaccharides and therefore prevents lactose digestion and absorption across the intestinal wall. Lactase deficiency is most common in blacks. The undigested lactose remains in the intestine where bacterial fermentation causes gases to form. The osmotic gradient in the intestine also increases, which causes irritation and osmotic diarrhea.

Conjugated bile acids or bile salts are necessary for the digestion and absorption of fats. When bile from the liver enters the duodenum, the bile salts aggregate with fatty acids and monoglycerides to form micelles. Micelle formation solubilizes fat molecules and allows them to pass through the unstirred layer at the brush border. Advanced liver disease, which causes bile salt deficiency, obstruction of the common bile duct, intestinal immotility, and diseases of the ileum, leads to poor intestinal absorption of fat and fat-soluble vitamins A, D, E, and K. Increased fat in the stool leads to diarrhea and decreased plasma proteins. The loss of fat-soluble vitamins causes night blindness, bone demineralization, and bleeding abnormalities.

6. **Compare ulcerative colitis and Crohn disease**.
   Study text pages 1471 through 1474; refer to Figures 39-11 through 39-13 and Table 39-6.
   Ulcerative colitis and **Crohn disease** are chronic relapsing inflammatory bowel diseases of unknown etiology.

Both diseases are associated with genetic factors, alterations in epithelial cell barrier functions, immune reactions to intestinal bacteria, and abnormal T-cell reactions.

7. **Characterize diverticular disease, appendicitis, and irritable bowel disease.**
   Study text pages 1474 through 1476; refer to Figure 39-14.
   Diverticulae are herniations or saclike outpouchings of mucosa through the muscle layers of the colon wall. **Diverticulosis** is asymptomatic diverticular disease. **Diverticulitis** represents symptomatic inflammation. The most frequent site of diverticula is the sigmoid colon at weak points in the colon wall where arteries penetrate the muscularis. Habitual consumption of a low-residue diet reduces fecal bulk and reduces the diameter of the colon. According to the law of Laplace, wall pressure increases as the diameter of the lumen decreases. Pressure within the narrow lumen can increase enough to rupture the diverticula and cause abscess formation or peritonitis. An increase of dietary fiber intake frequently relieves symptoms. Surgical resection may be required if there are severe complications.

Appendicitis is an inflammation of the vermiform appendix. Obstruction of the lumen with feces, tumors, or foreign bodies followed by bacterial infection is the most likely cause of appendicitis. The obstructed lumen does not allow drainage of the appendix, and as mucosal secretion continues, intraluminal pressure increases. The increased pressure decreases mucosal blood flow and the appendix becomes hypoxic. The mucosa ulcerates, which promotes bacterial inflammation and edema. Gangrene develops from thrombosis of the luminal blood vessels followed by perforation.

Comparison of Ulcerative Colitis and Crohn Disease

	Ulcerative Colitis	Crohn Disease
Family history	Less common	More common
Location of lesions	Large intestine, no "skip" lesions, mucosal layer involved	Large or small intestine, "skip" lesions common, entire intestinal wall involved
Granulomas	Rare	Common
Anal and perianal fistulas and abscesses	Rare	Common
Narrowed lumen and possible obstruction	Rare	Common
Abdominal pain	Common, mild to severe	Common, mild to severe
Diarrhea	Common	Common
Bloody stools	Common	Less common
Abdominal mass	Rare	Common
Small intestine malabsorption	Rare	Common
Steatorrhea	Rare	Common
Cancer risk	Increased	Not increased
Treatment	Steroids, salicylates Immunosuppressives, broad-spectrum antibiotics, possible surgical resection	Similar to ulcerative colitis; surgery for strictures, fistulas, obstruction, and perforation

Epigastric or periumbilical pain is the typical symptom of an inflamed appendix. Right lower quadrant pain that exhibits rebound tenderness is associated with extension of the inflammation to the surrounding tissues. Nausea, vomiting, and anorexia follow the onset of pain. Leukocytosis and a low-grade fever are common. Perforation, peritonitis, and abscess formation are the most serious complications of appendicitis.

Appendectomy and antibiotics are the treatment for simple or perforated appendicitis. This surgery is the most common surgical procedure of the abdomen.

Irritable bowel syndome (IBS) is a functional disorder characterized by lower abdominal pain, predominant or alternating diarrhea/constipation, gas bloating, and nausea. There is no cure for IBS. Symptomatic treatment includes laxatives and fiber, antidiarrheals, antispasmodics, antidepressants, analgesics, and serotonin agonists or antagonists.

8. **Distinguish between acute and chronic mesenteric insufficiency.**
   Study text page 1477.
   Acute occlusion of mesenteric artery blood flow results from dissecting aortic aneurysms or emboli arising from cardiac alterations. The ischemic and damaged intestinal mucosa cannot produce enough mucus to protect itself from digestive enzymes. Mucosal alteration causes fluid to move from the blood vessels into the bowel wall and peritoneum. Fluid loss causes hypovolemia and further decreases in intestinal blood flow. As intestinal infarction progresses, shock, fever, bloody diarrhea, and leukocytosis develop. Abdominal pain may be severe. Bacteria invade the necrotic intestinal wall, causing gangrene and peritonitis.

   Chronic mesenteric insufficiency can develop from any condition that decreases arterial blood flow. Elderly individuals with arteriosclerosis are particularly susceptible. Colicky abdominal pain after eating is the cardinal symptom of chronic mesenteric insufficiency. Progressive vascular obstruction eventually causes continuous abdominal pain and necrosis of the intestinal tissue. Chronic segmental ischemia may lead to strictures and destruction.

   Diagnosis of mesenteric artery occlusion is based on clinical manifestations and laboratory findings. After angiography, a vasodilating agent may be injected to improve circulation. Surgery is required to remove necrotic tissue or repair sclerosed vessels.

9. **Describe obesity.**
   Study text pages 1477 through 1480; refer to Figure 39-15.
   Obesity is defined as a body mass index (BMI) greater than 30. It is a major cause of morbidity, death, and high health care cost in the United States and the Western World. Three leading causes of death in the United States are associated with obesity: cardiovascular disease, type 2 diabetes mellitus, and cancer. The most frequent cancers involve the colon, breast in postmenopausal women, endometrium, prostate, kidney, and esophagus. Obesity is also a risk factor for hypertension, stroke, hepatobiliary disease, including gallstones and nonalcoholic steatohepatitis, osteoarthritis, and sleep apnea. Visceral obesity is associated with a higher incidence of cardiovascular disease.

Genotype and gene–environment interactions are important predisposing factors, and both single-gene syndromes and numerous susceptibility genes influence the development of obesity. Single-gene defects include the melanocortin receptor gene, leptin gene (also known as the obesity gene), and leptin receptor gene. All single-gene defects are directly or indirectly related to leptin.

Many different circulating hormones control appetite and body weight. The sources of these include insulin from the beta cells of the pancreas, ghrelin from the stomach, peptide YY from the intestines, and leptin, adiponectin, and resistin from adipodocytes of adipose tissue. These hormones circulate in the blood at concentrations proportional to body fat mass and serve as peripheral signals to the arcuate nucleus (ARC) in the hypothalamus, where appetite and metabolism are regulated. The ARC has two sets of neurons with opposing effects that interact to regulate food intake and energy metabolism. One set of neurons produces the molecules neuropeptide Y (NPY) and agouti-related protein (AGRP), which stimulate eating, decrease metabolism, and promote catabolism. Another set of neurons synthesizes pro–melanocortin-producing peptide (PROP), which is then processed to alpha-melanocyte–stimulating hormone (α-MSH) and cocaine- and amphetamine-regulated transcript (CART). These neurons are collectively known as α-MSH/CART neurons, which inhibit eating. Both sets of neurons express their effects by activating second order neurons in the hypothalamus that increase or decrease appetite and energy metabolism. Leptin and insulin decrease appetite by inhibiting NPY/AGRP neurons and stimulating PROP-α-MSH/CART neurons. Ghrelin stimulates appetite by activating NPY/AGRP-expressing neurons. Peptide YY (PYY) inhibits these neurons and decreases appetite. Molecules that stimulate eating are called *orexins,* and molecules that inhibit eating are called *anorexins*. Peripheral effects of these signaling pathways are transmitted via the autonomic nervous system and endocrine system to regulate appetite, food intake, and energy metabolism.

Obesity is a chronic disease with various approaches to treatment including correction of metabolic abnormalities, individually tailored weight reduction diets, and exercise programs. A combination of weight reduction and exercise is the most effective treatment. Self-motivation and support systems are critical aspects of treatment. Additional treatments, such as psychotherapy, behavioral modification, medications, and gastric bypass or gastric banding are also prescribed and when successful result in a significant reduction in comorbidities and a decrease in insulin resistance.

10. **Describe disorders of undernutrition.**
    Study text pages 1480 through 1482.
    Many young adults and adolescents in the United States are affected by two complex and related eating disorders: anorexia nervosa and bulimia. Anorexia nervosa is characterized by refusal to eat because of distorted body image perceptions that one is too fat. As the disease progresses, fat and muscle depletion give the individual a skeleton-like appearance. The loss of 25% to 30% of ideal body weight can eventually lead to death caused by starvation-induced

283

cardiac failure. Treatment objectives for anorexia nervosa include reversing the compromised physical state, promoting insights and knowledge about the disorder, and modifying food habits. Fluoxetine administration may improve weight gain and reduce obsessions.

Bulimia is characterized by binging or the consumption of normal-to-large amounts of food followed by self-induced vomiting or purging of the intestines with laxatives. Although individuals with bulimia are afraid of gaining weight, their weight usually remains within normal range. Because of negative connotations associated with vomiting and purging, individuals who have bulimia often binge and purge secretly. Bulimics may binge and purge as often as 20 times a day. Continual vomiting of acidic chyme can cause pitted teeth, pharyngeal and esophageal inflammation, and tracheoesophageal fistulas. Overuse of laxatives can cause rectal bleeding. Individual or group cognitive behavior change is the focus of treatment. Antidepressants may be of some benefit.

Starvation can be either short or long term. Therapeutic short-term starvation is part of many weight-reduction programs, and therapeutic long-term starvation is used in medically controlled environments to facilitate rapid weight loss in morbidly obese individuals. Pathologic long-term starvation can be caused by poverty or chronic diseases such as cardiovascular, pulmonary, hepatic, and digestive disorders, malabsorption syndromes, and cancer.

Short-term starvation consists of several days of total dietary abstinence or deprivation. Glucose is the preferred energy source for cells. Once all available energy has been absorbed from the intestine, glycogen in the liver is converted to glucose through glycogenolysis or the splitting of glycogen into glucose. This process peaks within 4 to 8 hours after glycogenolysis and gluconeogenesis in the liver begins by the formation of glucose from noncarbohydrate molecules. Both of these processes deplete stored nutrients and thus cannot meet the body's energy needs indefinitely. Proteins continue to be catabolized in gluconeogenesis to a minimal degree to provide carbon for the synthesis of glucose.

The main characteristics of **long-term starvation** are decreased dependence on gluconeogenesis and increased use of products of lipid and pyruvate metabolism for cellular energy sources. Absolute deprivation of food causes **marasmus** or protein energy malnutrition. Carbohydrate intake without protein intake is termed **kwashiorkor.**

Once the supply of adipose tissue is depleted, proteolysis begins. The breakdown of muscle protein is the last process to supply energy for life. Death results from severe alteration in electrolyte balance and loss of renal, pulmonary, and cardiac function.

Adequate ingestion of appropriate nutrients is the obvious treatment for starvation. Starvation caused by chronic disease, long-term illness, or malabsorption is treated by enteral or parenteral nutrition.

11. **Describe the complications, causes, and manifestations of liver disorders.**
    Study text pages 1482 through 1488; refer to Figures 39-16 through 39-19 and Table 39-8. See the table on page 285.

12. **Compare the viral hepatitis types.**
    Study text pages 1419 through 1422; refer to Figures 39-20 and 39-21 and Table 39-9. See the table above.

The pathologic lesions of hepatitis display hepatic cell necrosis, scarring, Kupffer's cell hyperplasia, and infiltrations by monocytes. Cellular injury is promoted by cell-mediated immune mechanisms, cytotoxic T cells, T regulatory cells, and natural killer cells. The inflammatory process damages and obstructs bile canaliculi.

The clinical manifestations of the different types of hepatitis are very similar and usually consist of three phases: the prodromal, icteric, and recovery phases. The **prodromal phase** of hepatitis begins about 2 weeks after exposure and ends with appearance of jaundice. Fatigue, anorexia, malaise, nausea, vomiting, headache, hyperalgia, cough, and low-grade fever precede the onset of jaundice. The infection is highly transmissible during this phase.

The **icteric phase** begins about 1 to 2 weeks after the prodromal phase and lasts 2 to 6 weeks. Hepatocellular destruction that prevents bilirubin conjugation and intrahepatic bile stasis causes jaundice or icterus. The icteric phase is the actual phase of illness. The liver is enlarged, smooth, and tender, and percussion over the liver causes pain. During the icteric phase, gastrointestinal and respiratory symptoms subside, but fatigue and abdominal pain may persist or unconjugated fractions increase.

The posticteric or **recovery phase** begins with resolution of jaundice at about 6 to 8 weeks after exposure. In most cases, liver function returns to normal within 2 to 12 weeks after the onset of jaundice.

Fulminant hepatitis is a clinical syndrome resulting in severe impairment or necrosis of liver cells and potential liver failure. It may occur as a complication of hepatitis C or hepatitis B and is compounded by infection with the delta virus. Acetaminophen overdose is a leading cause of liver failure in the United States. It usually develops 6 to 8 weeks after the initial symptoms of hepatitis or a metabolic liver disorder. Treatment of fulminant hepatitis is supportive. The hepatic necrosis is irreversible. Liver transplantation may be lifesaving. Survivors usually do not develop cirrhosis or chronic liver disease.

13. **Describe cirrhosis and describe its various types.**
    Study text pages 1491 through 1494; refer to Figures 39-22 and 39-23 and Table 39-9. See the table on page 286.

Cirrhosis is an irreversible inflammatory disease that disrupts liver structure and function. Structural changes result from fibrosis, which is a consequence of inflammation. The parenchyma of the liver becomes distorted and biliary channels may be altered or obstructed leading to jaundice. Obstruction caused by cirrhosis can cause portal hypertension. These vascular changes compromise liver function further, and the process of regeneration fails as hypoxia, necrosis, and atrophy ultimately cause liver failure.

14. **Compare cholelithiasis to cholecystitis.**
    Study text pages 1494 and 1495; refer to Figures 39-24 and 39-25.

Obstruction and inflammation are the most common disorders of the gallbladder. Obstruction is caused by

Liver Disease Complications

Complication	Causes	Manifestations
Portal hypertension	Obstruction or impeded blood flow in portal venous system or vena cava, cirrhosis, viral hepatitis, parasitic infection, hepatic vein thrombosis, right side heart failure	Esophageal and stomach varices with vomiting of blood, splenomegaly with thrombocytopenia, ascites with diaphragm displacement, hepatic encephalopathy with cognitive impairment and tremor
Ascites	Portal hypertension and reduced serum albumin levels increase capillary hydrostatic pressure, which pushes water into the peritoneal cavity, cirrhosis, heart failure, constrictive pericarditis, abdominal malignancies, nephrotic syndrome, malnutrition	Abdominal distention, displaced diaphragm with dyspnea, peritonitis
Hepatic encephalopathy	Blood that contains toxins such as ammonia is shunted from gastrointestinal tract to systemic circulation, toxins reach brain	Subtle changes in cerebral function, confusion, tremor of hands, stupor, convulsions, coma
Jaundice Hemolytic (unconjugated bilirubin)	Excessive hemolysis of red blood cells because of immune reactions, infections, toxic substances, or transfusions of incompatible blood	Dark urine, light-colored stools, anorexia, malaise, fatigue, pruritus
Obstructive (conjugated bilirubin)	Obstruction of bile flow by gallstones or tumor prevent flow into duodenum, drugs	
Hepatocellular (conjugated and unconjugated bilirubin)	Intrahepatic disease, obstruction by bile calculi, genetic enzyme defects, infections	
Hepatorenal syndrome	Alcoholic cirrhosis and fulminant hepatitis, decrease in blood volume, intravasoconstriction because the liver may fail to remove excessive vasoactive substances from the blood	Oliguria, jaundice, ascites, gastrointestinal bleeding

gallstones, which are aggregates of substances in the bile. The gallstones may remain in the gallbladder or enter the cystic duct. If gallstones become lodged in the cystic duct, they obstruct the flow of bile into and out of the gallbladder and cause inflammation. Gallstone formation is termed **cholelithiasis,** and inflammation of the gallbladder or cystic duct is known as **cholecystitis.**

Gallstones are of two types: cholesterol and pigmented. Cholesterol stones are the most common. Cholesterol gallstones form in bile that is supersaturated with cholesterol produced by the liver. Usually within the gallbladder, supersaturation sets the stage for cholesterol crystal formation and aggregation into "macrostones." If the stones become lodged in the cystic or common duct, they cause pain and cholecystitis.

The reason the hepatocytes secrete bile that is supersaturated with cholesterol may involve cholesterol synthesis or decreased secretion of bile acids that promote cholesterol solubility. Pigmented stones occur later in life and are associated with cirrhosis. Pigmented stones are created by

cholesterol, calcium bilirubinate, or pigmented polymers and are associated with biliary infection and increased amounts of unconjugated bilirubin in bile. The unconjugated bilirubin precipitates in the gallbladder or bile ducts as stones. Risk factors for cholelithiasis include obesity, middle age, female gender, American Indian ancestry, and gallbladder, pancreatic, or ileal disease.

Epigastric and right hypocondrium pain and jaundice are the cardinal manifestations of cholelithiasis. Vague symptoms include heartburn, flatulence, epigastric discomfort, and fatty food intolerances. Biliary colic pain is caused by the lodging of one or more gallstones in the cystic or common duct. The pain can be intermittent or steady and located in the right upper quadrant with radiation to the mid-upper back. Jaundice indicates that the stone is located in the common bile duct.

Laparoscopic cholecystectomy is the preferred treatment for gallstones that cause obstruction or inflammation. An alternative treatment is the administration of drugs that dissolve the stones.

285

Characteristics of Viral Hepatitis

	Hepatitis A	Hepatitis B	Hepatitis C	Hepatitis D	Hepatitis E	Hepatitis G
Transmission route	Fecal-oral, parenteral, sexual	Parenteral, sexual	Parenteral	Parenteral, fecal-oral, sexual	Fecal-oral	Parenteral, sexual
Incubation period	30 days	60-180 days	35-60 days	30-180 days	15-60 days	Unknown days
Carrier state	No	Yes	Yes	Yes	No	Yes
Severity	Mild	Severe, may be prolonged	Unknown	Severe	Severe in pregnant women	Unknown
Chronic hepatitis	No	Yes	Yes	Yes	No	Unknown
Prophylaxis	Hygiene, immune serum globulin	Hygiene, HBV vaccine	Hygiene, screening blood, interferon and ribavirin may prevent progression to fibrosis	Hygiene, HBV vaccine	Hygiene, safe water	

NOTE: Treatment is supportive, physical activity is restricted, low-fat and high-carbohydrate diet is recommended, and interferon is useful in chronic B and C types.

Types of Cirrhosis of the Liver

Type	Cause	Manifestations
Alcoholic cirrhosis	Toxic effects of chronic and excessive alcohol intake, alcohol is oxidized by the liver to acetylaldehyde, which damages hepatocytes	Typical,* decreased sexual function
Primary biliary cirrhosis	Unknown, possibly an autoimmune mechanism that scars ducts	Typical, but may be asymptomatic, circulating IgG
Secondary biliary cirrhosis	Obstruction by neoplasms, strictures, or gallstones scars the ducts proximally	Typical, pruritus
Postnecrotic cirrhosis	Viral hepatitis due to hepatitis C, drugs or other toxins, consequence of chronic and severe liver disease	Typical, small and distorted liver

*Typical manifestations include nausea, anorexia, fever, abdominal pain, hepatomegaly, splenomegaly, jaundice, ascites, and complications identified in objective 11.

Cholecystitis can be acute or chronic and is almost always caused by the lodging of a gallstone in the cystic duct. Obstruction causes the gallbladder to become distended and inflamed, followed by decreased blood flow, ischemia, necrosis, and possible perforation. Fever, leukocytosis, rebound tenderness, and abdominal muscle guarding are common findings. Serum bilirubin and alkaline phosphatase levels may be elevated. Persistent symptoms with recurrent attacks require cholecystectomy.

15. Describe the pathogenesis of pancreatitis.

Study text pages 1495 through 1497; refer to Figure 39-26.

Pancreatitis, or inflammation of the pancreas, is a relatively rare but potentially serious disorder. It is believed that **acute pancreatitis** develops because of an injury or disruption of the pancreatic ducts or acini that permits leakage of pancreatic enzymes into pancreatic tissue. The leaked enzymes initiate autodigestion and acute pancreatitis. Bile reflux into the pancreas occurs if gallstones obstruct the common bile duct; the refluxed bile also injures pancreatic tissue. The activated trypsin, elastase, and lipases destroy tissue and cell membranes, which causes edema, vascular damage, hemorrhage, and necrosis. Toxic enzymes also are released into the bloodstream and cause injury to vessels and other organs such as the lungs and kidneys. **Chronic pancreatitis** is caused by chronic alcohol abuse. Elevated serum amylase is a characteristic diagnostic feature as is the ratio of amylase clearance to creatine clearance by the kidney helpful for diagnosis.

286

Mild to severe epigastric or midabdominal pain is the cardinal symptom of acute pancreatitis. The pain may radiate to the back because of the retroperitoneal location of the pancreas. The pain is caused by distended pancreatic ducts and capsule, chemical irritation and inflammation of the peritoneum, and irritation or obstruction of the biliary tract. Fever and leukocytosis accompany the inflammatory response. Nausea and vomiting are caused by hypermotility or paralytic ileus secondary to the pancreatitis or peritonitis. Hypotension and shock frequently occur because plasma volume is lost as enzymes and kinins released into the circulation increase vascular permeability and dilate vessels. The results are hypovolemia, hypotension, and myocardial insufficiency. Flank or periumbilical ecchymosis indicates a poor prognosis.

The goal of treatment for acute pancreatitis is to stop the process of autodigestion and prevent systemic complications. Narcotic medications are needed to relieve pain. Parenteral fluids are given to restore blood volume and prevent hypotension and shock. For chronic pancreatitis, a fat-free diet and oral enzyme replacements preven malasorption and weight loss. Surgical drainage or partial resection of the pancreas may be required to relieve pain and prevent cystic rupture. Chronic pancreatitis is a risk factor for pancreatic cancer.

To correct enzyme deficiencies and prevent malabsorption, oral enzyme replacements are taken before and during meals. Multiple organ failure accounts for most deaths in severe pancreatitis.

16. Characterize the various cancers of the digestive system.

Study text pages 1498 through 1505; refer to Figures 39-27 through 39-32 and Tables 39-10 and 39-11. See the table below.

PRACTICE EXAMINATION

Multiple Choice
Circle the correct answer for each question.
1. During vomiting, there is:
   a. forceful diaphragm and abdominal muscle contractions, airway closure, esophageal sphincter relaxation, and deep inspiration.
   b. deep inspiration, airway closure, forceful diaphragm and abdominal muscle contractions, and esophageal sphincter relaxation.
   c. airway closure, forceful diaphragm and abdominal muscle contractions, deep inspiration, and esophageal sphincter relaxation.
   d. esophageal sphincter relaxation, forceful diaphragm and abdominal muscle contractions, deep inspiration, and airway closure.

Cancers of the Digestive System

Type and Location	Risks	Manifestations

Esophagus
  Squamous cell carcinoma
  Adenocarcinoma
	Malnutrition, alcohol, tobacco, chronic reflux	Chest pain, dysphagia

Stomach
  Adenocarcinoma
  Squamous cell carcinoma
	Dietary salty foods, nitrates, nitrosamines, gastric atrophy, *H. pylori* infection	Anorexia, malaise, weight loss, upper abdominal pain, vomiting, occult blood, symptoms of organ involved in metastasis from stomach

Colorectal Adenocarcinoma (left colon grows in ring: right colon grows in mass)	Chromosomal deletions, polyps, diverticulitits, ulcerative colitis, high refined CHO, low-fiber/high-fat diet	Pain, anemia, bloody stool surface, mass right colon, obstruction left colon, distention, elevated CEA

Liver
  Hepatocarcinoma
  Cholangiocarcinoma
	HBV, HCV, HDV, cirrhosis, intestinal parasites, aflatoxin, smoking, alcohol consumption	Pain, anorexia, bloating, weight loss, portal hypertension, ascites, +/− jaundice, elevated serum proteins and liver enzymes

Gallbladder
  Secondary metastases
  Adenocarcinoma
  Squamous cell carcinoma
	Cholelithiasis, cholecystitis	Steady upper right quadrant pain, diarrhea, anorexia, vomiting, +/− jaundice

Pancreas Adenocarcinoma	Chronic pancreatitis, cigarette smoking, alcohol, diabetic women	Weight loss, weakness, nausea, vomiting, abdominal pain, depression, +/− jaundice, possible hypoglycemia if an insulin-secreting tumor

NOTE. Genetic factors are important as causes of digestive system cancers. Two genes are particularly notable: *p53* and *K-ras*. *p53* is involved in esophageal, gastric, colorectal, liver, gallbladder, and pancreatic cancers. *K-ras* is associated with colorectal, gallbladder, and pancreatic cancers. Treatment for esophageal, stomach, gallbladder, and pancreatic cancer is essentially surgical. Liver neoplasms are treated by surgery and chemotherapy. Colorectal cancer therapy uses surgery, radiation, and chemotherapy. Pancreatic cancer mortality is near 100%, so treatment is palliative.

287

2. Achalasia:
   a. manifests as regurgitation of chyme.
   b. has denervation of smooth muscle in the esophagus.
   c. occurs in response to sedentary lifestyle.
   d. results in esophageal sphincter relaxation.
3. Osmotic diarrhea is caused by:
   a. nonabsorbable intestinal contents.
   b. bacterial enterotoxins.
   c. ulcerative colitis.
   d. Crohn disease.
4. Melena is:
   a. bloody vomitus.
   b. gaseous bowel distention.
   c. blood in the stool.
   d. loss of appetite.
   e. black, tarry stools.
5. A common manifestation of hiatal hernia is:
   a. gastroesophageal reflux.
   b. diarrhea.
   c. belching.
   d. vomitus without bile.
6. Gastroesophageal reflux is:
   a. caused by rapid gastric emptying.
   b. excessive lower esophageal sphincter functioning.
   c. associated with abdominal surgery.
   d. caused by lower esophageal sphincter incompetence.
7. Intestinal obstruction causes:
   a. decreased intraluminal tension.
   b. hyperkalemia.
   c. decreased nutrient absorption.
   d. epigastric fullness.
8. Peptic ulcers may be caused by:
   a. nonsteroidal antiinflammatory drugs (NSAIDs).
   b. *H. pylori.*
   c. habitual alcohol consumption.
   d. mucus secretion.
   e. a, b, and c are correct.
9. Gastric ulcers:
   a. may lead to malignancy.
   b. occur at a younger age than duodenal ulcers.
   c. always have increased acid production.
   d. exhibit nocturnal pain.
   e. Both a and c are correct.
10. Duodenal ulcers:
    a. occur four times more frequently in females than in males.
    b. may be complicated by hemorrhage.
    c. are associated with sepsis.
    d. may cause inflammation and scar tissue formation around the sphincter of Oddi.
11. In malabsorption syndrome, flatulence and abdominal distention are likely caused by:
    a. protein deficiency and electrolyte imbalance.
    b. undigested lactose fermentation by bacteria.
    c. fat irritating the bowel.
    d. impaired absorption of amino acids and accompanying edema.
12. The characteristic lesion of Crohn disease is:
    a. found in the colon.
    b. precancerous.
    c. granulomatous.
    d. malignant.
13. Which gene is most often associated with digestive system cancers?
    a. *K-ras*
    b. *p53*
    c. *p16*
    d. *APC*
14. A 14-year-old boy has been admitted to the emergency department with acute-onset abdominal pain in the lower right quadrant. Abdominal rebound tenderness is intense, and he has a fever and leukocytosis. This individual most likely has:
    a. acute appendicitis.
    b. diverticulitis.
    c. ulcerative colitis.
    d. cholelithiasis.
    e. cholecystitis.
15. The control of appetite and body is influenced by many different hormones. Leptin:
    a. decreases the appetite.
    b. stimulates NPY/AGRP neurons.
    c. stimulates appetite.
    d. sets the hypothalamus thermostat.
16. Short-term starvation involves:
    a. glycogenolysis.
    b. gluconeogenesis.
    c. proteolysis.
    d. Both a and b are correct.
    e. a, b, and c are correct.
17. The most common manifestation of portal hypertension is:
    a. rectal bleeding.
    b. cirrhosis.
    c. intestinal bleeding.
    d. duodenal bleeding.
    e. vomiting of blood from esophageal bleeding.
18. Hepatic encephalopathy is manifested by:
    a. ascites.
    b. splenomegaly.
    c. dark urine.
    d. oliguria.
    e. cerebral dysfunction.
19. Acute occlusion of mesenteric artery blood results from:
    a. dissecting aortic aneurysms.
    b. chronic segmental ischemia.
    c. arteriosclerosis.
    d. necrosis of intestinal tissue.
20. Which type of jaundice is due to genetic enzyme defects?
    a. Obstructive
    b. Hemolytic
    c. Hepatocellular
    d. Both a and c are correct

21. Which most often causes postnecrotic cirrhosis?
    a. Malnutrition
    b. Alcoholism
    c. Hepatitis C
    d. Autoimmunity
    e. Biliary obstruction
22. Diverticulitis:
    a. manifests as pain in the right lower quadrant.
    b. is asymptomatic.
    c. commonly involves the transverse colon.
    d. is inflammation of diverticular outpouchings of mucosa through muscle layers of the colon.
23. In pancreatitis:
    a. tissue damage likely results from release of pancreatic enzymes.
    b. cholesterol intake is causative.
    c. diabetes is uncommon in chronic pancreatitis.
    d. the cause is bacterial infection.
24. A complication of ulcerative colitis not seen with Crohn disease is:
    a. gangrene and rupture.
    b. obstruction.
    c. intestinal malabsorption
    d. increased risk for adenocarcinoma of the colon.
25. Excessive ingestion of NSAIDs and aspirin can cause:
    a. acute gastritis.
    b. esophagitis.
    c. stress ulcers.
    d. gastric atrophy.

CASE STUDY 1

Dr. R. is a 55-year-old male professor whose department chair is an unrelenting harasser. Dr. R.'s family investments have failed and his early planned retirement is no longer possible. Persistent upper abdominal pain for the last 2 months has convinced him that he needs a diagnostic work-up.

At the physician's office, Dr. R. revealed a history of smoking one pack of cigarettes a day for 25 years. His eating habits are irregular. However, he indicated a pain-antacid-relief pattern. The pain was more intense right after eating. He frequently takes aspirin for headaches and to relieve rheumatoid stiffness while golfing. His family and remaining histories were unremarkable except that he had lost 10 pounds during the last 6 weeks.

Questions

Which type of peptic ulcer do you suspect?

How could your suspicion be confirmed?

At a physician's office, D.K., a 33-year-old man states, "I have had several days of increasing fatigue and loss of appetite, and now I have a fever and abdominal and muscle discomfort." He admits to IV drug use.

Physical examination reveals right upper quadrant tenderness with hepatomegaly; a nonpalpable spleen; fever; no jaundice, rashes, nor ecchymoses; no ascites; no blood on rectal exam; no joint involvement; and no confusion nor neurological symptoms.

Questions

What laboratory tests would you choose and why?

What information obtained from the history, physical examination, and laboratory results differentiates one possible diagnosis from another?

40 Alterations of Digestive Function in Children

FOUNDATIONAL KNOWLEDGE OBJECTIVES

a. Describe the structure and function of the gastrointestinal tract and the accessory organs of digestion.
Refer to Figure 38-1.

> **MEMORY CHECK!**
>
> See this workbook's narrative for Foundational Knowledge Objective **a** in Chapter 39.

LEARNING OJECTIVES

After studying this chapter, the learner will be able to do the following:

1. Describe the pathophysiology and treatment of cleft lip and palate.
Study text pages 1516 through 1518; refer to Figure 40-1.

Cleft lip is caused by incomplete fusion of the nasomedial or intermaxillary process during the second month of embryonic development. Cleft lip may occur with or without cleft palate. The defect in cleft lip usually is beneath one or both nostrils and may involve the external nose, the nasal cartilages, the nasal septum, and the alveolar processes. It also may be associated with a flattening and broadening of the facial features.

Cleft palate is frequently associated with cleft lip, but it can occur alone. The defect may affect only the uvula and soft palate, but it may extend forward toward the nostrils through the hard palate. If it extends through the hard palate, open communication between the structures of the nasopharynx and the oral cavity leads to frequent sinusitis and otitis media. Children with orofacial cleft are at risk for *Streptococcus mutans* and *Lactobacillus* colonization, which can increase caries in the primary dentition.

In most cases, cleft lip and cleft palate are caused by genetic and environmental factors, and each contributes only a minor developmental defect. These factors reduce the amount of neural crest mesenchyme that migrates into the area that will develop into the embryo's face. Another major difficulty seen with cleft lip or palate is poor feeding. Because suckling involves both the tongue and pressure against the palate, the infant with isolated cleft lip but an intact palate may breast- or bottle-feed

without great difficulty. On the other hand, cleft palate may significantly interfere with breast- or bottle-feeding. Bottle-feeding may require large, soft nipples with an oversized opening. Breast-feeding may be impossible for some infants with cleft palate without a prosthesis for the roof of the mouth.

Treatment is surgical correction, and it is usually accomplished in stages. Supportive therapy may include prosthodontics and orthodontics, otolaryngology procedures, and speech and occupational therapy.

2. Describe the structural defects of esophageal atresia and tracheoesophageal fistula.
Study text pages 1518 and 1519; refer to Figure 40-2.

Congenital malformations of the esophagus occur in approximately 1 in 3000 to 4500 births. **Esophageal atresia** is a condition in which the esophagus ends in a blind pouch and may be accompanied by a connection between the esophagus and the trachea called a **tracheoesophageal fistula (TEF).** These conditions develop from aberrant differentiation of the trachea at 4 to 6 weeks of embryonic development. The blind esophageal pouch in atresia fills rapidly with secretions or food and overflows, which leads to persistent drooling, poor feeding, and aspiration. TEF generally causes immediate aspiration and respiratory distress on the first feeding. Thirty percent of children with this anomaly have other associated congenital defects, particularly cardiovascular defects. If the fistula is small, diagnosis may not be made until recurrent aspiration and pneumonias become problematic.

Diagnosis is confirmed by the inability to pass a catheter into the stomach when the x-ray shows the catheter coiled at the level of the defect. Treatment is surgical correction.

3. Describe the structural defect and pathophysiology associated with pyloric stenosis; note the consequence of intestinal malrotation.
Study text pages 1519 and 1520.

Pyloric stenosis is an obstruction of the pylorus because of hypertrophy of the pyloric sphincter. Obstruction becomes evident between 1 to 2 weeks and 3 to 4 months of age. Boys are affected five times more frequently than girls, and whites are more frequently affected than Asians or blacks. Pyloric stenosis is seen more frequently in full-term than in premature infants, and in children with Down syndrome. Increased gastrin

291

secretion in the mother tends to increase the probability of pyloric stenosis and may be linked to maternal stress; hereditary factors also may be involved.

Generally stenosis is manifested in a previously healthy infant who begins to have marked forceful projectile vomiting at 2 to 3 weeks of age that does not resolve. Weight loss, electrolyte imbalances, and dehydration follow and may end in death if intervention is not provided.

Pyloric stenosis is suspected on clinical manifestation and confirmed by ultrasonography or an upper gastrointestinal series that demonstrates the lesion. A small, muscular "olive" at the site of the hypertrophic pylorus may be palpable in the left upper quadrant of the abdomen. Treatment is surgical release of the hypertrophic fibers or pyloromyotomy after stabilization of the infant's fluid and electrolyte balance.

Intestinal malrotation of the intestine, which is an obstructing bend and twisting of the bowel on itself may partly or completely occlude the gastrointestinal tract and its blood vessels. Treatment consists of opening the abdomen and reducing the twisted bowel manually and resection of necrotic bowel followed by an anastomosis.

4. Describe meconium ileus.

Study text pages 1520 and 1521.

Meconium (intestinal secretions and amniotic fluid) is a substance that fills the entire intestine before birth. **Meconium ileus** is the intestinal obstruction caused by the meconium in the newborn. The cause is usually a lack of digestive enzymes during fetal life.

Abdominal distention usually develops during the first days of life, and the infant, unable to pass meconium, begins to vomit. Ten to fifteen percent of children with cystic fibrosis have meconium ileus as neonates.

The treatment in cases without volvulus or perforation is a hyperosmolar enema performed using fluoroscopy to evaluate the meconium. Enterotomy and irrigation are reserved for enema failures and difficult cases.

5. Describe congenital aganglionic megacolon or Hirschsprung disease.

Study text pages 1521 and 1522; refer to Figure 40-3.

Congenital aganglionic megacolon or **Hirschsprung disease** is a condition that is generally associated with the failure of the parasympathetic nervous system to produce intramural ganglion cells in the enteric nerve plexuses. This failed innervation causes a section of the colon to be immotile and creates a functional intestinal obstruction in the affected area. This section becomes distended with feces, and the resulting condition is called "megacolon." The distal rectum is always involved. Hirschsprung disease accounts for one third of all intestinal obstructions in infants and occurs in 1 in 5000 births, with a greater incidence in boys. Either a dominant gene pattern or a recessive gene pattern coupled with multiple interacting factors has been implicated as causative. Clinical manifestations are mild to severe chronic constipation, although diarrhea may be the first sign, because only liquid may pass the aganglionic section. Severe edema of the colon begins to obstruct blood and lymphatic flow,

thereby causing enterocolitis and tissue destruction. Bacteria can infiltrate the bowel wall from the lumen and may cause gram-negative sepsis. Severe fluid and electrolyte imbalance caused by diarrhea may become life-threatening.

Measurement of rectal pressures or rectal manometry is frequently helpful during diagnosis. Diagnosis is confirmed by rectal biopsy that demonstrates the aganglionic bowel. Definitive treatment consists of resection of the aganglionic segment and constant attention to bowel hygiene thereafter.

6. Describe intussusception.

Study text pages 1522 and 1523; refer to Figure 40-5.

Intussusception is the telescoping or invagination of one portion of the intestine into another; this causes an intestinal obstruction. The most commonly affected area is the ileum, which invaginates into the cecum through the ileocecal valve. Collapse is in the direction of peristaltic flow. Between 80% and 90% of intestinal obstructions in infants and children are caused by intussusception, and males are more commonly affected than females. Intussusception generally occurs between 3 and 36 months of age; 70% of cases occur in infants who are younger than 1 year. The pathophysiology of intussusception is like that of megacolon, because the telescoping bowel obstructs blood and lymphatic flow, which causes rapid edema and tissue exudation. Gangrene may follow.

The disorder is usually accompanied by passage of dark and gelatinous or "currant jelly" stools. Diagnosis is made with the clinical manifestations of intestinal obstruction, and it is confirmed by lower gastrointestinal ultrasound. Reduction of the intussusception must be done immediately, and it is frequently performed using hydrostatic pressure of the contrast media used for x-ray or an enema to push the invaginated bowel segment from its intussusception. This is successful 45% to 70% of the time, although some children require surgery to correct the intussusception or related complications. This condition is fatal if untreated.

7. Describe the pathophysiology and potential complications related to gastroesophageal reflux disease.

Study text pages 1523 and 1524.

Gastroesophageal reflux disease (GERD) is the return of gastric contents into the esophagus because of poor function of the lower esophageal sphincter. GER is more common in premature than in term newborn infants and usually resolves by 6 to 12 months of age without significant effect on the infants. GER causes significant problems for children with cerebral palsy and cystic fibrosis. The cause of GER is unknown, although delayed maturation of the sphincter or impaired hormonal or neurotransmitter response mechanisms are suspected. Other factors include the location of the gastroesophageal junction and the angle of the junction and mucosal gathering.

Clinical manifestations include forceful vomiting with an 85% occurrence within the first week of life, aspiration pneumonia in one third of those affected, and poor weight gain. Esophagitis may result from exposure of the esophagus to acidic gastric contents that may

292

cause either strictures or anemia from prolonged occult blood loss.

Eosinophilic esophagitis in children is considered an atopic disease involving both immediate and delayed hypersensitivity reaction to food ingestion. Dysphagia, food impaction, and vomiting are common. Treatment includes elimination diets and corticosteroids.

Diagnosis may be made from clinical manifestations or confirmed by barium swallow or esophageal pH probe studies that demonstrate reflux with an abrupt drop in esophageal pH during the reflux episodes. Mild GER resolves without treatment, although some children require elevated prone positioning after feedings to help reduce reflux. Pharmacologic therapies include medication to increase lower gastrointestinal motility and to increase gastric emptying time in an effort to decrease the opportunity for reflux of gastric contents; medications that decrease gastric acidity can be used. Surgical correction or fundoplication is rarely required.

8. **Describe the gastrointestinal abnormalities associated with cystic fibrosis.**

Study text pages 1524 and 1525; refer to Table 40-1.

Cystic fibrosis (CF) is a multisystem disease that is primarily manifested in the pancreas. The classic triad of pathophysiology of cystic fibrosis includes pancreatic enzyme deficiency that leads to maldigestion, overproduction of mucus in the respiratory tract that leads to chronic obstructive pulmonary disease, and elevated levels of sodium and chloride in perspiration. Very viscous exocrine secretions tend to obstruct glandular ducts. Although pancreatic function may range from normal to a virtual absence, 85% of children with CF have pancreatic insufficiency. The lack of pancreatic enzymes results in maldigestion of proteins, carbohydrates, and fats and leads to chronic malnutrition. Pancreatic ducts also may be blocked with viscous secretions that eventually may damage pancreatic beta cells and lead to diabetes mellitus because of insulin deficiency. Maldigestion of fats causes fatty stools; other complications include anemia, biliary cirrhosis, vitamin B_{12} deficiency, vitamin K deficiency, and rectal prolapse because of the passage of large, bulky stools.

Pancreatic enzyme function may be estimated by 72-hour fecal fat measurement; fecal content of trypsin and chymotrypsin may also be measured. Pancreatic enzyme replacement may be administered with meals, and a high-calorie/high-protein diet is usually prescribed.

9. **Describe gluten-sensitive enteropathy.**

Study text pages 1525 through 1527; refer to Figures 40-6 and 40-7.

Gluten-sensitive enteropathy, which was formerly called celiac sprue or celiac disease, is the loss of mature villous epithelium caused by the ingestion of gluten, which is the protein component of cereal grains. In individuals with this condition, the gluten is toxic to the intestinal epithelial cells. Pathogenesis appears to involve dietary, genetic, and immunologic factors. The disease occurs mostly in whites.

Diarrhea is an early sign of this enteropathy in most infants. The stools are pale, bulky, greasy, and foul-smelling;

they may contain oil droplets. Vomiting and abdominal pain are prominent in infants but unusual in older children. Anorexia is prevalent, and growth is usually diminished. Consequences of malabsorption such as rickets, tetany, frank bleeding, or anemia may be obvious. The child may bleed easily.

An intestinal biopsy is required to detect the classic mucosal changes caused by gluten-sensitive enteropathy. Serum IgA and IgG antibodies to gluten may also be diagnostic.

Treatment requires the immediate and permanent institution of a diet that is free of wheat, rye, barley, oats, and malt. Lactose (milk sugar) is also excluded because lactose intolerance is presumed. Infants are given vitamin D, iron, and folic acid supplements to treat deficiencies.

10. **Compare kwashiorkor to marasmus.**

Study text page 1528.

Kwashiorkor and **marasmus** are common types of malnutrition in children; they are collectively known as **protein energy malnutrition** (PEM), and both are states of long-term starvation. Kwashiorkor is a severe protein deficiency, and marasmus is a severe deficiency of all nutrients. Both are problems in impoverished populations.

In kwashiorkor, protein synthesis is reduced in all tissues. Physical and mental growth are stunted. The lack of sufficient plasma proteins results in generalized edema. The liver swells with stored fat because no hepatic proteins are synthesized to form and release lipoproteins. Kwashiorkor also causes malabsorption, reduced bone density, and impaired renal function.

In **marasmus,** metabolic processes including liver function are preserved, but growth is severely retarded. Caloric intake is too low to support protein synthesis for growth or the storage of fat. Muscle and fat wasting occurs. Anemia is common and may be severe. The presence of subcutaneous fat, hepatomegaly, and fatty liver distinguishes kwashiorkor from marasmus.

11. **Describe failure to thrive.**

Study text pages 1528 and 1529.

Failure to thrive (FTT) is the inadequate physical growth of an infant or child and has either an organic or nonorganic cause. Organic failure to thrive is caused by genetic, anatomic, or pathophysiologic factors. Nonorganic failure to thrive is caused by nutritional deficits associated with inadequate nurturing.

In organic problems, management of FTT consists of treating the cause. Management of nonorganic FTT involves the immediate total care of the infant or child.

12. **Describe necrotizing enterocolitis.**

Study text pages 1529 and 1530.

Necrotizing enterocolitis is a disorder of neonates, particularly premature infants. Reduced mucosal blood flow leading to hypoxic injury to intestinal mucosa is thought to be the cause. This injury allows bacteria to invade the mucosa and submucosa, and release of inflammatory mediators causes necrosis and even perforation of the intestinal wall.

Treatments include cessation of feeding, gastric section to decompress the intestines, fluid and electrolyte maintenance, and antibiotic administration to control sepsis. Surgical resection is the treatment of choice for intestinal perforation.

13. Describe childhood diarrhea.

Study text page 1530.

Diarrhea in children is similar to that for adults. **Prolonged diarrhea** is more dangerous in children because they have much smaller fluid reserves than adults. Therefore, dehydration can develop rapidly. **Infectious diarrhea** in newborns is usually associated with nursery epidemics involving gram-negative pathogens and staphylococci. **Acute diarrhea** in children is most synonymous with acute viral or bacterial gastroenteritis and tends to be self-limiting. **Chronic diarrhea**, persisting more than 4 weeks, is caused by abnormal colonic motility, lactose intolerance, parasitic infestation, impaired absorption, and antibiotic use.

14. Describe physiologic jaundice of the newborn.

Study page 1534.

Physiologic jaundice of the newborn is usually a transient, benign icterus that occurs during the first week of life in otherwise healthy, full-term infants. It is caused by mild unconjugated (indirect reacting) hyperbilirubinemia. A high level of indirect hyperbilirubinemia (15 mg/dl) is considered pathologic. There is a risk of brain damage, **kernicterus,** because the bilirubin passes into brain cells and is toxic with persistent high indirect hyperbilirubinemia.

Physiologic jaundice is usually treated by ultraviolet light. **Pathologic jaundice** requires an exchange transfusion.

15. Identify other childhood liver disorders.

Study text pages 1531 through 1533.

Biliary atresia is a congenital malformation of the bile ducts that obstructs bile flow, causing jaundice, cirrhosis, and liver failure. It is the most common reason for liver transplantation in children. **Acute hepatitis** is similar in both children and adults but is milder in children. Hepatitis A is the most common form observed in children. **Cirrhosis** is rare in children but can develop from chronic liver disease. Thrombosis of the portal vein is the most common cause of **portal hypertension** in children, and splenomegaly is the most common sign.

16. Identify common childhood metabolic disorders injurious to the liver.

Refer to Table 40-2.

The three most common metabolic disorders that cause liver damage in children are galactosemia (galactose cannot be converted to glucose), fructosemia (fructose, sucrose, or honey cannot be metabolized), and Wilson disease (impaired copper transport in blood). All three are inherited as genetic traits and permit the accumulation of toxins in the liver.

PRACTICE EXAMINATION

Fill in the Blanks

Supply the correct response for each statement.

1. _____ is seen more frequently in full-term than in premature infants, and in children with Down syndrome.

2. _____ is often associated with esophageal atresia.

3. _____ permits the accumulation of toxins in the liver.

4. _____ involves ileum invagination into the cecum through the ileocecal valve.

5. In jaundice of the newborn, _____ development is a possibility.

6. Increased _____ in pregnant women may contribute to pyloric stenosis in their infants.

7. Diabetes mellitus may be a complication of _____.

8. Stools are pale, bulky, greasy, and foul-smelling in _____.

9. _____ is the result of faulty innervation of the colon.

10. Protein synthesis is reduced in all tissues in _____ malnutrition.

11. Nutritional deficits associated with inadequate nurturing cause _____.

12. Stress and anoxia of the bowel wall in neonates result in _____.

13. Congenital aganglionic megacolon is diagnosed by rectal manometry and rectal _____.

14. A pH probe will demonstrate a(n) _____ in esophageal pH during a period of reflux.

15. Cleft palate is frequently complicated by communication between the _____ and the _____ cavities.

16. _____ may be a complication of cystic fibrosis secondary to the passage of large stools.

Matching

Match the description with the alterations (answer may be used more than once).

_____ 17. Absence of intramural ganglion cells in the enteric nerve plexuses.

_____ 18. Acute onset of abdominal pain and distention

_____ 19. Thick, tarry plug obstructs the duodenum, jejunum, and ileum.

_____ 20. May initially present with diarrhea

_____ 21. Food regurgitation

_____ 22. May contribute to aspiration pneumonia

_____ 23. Incompetent lower esophageal sphincter

_____ 24. "Currant jelly" stools

_____ 25. Enema may be treatment.

a. congenital aganglionic megacolon

b. meconium ileus

c. intussusception

d. gastroesophageal reflux

e. esophageal atresia

CASE STUDY

Baby B. is a male term infant born vaginally to a 21-year-old white woman; he is her first child. The pregnancy was complicated by moderate maternal hypertension during the last week of pregnancy. The mother was taking no medication, and the family history is normal. A nurse practitioner is called to see the infant 4 hours after birth because he is feeding poorly; he initially took some glucose water after birth and has been "spitty" and "drooling" since then. Baby B.'s initial physical examination is essentially normal, although he does have moderate amounts of saliva frequently spilling from his mouth that occasionally require suctioning. He is not experiencing respiratory distress.

Question

Because Baby B. is not in respiratory distress, what can be done to determine why he is having difficulty dealing with his secretions?

41 Structure and Function of the Musculoskeletal System

PREREQUISITE KNOWLEDGE OBJECTIVES

After reviewing the primary text where referenced, the learner will be able to do the following:

1. **Identify the function and structural elements of bone.**
   Review text pages 1540 through 1545; refer to Figures 41-1 and 41-2 and Tables 41-1 through 41-5.
2. **Describe the features of compact and spongy bone; classify bones.**
   Review text pages 1545 through 1547; refer to Figures 41-3 through 41-5.
3. **Describe the process of bone remodeling and healing.**
   Review text pages 1547 and 1548; refer to Figure 41-6.
4. **Structurally and functionally, classify joints; characterize articular cartilage.**
   Review text pages 1548 through 1554; refer to Figures 41-7 through 41-14.
5. **Describe the arrangements of muscle fibers in skeletal muscles; explain the structure and function of a motor unit.**
   Review text pages 1554 through 1557; refer to Figures 41-15 through 41-17 and Tables 41-6 and 41-7.
6. **Describe skeletal muscle contraction at the molecular level.**
   Review text pages 1557 through 1561; refer to Figures 41-18 and 41-19 and Tables 41-6 and 41-7.
7. **Identify the energy sources for muscular contraction.**
   Review text pages 1561 and 1562; refer to Table 41-8.
8. **Describe the types of skeletal muscle contractions and the interaction between groups of muscles.**
   Review text pages 1562 and 1563.
9. **Identify the tests of musculoskeletal function.**
   Review text pages 1563 and 1564.
10. **Describe the changes in the musculoskeletal system that accompany normal aging.**
    Review text page 1564.

PRACTICE EXAMINATION

Multiple Choice
Circle the best answer for each question.

1. Sialoprotein:
   a. promotes resorption.
   b. binds calcium.
   c. stabilizes the basement membrane of bones.
   d. promotes calcification.
2. Osteoprotegerin (OPG):
   a. increases bone loss.
   b. prevents bone resorption.
   c. provides a lattice framework of spongy bones.
   d. triggers osteoclast proliferation.
3. A function of the epiphyseal plate that is *not* a function of the articular cartilage is to:
   a. enable the articulation of bones.
   b. enable a bone to increase in length.
   c. repair damaged bone tissue.
   d. provide sensory nerves to bone.
4. The remodeling of bone is done by basic multicellular units that consist of bone precursor cells. Precursor cells:
   a. differentiate into osteoclasts and osteoblasts.
   b. are located on the free surfaces of bone and along vascular channels.
   c. enable the formation of new trabeculae in compact bone.
   d. Both a and b are correct.
5. Joints are classified functionally and structurally. Which of the following is a proper functional and structural relationship?
   a. Amphiarthrosis/fibrous
   b. Diarthrosis/synovial
   c. Synarthrosis/synchondrosis
   d. Diarthrosis/fibrous
   e. Synarthrosis/cartilaginous
6. In older individuals, the bone remodeling cycle:
   a. is faster, because osteoclastic activity is enhanced.
   b. is enhanced, because mineralization increases.
   c. has more precursor cells.
   d. has fewer precursor cells, because the bone marrow becomes infiltrated with fat.
   e. Both a and b are correct.

297

7. Which of the following is *not* included in a motor unit?
   a. Muscle fibers
   b. Motor nerve axons
   c. Anterior horn cell
   d. Upper motor neuron
8. The perimysium is to a fasciculus as the:
   a. periosteum is to a bone.
   b. muscle is to epimysium.
   c. myofibril is to a muscle fiber.
   d. epimysium is to the endomysium.
   e. muscle cell is to the endomysium.
9. Which of the following is *not* a characteristic of type I muscle fibers?
   a. Sparse capillary supply
   b. Slow contraction speed
   c. High resistance to fatigue
   d. Profuse capillary supply
   e. Oxidative metabolism.
10. Which protein is found in the thick myofilaments?
    a. Actin
    b. Myosin
    c. Troponin
    d. Tropomyosin
    e. a, c, and d are correct.
11. An important function of the transverse tubule is to:
    a. provide organic nutrients to muscle fibers.
    b. initiate fiber contraction.
    c. enable the regeneration of muscle fibers.
    d. carry the electrical action potential deeper into the muscle fiber.
12. The ion necessary for coupling is:
    a. sodium.
    b. calcium.
    c. potassium.
    d. magnesium.
    e. phosphate.
13. Aerobic respiration:
    a. permits the body to have brief periods during which it does not require oxygen.
    b. causes an increase in the amount of lactic acid.
    c. yields more molecules of ATP than anaerobic respiration.
    d. uses more glycogen to produce ATP than anaerobic respiration.
    e. leads to oxygen debt.

14. Repayment of oxygen debt:
    a. converts lactic acid to glycogen.
    b. replenishes ATP stores.
    c. replenishes phosphocreatine stores.
    d. Both b and c are correct.
    e. a, b, and c are correct.
15. The strength of muscle contraction depends on the:
    a. extent of the load.
    b. initial length of muscle fibers.
    c. recruitment of additional motor units.
    d. nerve innervation ratios.
    e. All of the above are correct.
16. Attempting to push an object that is too heavy to move is an example of which kind of contraction?
    a. Isotonic
    b. Concentric
    c. Flaccid
    d. Tetanic
    e. Isometric
17. Which of the following does *not* happen with muscle as individuals grow older?
    a. A reduction in the size of motor units occurs.
    b. Up to 30% of skeletal muscles may be lost by age 80.
    c. The synthesis of acetylcholine increases to compensate for muscle bulk loss.
    d. All of the above occur with advancing age.
18. Which of the following is *not* a function of the skeletal system?
    a. Supports tissues
    b. Binds organs together
    c. Protects CNS structures
    d. Participates in blood cell formation
19. Alphabetize the sequence of the stages of bone healing in fractures and surgical injuries.
    a. Procallus formation
    b. Callus formation
    c. Hematoma formation
    d. Callus replacement with lamellar or trabecular bone
    e. Periosteum and endosteum remodeling

Matching

Match the appropriate microscopic feature of muscle fibers with each description.

_____ 20. Sarcomere

_____ 21. Sarcolemma

_____ 22. Sarcoplasmic reticulum

a. membrane that covers the muscle fiber

b. flattened, tube-like network

c. stacks of myofilaments; unit of contraction

d. calcium transport system

e. tube-like structure that runs perpendicular to muscle fibers

Match the appropriate structure or descriptor with each microscopic feature of bone.

_____ 23. Volkmann canals

_____ 24. Trabecula

_____ 25. Lamellae

a. small canals that connect bone cells

b. concentric rings

c. cavities where bone cells are housed

d. contains blood vessels

e. irregular meshwork

Chapter **41** **Structure and Function of the Musculoskeletal System**

42 Alterations of Musculoskeletal Function

FOUNDATIONAL KNOWLEDGE OBJECTIVES

a. Describe the processes that maintain bone integrity.
Review text pages 1547 and 1548; refer to Figure 41-6.

MEMORY CHECK!

- Bone contains three types of cells: osteoblasts (bone forming), osteocytes (mature), and osteoclasts (resorptive). **Osteoblasts bring abut new bone formation by synthesis of osteoid ((nonmineralized bone matrix). Mineralization of bone matrix occurs by concentrating some growth factors found in the matrix and by facilitating the deposit and exchange of calcium and other ions at the site.**
- Osteoblasts and osteoclasts cooperate to maintain normal bone development. Receptor activator of nuclear factor ligand (RANKL) is a cytokine needed for the formation and activation of osteoclasts and increase bone loss. Osteoprotegerin (OPG) decreases bone loss. When RANKL binds to its receptor RANK on osteoclast precursor cells, it triggers their proliferation and increases bone resorption. OPG acts as a decoy by binding to RANK and thus prevents RANKL from binding to RANK so that bone resorption does not occur.
- The internal structure of bone is maintained by a remodeling process in which existing bone is resorbed and new bone is laid down to replace it. Remodeling is accomplished by clusters of bone cells made up of bone precursor cells located on the free surfaces of bones and along the vascular channels and marrow cavities. The precursor cells differentiate into osteoclasts and osteoblasts.
- In the first phase of the remodeling cycle, a stimulus such as a hormone, drug, vitamin, or physical stressor activates the osteoclasts. In phase two, the osteoclasts resorb bone and leave in its place an elongated cavity termed a resorption cavity. The resorption cavity in compact bone follows the longitudinal axis of the haversian system, whereas in spongy bone the resorption cavity parallels the surface of the trabeculae. In phase three, new bone or secondary bone is laid down by osteoblasts lining the walls of the resorption cavity. In compact bone, successive layers are laid down until the resorption cavity is reduced to a narrow haversian canal around a blood vessel. This process destroys old haversian systems and forms new haversian systems. New trabeculae are formed in spongy bone.
- The remodeling process just described is capable of repairing microscopic bone injuries, but gross injuries such as fractures and surgical wounds heal via a different process. In bone wound healing, the stages are as follows:
  1. Hematoma formation occurs when damaged vessels hemorrhage. Fibrin and platelets within the hematoma form a meshwork. Hematopoietic growth factors such as platelet-derived growth factor and transforming growth factor are involved in this stage.
  2. Procallus formation occurs as fibroblasts, capillary buds, and osteoblasts move into the wound and produce granulation tissue; this is the procallus. Enzymes and growth factors aid in this stage of healing.
  3. Callus formation occurs as osteoblasts in the procallus form membranous or woven bone. Enzymes increase the phosphate content, and it joins with calcium as a deposit of mineral that hardens the callus.
  4. Osteoblasts continue to replace the callus with either lamellar bone or trabecular bone.
  5. Synthesis of type I bone collagen predominates at this stage. This final remodeling stage is vital to ensure good mechanical properties for weightbearing and mobility.

b. **Describe the types of joints.**
   Review pages 1548 through 1554; refer to Figures 41-7 through 41-14.

MEMORY CHECK!

- Joints are classified by the degree of movement they permit or by the connecting tissues that hold them together. Based on movement, a joint is classified as a (1) synarthrosis or an immovable joint, (2) an amphiarthrosis or a slightly movable joint, or (3) a diarthrosis or a freely movable joint. On the basis of connective structures, joints are classified as fibrous, cartilaginous, or synovial.
- A joint united directly to bone by fibrous connective tissues is called a fibrous joint. Generally, fibrous joints are synarthroses, or immovable joints, but many fibrous joints allow some movement. The degree of movement depends on the distance between the bones and the flexibility of the fibrous connective tissue.
- There are two types of cartilaginous joints or amphiarthroses. A symphysis is a cartilaginous joint in which bones are united by a pad or disk of fibrocartilage. The articulating surfaces are usually covered by a thin layer of hyaline cartilage and a thick pad of fibrocartilage that acts as a shock absorber and stabilizer. Examples of symphyses are the symphysis pubis and the intervertebral disks. A synchondrosis is a joint in which hyaline cartilage connects the two bones. The joints between the ribs and the sternum are synchondroses. Slight movement at the synchondroses between the ribs and the sternum allows the chest to move outward and upward during breathing.
- Synovial joints or diarthroses are the most movable and complex joints in the body. A synovial joint consists of a fibrous joint capsule or articular capsule, a synovial membrane, a joint cavity or synovial cavity, synovial fluid, and an articular cartilage. The joint capsule consists of parallel, interlacing bundles of dense, white fibrous tissue. It has a rich supply of nerves, blood vessels, and lymphatic vessels. The nerves are sensitive to the rate and direction of motion, compression, tension, vibration, and pain.
- The synovial membrane is the smooth, delicate inner lining of the joint capsule. It lines the nonarticular portion of the synovial joint and any ligaments or tendons that traverse the joint cavity. The synovial membrane is capable of rapid repair and regeneration.
- The joint cavity or synovial cavity is an enclosed, fluid-filled space between the articulating surfaces of the two bones that enables the two bones to move "against" one another. Synovial fluid within the cavity lubricates the joint surfaces, nourishes the pad of the articular cartilage, and contains free-floating synovial cells and various leukocytes that phagocytose joint debris and microorganisms.
- Articular cartilage is a layer of hyaline cartilage that covers the end of each bone. The functions of articular cartilage are to reduce friction and to distribute the weightbearing forces. Articular cartilage has no blood vessels, lymph vessels, or nerves. Therefore, it is insensitive to pain and regenerates slowly and minimally after injury. Regeneration occurs primarily at sites where the articular cartilage meets the synovial membrane.

c. **Define terms associated with muscle fibers.**
   Review text pages 1554 through 1557; refer to Figures 41-15 through 41-17.

MEMORY CHECK!

- Each anterior horn cell, its axon, and the innervated muscle fibers is called a motor unit. The motor unit behaves as a single entity and contracts as a whole when it receives an adequate electrical impulse. A muscle fiber is a single muscle cell. This long cell is cylindrical in structure surrounded by a membrane capable of excitation and impulse propagation. The muscle fiber contains bundles of myofibrils in a parallel arrangement along the longitudinal axis of the muscle. The myofibrils contain sarcomeres that are the actual contracting units. The sarcomeres consist of actin and myosin, which are the contractile proteins.

Continued

- Besides the myofibrils, the major components of the muscle fiber include the muscle membrane, sarcotubular system, sarcoplasm, and mitochondria. The muscle membrane is a two-part membrane. It includes the sarcolemma, which contains the plasma membrane of the muscle cell and the cell's basement membrane. At the motor nerve endplate, where the nerve impulse is transmitted, the sarcolemma forms the highly convoluted synaptic cleft. The protein systems of the sarcolemma transport nutrients and synthesize proteins. They also provide the sodium-potassium pump and include the cell's cholinergic receptor. The basement membrane serves as the cell's microskeleton and maintains the shape of the muscle cell.
- The sarcoplasm is the cytoplasm of the muscle cell and contains numerous enzymes and proteins that are responsible for the cell's energy production, protein synthesis, and oxygen storage. Unique to the muscle is the sarcotubular system, which includes the transverse tubules and the sarcoplasmic reticulum. The sarcoplasmic reticulum is involved in calcium transport that initiates muscle contraction at the sarcomere. The sarcoplasmic reticulum is composed of tubules that run parallel to the myofibrils and are termed sarcotubules. The transverse tubules are closely associated with the sarcotubules and run across the sarcoplasm and communicate with the extracellular space. Both tubules allow for intracellular calcium uptake, regulation, release during muscle contraction, and storage of calcium during muscle relaxation.

d. **Identify the major events of muscle contraction and relaxation.**
   Review text pages 1557 through 1561; refer to Figures 41-18 and 41-19 and Tables 41-6 and 41-7.

Excitation and Contraction

A nerve impulse reaches the end of a motor neuron and releases acetylcholine
↓
Acetylcholine diffuses across the neuromuscular junction and binds to acetylcholine receptors on the muscle fiber
↓
Stimulation of acetylcholine receptors initiates an impulse that travels along the sarcolemma, through the T-tubules, and to the sarcoplasmic reticulum
↓
Calcium is released from the sarcoplasmic reticulum into the sarcoplasm; calcium binds to troponin molecules in the thin myofilaments
↓
Tropomyosin molecules shift to expose actin's active engagement sites
↓
Energized myosin cross-bridges of the thick myofilaments bind to actin and use their ATP energy to pull the thin myofilaments toward the center of each sarcomere
↓
As the thin filaments slide past the thick myofilaments, the entire muscle fiber shortens

Relaxation

After the impulse passes, the sarcoplasmic reticulum begins actively pumping calcium back into the sarcoplasm
↓
As calcium leaves the troponin molecules of the thin myofilaments, tropomyosin returns
↓
Myosin cross-bridges cannot bind to actin and can no longer sustain the contraction
↓
The thick and thin myofilaments are no longer connected, so the muscle fiber returns to its longer, resting length

After studying this chapter, the learner will be able to do the following:

1. **Compare the types of fractures; describe the causes, manifestations, and treatment of fractures.**

   Study text pages 1568 through 1572; refer to Figures 42-1 through 42-5 and Table 42-1.

   Fractures are classified as complete or incomplete and open or closed. In a **complete** fracture, the bone is broken all the way through, whereas in an **incomplete** fracture, the bone is damaged but remains in one piece. Complete or incomplete fractures also are considered **open** if the skin is broken or **closed** if it is not. Fractures also are classified according to the direction of the fracture line. A fracture wherein the bone breaks into two or more fragments is termed a **comminuted** fracture.

   The signs and symptoms of a fracture include unnatural alignment, swelling, muscle spasm, tenderness, pain, and impaired sensation. The immediate pain of a fracture is severe and usually due to the traumatic injury. Subsequent pain often is produced by muscle spasm. Numbness is caused by the pinching of a nerve by the trauma or by bone fragments. Pathologic fractures are not usually associated with trauma or trauma-related pain. Stress fractures are painful because of accelerated remodeling and are usually relieved by rest. Range of motion in the joint is limited, and movement may evoke audible clicking sounds or crepitus.

   Fracture treatment involves realigning the bone fragments to their normal or anatomic position and holding the fragments in place so that bone union can occur. Several methods are available to reduce or align a fracture, including closed manipulation, traction, and open surgical reduction. Splints and plaster casts are used to immobilize and hold a reduction in place. External fixation can be used to reduce and immobilize open fractures. Proximal and distant to the break, pins are placed in the bone and then stabilized by clamps and rods. Improper reduction or immobilization of a fractured bone may result in nonunion, delayed union, or malunion.

   Treatment of delayed union and nonunion includes modalities designed to stimulate new bone formation. Electric current devices, electromagnetic field generations, and low-density ultrasound have been effective in stimulating bone formation. Gene therapy also is showing promise. Large bone defects can be filled with bone grafts or synthetic materials, such as calcium phosphate cement.

2. **Define terms associated with musculoskeletal system stress.**

   Study text pages 1572 through 1576; refer to Figures 42-6 through 42-8 and Tables 42-2 through 42-4.

   Dislocation is the temporary displacement of two bones in which the articular cartilage loses contact entirely. If the contact between the surfaces is only partially lost, the injury is called subluxation. Dislocations and **subluxations** are often accompanied by fracture. As the bone separates from the joint, it may bruise or tear adjacent nerves, blood vessels, ligaments, supporting structures, and soft tissue.

   A tear in a tendon is a **strain.** Major trauma or excessive stress can tear a tendon at any site in the body. The tendons of the hands, feet, knee, upper arm, thigh, ankle, and heel are frequently injured sites. Ligament tears are known as **sprains.** Ligament tears and ruptures can occur at any joint

Types of Fractures

Type	Characteristics	Cause
Common Complete Fractures		
Open fracture	Communicating wound between bone and skin	Moderate to severe energy that exceeds to tissue tolerance
Oblique fracture	Fracture line at 45-degree angle to long axis of bone	Angulation and compressive energy
Spiral fracture	Fracture line encircling bone	Twisting energy with distal part unable to move
Transverse fracture	Fracture line perpendicular to long axis of bone	Energy directly toward bone
Impacted fracture	Fracture fragments pushed into one another	Compressive energy directly to distal fragment
Pathologic fracture	Fracture occurs at any point in the bone	Minor energy to already weakened bone
Common Incomplete Fractures		
Greenstick fracture	Break of the cortical bone on the convex side of a bent bone only with spongy bone splintering	Minor direct or indirect energy in children or elderly
Stress fracture	Microfracture	Bone is subjected to repeated stress beyond its strength; muscles are stronger than bone

but are most common in the wrist, ankle, elbow, and knee joints. A complete separation of a tendon or ligament from its attachment is an **avulsion.** An avulsion is the result of abnormal stress on the ligament or tendon and is commonly seen in young athletes, especially sprinters, hurdlers, and runners.

Trauma can also cause painful inflammation of tendons, or **tendinitis,** and bursae, or **bursitis. Tendinosis** results from trauma and repetitive stress causing degradation of collagen fibers and pain. Tendinitis and tendinosis are collectively known as **tendinopathy.** Besides trauma, causes of tendinitis include crystal deposits, postural misalignment, and hypermobility in a joint. **Epicondylitis** is inflammation of a tendon where it attaches to a bone. Examples of epicondylitis include tennis elbow, which is an inflammation of the lateral epicondyle of the humerus, and medical epicondylitis, which is referred to as golfer's elbow. Epicondylitis is related to work activities involving repetitive cyclic flexion and extension of joints. **Bursitis** occurs primarily in the middle years and is caused by repeated trauma. Septic bursitis is caused by wound infection or bacterial infection of the skin overlying the bursae. The shoulder is a common site of bursitis.

Muscle strain is often the result of sudden, forced motion causing the muscle to become stretched beyond its normal capacity. Muscles are injured more often than tendons in young people; the opposite is true in older populations. Regardless of the cause of trauma, skeletal muscle cells usually are able to regenerate, although regeneration may take up to 6 weeks.

Myositis ossificans is a complication of localized muscle injury and thought to be caused by scar tissue calcification and subsequent ossification. An example is seen in football players after injury to thigh muscles.

Rhabdomyolysis or **myoglobinuria** can be a life-threatening complication of severe muscle trauma manifested by excess myoglobin, an intracellular muscle protein, in the urine. Muscle damage releases the myoglobin. The most severe form is often called **crush syndrome.** Less severe and more localized forms are called compartment syndromes, which can lead to Volkmann ischemic contracture in the forearm or leg. Crush syndrome first gained notoriety in injuries seen following the London air raids in World War II. More recently, it has been reported in individuals found unresponsive because of drug overdoses and those who are immobile for long periods of time. Myoglobinuria can also be seen following viral infections, administration of certain anesthetic agents, strychnine poisoning, tetanus, excessive muscular activity, heatstroke, electrolyte disturbances, fractures, status epilepticus, electroconvulsive therapy, and high-voltage electrical shock.

3. **Differentiate among osteoporosis, osteomalacia/ rickets, Paget disease, and osteomyelitis.**
   Study text pages 1576 through 1580 and 1582 through 1588; refer to Figures 42-9 through 42-16. See table on page 306.
   RANKL, a member of the tumor necrosis factor (TNF) family, is expressed by osteoblasts and their immature precursors and is necessary for osteoclast development.

RANKL activates the receptor **RANK,** which is expressed on osteoclasts and their precursors, and suppresses apoptosis, which leads to activation and prolongation of osteoclast survival. The effects of RANKL are blocked by **osteoprotegerin (OPG),** which is a glycoprotein that acts as a decoy or soluble receptor antagonist for RANKL that prevents it from binding and activating RANK. The balance between RANKL and OPG is regulated by cytokines and hormones, and alterations of the **RANKL/RANK/ OPG** can lead to dysregulation and pathologic conditions, including osteoporosis, immune-mediated bone diseases, malignant bone disorders, and inherited skeletal diseases.

4. **Classify bone tumors by tissue of origin, whether benign or malignant, and their pattern of bone destruction.**
   Study text pages 1588 through 1590; refer to Figure 42-17 and Tables 42-5 and 42-6. See the diagram on page 306.
   Bone tumors may originate from bone cells, cartilage, fibrous tissue, marrow, or vascular tissue. On the basis of mesodermal tissue of origin, bone tumors are classified as osteogenic, chondrogenic, collagenic, or myelogenic. The mesoderm contributes to primitive fibroblasts and reticulum cells. The fibroblast is the progenitor of the osteoblast, the chondroblast, and the fibrous connective tissue cell.

   Benign bone tumors destroy small areas of bone, tend to be limited to the anatomic confines of the host bone, and have a well-demarcated border. Benign bone tumors push against neighboring tissue, have a symmetric, controlled growth pattern, and tend to compress and displace neighboring normal bone tissue, which weakens the bone's structure until it leads to pathologic fracture.

   The geographic pattern, the moth-eaten pattern, and the permeative pattern are patterns of bone destruction in bone tumors. The latter two are malignant lesions; the first is benign. Tumors exhibiting the geographic pattern have well-defined margins that can be easily separated from the surrounding normal bone. There is a uniform and well-defined lytic area in the bone of these benign lesions.

   In the moth-eaten pattern, the tumorous lesion has a less-defined or demarcated margin that cannot be easily separated from normal bone. Areas of partially destroyed bone adjacent to completely lytic areas are found. This pattern of bone destruction is characteristic of rapidly growing, malignant bone tumors. An aggressive, malignant tumor causes the permeative pattern of bone destruction. The margins of the tumor are poorly demarcated, and abnormal bone merges with surrounding normal bone tissue. Malignant bone tumors tend to be large and aggressive in their bone destruction, to invade surrounding tissue, and to metastasize.

5. **Characterize the common types of bone tumors.**
   Study text pages 1590 through 1592; refer to Figures 42-18 through 42-20.
   Osteosarcomas or osteogenic tumors account for 38% of bone tumors and occur more frequently in males than in females. Adolescents and young adults are the predominant victims. In the 50- to 60-year-old age group, individuals with a history of radiation therapy for other malignancies also develop osteosarcomas.

305

Common Disorders of Bone

Disorder	Cause	Pathophysiology	Manifestations
Osteoporosis	Decreased levels of estrogen and testosterone, reduced physical activity lessens muscle stress on bone, inadequate vitamins C and D, insufficient dietary magnesium and calcium, corticosteroid use, other drugs	Reduced bone mass or density, imbalance in bone resorption and formation, alteration in the RANKL/RANK/OPG system*	Pain and bone deformity, fracture, increased radiolucency
Osteomalacia (adult) Rickets (children)	Deficiency of vitamin D lowers absorption of calcium from intestines, low serum phosphate	Inadequate and delayed mineralization, osteoid tissue is not mineralized	Pain, bone fractures, vertebral collapse, radiolucent bands perpendicular to bone surface, pseudofracture
Paget disease	Unknown	Excessive resorption of spongy bone followed by accelerated formation of softened bone	Thickening of bones, radiographic findings of irregular bone trabeculae with thickened and disorganized patterns
Osteomyelitis	Most often a staphylococcal infection, contaminated open wound or hematogenous bone infection	Acute inflammation of marrow and cortex, impaired blood supply leads to necrosis	Acute and chronic inflammation, fever, pain, lymphadenopathy, necrotic bone by radiographic imaging

*The cytokine receptor activator of nuclear factor kappa B ligand (RANKL), its receptor RANK, and its decoy receptor osteoprotegerin (OPG) are involved in osteoclast biology. Anti-RANKL therapy, a monoclonal antibody, reduces bone resorption. Treatment generally involves nutrient dietary supplements; sex hormones or modulators for osteoporosis; and antibiotics, surgical débridement, and hyperbaric oxygen therapy for osteomyelitis.

Osteosarcoma is a malignant bone-forming tumor that is large and destructive and most often found in bone marrow; it has a moth-eaten pattern of bone destruction. Osteosarcomas always contain osteoid and callus and also may contain chondroid and fibrinoid tissue. The osteoid is deposited between the trabeculae of the callus. The "streamers" of osteoid infiltrate the normal compact bone, destroy it, and replace it with dense callus and masses of osteoid. The bone tissue never matures to compact bone. Ninety percent of osteosarcomas are located in the metaphyses of long bones. Fifty percent of osteosarcomas occur around the

Origin of Benign and Malignant Bone Tumors

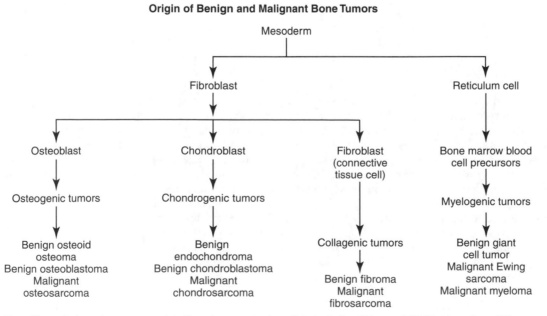

NOTE: Diagnosis depends on serum metabolite and enzyme levels, radiologic studies, CT scans, MRI, blood counts, and biopsy.

Chapter 42 Alterations of Musculoskeletal Function

knee area. The tumor breaks through the cortex, lifts the periosteum, and forms a soft tissue mass that is not covered by new bone.

Common initial symptoms are pain and swelling; pain is usually worse at night. Systemic symptoms are uncommon. Surgery is a major treatment of choice. The location of the tumor, its size, malignancy grade, and evidence of metastasis dictate the type and extent of surgery. Preoperative chemotherapy has increased the number of individuals whose limbs can be saved. Chemotherapy can be given both preoperatively and postoperatively.

Chondrosarcoma, a chondrogenic tumor, is a tumor of middle-aged and older adults. A chondrosarcoma is a large, ill-defined malignant tumor that infiltrates trabeculae in spongy bone. It occurs most often in the metaphysis or diaphysis of long bones. The tumor contains large lobules of hyaline cartilage that are separated by bands of fibrous tissue and anaplastic cells. It expands and enlarges the contour of the bone, causes extensive erosion of the cortex, and expands into the soft tissues.

Symptoms associated with the chondrosarcoma have an insidious onset. Local swelling and pain are usual symptoms. At first, the pain is intermittent; then, it gradually intensifies and becomes constant. Surgical excision is generally regarded as the treatment of choice; however, individuals demonstrate recurrences and so amputation is considered.

Fibrosarcoma, a malignant collagenic tumor, is seen in middle-aged adults. It is a solitary tumor that most frequently affects the metaphyseal region of the femur or tibia. The tumor is composed of a firm, fibrous mass of tissue containing collagen, malignant fibroblasts, and occasional osteoclast-like giant cells.

Pain and swelling are the usual symptoms and indicate that the tumor has broken through the cortex. Local tenderness, a palpable mass, limitation of motion, or a pathologic fracture are other symptoms and signs. Radical surgery and amputation are the treatments of choice for fibrosarcoma.

Giant cell tumors originate from myelogenic tissue and have a wide age distribution, with the majority found in persons between 20 and 40 years of age. Unlike most other bone tumors, giant cell tumors affect females more frequently than males.

The giant cell tumor is a solitary, circumscribed tumor that causes extensive bone resorption because of its osteoclastic origin. The tumor is rich in osteoclast-like giant cells and anaplastic stromal cells and is found in the center of the epiphysis in the femur, tibia, radius, or humerus. The tumor has a slow, relentless growth rate and is usually contained within the original contour of the affected bone. It may extend into the articular cartilage. It has recurrence rate as high as 80%.

The most common symptoms associated with the giant cell tumor are pain, local swelling, and limitation of movement. Cryosurgery and resection of the tumor decrease recurrence and are more successful treatments than curettage and radiation; amputation may be necessary but is not common.

6. **Compare osteoarthritis to rheumatoid arthritis.**
   Study text pages 1592 through 1600; refer to Figures 42-24 through 42-27 and Table 42-7. See the table on page 308.
7. **Characterize ankylosing spondylitis and gout.**
   Study text pages 1600 through 1606; refer to Figures 42-28 through 42-32 and Table 42-8.

Ankylosing spondylitis (AS) is a chronic, inflammatory joint disease characterized by stiffening and fusion or ankylosis of the spine and sacroiliac joints. Like rheumatoid arthritis, ankylosing spondylitis is a systemic, immune inflammatory disease. The disease is strongly associated with the presence of histocompatibility antigen HLA-B27 on the chromosomes of affected individuals; this suggests a genetic predisposition to the disease. In ankylosing spondylitis, the primary pathologic site is at the point where ligaments, tendons, and the joint capsule are inserted into bone rather (cartilage is the primary target) than in the synovial membrane as in rheumatoid arthritis. The end result of ankylosing spondylitis is fibrosis, ossification, and fusion of the joint.

Ankylosing spondylitis begins with inflammation of fibrocartilage in cartilaginous joints, particularly in the vertebrae. As inflammatory cells infiltrate and erode fibrocartilage in joint structures, repair begins to occur. Repair begins with the proliferation of fibroblasts. The collagen synthesized by fibroblasts becomes organized into fibrous scar tissue. Eventually, the scar tissue calcifies and ossifies. With time, all the cartilaginous structures of the joint are replaced by ossified scar tissue and the joints fuse or lose flexibility.

The most common symptoms of early ankylosing spondylitis are low back pain and stiffness. The pain, initially, is insidious but progressively becomes persistent. Forward flexion, rotation, and lateral flexion of the spine are restricted and painful. As the disease progresses, the individual becomes increasingly stooped. The thoracic spine becomes rounded, the head and neck are held forward on the shoulders, and the hips are flexed. Along with low back pain, many individuals may have peripheral joint involvement, uveitis or inflammation of eye structures, fibrotic changes in the lungs, cardiomegaly, aortic incompetence, amyloidosis, and Achilles tendinitis.

Treatment of individuals with ankylosing spondylitis consists of physical therapy to maintain skeletal mobility and prevent the natural progression of contractures. Anti-inflammatory and analgesic medications are prescribed to suppress some of the pain and stiffness and to facilitate exercise. Drugs blocking the inflammatory effects of TNF can be used for individuals with severe AS. Surgical procedures and radiotherapy are sometimes used to provide relief for individuals with end-stage disease or intolerable deformity.

Gout is a metabolic disorder that disrupts the body's control of uric acid production or excretion. High levels of uric acid accumulate in the blood and in other body fluids, including synovial fluid. When the uric acid reaches a certain concentration in fluids, it crystallizes. The crystals are deposited in connective tissues throughout the body.

307

Comparison of Osteoarthritis and Rheumatoid Arthritis

	Osteoarthritis (OA)	Rheumatoid arthritis (RA)
Pathologic feature	Inflammatory, loss of proteoglycans and collagen fibers from articular cartilage in synovial joints, bone sclerosis, bone spurs	Inflammatory; damage or destruction of synovial membrane, extends to articular cartilage joint capsule and surrounding ligaments and tendons; pannus
Onset age	>40, increases with age, equal sex distribution until age 55, then men	Middle age, prevalence in females
Cause	Joint stress, congenital abnormalities, joint instability, collagenases	Genetics, environmental microbes, autoimmunity, estrogen, released TNF-α and IL-1, RANKL
Joints affected	Peripheral and central, weightbearing	Phalangeal, wrists, knee
Joint fluid	Proteoglycans/fragments, normal mucin, few cells	Inflammatory exudates, poor mucin
Manifestations	Pain, stiffness, enlargement, tenderness, limited motion, muscle wasting, dislocation, deformity	Same as OA with systemic involvement, subcutaneous nodules, deviation of joints, rheumatoid factor (RF) and circulating immune complexes

NOTE: Conservative treatment for OA includes rest and support for weightbearing joints: analgesics and anti-inflammatory agents. For RA, conservative treatment includes disease-modifying antirheumatic drugs (DMARDs) and biologic response modifiers (BRMs), and anti-inflammatory drugs. Surgery for OA and RA can correct deformities or create new joints.

When crystallization occurs in synovial fluid, painful inflammation of the joint develops. This condition is known as **gouty arthritis.** With time, crystal deposition in subcutaneous tissues causes the formation of small, white nodules or **tophi** and their inflammatory sequelae.

The pathophysiology of gout is closely linked to purine metabolism, cellular metabolism of purines, and kidney function. Uric acid is a breakdown product of purine nucleotides. Some individuals with gout have an accelerated rate of purine synthesis and other individuals breakdown purine nucleotides at an accelerated rate. Both conditions result in an overproduction of uric acid. A deficiency of the enzyme hypoxanthine guanine phosphoribosyl transferase (HGPRT) leads to the increased production of uric acid.

Kidney function is involved in the pathophysiology of gout because most uric acid is eliminated from the body through the kidneys. Urate undergoes both reabsorption and excretion within the renal tubules. Sluggish urate excretion by the kidney may be caused by decreased glomerular filtration of urate or an acceleration in urate reabsorption.

The presence of urate crystals anywhere triggers the acute inflammatory response as the neutrophils are attracted to phagocytose the crystals. Tissue damage occurs when the phagocytizing neutrophils release the contents of their digestive lysosomes. Lysosomal contents are released from neutrophils as they die following their life span of about 2 days, leakage after injury by biochemical reactions with ingested urate crystals, or through rupture of neutrophils during attempts to ingest exceptionally large urate crystals.

Attacks of gouty arthritis occur abruptly, usually in a peripheral joint. The primary symptom is severe pain. Approximately 50% of the initial attacks occur in the metatarsophalangeal joint of the great toe. Other involved joints are the heel, ankle, instep of the foot, knee, wrist, or elbow.

The helix of the ear is the most common site of tophi, which are the diagnostic lesions of chronic gout. Each tophus consists of a deposit of urate crystals surrounded by a granuloma made of mononuclear phagocytes that have developed into epithelial giant cells. Tophaceous deposits appear in other areas and produce irregular swellings of the fingers, hands, knees, and feet. Although the tophi themselves are painless, they often cause progressive stiffness and persistent aching of the affected joint.

Acute gouty arthritis is treated with anti-inflammatory drugs. The individual should have a low-purine diet and high fluid intake to increase urinary output. Antihyperuricemic drugs can be given to reduce serum urate concentrations.

8. **Describe examples of secondary muscular dysfunction.**

Study text pages 1606 through 1609; refer to Figure 42-33 and Tables 42-9 through 42-11.

Muscular symptoms can arise from causes unrelated to the muscle itself. These secondary muscular phenomena include contracture, stress-related muscle tension, and immobility.

Several conditions cause the muscle fibers to shorten without contracting; this is called a **contracture.** A physiologic muscle contracture occurs without muscle action potential in the sarcolemma and is explained as failure of the calcium pump even in the presence of plentiful adenosine triphosphate (ATP). A physiologic contracture is seen in McArdle disease, which is an enzyme deficiency, and in malignant hyperthermia. The contracture is usually temporary if the underlying pathology can be corrected.

A pathologic contracture is considered a permanent muscle shortening due to muscle spasm or weakness. It is associated with plentiful ATP and will occur in spite of a normal action potential. The most common form of contracture is seen in muscular dystrophy and central nervous system (CNS) injury. Contractures may also develop secondary to scar tissue contraction in the flexor tissues of a joint.

Stress-induced muscle tension has been associated with chronic anxiety as well as a variety of stress-related muscular symptoms including neck stiffness, back pain, and headache. The underlying pathophysiology presumably is caused by increased activity of the reticular-activating system and increased firing of the efferent loop of the gamma fibers that produce further muscle contraction and increased muscle tension.

Progressive relaxation training and biofeedback are possible ways to treat muscle tension. The hope is to enhance the individual's ability to relax specific muscle groups in order to relieve tension. This could reduce CNS and autonomic nervous system (ANS) arousal.

Fibromyalgia is a chronic musculoskeletal syndrome characterized by increased sensitivity to touch, the absence of systemic or localized inflammation, and fatigue and sleep disturbances. Because the symptoms are vague, fibromyalgia has often been misdiagnosed or completely dismissed by clinicians.

The etiology of fibromyalgia unlikely is caused by a single factor. The most common precipitating factors include viral illnesses, physical traumas, or stress. Low hypothalamic-pituitary axis (HPA) and locus ceruleus–norepinephrine (LC/NE) activity may be associated with fibromyalgia. Rheumatoid arthritis (RA) or systemic lupus erythematosus (SLE) may coexist if not initially present with fibromyalgia.

The prominent symptom of fibromyalgia is chronic pain. The majority of women experience pain and fatigue during more than 90% of their wakefulness. Fatigue is most notable when arising from sleep and during midafternoon. Headaches, symptoms of irritable bowel syndrome, and sensitivity to cold are reported in 50% of individuals. Almost 25% of individuals seek psychological support for depression. Anxiety, particularly in regard to their diagnosis and future, is almost universal. The only finding on examination is the presence of multiple tender points.

No one regimen of medication has proved successful for fibromyalgia. Amitriptyline can significantly improve pain tolerance, morning stiffness, and sleep quality but not tender points.

The term **disuse atrophy** describes the pathologic reduction in normal size of muscle fibers following inactivity due to bed rest, trauma, casting, or local nerve damage. Atrophy may be prevented by frequent forceful isometric muscle contractions and passive lengthening exercises.

9. Distinguish between muscle membrane abnormalities.
Study text page 1609.

The hyperexcitable membrane seen in myotonic disorders and the intermittently unresponsive membrane seen in the periodic paralyses are defects in the plasma membrane of the muscle fiber. **Myotonia** is a delayed relaxation after voluntary muscle contraction such as gripes, eye closure, or muscle percussion. It is due to the prolonged depolarization of the muscle membrane. Myotonia is seen mostly in inherited disorders. Its symptoms are mild except in myotonic muscular dystrophy where there is progressive atrophy of skeletal muscles. Myotonia is treated by drugs that reduce muscle fiber excitability.

In **periodic paralysis,** the muscle membrane is unresponsive to neural stimuli. Periodic paralysis is triggered by exercise and any process or medication that alters serum potassium. The disorder is often inherited in an autosomal dominant pattern. The flaccid paralysis does not affect the respiratory muscles. Hypokalemic periodic paralysis is triggered by high-carbohydrate meals, prolonged bed rest, or emotional stress. Oral and intravenous potassium can relieve acute attacks. A low-salt diet and diuretic drugs are useful for long-term therapy.

10. Compare the metabolic, inflammatory, and acquired toxic myopathies.
Study text pages 1610 through 1613; refer to Figures 42-34 through 42-36. See the table on page 310.

11. Identify the incidence, manifestations, treatment, and prognosis of rhabdomyosarcoma; note the status of other muscle tumors.
Study text page 1613.

The malignant tumor of striated muscle is a **rhabdomyosarcoma.** The incidence of rhabdomyosarcoma ranges from 10% to 20% of all soft tissue cancers and is highly malignant. These tumors are located in the muscle tissue of the head, neck, and genitourinary tract 75% of the time. The remainder are in the trunk and extremities.

The diagnosis of rhabdomyosarcoma is made by incisional biopsy and histologic examination of the specimen. Pleomorphic, embryonal, and alveolar types can be differentiated. The pleomorphic type is a highly malignant tumor of the extremities of adults.

Treatment consists of a combination of surgical excision, radiation therapy, and systemic chemotherapy. Cure in cases with distant metastasis is unlikely.

Metastatic tumors in muscles are rare in spite of the extensive vascular supply of skeletal muscles. It is likely that local pH or metabolic changes prevent metastatic involvement from other tumors.

309

Myopathies

Type	Causes	Manifestations
Metabolic Myopathy	Altered thyroid hormone levels change muscle protein synthesis and electrolyte balance	
	Thyrotoxicosis	Proximal weakness, paresis of extraocular muscles
	Hypothyroidism	Flabby and weak muscles, sluggish movements
McArdle disease	Absence of muscle phosphorylase, inability to catabolize glycogen or produce lactic acid	Exercise intolerance, fatigue, painful muscle cramps, muscle weakness and wasting
Acid maltase deficiency	Autosomal recessive; absence of acid maltase, accumulation of glycogen in lysosomes of muscle and other cells	Adult: similar to muscular dystrophy or polymyositis, severe respiratory muscle weakness
Pompe disease (infantile form of acid maltase deficiency)		Infant: hypotonia; areflexia; enlarged heart, tongue, and liver; early death
Myoadenylate deaminase deficiency	Absence of myoadenylate deaminase, inability to form phosphocreatine and ATP during exercise	Exercise intolerance
Carnitine palmitoyl transferase (CPT) and carnitine deficiency	Absence of CPT and carnitine; fatty acid byproducts and energy are not transported to myofibrils	CPT: mild muscular symptoms, episodes of renal failure because of myoglobinuria Carnitine: progressive muscle weakness
Inflammatory Myopathy	Infectious Tuberculosis and sarcoidosis Trichinosis Viral infections	Granulomas in muscle and other tissues Larvae from infected pork migrate to host lymphatics: pain, rash, and muscle stiffness Muscle pain and tenderness similar to symptoms of influenza
Polymyositis (generalized muscle inflammation) Dermatomyositis (polymyositis with skin lesions)	Cell-mediated (cytotoxic T cells) and humoral (autoantibodies) immune factors, human leukocyte antigen (HLA) genetic markers	Necrosis of muscle fibers; malaise; fever; muscle swelling, pain, and tenderness; lethargy; symmetric proximal muscle weakness; both diseases show dysphagia, vasculitis, Raynaud phenomenon, cardiomyopathy, fibrosis, coexisting pulmonary collagen disorders; dermatomyositis exhibits skin rash, calcinosis, and eyelid edema
Toxic Myopathy	Alcohol abuse; direct toxic effect and nutritional deficiency cause necrosis of muscle fibers	Benign cramps and pain, severe weakness, myoglobinuria and renal failure
	Antimalarial and amebicidal agents impair lysosomal processes	Generalized muscle weakness Myoglobinuria
	Sedatives and narcotics Repeated therapeutic drug injection	Local muscle fiber necrosis, fibrotic bands

Multiple Choice

Circle the correct answer for each question.

1. Tendinosis is:
   a. painful because of degradation of collagen fibers caused by repetitive stress on tendons.
   b. painful because of inflammation of tendons.
   c. a torn tendon.
   d. a complete separation of a tendon.
   e. inflammation of a tendon where it attaches to a bone.

2. In an oblique fracture, the energy or force is:
   a. twisting with the distal part unable to move.
   b. compressive and at an angle.
   c. directly to an already weakened bone.
   d. directly to the distal fragment.

3. Which is a definite sign of a fracture?
   a. Abrasion
   b. Shock
   c. Muscle spasm
   d. Unnatural alignment
   e. All of the above are correct.

4. Compartment syndromes:
   a. involve large compartments of hemorrhage.
   b. are caused by wound infection.
   c. lead to muscle ischemia.
   d. may result from myoglobinuria.
   e. Both b and c are correct.

5. The most common cause of osteomyelitis is:
   a. hematogenous spread of infection.
   b. rheumatoid disease.
   c. direct contamination of an open wound.
   d. deficiency of calcium.
   e. deficiency of vitamin D.

6. Osteoporosis is:
   a. inadequate mineralization.
   b. impaired synthesis of bone organic matrix.
   c. reduced bone mass or density.
   d. formation of sclerotic bone.
   e. None of the above is correct.

7. Osteomalacia causes:
   a. loss of bone matrix.
   b. inadequate mineralization.
   c. radiolucency.
   d. All of the above are correct.
   e. Both b and c are correct.

8. Bone tumors may originate from all *except:*
   a. epithelial tissue.
   b. cartilage.
   c. fibrous tissue.
   d. vascular tissue.
   e. mesoderm.

9. In benign bone tumors, there is:
   a. a uniform and well-defined lytic area.
   b. a moth-eaten pattern of bone destruction.
   c. abnormal bone merging with surrounding normal bone tissue.
   d. an area of partially destroyed bone adjacent to completely lytic areas.

10. An osteosarcoma is a(n):
    a. collagenic, malignant bone tumor.
    b. myelogenic, benign bone tumor.
    c. myelogenic, malignant bone tumor.
    d. osteogenic, benign bone tumor.
    e. osteogenic, malignant bone tumor.

11. The major symptom of bone cancer is a:
    a. flattering gait.
    b. persistent pain that worsens at night.
    c. lack of sensation.
    d. general swelling over a bone.
    e. coolness over a bone.

12. Giant cell tumors:
    a. affect males more frequently than females.
    b. are located in the diaphysis of a long bone.
    c. have extensive osteoblastic activity.
    d. have high recurrence rates.
    e. are multifocal.

13. Osteoporosis pathogenesis involves:
    a. nonmineralized osteoid tissue.
    b. excessive resorption of spongy bone.
    c. marrow and cortical inflammation.
    d. alteration in the OPG/RANKL/RANK system.

14. Rheumatoid arthritis begins with:
    a. inflammatory destruction of the synovial membrane and subsynovial tissue.
    b. inflammation of ligaments.
    c. destruction of the articular cartilage.
    d. softening of the articular cartilage.
    e. destruction of the joint capsule.

15. In gout:
    a. the pathogenesis is formation of monosodium urate crystals in joints and tissues.
    b. metatarsophalangeal joints are usually involved.
    c. affected individuals likely have an inherited enzyme (HGPRT) defect.
    d. the hyperuricemia can be the result of acquired chronic disease or a drug.
    e. All of the above are correct.

16. RANKL is:
    a. expressed on osteoclasts.
    b. necessary for osteoclast development.
    c. suppressive of apoptosis.
    d. a glycoprotein that activates RANK.

17. Myotonia is all *except:*
    a. delayed relaxation after voluntary muscle contractions.
    b. prolonged depolarization of the muscle membrane.
    c. mostly inherited.
    d. unresponsiveness to neural stimulation.
    e. progressive atrophy of skeletal muscle.

18. Rhabdomyosarcomas have:
    a. a poor prognosis.
    b. aggressive invasion.
    c. early, widespread dissemination.
    d. two age peaks, at 6 years and the teens.
    e. All of the above are characteristics of this sarcoma.

19. Which contributes to osteoarthritis?
    a. Collagenases
    b. Rheumatoid factor
    c. Circulating immune complexes
    d. Infections
20. Which of the following is *not* true of ankylosing spondylitis?
    a. It is a systemic immune inflammatory disease.
    b. It is characterized by stiffening or fusion of the spine.
    c. It causes instability of synovial joints.
    d. It begins with inflammation of fibrocartilage.
    e. It is manifested early by low back pain and stiffness.

21. Fibromyalgia:
    a. exhibits systemic inflammation.
    b. is characterized by increased sensitivity to touch.
    c. manifests acute pain.
    d. fatigue is most notable in the late evening.
    e. Both b and d are correct.
22. Myotonia is:
    a. hypertrophy of skeletal muscles.
    b. triggered by exercise.
    c. inherited as an autosomal dominant trait.
    d. due to prolonged depolarization of the muscle membrane.

Matching

Match the myopathy with the cause.

_____ 23. McArdle disease

_____ 24. Acid maltase deficiency

_____ 25. Polymyositis

a. hypothyroidism

b. hyperparathyroidism

c. accumulation of glycogen in lysosomes

d. unable to catabolize glycogen

e. immune system abnormality

CASE STUDY 1

Mrs. B. is a 52-year-old homemaker who complained that, "Both knees and hands have hurt for several years but are getting worse." The pain has progressively worsened and persists during rest and limits her walking, climbing stairs, and weightbearing. Her physical examination showed slight ulnar deviation of the digits and swelling of the metacarpal, phalangeal, and proximal interphalangeal joints with limited range of motion and some instability of both knees. Laboratory studies revealed the following:

CBC = normal, except for mild anemia

Rheumatoid factor = high titer

Synovial fluid analysis = turbid appearance

Radiographic examination of knees = joint narrowing on both knees, thinning of the articular cartilage, cystic areas, and bony spurs

Question

Which arthritis is Mrs. B. experiencing?
Explain your answer.

A 64-year-old female, Mrs. C.S., complains of constant back pain lasting for 4 to 6 weeks that is aggravated by activity. A review of her history and activities reveal no previous injury to her back nor bone fractures, no relief of pain when changing positions, and postmenopausal since age 48. When asked if she takes hormone replacement therapy, she replied "No, I am afraid of getting breast cancer because my mother had it and my sister has it, but my last year's mammogram was normal". She added that she was taking inhaled corticosteroids for chronic asthma; occasionally, an acute attack required systemic corticosteroids therapy and she takes no dietary supplements. Mrs. C.S. exercises little and drinks several caffeinated beverages daily.

The physical examination shows tenderness and decreased range of motion in lumbar region and no kyphosis. A radiograph of the lumbosacral spine shows osteopenia and a fracture of L2. Blood chemistries are normal with no rheumatoid factor present.

Question

What likely caused the osteopenia and what is your plan for treatment?

313

43 Alterations of Musculoskeletal Function in Children

FOUNDATIONAL KNOWLEDGE OBJECTIVE

a. Describe the processes of bone and muscle growth from birth to maturity.
Review text pages 1618 through 1620; refer to Figure 43-1.

MEMORY CHECK!

- Until adult stature is reached, growth in the length of bone occurs at the epiphyseal plate through endochondral ossification. Cartilage cells in the proximal layer of the epiphyseal plate multiply and enlarge and then are destroyed and replaced by bone at the metaphyseal side of the plate. In the shaft of new bone, the slow-growing bone is produced by accretion and is compact and dense. The longitudinal growth rate of the extremities is greater at birth than at any other time. Growth in the diameter of bone occurs by deposition of new bone on an existing bone surface. Bone matrix is laid down by osteoblasts on the periosteal surface and subsequently becomes calcified. While bone resorption occurs on the endosteal surface, endosteal resorption increases the diameter of the medullary cavity and its spongy bone. When the skeleton is mature, the epiphyseal plate is replaced by bone. This epiphyseal closure that unites the diaphysis and epiphysis (physical closure) occurs earlier in females than males because of the accelerating influence of estrogens on cartilage growth and matrix formation. Throughout life, bone is constantly being destroyed and reformed. The process is at its maximum in children about $2\frac{1}{2}$ years of age. Peak bone mass is achieved by the mid to late 20s and slowly decreases throughout life.
- The axial skeleton changes shape with growth. In a newborn, the entire spine is concave anteriorly; the child's natural posture is "curled up." In the first 3 months of life, as the ability to control the head develops, the upper or cervical spine begins to "arch" or become convex anteriorly. The normal arch in the spine begins to develop with sitting. The appendicular skeleton, or the extremities, grows faster during childhood than does the axial skeleton. The neonate has a relatively large head and long spine with disproportionately shorter limbs than an adult. By age 1 year, 50% of the total growth of the spine has occurred.
- After birth, the muscle fibers enlarge by accumulating cytoplasm. Between birth and maturity, the number of muscle nuclei in the body increases 14 times in boys and 10 times in girls. Muscle fibers reach their maximal size in girls about the age of 10 years and in boys by the age of 14 years. The length of a muscle fiber is the direct consequence of the range of movement it is called on to perform. In the infant, muscle accounts for approximately 25% of total body weight compared with 40% in the adult. The respiratory and facial muscles are well developed at birth so that the infant can perform the vital functions of breathing and sucking. Other muscle groups such as the pelvic muscle take several years to develop fully. Throughout life, the weight of the skeletal muscles can be increased by exercise. Visceral muscle fibers increase both in number and size; fiber enlargement alone can increase the bulk of visceral muscle by as much as eight times. Cardiac muscle also grows mainly by enlargement of existing fibers.

LEARNING OBJECTIVES

After studying this chapter, the learner will be able to do the following:

1. **Describe common congenital musculoskeletal defects in children.**
Study text pages 1620 through 1624; refer to Figures 43-2 through 43-4 and Table 43-1.

The most common congenital defect of the upper extremity is **syndactyly,** or webbing of the fingers. True syndactyly involves fusion of the bones and nails as well

as soft tissue; it may be associated with abnormalities of bone or neurovascular units.

Corrective surgery is deferred until the child is 6 to 12 months of age. Extra digits are best removed during the neonatal period.

Developmental dysplasia of the hip (DDH), formerly known as congenital hip dislocation, is an anomaly of the development of the proximal femur, acetabulum, or both. The hip may be subluxed, dislocatable, or dislocated. The subluxed femur maintains contact with the

315

acetabulum but is not well seated within it. Subluxation leads to early osteoarthritis. Incidence is approximately 1 in 1000 live births, with girls being affected at a rate of 6:1 compared with boys.

The exact cause of this disorder is unknown and is probably multifactorial. Risk factors include breech presentation, family history, first pregnancy, and deficient volume of amniotic fluid. Presence of other lower extremity deformities may increase the risk of DDH. Clinical findings include leg length discrepancy, limitation of hip abduction, asymmetry of gluteal folds, positive **Ortolani** and **Barlow signs,** positive Trendelenburg sign, abnormal gait, and pain. Treatment generally consists of bracing the joint in flexion and abduction. Surgery is occasionally required.

Metatarsus adductus is the most common congenital defect of the foot and is believed to be due to intrauterine positioning of the feet. In this deformity, the bones of the forefoot are inwardly rotated and may be easily flexed back into position or may be fairly fixed. Most cases are self-correcting, but the more fixed forms required physical therapy or serial casting.

In **equinovarus** or **clubfoot,** the forefoot is abducted and the hindfoot is adducted and inverted. The entire foot points downward. There are three types of equinovarus: positional, idiopathic congenital, and teratologic. Positional equinovarus appears secondary to intrauterine position while teratologic equinovarus is either neuromuscular (spina bifida) or syndromic (diastrophic dwarfism). The foot is in rigid fixation. Treatment consists of early Ponseli serial casting and frequently requires surgery for full correction.

Congenital myopathies are rare and generally exhibit mild defects in muscular development. The defects include congenital absence of muscles, hypoplasia or hyperplasia of muscles, faulty intrinsic development leading to disfigurement of fibers, and presenile degeneration. Diagnosis is confirmed by muscle biopsy and histologic appearance. Treatment is nonspecific and usually requires aggressive physical therapy programs to maximize potential.

2. **Describe the pathophysiology and common clinical features related to osteogenesis imperfecta; characterize rickets.**

Study text pages 1624 and 1625; refer to Figures 43-5 and 43-6 and Table 43-2.

Osteogenesis imperfecta is primarily a defect in collagen production resulting in easily fractured, "brittle" bones. Incidence is approximately 1 in 30,000 live births, and it is usually inherited by the autosomal dominant route but may be autosomal recessive. Types I and IV are inherited as autosomal dominant traits. Types II and III are more severe than types I and IV and are characterized by autosomal recessive patterns.

In the most severe form, fractures may occur in utero but usually do not become a problem until the child walks. Other clinical features include osteoporosis and bowed or deformed limbs. Short stature, curvature of the spine, or a bluish discoloration of the sclera also may be a feature.

Diagnosis is based on clinical findings and serologic tests. Alkaline phosphatase is elevated in all forms of the disease. Prenatal diagnosis is available through ultrasound and chorionic villus sampling. No clear benefits have been demonstrated for most therapies, bisphosphonate therapy shows promise in type III.

Rickets is caused by deficiencies in vitamin D, calcium, and usually phosphorus. It is characterized by failure of bones to become mineralized, resulting in skeletal deformity. Children with rickets often are listless and irritable and have muscle weakness. Parietal flattening occurs in the skull, calvaria become soft, cartilaginous attachments of the ribs become prominent, and the long bones of the extremities may be bowed.

3. **Describe scoliosis.**

Study text pages 1625 through 1628; refer to Figure 43-7.

Scoliosis, or lateral curvature of the spine, may be classified as (1) nonstructural occurring from causes extrinsic to the spine, such as posture, pain, or leg length discrepancy; (2) structural that is associated with vertebral rotation; or (3) idiopathic. Idiopathic scoliosis may be further classified as infantile, juvenile, or adolescent, according to age of onset. Adolescent idiopathic scoliosis is the most common. Girls most frequently have severe curvature and require treatment.

Pathophysiologic change includes shortening of ligaments on the concave side of the curve; this eventually results in vertebral deformity. The deformity is due to unequal stress on the epiphyseal centers of the vertebral bodies. Eventually, progressive deformity of the vertebral column and ribs develops. The curvature progresses most rapidly during times of rapid skeletal growth. In curvature greater than 50 degrees, the spine is mechanically unstable and the curvature will probably progress throughout life. Curvature greater than 60 degrees results in pulmonary dysfunction.

Clinical manifestations include asymmetry of hip and shoulder height, shoulder and scapular prominence, rib prominence, and posterior humping of ribs or hips. These findings are noted when the child bends forward from the waist. Diagnosis is confirmed by radiography. Treatment includes bracing of curvatures between 25 and 35 degrees in the skeletally immature but is not effective in curvatures greater than 40 degrees or in the skeletally mature. These individuals require surgery and instrumentation of the vertebrae.

4. **Describe the pathophysiology and common pathogens related to osteomyelitis in children.**

Study text pages 1628 through 1630; refer to Figures 43-8 and 43-9.

Osteomyelitis is an inflammation of the bone that occurs most frequently between 3 and 12 years of age, with a predilection for boys. In this disorder, bacteria enter the bone through the bloodstream and lodge in the medullary cavity. This is frequently where the process is halted by the immune system because of a rich supply of phagocytes in this area. In other cases, however, bacteria invade the epiphyseal plate where phagocytes are absent, and resultant infection develops. Osteomyelitis may be preceded by trauma, which may then predispose to infection. The infection usually begins as a bloody abscess in the metaphysis of the bone that ruptures under the periosteum and spreads along the shaft or into the medullary cavity. The microorganism usually gains access to the subperiosteal space through the metaphysis, which is the path of least resistance because of the porous nature of the bone in that area.

If infection occurs near a joint, the accumulated pressure of inflammatory products may cause pus and bacteria to rupture through the bone and into the joint space, causing **secondary suppurative arthritis.** The spread of infection into joint spaces is also aided because the epiphyseal plates in infants less than 1 month of age are penetrated by capillaries that communicate directly into joints. Severe infection in infants and young children rapidly leads to permanent damage of the joints and disruption of the blood supply to the bone with subsequent growth arrest.

The most common etiologic agents in osteomyelitis are *Staphylococcus aureus*, group B streptococci, and *Escherichia coli. S. aureus* is the common agent in older children; *Haemophilus influenzae* is the agent in children younger than 5 years. Gram-negative microbes account for increasing numbers of vertebrae infections; salmonella infections are associated with sickle cell disease.

Clinical presentation of the illness tends to be somewhat variable. Osteomyelitis is frequently abrupt in onset in young children and infants as the child displays signs of toxicity, fever, and refusal to move the affected limb. This process may be more subacute in older children and adults and may involve the vertebrae, whereas in young children and infants, it usually involves the long bones.

Diagnosis is usually confirmed by (1) an elevated white blood cell count, erythrocyte sedimentation rate, and C-reactive protein (CRP); (2) radiologic imaging, although findings on plain radiographs may take 2 weeks to become apparent; and (3) culture aspirations of the blood and affected tissues. Treatment includes long-term, appropriate intravenous antibiotic therapy and surgical intervention where warranted.

5. **Describe the features of juvenile rheumatoid arthritis.**

   Study pages 1630 and 1631.

   The basic pathophysiology of **juvenile rheumatoid arthritis (JRA)** is the same as that of adult rheumatoid arthritis, but JRA differs in the following points:

   a. Mode of onset has three distinct forms:
      ■ Arthritis in fewer than five joints (pauciarticular)
      ■ Arthritis in more than five joints (polyarthritis)
      ■ Systemic disease (most common)
   b. The large joints are predominantly affected.
   c. Subluxation and ankylosis of the cervical spine are common.
   d. Joint pain is not as severe as the adult type.
   e. Chronic uveitis is common.
   f. Serologic tests often detect antinuclear antibody.
   g. Serologic tests seldom detect rheumatoid factor.

   h. Rheumatoid nodules are not limited to subcutaneous tissue but are found in the heart, lungs, eyes, and other organs.

   Treatment for children with JRA is supportive but not curative, its aim being to control inflammation and other clinical manifestations of the disease and to minimize deformity.

6. **Describe the pathophysiology, evaluation, and treatment of Legg-Calvé-Perthes disease and Osgood-Schlatter disease.**

   Study text pages 1631 and 1632; refer to Figure 43-10.

   Legg-Calvé-Perthes disease (LCP) is a result of interrupted blood supply to the femoral head. It commonly occurs between 3 and 10 years of age with a peak incidence at 6 years. It is most frequently seen in boys and is self-limiting in nature, running its course in 2 to 5 years. The deformation that results is permanent. In this process, interruption of blood flow to the femoral head results in necrosis of the femoral head. Inflammation and new bone formation follow over time with a resultant flattening of the femoral head and distortion of the hip joint. The first necrotic stage lasts only a few weeks; however, the healing phase lasts from 2 to 4 years.

   The etiology of LCP is unknown, although familial occurrence is known as is a history of antecedent trauma. It is probable that an earlier synovitis causes increased hydrostatic pressure within the joint and interferes with blood flow. Birth weight tends to be low in children with LCP disease and skeletal maturation is delayed as well.

   Presentation of LCP disease may be fairly incipient, with the child complaining of lower extremity pain for weeks to months. A limp then follows, known as the Trendelenburg gait or an abductor lurch. The child frequently demonstrates pain when the hip is externally rotated while in extension.

   Diagnosis is confirmed by radiologic imaging, and treatment is accomplished with anti-inflammatory medications and bed rest for episodes of synovitis and avoidance of activities that stress the hip.

   Osgood-Schlatter disease consists of osteochondrosis of the tubercle of the tibia and often tendinitis of the patella. The mildest form of Osgood-Schlatter disease causes ischemic (avascular) necrosis in the region of the bony tibial tubercle, with hypertrophic cartilage formation during the stages of repair. In more severe cases, the abnormality involves a true apophyseal separation of the tibial tubercle with avascular necrosis. The child complains of pain and swelling in the region around the patellar tendon and tibial tubercle, which becomes prominent and is tender to direct pressure.

   The goal of treatment for Osgood-Schlatter disease is to decrease the stress at the tubercle. Often a period of 4 to 8 weeks of restriction from strenuous physical activity, especially activities requiring deep knee bending, is sufficient. If relief from pain is not achieved, a cast or knee immobilization is required, a situation that is particularly difficult if the condition is bilateral.

7. Describe cerebral palsy.

Study text pages 1632 and 1633.

Cerebral palsy (CP) is a static disorder of muscle tone and balance caused by an ischemic insult to the brain, usually perinatally. The incidence presently is 3% to 5% but is increasing with successful resuscitation of premature infants.

The diagnosis of CP can be quite subtle but is often made when gross motor milestones are not met by predicted ages. In some infants, diagnosis can be made as early as 4 months. Cognitive involvement is widely variable and is dependent on the amount of central nervous system involvement. There are classic patterns: hemiplegia involves one side of the body, diplegia usually involves the lower extremities only, and quadriplegia involves all four extremities. Quadriplegic involvement is most often associated with cognitive involvement, seizure disorder, and aphasia.

Treatment of cerebral palsy is multifaceted and undergoing constant evolution. Physical and occupational treatments and surgery are used to maximize a child's function.

8. Describe the pathophysiology, evaluation, and treatment of Duchenne muscular dystrophy; identify features of other muscular dystrophies.

Study text pages 1633, 1634, 1636, and 1637; refer to Figures 43-11 and 43-12 and Table 43-4.

The muscular dystrophies are genetically transmitted diseases characterized by progressive atrophy of groups of muscles without involvement or degeneration of neural tissue.

Duchenne muscular dystrophy is an X-linked inherited disorder that is caused by a deletion of a segment of DNA. This deletion results in an absence of dystrophin that is found in normal muscle cells. The lack of dystrophin apparently causes loss of muscle bulk and fibers. In the late stages, interstitial connective tissue and fat may replace muscle fibers.

The disease is frequently diagnosed at approximately 3 years of age when parents notice slow motor development, problems with coordination and walking, and generalized weakness. Weakness always begins in the pelvic girdle, and hypertrophy is present in the calf muscles of approximately 80% of affected children. Gower sign, a peculiar manner of standing up from a sitting position by climbing up the legs, is often evident. Within 3 to 5 years, the shoulder girdle muscle becomes involved with constant progression of the illness until cardiac involvement is seen. Pulmonary and cardiac failure may follow by the late teens.

Diagnosis is confirmed by serum enzyme studies and electromyography. Creatine phosphokinase (CPK) may be 10 times normal, and histologic examination of biopsied muscle fibers will be abnormal as well. Treatment is chiefly supportive, with the goal being to preserve function of remaining muscle groups for as long as possible.

Other less frequently occurring types of muscular dystrophy exist. Most are genetically transmitted and characterized by progressive atrophy of symmetric groups of skeletal muscles without involvement or degeneration of neural tissue. Insidious loss of strength with increasing disability and deformity occur in all forms of these disorders.

9. Characterize the childhood malignancies of osteosarcoma and Ewing sarcoma.

Study text pages 1637 through 1639.

Fortunately, most pediatric tumors are benign. These lesions include nonossifying fibroma, chondroma, simple bone cyst, aneurysmal bone cyst, aneurysmal bone cyst, osteoid osteoma, and fibrous dysplasia.

Malignant **osteosarcoma** accounts for 60% of the bone tumors in children and originates in bone-producing mesenchymal cells. Most of these neoplasms occur between the ages of 10 and 18.

Deletion of a tumor suppression gene on the long arm of chromosome 13 has been identified as part of the mechanism of causation. The oncogene *src* also has been associated with osteosarcoma.

The most common complaint is pain. Symptoms may also include cough, dyspnea, and chest pain when lung metastasis occurs.

Surgery and chemotherapy are the primary treatments for osteosarcoma. Chemotherapy is an important component of treatment because as many as 80% of children treated with surgery alone eventually develop metastatic disease. The tumor is resistant to radiation.

Ewing sarcoma is the second most common but most lethal malignant bone tumor of childhood. It probably originates from cells within the bone marrow space and does not involve bone-forming cells. Its incidence is greatest between 5 and 15 years of age; it is rare after age 30. The most common site of this tumor is the marrow of the femur, followed by the marrow of the pelvis and then the humerus.

The most common symptom is pain that increases in severity. A soft-tissue mass is often present. Ewing sarcoma metastasizes early to nearly every organ. The most common sites are the lung, other bones, lymph nodes, liver, spleen, and central nervous system.

Treatment is preoperative chemotherapy followed by radiation or surgical resection or both and continued chemotherapy for 12 to 18 months afterward. Involved sites with the best prognosis are the extremities; the worst prognosis involves tumors of the trunk and the pelvis.

10. Describe rhabdomyosarcoma of childhood.

Study text pages 1639 and 1640; refer to Table 42-6.

Rhabdomyosarcoma (RMS) is the most common sarcoma of childhood and accounts for more than 50% of soft-tissue tumors but less than 3% of all childhood cancers. RMS arises from embryonal cells that normally differentiate into mature striated muscle.

RMSs are located, in descending order of frequency, in the (1) head and neck, (2) trunk, (3) extremities, and (4) genitourinary tract. More than two thirds are diagnosed by 10 years of age, with males affected more often than females. RMS has been associated with mutation of *p53* (a tumor suppressor gene). Three oncogenes (*src*, H/K-ras, and *c-myb*) also are likely involved.

318

RMS generally appears as firm, fleshy, grayish white masses. Depending on the phase of differentiation of the rhabdomyoblast, these tumors may have round or spindle-shaped, tadpole-shaped, or multinucleated giant cells. They spread by rapid local infiltration and via the bloodstream and lymphatic system. The sites of metastases include the lungs, lymph nodes, bone marrow, liver, brain, and bone. Twenty percent of children with RMS have metastatic disease at diagnosis.

The tumors are usually painless and are detected by the presence of a palpable or visible mass. Deep-seated tumors cause functional impairment.

RMS is treated by a combination of surgery, radiation, and chemotherapy. Children with localized disease have long-term survival rates of 70% to 80%. In widespread disease, long-term survival rates drop to 20%.

Practice Examination

Fill in the Blanks

Supply the correct response for each statement.

1. Type I osteogenesis imperfecta is an autosomal _____ trait.

2. Developmental dysplasia of the hip is recognized due to limited hip _____.

3. Osteogenesis imperfecta is a defect in _____ production resulting in bone that is brittle and breaks easily.

4. _____ is a positional deformity of the foot that may be self-correcting.

5. Legg-Calvé-Perthes disease may be suspected when a positive _____ is observed.

6. _____ is an infection of bone that can be spread through the blood.

7. Treatment of equinovarus consists of early _____ serial casting.

8. Most pediatric tumors are _____.

9. Muscular dystrophies are characterized by defective _____ metabolism.

10. Cerebral palsy (CP) is a static disorder of muscle tone and balance caused by an ischemic insult to the _____, usually perinatally.

11. The disease process of Legg-Calvé-Perthes results in _____.

12. Gluteal folds in developmental dysplasia of the hip may be _____.

13. Duchenne muscular dystrophy results from a lack of _____ in muscle cells.

14. DDH is treated by bracing the hips in _____ and _____.

15. Osteosarcoma may be caused by a deletion of a _____ on chromosome 13.

Matching

Match the alteration with the outcome (choices can be used more than once).

_____ 16. Fractures present at birth

_____ 17. Elevated serum CPK

_____ 18. Positive Barlow or Ortolani maneuver or both

_____ 19. Gower sign

_____ 20. Antalgic abductor lurch

_____ 21. Subluxed, dislocated, dislocatable

_____ 22. Pain in external rotation with affected limb

_____ 23. Frequently caused by *S. aureus*

_____ 24. Defect in collagen synthesis

_____ 25. Lateral curvature of the spine

a. scoliosis

b. osteogenesis imperfecta

c. osteomyelitis

d. Legg-Calvé-Perthes disease

e. developmental hip dysplasia

f. Duchenne muscular dystrophy

Bobby is a 3-year-old white boy who was brought to a pediatrician's office where his mother states, "Bobby is clumsy, frequently falls, and has difficulty in climbing stairs." On physical examination, Bobby tends to walk on his toes, exhibits a positive Gower sign, and appears to have hypertrophy of calf muscles.

Questions

What disease is suspected?

How could the diagnosis be confirmed?

44 Structure, Function, and Disorders of the Integument

FOUNDATIONAL KNOWLEDGE OBJECTIVES

a. **Describe the skin and its layers**.
   Review text pages 1644 through 1646; refer to Figure 44-1 and Table 44-1.

MEMORY CHECK!

- The skin is the largest organ of the body; it covers the entire body and accounts for approximately 20% of the body's weight. Outer skin serves as a barrier against microorganisms, ultraviolet radiation, and loss of body temperature. It is involved in the production of vitamin D, and its touch and pressure receptors provide important protective functions and pleasurable sensations. The skin has three major layers: a superficial **epidermis,** a deeper **dermis,** and a **subcutaneous** layer.
- The subcutaneous tissue is an underlying layer of connective tissue that contains macrophages, fibroblasts, and fat cells. The lobules are separated by fibrous walls of collagen and large blood vessels.
- The epidermis grows continually by shedding its superficial layer of stratum corneum, which consists of keratinocytes and melanocytes. **Keratinocytes** produce keratin, which is a scleroprotein. Keratin is the main constituent of skin, hair, and nail cells. Keratinocytes are formed in the basal layer or stratum basale; they move upward and differentiate to form the spinous layer (stratum spinosum). Together, these two layers form the germinative layer (stratum germinativum). The cells enlarge and then become flattened, stacked, and cornified as they move to the skin surface to become the stratum corneum. Cornification (keratinization) of this layer prevents the dehydration of deeper skin layers.
- The **melanocytes** are usually located near the base of the epidermis. They synthesize and secrete the pigment melanin when exposed to sunlight in response to the melanocyte-stimulating hormone of the pituitary gland. Melanin provides a protective shield against ultraviolet radiation and determines skin color. Other cells contribute to the function of the epidermis. **Langerhans cells** migrate to the dermis from the bone marrow to provide protection against environmental antigens. **Merkel cells** are associated with touch receptors and function when stimulated by deformation of the epidermis.
- The dermis is composed of connective tissue that contains collagenous and elastic fibers. Their arrangement permits the skin to be mobile, to stretch, and to contract with body movement. Hair follicles, sebaceous glands, sweat glands, blood vessels, lymphatic vessels, and nerves are contained in the dermis. Projections of the papillary dermis interface with the epidermis and are known as **rete pegs**. The cells of the dermis include fibroblasts, mast cells, and macrophages. Fibroblasts secrete the connective tissue matrix. Mast cells release histamine and play a role in hypersensitivity reactions in the skin. Histiocytes and macrophages are phagocytic for pigments and the debris of inflammation.
- The dermal appendages include the nails, the hair, the sebaceous glands, and the eccrine and apocrine sweat glands. The **nails** are protective keratinized plates that appear at the ends of the fingers and toes. **Hair follicles** arise from the matrix that is located deep within the dermis. Hair growth begins in the bulb, with cellular differentiation occurring as the hair progresses up the follicle. Hair is fully cornified by the time it emerges at the skin surface. The **sebaceous glands** open onto the surface of the skin through a canal and secrete sebum, which is composed primarily of lipids and lubricates the skin and hair and prevents drying.
- The **eccrine sweat glands** are distributed over the body and are important in the cooling of the body through evaporation. The **apocrine sweat glands** are fewer in number and are located in the axillae, scalp, face, abdomen, and genital area.
- The blood supply to the skin is provided by the papillary capillaries (the plexus) of the dermis. Arteriovenous anastomoses in the dermis facilitate the regulation of body temperature. Heat loss can be regulated by varying blood flow through the skin by opening or closing the arteriovenous anastomoses to modify evaporative heat loss through sweat. The sympathetic nervous system regulates both vasoconstriction and vasodilation, because there are only adrenergic receptors in the skin. The lymphatic vessels of the skin arise in the dermis and drain into larger subcutaneous trunks; these vessels remove cells, proteins, and immunologic mediators.

b. Identify the changes that occur in the skin during aging.
  Review text pages 1646 and 1647.

MEMORY CHECK!

- Structurally, the skin becomes thinner, drier, and wrinkled, and it changes in pigmentation during aging. Fewer melanocytes decrease the skin's protection against ultraviolet radiation. Fewer Langerhans cells decrease the skin's immune response during aging. The thickness of the dermis decreases, and the skin becomes translucent and assumes a paper-thin quality. Loss of the rete pegs gives the skin a smooth, shiny appearance. The decreased vasculature probably contributes to the atrophy of eccrine, apocrine, and sebaceous glands, so the skin becomes drier. Loss of elastin fibers is associated with wrinkling. The collagen fibers become less flexible and decrease the ability of the skin to stretch and regain shape. Decreased cell generation, blood supply, and depressed immune responses delay wound healing in aging skin.
- Graying of hair is due to a loss of melanocytes from hair bulbs, and thinning hair occurs from a gradual decline in the number of hair follicles. As the barrier function of the stratum corneum is reduced, there is increased permeability and decreased clearance of substances from the dermis; the accumulation of such substances can cause skin irritation. Temperature regulation is less effective in the elderly, and there is increased risk for both heatstroke and hypothermia. The pressure and touch receptors and free nerve endings all decrease in number and reduce sensory perception.

c. Summarize diagnostic skin procedures.
  Refer to Table 44-2.

After studying this chapter, the learner will be able to do the following:
1. **Distinguish among the various skin lesions.**
    Refer to Tables 44-3 and 44-4.

Basic Lesions of the Skin*

Type	Characteristics	Example/Disease
Macule	A flat, circumscribed discolored lesion	Hyperpigmentation, erythema, telangiectasias, purpura
Papule	Lesions 1 cm or less in diameter because of infiltration or hyperplasia of dermis	Verruca (warts), lichen planus, nevus
Patch	Flat, irregular lesion larger than a macula	Vitiligo
Plaque	Lesions with a large surface area, larger laterally than in height	Psoriasis, eczema
Wheal	Transient lesion with well-defined and often changing borders caused by edema of the dermis	Hives, angioedema
Nodule	Palpable circumscribed lesion 1 to 2 cm in diameter located in the epidermis, dermis, or hypodermis; smooth to ulcerated	Benign or malignant tumors, foreign body inflammation, calcium deposits
Tumor	A well-demarcated solid lesion greater than 2 cm in diameter	Fibroma, lipoma, melanoma, hemangioma
Vesicle and bulla	A fluid-filled, thin-walled lesion; a bulla is a vesicle greater than 0.5 cm in diameter	Herpes zoster, impetigo, pemphigus, second-degree burns
Pustule	Lesion containing an exudate of white blood cells	Acne, pustular psoriasis
Cyst	An encapsulated mass of dermis or subcutaneous layers, solid or fluid filled	Sebaceous cyst
Comedone	Plugged hair follicle	Blackhead, whitehead
Telangiectasia	Dilated, superficial blood vessels	Rheumatoid arthritis, hepatitis
Scale	Accumulation of loose stratum corneum from cellular retention or cellular overproduction	Psoriasis
Lichenification	Thickening, toughening of the skin with accentuation of skin lines caused by scratching	Chronic dermatitis
Keloids	Elevated, irregular, progressively grows beyond the boundaries of wound; excessive collagen formation during healing	Burns, autosomal patterns dominate in dark-pigmented skin
Scar	Thin or thick fibrous tissue	Healed laceration, burn, surgical incision
Excoriation	Loss of epidermis with exposed dermis	Scratches
Fissure	Linear crack or break exposing dermis	Athlete's foot, cheilosis
Erosion	Moist, red break in epidermis, follows rupture of vesicle or bulla, larger than fissure	Chickenpox, diaper dermatitis
Ulcer	Loss of epidermis and dermis	Pressure sores,* basal cell carcinoma
Atrophy	Thinning of the epidermis or dermis caused by decreased connective tissue	Thin facial skin in elderly, striae of pregnancy
Petechiae	A circumscribed area of blood less than 0.5 cm in diameter	Thrombocytopenia
Purpura	A circumscribed area of blood greater than 5 cm in diameter	Bruises
Burrow	A narrow, raised, irregular channel	Parasitic burrowing

*Pressure ulcers develop from continuous pressure and shearing forces that occlude capillary blood flow with subsequent ischemia and necrosis. Areas at greatest risk are pressure points over bony prominences, such as the greater trochanter, sacrum, ischia, and heels.

2. Identify stimuli for pruritus.

Study text pages 1654 and 1655.

Pruritus, which is also called itching, is a symptom associated with many primary skin disorders and systemic diseases. The condition may be localized or generalized, and it may move from one location to another.

Multiple mediators can produce itching, including neuropeptides, serotonin, prostaglandins, bradykinin, or acetylcholine. Itch is carried by specific unmyelinated C-nerve fibers. Substance P, which is a neurotransmitter, causes histamine release and wheal formation with itching when injected into the skin. Small C-receptors are also sensitive to histamine released from dermal mast cells. Lymphocytes present in itching skin may be involved in the pathogenesis of itching.

The management of pruritus depends on the cause; the primary condition must be treated. Symptomatic relief can be obtained from antihistamines, tranquilizers, emollients, and topical steroids in some cases. Phototherapy with narrow band UVB and vagal nerve stimulation are emerging therapies.

3. Identify the cause and lesions of inflammatory and papulosquamous disorders of the skin.

Study text pages 1655 through 1660; refer to Figures 44-5 through 44-14.

Inflammatory and Papulosquamous Skin Disorders

Disorder	Cause	Lesions
Inflammatory Disorders		
Allergic contact dermatitis	Allergen binds to carrier protein to form a sensitizing antigen, T-cell hypersensitivity	Pruritic (itching) vesicles
Atopic dermatitis	IgE, T lymphocytes, and monocytes interact	Red, weeping crusts, lichenification
Stasis dermatitis	Venous stasis and edema	Initial erythema and pruritus; then, scaling, petechiae, and hyperpigmentation
Irritant contact dermatitis	Nonimmunologic inflammation, due to chemicals	As above
Seborrheic dermatitis	Inflammatory cytokines from T cells	Scaly plaques with mild pruritus
Papulosquamous Disorders		
Psoriasis*	Autoimmune T cell mediated, inflammatory cytokines from T cells, B cells, and macrophages	Thick, silvery, scaly, erythematosus, plaque surrounded by normal skin; rapid shedding of epidermis, pruritic
Pityriasis rosea	Unknown (virus?)	Pruritus, demarcated salmon-pink scale within a plaque
Lichen planus	Unknown, hepatitis virus (exposure to drugs?)	Nonscaling, violet-colored pruritic papules
Acne vulgaris	Increased activity of sebaceous glands or sebum inability to escape through the narrow opening	Comedones
Acne rosacea	Unknown, associated with chronic flushing and sensitivity to sun	Erythema, papules, pustules, telangiectasia
Systemic lupus erythematosus (SLE)	Genetic or autoimmunity	Systemic manifestations of connective tissue degeneration; stiffness and pain in hands, feet, or large joints; patchy atrophy of skin with diffuse facial erythematous rash in a butterfly pattern over the nose and face
Discoid lupus erythematosus (subset of SLE)	Immune response to unknown antigen; response to UV light with development of self-reactive T and B cells, preinflammatory cytokines, and decreased regulatory T cells	Cutaneous manifestations of elevated red plaque with brown scale, hair loss, urticaria (hives), telangiectasia

*Guttate psoriasis follows streptococcal respiratory infections. Pustule psoriasis appears as noninfectious blisters of pus. Erythrodermic psoriasis is often accompanied by itching. Psoriatic arthritis is associated with arthritis of hand, feet, knee, and ankle joints.

324

4. **Contrast the vesiculobullous disorders of pemphigus and erythema multiforme.**
   Study text pages 1660 through 1662; refer to Figures 44-15 and 44-16.
   Pemphigus is a rare, chronic, blister-forming disease of the skin and oral mucous membranes with several different types that include pemphigus vulgaris, pemphigus foliaceus, and pemphigus erythematosus. The blisters form in the epidermis and occur deeply in pemphigus vulgaris and superficially in pemphigus foliaceus and pemphigus erythematosus.

   Pemphigus is an autoimmune disease caused by circulating IgG or IgA autoantibodies and C3 complement. Serum autoantibodies are formed, and these react with the intracellular cement, which is the substance that holds the epidermal cells together. The antibody reaction likely causes the intraepidermal blister formation and acantholysis, which is the loss of cohesion between epidermal cells.

   Pemphigus vulgaris is the most common form of the disease. Oral lesions precede the onset of skin blistering, which is more prominent on the face, scalp, and axilla. Over time, flaccid bullous lesions appear, and these rupture easily and leave crusty, denuded skin. In the less severe forms of **pemphigus foliaceus** and **pemphigus erythematosus,** oral lesions are usually absent, and erythema with localized crusting, scaling, and occasional bullae develops. **Bullous pemphigoid** is a blistering disease that resolves rapidly.

   In the diagnosis of pemphigus, immunofluorescence demonstrates the presence of antibodies at the site of blister formation. The primary treatment for pemphigus is systemic corticosteroids, usually in high doses, to suppress the immune response during acute episodes or when there is widespread involvement.

   Erythema multiforme is an acute, recurring, inflammatory disorder of the skin and mucous membranes. It is associated with allergic or toxic reactions to drugs or microorganisms such as *Mycoplasma pneumoniae* and herpes simplex. Immune complex formation and deposition of C3, IgM, and fibrinogen around the superficial dermal blood vessels, basement membrane, and keratinocytes can be observed in most individuals with erythema multiforme. The characteristic "bull's eye" lesion occurs on the skin surface, with a central erythematous region surrounded by concentric rings or alternating edema and inflammation. A vesiculobullous form is characterized by mucous membrane lesions and erythematous plaques on the extensor surfaces of the extremities.

   The most common forms expressed in children and young adults are **Stevens-Johnson syndrome** and toxic epidermal necrolysis, wherein there are numerous erythematous, bullous lesions on both the skin and the mucous membranes. The bullous lesions form erosions and crusts when they rupture. The mouth, air passages, esophagus, urethra, and conjunctiva may be involved. Severe forms of the disease involving the lung or kidney can be fatal. Mild forms of the disease require no treatment, because they are self-limiting; underlying infections should be treated.

5. **Identify the causes and lesions of cutaneous infections.**
   Study text pages 1662 through 1665; refer to Figures 44-17 through 44-21 and Tables 44-6 and 44-7. See the table on page 326.

6. **Contrast vasculitis, urticaria, and scleroderma.**
   Study text pages 1665 through 1667; refer to Figures 44-22 through 44-24.
   Vasculitis, which is also called angiitis, is an inflammation of the blood vessels. Cutaneous vasculitis develops from the deposit of immune complexes in small blood vessels as a response to drugs, allergens, or streptococcal or viral infection. The deposit of immune complex likely activates complement, which is chemotactic for polymorphonuclear leukocytes. The lesions appear as palpable purpura and progress to hemorrhagic bullae with necrosis and ulceration because of occlusion of the vessel. Identifying and removing the antigen is the first step in treatment. Prednisone may be used if symptoms are severe.

   Urticarial lesions are most commonly associated with type I hypersensitivity reactions to drugs, certain foods, intestinal parasites, or physical agents. The lesions are mediated by histamine release, which causes the endothelial cells of skin blood vessels to contract and increase their permeability. The fluid from the vessel appears as wheals, welts, or hives. Antihistamines usually reduce the hives and provide relief from itching. Corticosteroids, epinephrine, or β-adrenergic agonists may be required for treatment of severe attacks. Chronic urticaria is likely an autoimmune disease.

   Scleroderma is sclerosis of the skin that may remain localized to the skin, or it may affect the visceral organs. If systemic, scleroderma involves the connective tissue and affects the kidneys, gastrointestinal tract, and lungs. The cutaneous lesions can cover the entire skin, but they are most often on the face, hands, neck, and upper chest.

   The lesions exhibit massive deposits of collagen with fibrosis, inflammatory reactions, vascular changes in the capillary network with decreased capillary loops, and dilation of the remaining capillaries. Autoimmunity and an immune reaction to toxic substances are possible initiating mechanisms of the disease. Autoantibodies often can be recovered from the skin and serum of individuals with scleroderma.

   In individuals with this condition, the skin is hard, hypopigmented, taut, and tightly connected to the underlying tissue. An immobile, mask-like appearance with incomplete opening of the mouth is caused by the tightness of the facial skin. The fingers become tapered and flexed, and fingertips are lost from atrophy. Calcium deposits develop in the subcutaneous tissue and erupt through the skin. When progression to body organs occurs, death is caused by subsequent respiratory failure, renal failure, cardiac dysrhythmias, or obstructions or perforations of the esophagus or intestine. There is no specific treatment, and 50% of individuals die within 5 years of the onset of scleroderma.

325

Cutaneous Infections

Type	Cause	Lesions
Folliculitis	Bacterial infection of hair follicles usually by *Staphylococcus aureus*	Pustules with surrounding erythema
Furuncle	Infection from folliculitis spreading into dermis	Deep, red, firm, painful nodule changes to fluctuant and tender cystic nodule
Carbuncle	Collection of infected hair follicles	Erythematous, painful mass that drains through many openings
Cellulitis	Infection of dermis and subcutaneous tissue; extension from skin wound, ulcer, furuncle, or carbuncle	Erythematous, swollen, and painful area
Erysipelas	Group A streptococci	Systemic manifestations, red spots progress to pruritic vesicles
Impetigo	Coagulase positive staphylococci, β-hemolytic streptococci	Serous and purulent vesicles that rupture and crust
Herpes simplex virus (HSV-1)	Primary and secondary infectious (sensory nerve ganglion latency) on nongenital sites	Clusters of vesicles on a type 1 erythematous base that become purulent and crusty ("cold sore" or "fever blister")
Herpes simplex virus type 2 (HSV-2)	Primary and secondary infection (sensory nerve ganglion latency) genital herpes	Vesicles that progress to painful ulceration, pruritus, and weeping more commonly transmitted sexually
Herpes varicella-zoster virus	Varicella (chickenpox), primary infection	Varicella: pink papules with reddened halo that is dry and crusty
	Zoster (shingles), secondary infection	Zoster: erythema followed by grouped vesicles along a unilateral dermatome that later crusts
Warts (verrucae)	Human papillomavirus	Round, elevated with a rough, grayish surface
Venereal warts	Human papillomavirus	Sexually transmitted; causes cervical cancer
Tinea capitis (scalp) Tinea pedis (athlete's foot) Tinea corporis (ringworm) Tinea cruris ("jock itch")	Dermatophytes (fungi) that invade and thrive on keratin	Scaling and erythema, vesicles and fissures
Candidiasis	*Candida albicans* (yeastlike fungus) changes from a skin and mucous membrane commensal to an opportunistic pathogen	Thin-walled pustule with inflammatory pruritic base

NOTE: There are eight types of DNA herpes simplex virus (HSV). Among the eight types are included cytomegalovirus; Epstein-Barr; and human types 6, 7, and 8 (Kaposi sarcoma–associated). The varicella vaccine may boost immunity in the elderly.

7. Identify diseases caused by insect bites.

Study text pages 1667 and 1668.

Ticks are significant vectors of transmitted diseases including Rocky Mountain spotted fever and other rickettsial diseases, tularemia, and Lyme disease. Ticks embed their heads in the skin to obtain blood. If mouthparts remain in the skin after tick removal, a persistent nodule may develop. As ticks feed, they enlarge to many times their normal size, and they may release toxins or transmit microorganisms. In most instances, tick bites cause only a papular urticaria.

Lyme disease is a multisystem inflammatory disease caused by *Borrelia burgdorferi* and transmitted by tick bites. The disease occurs in stages. Soon after the bite, a rash with or without flulike illness occurs. Within days to weeks, secondary erythema migrans, arthralgias, meningitis, neuritis, and carditis develop. Persistent infection continues for years and involves arthritis, encephalopathy, and polyneuropathy. Serologic tests may confirm the diagnosis subsequent to the presence or history of tick bite. Antibiotics are used for treatment with good success in the early stages, but the response may be slow. Vaccines are available for prevention.

Mosquitoes are responsible for malaria, yellow fever, dengue fever, filariasis, and St. Louis encephalitis. Mosquitoes can bite through thin, loose clothing and are attracted by warmth and perspiration. The edema, pruritus, and papular lesions are caused by the insertion of a blood tube by a female mosquito. Irritating salivary secretions also contain anticoagulants. Reactions vary depending on the sensitivity of the victim.

Several species of **flies** are bloodsuckers. The bite of a small female fly produces immediate pain, erythema, and vesicles. Itching and vesicular reactions may persist for weeks. The fiercest bloodsuckers are the larger types like the horseflies and deerflies; these produce painful, bleeding bites because of their large mouthparts. The bites produce urticaria that may be accompanied by weakness, dizziness, and wheezing.

8. Compare the benign lesions of the skin.

Study text pages 1668 and 1669; refer to Figures 44-25 through 44-27.

Seborrheic keratosis is a benign proliferation of basal cells that produces elevated smooth or warty lesions. Multiple lesions are seen on the chest, back, and face in older people. The color of the lesions varies; it may be tan to waxy yellow, flesh-colored, or dark brown-black, and the lesions are often oval and greasy-appearing, with a hyperkeratotic scale. Lesion size varies from a few millimeters to several centimeters. Cryotherapy with liquid nitrogen is an effective treatment, and the lesions usually slough within 2 to 3 weeks of treatment.

A **keratoacanthoma** is a benign, self-limiting tumor that arises from hair follicles. It usually occurs on sun-exposed surfaces, and it develops in individuals who are between 60 and 65 years of age. The lesion develops in stages. The proliferative stage produces a rapid-growing, dome-shaped nodule with a central crust. In the mature stage, the lesion is filled with whitish-colored keratin. The mature lesion requires differentiation from squamous cell carcinoma. The involution stage usually occurs over a 3- to 4-month period as the lesion regresses. Although the lesion will resolve spontaneously, it can be removed surgically.

Actinic keratosis is a premalignant lesion found on skin surfaces that have been exposed to the ultraviolet radiation of the sun. The lesions can progress to squamous cell carcinoma. The prevalence is highest in individuals with unprotected, light-colored skin. The lesions appear as pigmented patches of rough, adherent scale, and surrounding areas may have telangiectasia. Freezing with liquid nitrogen provides quick, effective treatment. Excisions provide tissue for biopsy.

Nevi, which are also called moles, are pigmented or nonpigmented lesions that form from melanocytes; they start developing when a person is between 3 and 5 years of age. During early development, the melanocytes accumulate at the junction of the dermis and epidermis and become macular lesions. Over time, the cells move into the dermis and become nodular and palpable. Nevi may appear anywhere on the skin, either singly or in groups, and they vary in size. Nevi may undergo transition to malignant melanoma; if irritated, they can be excised.

9. Describe malignant skin lesions.

Study text pages 1669 through 1673; refer to Figures 44-29 through 44-34; refer to Tables 44-8 and 44-9.

Cancerous Skin Lesions

Type	Cause	Growth Rate/Metastasis	Appearance
Basal cell carcinoma	Ultraviolet radiation exposed skin, *p53* gene	Slow growth/Almost never metastasize, invasive destruction	Smooth appearance with rolled border, depressed center, small surface blood vessels
Squamous cell	Ultraviolet exposed skin, *p53* gene	Moderate growth/Some metastasize	Rough, firm nodule with an indurated base, bleeding ulcer
Malignant melanoma	Genetic predisposition, solar radiation and hormones, precursor nevi	Fast growth/Highly invasive, rapid metastasis if thickness is greater than 1.5 mm	Nevi that exhibit asymmetry, steroid border irregularity, color variation, larger than 6 mm in diameter
Kaposi sarcoma	Herpes virus, angiogenic-inflammatory state, immunodeficient state, genetics—Black, Jewish, or Italian males	Slow spread through skin/Some aggressive change	Multifocal purplish, brown vascular macules that develop into plaques and nodules that may be painful and pruritic, may affect gastrointestinal and respiratory tracts

NOTE: Treatment consists of surgery, electrodesiccation, radiation, or cryosurgery. For malignant melanomas, wide and deep excisions and removal of lymph nodes are required. For basal cell and squamous cell skin cancers, cure is virtually assured with early detection and treatment. The survival is poor for malignant melanoma because it metastasizes quickly; prognosis is better if lesion is <1 mm in thickness. The general response to treatment of Kaposi sarcoma is poor. New antiretroviral therapies for AIDS are decreasing the incidence of KS.

10. Characterize frostbite.

Study text page 1673.

Frostbite is an injury to the skin that is caused by exposure to extreme cold. The mechanism of injury appears to be direct cold injury to cells, indirect injury from ice crystal formation, or impaired circulation from anoxia to the exposed area. Frozen skin becomes white or yellowish, is waxy, and has no sensation of pain. With mild frostbite during rewarming, there is redness and discomfort followed by a return to normal in a few hours.

Cyanosis and mottling develop and are followed by redness, swelling, and burning pain on rewarming in more severe cases. The most severe cases result in gangrene and loss of the affected part. Frostbite may be classified by depth of injury. Superficial frostbite includes partial skin freezing and is known as first-degree frostbite; full-thickness skin freezing is second-degree frostbite; full-thickness skin and subcutaneous freezing is third-degree frostbite. Immersion in a warm-water bath until the frozen tissue is thawed is the best treatment. Pain during the thawing period is severe and should be treated with potent analgesics. Gentle cleansing and avoidance of pressure on the skin should be maintained during healing. Amputation of necrotic tissue is delayed until a clear line of demarcation appears.

11. Define the terms used to describe disorders of the hair and nails.

Study text pages 1673 and 1674.

Male-pattern alopecia is an inherited form of irreversible baldness in which hair is lost in the central scalp and the recession of the temporofrontal hairline occurs. **Female-pattern alopecia** is a thinning of the central hair of the scalp that begins in women who are between 20 and 30 years of age. **Alopecia areata** is a patchy loss of hair that is usually associated with autoimmune T cell–mediated chronic inflammatory disease. **Hirsutism** is a male pattern of hair growth in women; it may be normal or the area of hair growth is androgenic sensitive. **Paronychia** is an inflammation of the cuticle that can be acute or chronic and that is usually caused by staphylococci, streptococci, or occasionally by *Candida*. **Onychomycosis** is a fungal infection of the nail plate; the plate turns yellow or white and accumulates hyperkeratotic debris.

PRACTICE EXAMINATION

Multiple Choice

Circle the correct answer for each question.

1. The major differentiating cell of the epidermis is the:
   a. mast cell.
   b. histiocyte.
   c. keratinocyte.
   d. melanocyte.
   e. fibroblast.

2. The dermis is composed of all of the following except:
   a. melanocytes.
   b. collagen.
   c. elastin.
   d. mast cells.
   e. fibroblasts.

3. Which of the following does not occur as the skin ages?
   a. Increased number of melanocytes
   b. Decreased number of Langerhans cells
   c. Loss of rete pegs
   d. Loss of elastin fibers
   e. Depressed immune response

4. The application of KOH and low heat to skin scrapings on a glass slide identifies:
   a. chronic bacterial infections.
   b. vasculitis.
   c. antibodies.
   d. fungi.
   e. None of the above is correct.

5. The cause of atopic dermatitis is:
   a. unknown.
   b. venous stasis.
   c. increased activity of sebaceous glands.
   d. mast cell, T cell, and monocyte interaction.
   e. nonimmunologic inflammation in response to chemicals.

6. The skin lesion of psoriasis is a:
   a. nonscaling, violet-colored, pruritic papule.
   b. comedone.
   c. pruritic vesicle.
   d. erythematous, butterfly-shaped rash.
   e. thick, scaly, erythematous plaque.

7. A circular, demarcated, salmon-pink scale within a plaque is characteristic of:
   a. psoriasis.
   b. seborrheic dermatitis.
   c. acne rosacea.
   d. pityriasis rosea.
   e. lichen planus.

8. The Nikolsky sign is seen in:
   a. herpes simplex infections.
   b. pemphigus.
   c. erythema multiforme.
   d. Stevens-Johnson syndrome.
   e. Both c and d are correct.

9. The cause of impetigo is:
   a. *Staphylococcus aureus.*
   b. group A streptococci.
   c. coagulase-positive staphylococci.
   d. β-hemolytic streptococci.
   e. All of the above are correct.

10. The usual, more common transmission mode of herpes simplex type 2 is by:
    a. fomites.
    b. kissing and touching.
    c. sexual encounters.
    d. contaminated food or water.
    e. b, c, and d are correct.
11. Of the benign tumors of the skin, keratoacanthomas are characterized by:
    a. the proliferation of basal cells.
    b. hyperkeratotic scales.
    c. origination from hair follicles.
    d. a proliferative stage that produces a nodule with a central crust.
    e. Both c and d are correct.
12. Which of the following are most likely to undergo malignant transition?
    a. Seborrheic keratosis and keratoacanthoma
    b. Seborrheic keratosis and actinic keratosis
    c. Nevi and keratoacanthoma
    d. Nevi and actinic keratosis
    e. None of the above is correct.
13. The likely cause of Kaposi sarcoma is:
    a. solar radiation.
    b. steroidal hormones.
    c. precursor nevi.
    d. immunodeficiency/herpesvirus association.
    e. keratinization.

14. Squamous cell carcinoma of the skin is manifested as:
    a. irregular pigmentation.
    b. elevated, firm lesions.
    c. a smooth, pearly lesion with multiple telangiectasia.
    d. multifocal, purplish brown macules.
15. An untreated basal cell carcinoma:
    a. metastasizes frequently.
    b. often involves regional lymphatics.
    c. usually ulcerates and involves local tissue.
    d. grows rapidly.
    e. eventually requires removal of nearby lymph nodes.
16. Which of the following malignant skin lesions metastasizes most quickly?
    a. Basal cell carcinoma
    b. Squamous cell carcinoma
    c. Malignant melanoma
    d. Kaposi sarcoma
17. Onychomycosis is:
    a. a fungal infection of the nail plate.
    b. caused by staphylococci or streptococci.
    c. an inflammation of the cuticle.
    d. None of the above is correct.

Matching

Match the lesion with its descriptor.

_____ 18. Macule

_____ 19. Pustule

_____ 20. Scale

_____ 21. Wheal

a. hardened, adherent serum

b. changed color, not raised or depressed

c. accentuated skin lines caused by scratching

d. exudate of white blood cells

e. flaky, accumulated stratum corneum

f. ridge-like, reddened elevation caused by edema and congestion

Match the lesion with the example of disease/disorder.

_____ 22. "Bull's eye"

_____ 23. Telangiectasia

_____ 24. Purpura

_____ 25. Dermatome-grouped vesicles

a. rheumatoid arthritis

b. bruise

c. erythema multiforme

d. shingles

e. psoriasis

f. pemphigus

Chapter **44** **Structure, Function, and Disorders of the Integument**

Mr. E. is a 36-year-old, fair-haired, light-skinned individual who owns a garden nursery. He had the habit of removing his shirt in order to obtain a "nice suntan" as he worked in his nursery. One evening as he was showering, his wife noticed that a mole on his back, under his belt, was getting larger and darker. She asked him to see a dermatologist; he said it was the same and decided not to see a physician. A very charismatic neighbor said, "I have a salve that will remove the mole and avoid the need for surgery." Mr. E. used the salve, but the mole became larger and darker and its border became irregular.

Questions

Should Mr. E. be concerned about the changes occurring in his mole; if so, why?

What therapy is best for Mr. E.?

What determines his prognosis?

45 Alterations of the Integument in Children

FOUNDATIONAL KNOWLEDGE OBJECTIVES

a. Identify the structures of the integumentary system and describe their function.
Refer to Figure 44-1 and Table 44-1.

MEMORY CHECK!

- See the study guide's narrative for Foundational Knowledge Objective **a** in Chapter 44.

b. Identify diagnostic skin procedures.
Refer to Table 44-2.

MEMORY CHECK!

- See the study guide's narrative for Foundational Knowledge Objective **c** in Chapter 44.

LEARNING OBJECTIVES

After studying this chapter, the learner will be able to do the following:

1. Describe acne vulgaris.
Study text pages 1680 and 1681; refer to Figure 45-1.

Acne vulgaris is the most common of the skin diseases and affects 85% of the population between the ages of 12 and 25 years. The incidence of acne is the same in both genders; severe disease affects males more often. Genetics may determine the susceptibility and severity of the disease. **Acne conglobata** is a highly inflammatory form of severe disfiguring acne with formation of communicating cysts and abscesses beneath the skin.

Acne develops primarily on the face and upper parts of the chest and back from sebaceous follicles. The follicles have many large sebaceous glands, a small vellus hair, and a dilated follicular canal that is visible on the skin surface as a pore. In **noninflammatory acne**, the comedones are open (blackheads) or closed (whiteheads) and the accumulated material causes follicular distension and thinning of follicular canal walls. **Inflammatory acne** develops in closed comedones when follicular walls

rupture and expel sebum into the surrounding dermis and initiate inflammation.

The causes are abnormal keratinization of follicular epithelium, excessive sebum production, and proliferation of *Propionibacterium acnes*. Androgenic hormones increase the size and productivity of the sebaceous glands. Sebum and bacterial accumulation produce inflammation of the dermis as the follicle ruptures.

Topical treatment, including benzoyl peroxide, salicylic acid, and tretinoin, is used because it is the least invasive. Use of systemic therapies, including antibiotics, sex hormones, and corticosteroids may be may be used if topicals fail. Acne surgery, including comedo extraction, intralesional steroids, and cryosurgery may be useful. Severe scarring may be treated with dermabrasion or subincision.

2. Differentiate between atopic and diaper dermatitis in infants and children.
Study text pages 1681 and 1682; refer to Figures 45-2 and 45-3.

Atopic dermatitis, or eczema, is an inflammation of the skin. There is an increased incidence of 75% to 80% in individuals who have allergies and reactive airways (asthma). Onset usually is in infancy, with 85% of cases occurring by 5 years of age. Positive allergy tests to food and inhaled allergens, increased serum IgE levels, and eosinophilia are common findings. Local cytokines and chemokines, abnormalities of memory and helper T cells, multiple roles of IgE, and infectious agents are all likely causal factors. Th2 cytokine expression also contributes to reduction in antimicrobial peptides and reduced filaggrin expression. Alterations in filaggrin protein leads to a defect of the epidermal barrier that causes transepidermal water loss and allows easy penetration of pathogens and allergens through the skin and a systemic hyperimmune response.

In infants, the rash appears primarily on the face, scalp, trunk, and extensor surfaces of the arms and legs. In older children, the rash tends to be on the neck, antecubital and popliteal fossae, and hands and feet. Lichenification is more common in adults with chronic eczema. Treatment includes avoiding known irritants, hydration of the skin, antihistamines to relieve pruritus, and topical steroids to decrease inflammation. Antibiotics or antifungal agents may be necessary for secondary skin infections.

Diaper dermatitis is an inflammation of the skin in the diaper area that is caused by many factors, including

331

lengthy exposure to wet and soiled diapers. It mostly is localized in the perineal area but may extend from the abdomen to the thighs and usually affects infants and young children. Diaper dermatitis is characterized by an erythematous rash of varying degrees of severity and often is complicated by a secondary fungal infection caused by the microorganism *Candida albicans*. The characteristic rash of *C. albicans* is very erythematous and papular and is associated with **papulovesicular satellite lesions.**

The best treatment is preventive by keeping the perineal area clean and dry with frequent diaper changes and routine hygiene. Topical barriers may become necessary once the rash develops. If *C. albicans* is present, a topical antifungal agent should be included in the treatment.

3. Categorize and characterize the infectious processes of impetigo.

Study text page 1683; refer to Figure 45-4.

Impetigo is a common contagious bacterial skin infection in children and is either a bullous or, more commonly, vesicular form.

4. Describe the etiology and pathophysiology of staphylococcal scalded-skin syndrome.

Study text page 1684; refer to Figure 45-5.

Staphylococcal scalded skin syndrome (SSSS) is the most serious staphylococcal infection affecting the skin and usually occurs in infants and children younger than 5 years. SSSS is caused by virulent group II staphylococci, which produce an exfoliative toxin that attacks desmoglein and adhesion molecules, causing a separation of the skin just below the granular layer of the epidermis. The toxins are usually produced at body sites other than the skin. Infection often begins in the throat or chest and arrives at the epidermis through the circulatory system. Newborns are at a high risk because of their lack of immunity.

The clinical symptoms begin with fever, malaise, rhinnorrhea, and irritability followed by generalized erythemas with exquisite tenderness of the skin. The erythema spreads from the face and trunk to cover the entire body except the palms, soles, and mucous membranes.

5. Compare tinea capitis and tinea corporis; describe thrush.

Study text pages 1684 and 1685; refer to Figure 45-6.

Diagnosis of fungal infections is confirmed by culture and histologic studies. Lesions are treated with oral or topical antifungals. Healing in uncomplicated cases usually requires 10 to 14 days.

Candida albicans is part of the normal skin flora in certain individuals that invades susceptible tissue sites if the predisposing factors are not eliminated. This organism penetrates the epidermal barrier because of its keratolytic proteases and other enzymes. *C. albicans* attracts neutrophils to skin sites of invasion and generates inflammation by activation of the complement system. Thrush is the presence of Candida in the mucous membranes of the mouth of infants and, less frequently, adults.

Thrush is characterized by white plaques or spots in the mouth that lead to shallow ulcers. The underlying

Characteristics of Impetigo

	Bullous	Vesicular
Etiologic agent	*Staphylococcus aureus* produces an exfoliative toxin	*Streptococcus pyogenes*, which can combine with staphylococci
Source	Other infected individuals or contaminated objects	Other infected individuals, contaminated objects, insect bites
Regional lymphadenitis	Uncommon	Common
Treatment	Systemic and topical antibiotics	Systemic and topical antibiotics
Potential complications	Uncommon	Acute glomerulonephritis

Comparison of Fungal Infections

	Tinea Capitis	Tinea Corporis
Etiologic agent	*Microsporum canis, Trichophyton tonsurans*	*Microsporum canis, Trichophyton mentagrophytes*
Source	*M. canis* from cats, dogs, or rodents; *T. tonsurans* from humans	*M. canis* and *T. mentagrophytes* from kittens or puppies
Lesion	Circular, slight erythema, scaling raised border	Oval or round with scale, central clearing mild erythema or ringworm
Diagnostic test	KOH examination	KOH examination
Treatment	Oral antifungals (topicals do not penetrate hair bulb)	Topical antifungals

mucous membrane is red and tender and may bleed when the plaques are removed. Treatment is with oral antifungal washes. Simultaneous treatment of nipple infection or vaginitis in the mother is helpful in reducing *C. albicans* surface colonization of the infant.

6. **Describe the infections in children caused by poxviruses, papovaviruses, and herpesviruses.**

Study text pages 1685 through 1688; refer to Figures 45-7 through 45-9 and Table 45-1.

Molluscum contagiosum is a contagious, viral disease characterized by a 1- to 5-mm diameter, pearlescent, dome-shaped lesions that may appear anywhere on the body but most frequently affect the face, trunk, and extremities. The lesions are not inflamed. It is self-limiting, although recurrence is common, particularly if the child manipulates the lesions. Treatment options include topical, oral, and surgical approaches although no treatment is universally effective.

Rubella, or 3-day measles, is a common communicable disease of children and young adults caused by an RNA virus that enters the bloodstream through the respiratory tract. The incubation period is between 14 and 21 days. A faint pink to red coalescing maculopapular rash develops on the face and spreads to the trunk and extremities 1 to 4 days after the prodromal symptoms. Women of childbearing age are immunized if their antibody titers are low, and pregnancy should be avoided for 3 months after vaccination because the attenuated virus may remain for this time period. Pregnant women who have rubella early in the first trimester may have a fetus develop congenital defects. There is no specific, only supportive, treatment. Recovery is spontaneous. Vaccination for rubella is usually combined with vaccines for mumps and measles (rubeola) This vaccine is identified as MMR.

Rubeola, or red measles, is a contagious disease of children transmitted by direct contact with droplets from infected persons. Rubeola is caused by an RNA paramyxovirus having an incubation period of 7 to 12 days. Prodromal symptoms are followed within 3 to 4 days by an erythematous maculopapular rash over the head that spreads distally over the trunk, extremities, hands, and feet. Early lesions blanch with pressure, but do not do so as the rash fades. Pinpoint white spots surrounded by an erythematous ring develop over the buccal mucosa and are known as Koplik spots. Most children recover completely, but measles encephalitis occurs in about 1 in 800 cases. There is no specific treatment for measles.

Roseola likely is a viral infection; it is seen most often in infants between the ages of 6 months and 2 years. There is a sudden onset of fever that lasts for 3 to 5 days. After the fever, an erythematous macular rash lasts for about 24 hours; it is primarily over the trunk and neck. Usually there is no treatment.

Chickenpox is a highly contagious disease of early childhood and is primarily spread by droplet transmission from an infected person to others. Household infection rates approach 90% in susceptible individuals. The incubation period is approximately 14 days, with infected persons contagious for approximately 24 hours prior to the onset of the rash and for 5 to 6 days after the rash appears. Chickenpox is usually an illness of late winter or early spring. The first signs of illness are pruritus or itching or the appearance of vesicles. There may be no prodromal symptoms.

Characteristically, the rash undergoes a process of maturation with lesions starting as macules that progress to superficial papules and vesicles, which then rupture and heal. The rash lasts for 4 to 5 days and may consist of up to 300 lesions distributed over the body. Complications from chickenpox are fairly rare but may include pneumonia due to the varicella virus. Treatment is symptomatic and consists of cool baths, wet dressings, and oral antihistamines.

Herpes zoster (shingles) occurs mainly in adults, but approximately 5% of cases are in children younger than 15 years. The chickenpox virus persists for life in sensory nerve ganglia and reactivates to cause herpes zoster. The zoster consists of groups of vesicles situated on an inflammatory base that follows the course of a sensory nerve. The base of the lesion appears hemorrhagic, and some may become necrotic and ulcerative. In children, the thorax is the site of distribution of the lesions. Therapy is similar to that for chickenpox unless it is disseminated zoster or there is ophthalmic involvement; then, acyclovir is indicated. A quadrivalent vaccine, MMRV, which combines the attenuated virus MMR vaccine with the addition of varicella (chicken pox) has been approved for children ages 1 to 12 years.

7. **Compare and contrast the infestations of scabies and lice; characterize flea and bedbug bites.**

Study text pages 1688 through 1690; refer to Figures 45-10 through 45-12. See the table on page 334.

Flea bites produce a pruritic wheal with a central puncture site and occur in clusters in areas of tight-fitting clothing. Bedbugs are blood-sucking parasites that live in cracks of floors, furniture, or bedding and feed at night. They produce pruritic wheals and nodules.

8. **Compare and contrast the congenital vascular disorders.**

Study text pages 1690 through 1692; refer to Figures 45-13 and 45-14. See the table on page 334.

9. **Describe other dermatoses seen in young children.**

Study text page 1692; refer to Figure 45-15.

Miliuria is characterized by small pruritic papules or vesicles resulting from prolonged sweating because of obstruction of sweat duct openings in infants. **Erythema toxicum neonatorum** is a benign accumulation of macules, papules, and pustules appearing at birth or 3 to 4 days later that spontaneously resolve within a few weeks.

Toxic epidermal necrolysis (TEN) is a severe, but rare, drug reaction to NSAIDs, sulfonamides, and anticonvulsants, resulting in epidermal apoptosis and detachment that is increasing in children. Blisters and bullae form; the entire epidermis may shed, leaving open, weeping, painful areas. Treatment requires intensive burn management, and the offending drug must be discontinued.

333

Insect Infestations

	Scabies (mite)	Pediculosis (lice)
Etiologic agent	*Sarcoptes scabiei*	*Pediculus capitis* (head) *Pediculus corporis* (body) *Phthirius pubis* (pubic)
Transmission	Contact with infested person or object (clothing, bedding)	Contact with infested person or object (hat, clothing)
Symptoms	Severe pruritus and burrows in the intertriginous areas	Pruritus, ova (nits) may be seen on hair shafts, mature lice may be seen
Cause of symptoms	Sensitization to larva buried in the skin	Irritation from toxic saliva from lice bites
Treatment	Permethrin/lindane, treatment of exposed persons and infected objects	Permethrin/lindane, treatment of exposed persons and infested objects

Vascular Disorders

	Strawberry Hemangioma	Cavernous Hemangioma	Port-Wine Stain	Salmon Patches
Description	Raised vesicular	Raised vesicular with larger mature vessels	Flat, becomes papular and cavernous	Macular, most common
Manifestations	At birth or emerges in 3 to 5 weeks	At birth	At birth or in a few days	At birth
Color	Bright red (capillary projections)	Bluish, in distinct border	Pink to dark reddish purple	Pink, distended dermal capillaries
Location	One lesion on head, neck, or trunk	Head, neck	Face and other body surfaces	Nape of neck, forehead, upper eyelid
Growth	Initially rapid then at child's rate of growth	Rapid first 6 months, matures at 1 year	Does not fade	Fades in 1 year
Involution	Begins by 12 to 16 months, complete by 5 to 6 years	Begins by 6 to 12 months, complete by 9 years	N/A	Macular, most common
Treatment	None	May require surgery, laser surgery, or liquid nitrogen depending on location of lesion	Crysosurgery, laser surgery	None

PRACTICE EXAMINATION

Fill in the Blanks

Supply the correct response for each statement.

1. Acne vulgaris is caused by keratinization of follicular epithelium and excessive _____.

2. Impetigo is contracted by _____ contact and contaminated objects.

3. Molluscum contagiosum is a _____ viral infection.

4. Atopic dermatitis is a form of _____.

5. Staphylococcal scalded-skin syndrome is a disease usually preceded by a(n) _____ infection.

6. Tinea capitis must be treated with _____ agents.

7. Salmon patches are common and _____ over time.

8. Port-wine stains _____ by adulthood.

9. Acute glomerulonephritis can be a complication of _____ impetigo.

10. The microorganism that causes bullous impetigo is _____.

Matching

Match the lesion or condition with the disorder (choices may be used more than once).

_____ 11. Viral skin infection contracted during the first decade of life

_____ 12. Positive allergy tests, increased IgE, and eosinophilia

_____ 13. Erythematous lesions in the perineal area with secondary papulovesicular lesions

_____ 14. Raised, erythemic, scaling lesions on the scalp

_____ 15. Dome-shaped lesions ranging from 1 cm to 5 cm on the extremities without pruritus

_____ 16. Macules, fever, itching, papules, and rupturing and healing vesicles

_____ 17. Crusted lesion

_____ 18. Mite burrowing in the stratum corneum

_____ 19. Present at birth or shortly after birth

_____ 20. Entire skin sloughing

_____ 21. Nits on hair shaft

_____ 22. Chronic condition with acute exacerbations, pruritus, thick leathery skin

_____ 23. Oval or circular lesions, peripheral spreading, central clearing (ringworm)

_____ 24. Action of an epidermolytic toxin

_____ 25. Parasitic in nature, epidemic in elementary schools

a. staphylococcal scalded-skin syndrome

b. tinea capitis

c. atopic dermatitis

d. pediculosis

e. diaper dermatitis with *Candida albicans*

f. chickenpox

g. erythema toxicum neonatorum

h. impetigo

i. molluscum contagiosum

j. scabies

k. tinea corporis

L.D. is a 4-year-old white boy who is brought to a physician assistant's office with a "runny" nose that started about 1 week ago but has not resolved. He has been blowing his nose quite frequently and "sores" have developed around his nose. His mother states, "The sores started as 'big blisters' that rupture; sometimes, a scab forms with a crust that looks like "dried maple syrup" but continues to seep and drain." She is worried because the lesions are now also on his forearm. L.D.'s past medical and family histories are normal. He has been febrile but is otherwise asymptomatic. The physical examination was unremarkable except for moderate, purulent rhinorrhea and 0.5- to 1-cm diameter weeping lesions around the nose and mouth and on the radial surface of the right forearm. There is no regional lymphadenopathy.

Questions

What is the likely name and cause of these lesions?

Why have these lesions spread to L.D.'s arm?

46 Shock, Multiple Organ Dysfunction Syndrome, and Burns in Adults

FOUNDATIONAL KNOWLEDGE OBJECTIVES

a. Establish the determinants of blood pressure.

MEMORY CHECK!

- See this study guide's narrative for Foundational Knowledge Objective **e** in Chapter 30.

b. Describe the skin and its layers.

MEMORY CHECK!

- See this study guide's narrative for Foundational Knowledge Objective **a** in chapter 44.

LEARNING OBJECTIVES

After studying this chapter, the learner will be able to do the following:

1. **Illustrate the impaired cellular metabolism that occurs in shock.**
   Study text pages 1696, 1697, and 1699; refer to Figure 46-1. See flow chart on page 338.

Shock is a condition in which the cells are not receiving adequate oxygen or unable to use oxygen. This failure results in the widespread impairment of cellular metabolism. Any factor that alters heart function, blood volume, or blood pressure can cause shock. Ultimately, shock, irrespective of its cause, progresses to organ failure and death unless compensatory mechanisms or clinical intervention reverse the process.

Without glucose, there is a shift to glycogenolysis (breakdown of glycogen to glucose), gluconeogenesis (glycogen formation from fatty acids and proteins rather than from glucose), and lipolysis (fat breakdown) as alternatives for fuel generation. Gluconeogenesis uses proteins necessary for cellular structure, function, repair, and replication leading to more impairment of cellular metabolism. Lipolysis decreases serum protein transport. Gluconeogenesis increases lactic acid, uric acid, and ammonia levels; interstitial edema; and impaired immunity. Anaerobic metabolism activates the inflammatory response, decreases circulatory volume, and decreases pH.

2. **Classify the different types of shock by etiology. Identify the mechanisms of vasodilation and proinflammatory mediators.**
   Study text pages 1699 through 1704 and 1706 and 1707; refer to Figures 46-2 through 46-7 and Table 46-1. See the table on page 338.

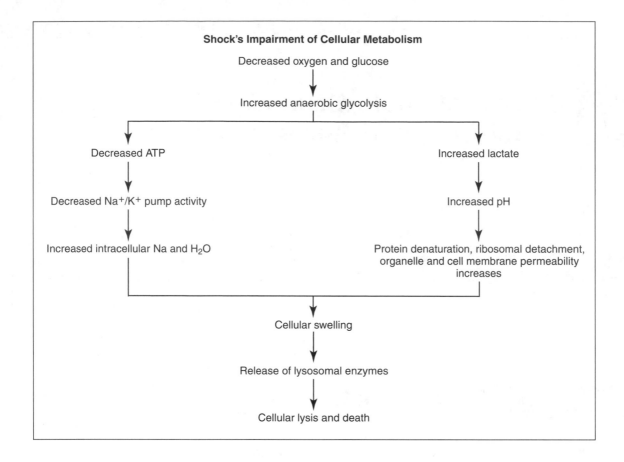

Types of Shock

Type	Etiology
Cardiogenic (heart failure)	Myocardial ischemia, myocardial infarction, congestive heart failure, myocardial or pericardial infections, arrhythmias, excessive right ventricular afterload, drug toxicity
Hypovolemic (insufficient intravascular fluid volume)	Loss of whole blood plasma or interstitial fluid, fluid sequestration
Neurogenic (neural alterations of vascular tone)	Imbalance of sympathetic or parasympathetic stimulation of vascular smooth muscle leading to vasodilation,* decreased systemic vascular resistance smooth muscle
Anaphylactic (immunologic alterations)	Hypersensitivity leads to vasodilation and peripheral pooling
Septic (infectious processes)	Bacteremia and triggering substances released by the bacteria including endotoxins from gram-negative bacteria, lipoteichoic acids and peptidoglycans from gram-positive bacteria, and superantigens cause the host to initiate a proinflammatory response; many proinflammatory mediators† promote vasodilation; then a compensatory host anti-inflammatory response with its mediators follows; now, a mixed antagonistic response between inflammatory and anti-inflammatory mediators leads the host into multiple organ dysfunction syndrome (MODS)

NOTE: Traumatic shock combines features of hypovolemic shock and septic shock.

*Vasodilation is caused by inactivation of vasodilatory mechanisms and failure of constrictor mechanisms. Unregulated nitric oxide causes dephosphorylation of myosin leading to vasodilation. Nitric oxide synthesis and metabolic acidosis activate the potassium channels of the plasma membrane of vascular smooth muscle. This prevents calcium, which mediates norepinephrine and angiotensin II–induced vasoconstrictors, from entering the cell.

†Proinflammatory mediators include tumor necrosis factor, IL-1, IL-6, IL-8, IL-15, platelet activating factor, arachidonic acid metabolites, leukemia inhibitory factor, nitric oxide, and many kinins. Anti-inflammatory mediators include IL-4, IL-10, IL-11, IL-13, transforming growth factor B, colony-stimulating factors, soluble tumor necrosis factor receptor, IL-1 receptor antagonist, protein C, and endogenous glucocorticoids.

3. **Briefly diagram the common events found in all types of shock, and relate the events to the signs and symptoms of shock. Identify treatments for different types.**

Refer to Figures 46-1 through 46-7.

Treatment for cardiogenic shock begins with treatment of heart failure or at least enhancement of cardiac output. If hypovolemia is the cause of shock, hemorrhage and other causes of fluid loss must be stopped. In neurogenic shock as a result of spinal cord trauma, stabilization of the spine and surrounding tissue is a beginning, and pain usually can be decreased to a level at which neurally mediated decreases of systemic vascular resistance (SVR) cease. The initial treatment for anaphylactic shock begins with eradication of the infective agent, usually with antimicrobials.

After the underlying cause or condition is corrected as far as possible, treatment thereafter is supportive. Intravenous fluid is administered to expand intravascular volume, except in cases of cardiogenic shock, which require diuresis to reduce preload. Supplemental oxygen is always given. Cardiotonic drugs are given early in cardiogenic shock and given later in other forms of shock. Steroid use in septic shock remains unproven, although there is evidence that low-dose therapy improves mortality. Stress ulcer prophylaxis and gastric tonometry (to measure splanchnic blood flow) are imperative because the gut is one of the drivers of the septic syndrome.

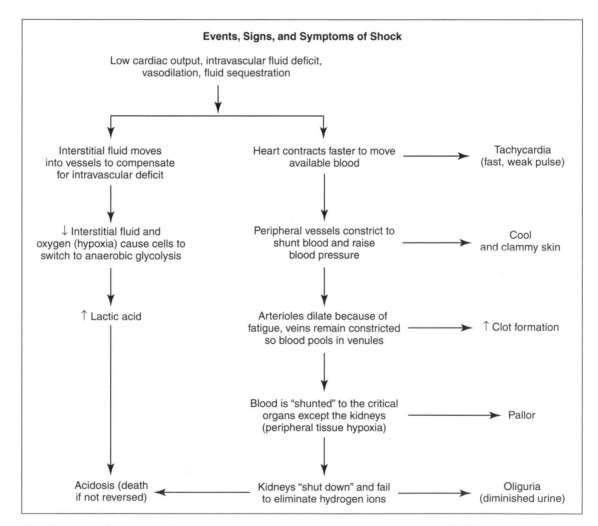

Events, Signs, and Symptoms of Shock

NOTE: The scoring of the severity of illness is accomplished by the sequential organ failure assessment (SOFA) and the predisposition-infection-response-organ (PIRO) dysfunction staging system.

4. Describe the pathophysiology and illustrate the sequence of events in multiple organ dysfunction syndrome.

Study text pages 1707, 1708, and 1710 through 1714; refer to Figure 46-8 and Table 46-2.

Multiple organ dysfunction syndrome (MODS) is the progressive failure of two or more organ systems resulting from a systemic inflammatory response after a severe illness or injury. The inflammatory response can be triggered by sepsis, necrotic tissue, surgical trauma, burns, adult respiratory distress syndrome, acute pancreatitis, and other severe injuries.

Primary MODS is the immediate local or mild systemic response to the triggering event or illness. It primes the inflammatory system. Secondary MODS is the uncontrollable, excessive **systemic inflammatory response syndrome (SIRS)** that develops after a latent period and results in organ dysfunction.

Multiple organ dysfunction involves the stress response; release of complement, coagulation, and kinin proteins; changes in the vascular endothelium; and numerous inflammatory processes mediated by substances released by activated neutrophils and macrophages. The consequences of the release of inflammatory mediators in MODS are vasodilation, increased vasopermeability, and selective vasoconstriction resulting in maldistribution of blood flow; hypermetabolism; myocardial depression; and hypoxic injury to cells. Cellular hypoxia and acidosis impair cellular metabolism, leading to organ dysfunction.

Clinical manifestations of the development of MODS are general during the first 24 hours: low-grade fever, tachycardia, tachypnea, dyspnea, and altered mental status. Over the next several days, beginning with the lungs, individual organ systems show signs of failure. People at greatest risk for developing MODS are elderly individuals, those with significant tissue injury or preexisting disease, and those in whom resuscitation from the initiating illness or injury has been delayed or inadequate. Mortality from MODS is very high: 45% to 55% for failure of two organ systems, 80% for failure of three or more organ systems, and nearly 100% if the failure of three or more organs persists longer than 4 days.

At present, the therapeutic management of MODS consists of prevention or removal of triggering mechanisms and support of individual organs. Surgery may be required to débride and drain the infectious process. A combination of powerful antibiotics, continous oxgenation, fluid therapy, and enteral feeding are required. Recent scientific knowledge about inflammatory mediators has led to many promising future therapies for MODS.

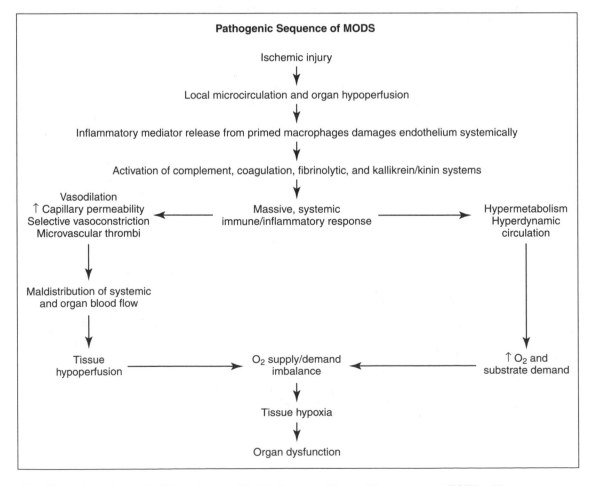

Pathogenic Sequence of MODS

Ischemic injury
↓
Local microcirculation and organ hypoperfusion
↓
Inflammatory mediator release from primed macrophages damages endothelium systemically
↓
Activation of complement, coagulation, fibrinolytic, and kallikrein/kinin systems
↓

Vasodilation
↑ Capillary permeability
Selective vasoconstriction
Microvascular thrombi
← Massive, systemic immune/inflammatory response → Hypermetabolism Hyperdynamic circulation
↓
Maldistribution of systemic and organ blood flow
↓
Tissue hypoperfusion → O₂ supply/demand imbalance ← ↑ O₂ and substrate demand
↓
Tissue hypoxia
↓
Organ dysfunction

NOTE: The scoring of the severity of illness is accomplished by the sequential organ failure assessment (SOFA) and the predisposition-infection-response-organ (PIRO) dysfunction staging system.

5. Identify organ failures and their manifestations observed in MODS.

Refer to Box 46-2 and the box below.

Organ Abnormalities Seen in Shock	
Organ Tissue	**Symptoms and Signs**
Brain	Lethargy, confusion, stupor
Kidneys	Azotemia, impaired drug excretion, oliguria, edema, acidosis
Lungs	Dyspnea, orthopnea, pulmonary hypertension, tachypnea, rales, pleural effusions
Liver	Jaundice, abdominal distention, muscle wasting, bleeding, enlargement, tenderness, ascites
Skin	Cold, pale, cyanotic, perspiring extremities, impaired heat loss, dependent pitting edema
Gut	Ascites, constant fullness, diarrhea, mucosal ulceration, bleeding

NOTE: The scoring of the severity of illness is accomplished by the sequential organ failure assessment (SOFA) and the predisposition-infection-response-organ (PIRO) dysfunction staging system.

6. Characterize burns according to the extent of injury.

Study text pages 1714 through 1717; refer to Figures 46-9 through 46-13 and Table 46-3.

7. Characterize the cardiovascular and cellular response to burn injury.

Study text pages 1717 through 1722; refer to Figures 46-14 through 46-19 and Table 46-4.

The immediate physiologic consequence of a major burn injury involves the profound, life-threatening hypovolemic shock that occurs in conjunction with cellular and immunologic disruption within a few hours of injury. The severity of burn shock is directly proportional to the extent of the total body surface area (TBSA) burned. Burns that involve 20% to 40% of TBSA in adults or 8% to 25% of TBSA in children require cardiovascular support with intravenous fluid.

Within minutes of a major burn injury, the capillary bed opens not only in the burn area but also in the entire capillary system; this increased capillary permeability leads to the ensuing **hypovolemic shock** and massive

Characteristics of Burn Injury

	First Degree	Second Degree		Third Degree
		Superficial Partial Thickness	**Deep Partial Thickness**	**Full Thickness**
Morphology	Destruction of epidermis only	Destruction of epidermis and some dermis	Destruction of epidermis and dermis	Destruction of epidermis, dermis, and subcutaneous tissue
Skin function	Yes	No	No	No
Tactile and pain sensors	Yes	Yes	Diminished	No
Blisters	Present after 24 hours	Present within minutes	May or may not appear, a flat dehydrated layer that lifts off in sheets	Blisters are rare: a flat dehydrated layer that lifts off easily
Appearance of wound after initial débridement	Skin peel after 24 to 48 hours, normal or slightly red	Red to pale ivory, moist surface	Mottled with areas of waxy white, dry surface	White, cherry red, or black; may contain visible thrombosed veins; dry, hard leathery surface
Healing time	3 to 5 days	21 to 28 days	30 days to many months, excision and grafting	Will not heal, may close from edges with secondary healing if wound is small; excision and grafting
Scarring	None	May be present, Influenced by genetic predisposition	Highest incidence, influenced by genetic predisposition	Scarring minimized by early excision and grafting, influenced by genetic predisposition

Chapter **46 Shock, Multiple Organ Dysfunction Syndrome, and Burns in Adults**

edema. If the profound hypovolemic shock is not treated, irreversible shock and death may occur within a few hours.

Burn shock resuscitation to replace normal intravascular volume involves the infusion of intravenous fluid at a rate faster than the loss of circulating volume fluid for 24 hours after burn injury. The massive edema associated with burn shock is an iatrogenic complication, but failure to administer resuscitation fluids results in irreversible hypovolemic shock and death. The most reliable criterion to use to determine the adequate resuscitation of burn shock is the urine output. If the individual does not have adequate urine output, sufficient fluid is not being administered. As burn shock ends, fluid administered remains in the circulating volume and is reflected as increased urine output.

Major burn injury affects the entire physiologic system; however, survival depends on its ultimate impact at the **cellular level.** The cellular response to burn injury has a metabolic response and an immunologic response. The cellular dysfunction of burn injury involves the disruption of transmembrane potential and sodium-potassium pump impairment and includes the loss of intracellular magnesium and phosphate and elevated serum lactate dehydrogenase (LDH) levels.

Metabolic reactions to the stress of a major burn injury involve systemic alterations of the sympathetic nervous system and other homeostatic regulators. Catecholamines are found in elevated amounts in both the serum and urine of burned individuals. Cortisol, glucagon, and insulin levels are elevated and increase gluconeogenesis, lipolysis, and proteolysis.

Burn injury induces an almost immediate **hypermetabolic state** that persists until wound closure; there is a persistent elevation of core body temperatures. Evaporative water loss and surface cooling are not the primary stimuli for the hypermetabolic state; rather, the hypermetabolism is related to an increase and resetting of the hypothalamic thermal regulatory set point. A reflex arc mobilizes neural and/or hormonal afferent stimuli to the hypothalamus, and this produces a catecholamine response that is manifested as hypermetabolism, hyperthermia, and hyperglycemia; gluconeogenesis is promoted. Vasodilation, increased capillary permeability, and edema facilitate healing of the local area by transporting both heat and glucose preferentially to the wound.

The extensive **evaporative water loss** may be 20 times normal during the early phase of injury. It is a heat-consuming process, and the energy need is met in part by increased visceral heat production. Hypothalamic function alterations cause the elevation of human growth hormone (hGH) serum levels and hyperglycemia.

A hepatic response to burn injury is characterized by alterations in the clotting factors. A **hypercoagulable** state develops, and this is manifested by elevated plasma fibrinogen concentration in the presence of shortened prothrombin time (PT) and activated partial thromboplastin time (PTT).

These systemic alterations occur because of the cutaneous inflammatory response process, and they are believed to facilitate wound repair. The neural component of this alteration is in response to a sympathetic reaction that releases catecholamines in large amounts.

In individuals who survive burn shock, **immunosuppression** and increased susceptibility to potentially fatal systemic burn wound sepsis develop. Chemical mediators released during immune response cause peripheral vasodilation, pulmonary vasoconstriction, increased capillary permeability, and local tissue ischemia in the burn wound.

The translocation of microbes and endotoxins across the intestinal wall may be a mechanism of infection that leads to septic shock following burn injuries and other major trauma. Natural resistance to infection in burn wounds depends on the nonspecific immune system and relies on the ability of phagocytic cells to leave the bloodstream, migrate to the site of infection, and ingest and kill microorganisms. The burned individual's serum contains an inhibitor of complement conversion that leads to decreased opsonization of bacteria and less polymorphonuclear neutrophil chemotaxis. Individuals with altered immunocompetence who are burned are at an additional risk for complications.

Treatment of major burns involves meticulous wound management, adequate fluids and nutrition, early surgical excision and grafting, modulation of the hypermetabolic state, and pain management. Skin replacement includes sheets of acellular dermal matrix that can be used with thin, meshed autografts or cultured epithelial autografts.

PRACTICE EXAMINATION

Multiple Choice
Circle the correct answer for each question.

1. Neurogenic shock is caused by all *except:*
   a. endogenous glucocorticoids.
   b. decreased vascular resistance.
   c. vasodilation.
   d. endotoxins.

2. Without glucose as a cellular fuel, there is a shift to:
   a. decreased lactate levels.
   b. better immunologic responses.
   c. gluconeogenesis
   d. lipogenesis.

3. Metabolic acidosis activates the plasma membrane potassium channels of vascular smooth muscle. This prevents _____ from entering the cell.
   a. nitric oxide
   b. vasoconstrictors
   c. norepinephrine
   d. angiotensin II
   e. b, c, and d are correct.

4. To compensate for intravascular fluid deficit, peripheral vessels constrict and cause:
   a. tachycardia.
   b. cool and clammy skin.
   c. clots.
   d. oliguria.

342

5. The pathogenic sequence of MODS is:
   1. organ hypoperfusion
   2. O_2 supply/demand imbalance
   3. SIR
   4. endothelia damage
   5. complement activation
   6. ischemic injury
      a. 1, 2, 3, 4, 5, 6
      b. 1, 3, 6, 2, 4, 5
      c. 3, 1, 6, 4, 2, 5
      d. 6, 1, 4, 5, 3, 2
      e. None of above is correct.

6. Shock is a complex pathophysiologic process that involves all of the following events *except:*
   a. decreased blood perfusion to the kidneys.
   b. acidosis.
   c. rapid heart rate.
   d. polyuria.
   e. anaerobic glycolysis.

7. In which of the following types of burn does skin function continue?
   a. First degree
   b. Superficial partial thickness
   c. Deep partial thickness
   d. Full thickness

8. A burn that destroys the epidermis and dermis is a:
   a. first-degree burn.
   b. superficial partial-thickness burn.
   c. deep partial-thickness burn.
   d. full-thickness burn.

9. Hypovolemic shock in severely burned individuals is the result of:
   a. dilation of the capillaries.
   b. increased capillary permeability.
   c. increased peripheral resistance.
   d. Both a and b are correct.
   e. a, b, and c are correct.

10. In individuals who survive burn shock, increased wound sepsis is due to:
    a. altered complement conversion.
    b. translocation of microbes and endotoxins across the intestinal wall.
    c. inability of phagocytes to migrate to the site of infection.
    d. a, b, and c are correct.
    e. Both b and c are correct.

Fill in the Blanks
Supply the correct response for each statement.
11. Shock impairs cellular _____.

12. Shock progresses to _____ unless compensation or intervention reverses the process.

13. Septic shock infectious processes promote _____.

14. Hypoxia causes cells to "switch" to _____.

15. In shock, blood is "shunted" to all of the critical organs except the _____.

16. Fluid sequestration can cause _____ shock.

17. Decreased Na^+/K^+ pump activity leads to increased _____ and _____.

18. The microcirculation, particularly its _____, has a central role in the pathogenesis of MODS.

19. Anaphylactic shock causes vasodilation and results in _____ and tissue edema.

20. Hypermetabolism initially is a compensatory mechanism to meet the body's increased demands for energy in _____.

21. When kidneys "shut down" in shock, _____ develops.

22. As peripheral vessels constrict to shunt blood to critical organs, _____ and _____ skin is observed.

23. In shock, interstitial fluid moves into vessels to compensate for _____ deficit.

24. Pooling of blood in venules leads to increased _____ formation.

25. _____ and _____ are the most common causes of MODS.

Chapter **46** **Shock, Multiple Organ Dysfunction Syndrome, and Burns in Adults**

Mr. K.S., a 30 year-old man, had a routine laparoscopic appendectomy. After discharge while at home, he experienced increasing abdominal girth, a fever, tachypnea with dyspnea, and tachycardia. His surgeon was unresponsive to telephone calls requesting an explanation of his distress; so, his wife took him to the emergency department of the hospital, where he was admitted as an in-patient. All his clinical signs were verified as well as pronounced ascites, hypotension, and diminished mental status.

Laboratory values were reported:

Low bicarbonate levels, neutrophilia with many band cells, bacteremia, elevated creatinine, and hyperglycemia.

Question

What do you suspect as the cause of these signs and symptoms and what needs to be done?

Mr. E. is a 26-year-old white man who sustained severe burns while welding an automobile gasoline tank that had been removed from a truck. Mr. E.'s friend, for whom the welding was being done, took him immediately to a regional burn center located 20 miles away. On admission to the burn unit, it was determined from information provided by his friend that Mr. E. neither smokes cigarettes nor drinks alcohol and likely has never been seriously ill or had any surgical operations. His family history was noncontributory.

Initial assessment revealed that Mr. E. had received full-thickness burns on his face, to both of his arms and hands bilaterally and circumferentially, and to the anterior trunk; the burned total body surface area (TBSA) was 35%.

Question

What are the immediate and major concerns of the burn unit?

47 Shock, Multiple Organ Dysfunction Syndrome, and Burns in Children

FOUNDATIONAL KNOWLEDGE OBJECTIVE

a. Identify the determinants of blood pressure.
See this study guide's narrative for Foundational Knowledge Objective **e** in Chapter 30.

b. Identify normal pediatric vital signs and circulating blood volumes.
Refer to Tables 47-1 and 47-5.

Learning Objectives

After studying this chapter, the learner will be able to do the following:

1. Describe childhood shock.
Study text pages 1727 and 1728.

Shock in children is most often the result of hemorrhage, severe dehydration, progressive heart failure, or sepsis. It also may complicate the care of the child with pulmonary failure, drug toxicity, electrolyte or acid-base imbalances, arrhythmia, or multiple organ failure.

Childhood shock is present when there are signs of poor systemic perfusion regardless of the blood pressure; shock may be present with normal, high, or low blood pressure. When blood pressure is appropriate for age but inadequate for tissue perfusion, the child is in **compensated shock.** If shock is associated with hypotension, the child is in **decompensated shock.** Oxygen delivery may be inadequate because arterial oxygen content or cardiac output is low, or there are increased metabolic requirements or impaired cellular utilization of oxygen. **Multiple-organ dysfunction syndrome (MODS)** can develop as a complication of sepsis, cardiopulmonary arrest, congenital heart disease, liver and bone

marrow transplants, or trauma, and the signs of organ failure develop within days.

2. Describe the types of shock in children and its treatment.
Study text pages 1728 through 1730 and 1732 through 1735 and 1737 through 1741; refer to Figure 47-1 and Tables 47-2 through 47-4 and 47-6 through 47-8.

Hypovolemic shock is the most common type of shock in children. **Relative hypovolemia** may be caused by an increase in the vascular space relative to intravascular volume. This relative hypovolemia is associated with **distributive shock** (the vasodilation of sepsis, anaphylaxis, neurogenic shock, or beta-adrenergic drug toxicity). **Neurogenic shock** is caused by loss of vasomotor tone after severe head or spinal cord injury. The translocation of extravascular fluid to a location that is neither intravascular nor intracellular, as is edema, is termed **"third spacing" of fluids.** Clinical manifestations of hypovolemic shock include tachycardia, cool extremities, delayed capillary refill, and oliguria. Neurogenic shock is characterized by warm skin, hypotension with low diastolic blood pressure, and poor systemic perfusion.

Cardiogenic shock is present when impaired myocardial function compromises cardiac output. It is observed after cardiovascular surgery or with inflammatory diseases of the heart, such as cardiomyopathy and myocarditis. It is also found in children with obstructive congenital heart disease and those with drug toxicity or severe electrolyte of acid-base imbalances. Adrenergic compensatory responses produce tachycardia, peripheral vasoconstriction, and constriction of the splanchnic arteries to divert flood flow from the skin, kidneys, and gut to maintain blood flow to the heart and brain. The child's

MEMORY CHECK!

Normal Pediatric Values

	Infant	Child	Adolescent
Heart rate (beats per min)	100–160	65–110	60–90
Respiratory rate (breaths per min)	30–60	18–30	12–16
Systolic blood pressure (mmHg)	87–105	97–112	112–128
Diastolic blood pressure (mmHg)	53–66	57–71	66–80
Circulating blood volume (ml/kg body weight)	75–80	70–75	65–70

extremities are cool with delayed capillary refill, and the skin may be mottled.

In **septic shock,** sepsis often is caused by nosocomial infections. Sepsis and its complications result from activation of biochemical and physiologic cascades that lead to formation or activation of cytokines and protein systems that result in vasodilation (TNF), increased capillary permeability (interleukins), maldistribution of blood flow, and cardiovascular dysfunction, causing an imbalance between proinflammatory and anti-inflammatory mediators. Tumor necrosis factor levels are directly related to mortality in newborns and children with meningitis and sepsis. Sepsis is a systemic response to infection presenting as systemic inflammatory response syndrome (SIRS). SIRS is present when the child demonstrates two or more of following: fever or hypothermia, tachycardia, tachypnea with respiratory alkalosis, and alterations in the white blood cell count. The newborn often develops hypothermia rather than fever as sign of infection and may develop bradycardia instead of tachycardia.

Treatment for childhood shock cautiously maximizes oxygen delivery while minimizing oxygen demand. The child should be kept warm. Immediate resuscitation that includes fluid replacement, administration of blood or blood components, and management of electrolyte and acid-base imbalances is essential.

3. Describe reperfusion and inflammatory injury.

Study text page 1737.

Reperfusion injury is cellular injury that is caused by the restoration of physiologic concentrations of oxygen to cells that have been exposed to injurious but nonlethal hypoxic conditions. Reperfusion injury generates highly **reactive oxygen intermediates** such as free oxygen radicals and superoxides that damage cell membranes, denature proteins, and disrupt chromosomes. The amount of free oxygen radicals produced is directly related to the severity and duration of the ischemic event. The process is most likely to affect endothelial cells of the microvasculature, which causes MODS and contributes to the compromise of organ perfusion following shock resuscitation.

An **ischemic insult** activates monocytes and macrophages and contributes to the release of inflammatory mediators or cytokines, including TNF, the interleukins (IL-1, IL-6, and IL-8) and platelet activating factor (PAF). These, in turn, contribute to vasodilation, increased capillary permeability, and altered platelet function. The ultimate result is a maldistribution of blood flow and a compromise in organ perfusion as seen in MODS. Signs of organ system failure include, but are not limited to, lactic acidosis, oliguria, and an acute alteration in mental status.

Acidosis may be the most sensitive indicator of inadequate systemic perfusion in children. The development of a metabolic acidosis indicates the presence of inadequate tissue oxygenation. Hypotension is a late sign of shock in infants and children and often indicates cardiovascular collapse.

4. Characterize the differences that exist in children related to the etiology of burn injury, growth and development, pathophysiology, and clinical course.

Study text pages 1741 through 1750; refer to Figures 47-2 through 47-12 and Table 47-9.

Burns in children are often the result of inadequate supervision, curiosity, inability to escape the burning agent, or intentional abuse. **Scald injuries** commonly are seen in the very young child and result from exposure to hot water or other hot liquids. A child's skin is thinner and more susceptible to injury than adult skin. The kitchen is a common site of burn injury; pulling over dishes or appliances containing hot liquids happens. It is estimated that from 6% to 20% are the result of **child abuse** by scalding. **Flame burns** that involve flammable liquids (notably gasoline), are more common in older children. Risk-taking factors in young males can lead to electrical burns.

The use of the standard rule of nines results in inaccurate calculation of the percentage of total body surface area (TBSA) burned in children. A modified rule of nines deducts 1% from the head and adds 0.5% to each leg for each year of life after 2 years of age.

Major thermal trauma involves all body systems, and the consequences of injury include shock, infection, hypermetabolism, organ failure, MODS, and functional limitations. These effects can be magnified in the pediatric population because of physiologic immaturity and age-related variations in treatment modalities. Infection, applying ice to the burn area, or trauma may convert a partial-thickness injury to a full-thickness one, especially in young children, who have thinner, more delicate skin.

Marked reduction in cardiac output occurs immediately after injury and is accompanied by an initial increase in systemic vascular resistance. Also, as fluid is lost to interstitial spaces, reduced cardiac output occurs. A compensation to overcome lower output is to increase the heart rate, which further reduces stroke volume and output. Now, organ failure results with possible death. The inefficient and labile peripheral circulation of the infant complicates management of the burn shock phase of treatment. Constriction of the chest and impairment of respiratory excursion can happen in the very young child because of the increased pliability of the rib cage. At times, chest wall scarring from burns limits thorax cage excursion at a later time.

Children younger than 2 years lack the ability to concentrate urine because of the immaturity of the renal system and are therefore at increased risk for dehydration. Because children have a relatively larger body surface area in relation to weight than adults, they require increased fluid during burn shock resuscitation to compensate for evaporative water losses.

A biphasic pattern of physiologic responses is evident in thermally injured children. The initial phase occurs during the immediate postburn period and continues for 3 to 5 days. This phase is characterized by reduced oxygen consumption, impaired circulation, and cellular shock. Following this phase and the restoration of volume, the metabolic response shifts to a catabolic or flow phase. This phase is characterized by hypermetabolism

346

with an increased oxygen consumption and an elevation of catecholamines, glucocorticoids, and glucagon. Glycogen stores are limited in children, making it difficult to meet the increased energy demands of the burn. Digestive malabsorption and increased intestinal permeability develop and limit nutrients.

Some children exhibit immunosuppression for a prolonged period after wound closure is achieved. Additionally, young children have an increased risk for microbial invasion. Endotoxins are observed very early after injury in the serum of burned individuals.

Although age is not a predictor of hypertrophic scarring, children have greater skin tension and an accelerated rate of collagen synthesis. The immature scar is the result of increased vascularity, an increase in the number of fibroblasts, reduced interstitial spaces, and abundant and altered ground substance. As the hypertrophic scar matures, collagen orients in a more parallel fashion, and vascularity decreases. Long-term scar and contracture management is necessary because of changes in body composition as the child grows and matures.

Children require greater fluid resuscitation for smaller burns than the adult population as a result of their limited physiologic reserves. Colloid replacement may be required in the very young child who fails to respond to fluid replacement. Resuscitation is considered complete when the child is able to maintain urine output for 2 hours with fluid rates at maintenance levels.

PRACTICE EXAMINATION

Fill in the Blanks

Supply the correct responses for each statement.

1. If shock is associated with hypotension, the child is in _____ shock.

2. A sign of shock in children may be _____ blood pressure.

3. If shock is associated with blood pressure appropriate for age, the child is in _____ shock.

4. Septic shock is associated with an imbalance between _____ mediators and _____ mediators.

5. _____ shock is caused by altered intravascular volume relative to vascular space.

6. _____ is a manifestation of hypovolemic shock.

7. When hypovolemic or cardiogenic shock is present, the extremities may feel _____.

8. In hypovolemia, despite warm ambient temperature, capillary refill time is _____.

9. If a child's heart rate exceeds 180 beats per minute, stroke volume is _____.

10. A child with cardiogenic shock may exhibit _____ skin.

11. TNF causes _____.

12. IL-1, IL-6, and IL-8 increase _____.

13. SIR is manifested in _____ shock.

14. _____ shock results in larger _____ and relative hypovolemia.

15. Signs of organ failure include _____, _____, and _____.

16. Shock is present whenever systemic perfusion is poor, regardless of _____.

17. The child is in _____ shock whenever impaired _____ function exists.

18. _____ may be the most sensitive indicator of inadequate systemic perfusion in children.

19. _____ injury is cellular injury that is caused by the restoration of physiologic concentrations of oxygen to cells that have been previously exposed to injurious but nonlethal hypoxic conditions.

20. _____ injuries are seen in very young children and result from exposure to hot water or other liquids.

21. A child's skin is _____ and more _____ to injury than adult skin.

22. Infection may convert a partial-thickness injury to a(n) _____ injury in young children.

23. Increased pliability of the rib cage in the very young child can impair _____.

24. Children who are younger than 2 years are unable to concentrate urine and are therefore at risk for _____.

25. As hypertrophic scars mature, _____ orients more parallel, and _____ decreases.

K.H. is a 5-month-old female infant whose parents returned from a long weekend vacation to find their daughter very weak. Her babysitter said, "Nearly all of the disposable diapers have been used because of frequent, watery stools for the last 3 days." During the last 12 hours, K.H. had eight watery stools and she was taken to an emergency department.

On physical examination, K.H. was lethargic, her anterior fontanel was depressed, and her eyes were sunken. Her skin was generally cool and gray, capillary refill was delayed, and peripheral pulses were weak. Her heart rate was 176 beats per minute, blood pressure was 90/58 mmHg, and respirations were 56 per minute.

Questions

Given the history and physical findings, which type of shock is likely?

Indicate compensatory attempts to maintain K.H.'s perfusion.

What therapy likely will be initiated on hospital admission?

Answer Key

CHAPTER 1

1. c
2. e
3. e
4. d
5. d
6. a
7. c
8. d
9. b
10. e
11. a, b, c, d, e
12. a, b, c, d
13. c, a, e, b, d
14. e
15. d
16. d
17. d
18. g
19. e
20. f
21. j
22. i
23. b
24. e
25. c

CHAPTER 2

1. d
2. c
3. d
4. a
5. a
6. a
7. a, c
8. d
9. c
10. b
11. d
12. a
13. e
14. c
15. a
16. d
17. b
18. e
19. b
20. d
21. a
22. c
23. e
24. xanthine oxidase
25. creatine kinase (CK)

CHAPTER 3

1. e
2. c
3. b
4. c
5. d
6. b
7. d
8. c
9. d
10. d
11. c
12. b
13. e
14. a
15. e
16. b
17. b
18. b
19. a
20. d
21. a
22. e
23. b
24. a
25. c

Case Study Analysis and Application

Potassium and chloride levels are low. The *potassium depletion* constitutes an emergency, because the individual could develop cardiac arrhythmias. The person should be admitted to the hospital for intravenous fluids with KCl and monitoring of blood pressure, pulse, and cardiac function.

CHAPTER 4

1. a
2. b
3. d
4. c
5. d
6. b
7. b
8. a, c, d
9. a
10. c
11. d
12. d
13. b
14. c
15. a
16. f
17. h

349

18. g
19. i
20. b
21. h
22. d
23. f
24. g
25. c

Case Study Analysis and Application

Down syndrome occurs when the chromosomes fail to divide properly. An extra chromosome 21 is present (trisomy 21), and this happens as a result of multiple factors. The risk of having a baby with Down syndrome for an older mother is greater than it is for younger mothers. The physical problems that the baby may have include heart septal anomalies, respiratory infections, and kidney defects. Every child with Down syndrome has some mental retardation, but most are trainable.

CHAPTER 5

1. T
2. T
3. T
4. T
5. F
6. F
7. T
8. T
9. T
10. F
11. F
12. T
13. T
14. F
15. F
16. T
17. T
18. F
19. T
20. T
21. F
22. g
23. c
24. b
25. c, h

Case Study Analysis and Application

Mrs. C.'s discharge diagnosis likely is *essential hypertension*. High sodium and fat intake, minimal exercise, smoking, sympathetic nervous system activity, and genetic factors have been implicated as causes of essential hypertension.

CHAPTER 6

1. d
2. b
3. a

4. a
5. b
6. b
7. d
8. c
9. a
10. c
11. d
12. b
13. d
14. b
15. c
16. b
17. d
18. d
19. a
20. Neutrophils
21. Macrophages
22. Eosinophils
23. Natural killer cells
24. Resolution
25. Granulation tissue

CHAPTER 7

1. a
2. d
3. b
4. b
5. b
6. c
7. d
8. a
9. d
10. e
11. d
12. d
13. b
14. c
15. a
16. c
17. b
18. a
19. b
20. d
21. Helper T cells
22. anamnestic
23. Regulatory T cells
24. Superantigens
25. secretory immune system

CHAPTER 8

1. d
2. a
3. d
4. a
5. a
6. c
7. c

350

8. a
9. d
10. a, c, d
11. d
12. b
13. c
14. a
15. c
16. d
17. b
18. d
19. c
20. d
21. c
22. a
23. b
24. d
25. e

Case Study Analysis and Application

A seasonal pattern to this patient's symptoms—a clear nasal discharge, itchy eyes, and high levels of allergen exposure as a teenager—likely promoted a humoral immunity. The probability of *allergic rhinitis* is high. Relief likely could be obtained by recommending oral antihistamines, steroid nasal sprays, or decongestants. A referral to an allergist to evaluate the allergens responsible for the symptoms is recommended. The initiation of hyposensitivity immunotherapy may be suggested to reduce the symptoms. If possible, known allergens should be avoided.

CHAPTER 9

1. a
2. d
3. c
4. d
5. a
6. b
7. d
8. b
9. d
10. b
11. d
12. c
13. b
14. d
15. a
16. b
17. b
18. f
19. c, g
20. h
21. i
22. c
23. e
24. a
25. d

Case Study Analysis and Application

A chest radiograph, a lymphocyte screen, and a test for antibody against HIV would be warranted. The chest radiogram would likely reveal diffuse infiltrates. In the CBC or lymphoid screen, the T_4 helper cell–to–T_8 suppressor cell ratio would be reduced below the normal 2:1 ratio. Circulating antibody against HIV would be present.

CHAPTER 10

1. a
2. b
3. c
4. b
5. d
6. c
7. c
8. c
9. a
10. a
11. a
12. a
13. a
14. c
15. d
16. corticoids
17. Stressors
18. stress response
19. exhaustion stage
20. alarm stage
21. IL-1
22. IL-2
23. NPY
24. IFN
25. Endorphins

CHAPTER 11

1. b
2. b
3. d
4. b
5. d
6. c
7. d
8. b
9. *Helicobacter pylori*
10. Transformation
11. apoptosis
12. pleomorphism
13. pituitary
14. telomerase, telomeres
15. d
16. c
17. d
18. d
19. e
20. b
21. d
22. a

351

23. e
24. c
25. b

CHAPTER 12

1. individual carcinogens
2. miRNAs
3. Developmental plasticity
4. Environmental tobacco smoke
5. Xenobiotics
6. meat
7. Hypomethylation
8. Adipose cells
9. mesothelium
10. melanoma, basal cell carcinoma, and squamous cell carcinoma
11. benzol
12. genetic
13. bystander cells
14. TNF
15. phase I activators
16. endogenous androgen
17. BMI
18. Epigenetic
19. breast, endometrial
20. ionizing radiation
21. antioxidants, oxygen-degrading
22. Methylation
23. long latency
24. HPV-16
25. Radon

CHAPTER 13

1. short-latency
2. functional
3. metastasized
4. leukemia
5. chemotherapy
6. cytotoxic agents
7. 0.9:1.0
8. histology
9. anatomical site
10. e
11. f
12. a
13. d
14. b
15. c
16. b
17. b
18. b
19. a
20. a
21. b
22. b
23. a
24. a
25. a

CHAPTER 14

1. c
2. d
3. c
4. a
5. c
6. a
7. b
8. b
9. b
10. c
11. a
12. d
13. c
14. a
15. d
16. c
17. b
18. e
19. a
20. c
21. a
22. c
23. a
24. a
25. b

CHAPTER 15

1. b
2. c
3. b
4. c
5. c
6. c
7. c
8. a
9. b
10. b
11. b
12. a
13. c
14. a
15. b
16. d
17. b
18. a
19. b
20. a
21. e
22. b
23. b
24. c
25. a

Case Study Analysis and Application

Mrs. D.'s history and response to medication were typical of *depression*. Depression causes sleep disturbances characterized by insomnia, early morning awakenings, or

352

multiple awakenings during the night. The improvement in the quality of sleep following antidepressants often occurs before other appropriate behavioral changes are seen. It seems likely that Mrs. D.'s insomnia may return, and an appropriate course of action might include seeking assistance from a sleep disorder center and/or a social worker, psychiatrist, or psychologist.

CHAPTER 16

1. d
2. a
3. b
4. a
5. e
6. d
7. b
8. a
9. d
10. c
11. c
12. b
13. a
14. b
15. d
16. b
17. c
18. b
19. b
20. d
21. Dyspraxia
22. hypotonia
23. Spinal shock
24. Anterograde amnesia
25. vigilance deficit

Case Study 1 Analysis and Application

Normal laboratory values and the normal CSF likely exclude the possibility of an infection, such as meningitis, or other causes that are known to precipitate seizures. The skull x-ray ruled out the possibility of a skull fracture. The absence of slow-wave activity on the electroencephalograph likely excludes intracranial pressure from brain masses. Because the electroencephalograph finding may be normal between seizures, the episodal pattern suggests a *generalized grand mal seizure*. A judicious administration of anticonvulsant medications is likely indicated.

Case Study 2 Analysis and Application

To conduct a focused history, with input from the son, looking for evidence of depression—an entity that overlaps dementia presentation—order a head CT to rule out any organic cause for the cognitive dysfunction, and serum chemistries to detect other organ disorders that can contribute to dementia. If the physician finds for Alzheimer disease, cholinesterase inhibitors or drugs blocking the activity of glutamate can be used. Treatment of AD is also directed at compensation techniques such as memory aids, maintaining cognition that is not impaired,

and improving the hygiene, nutrition, and health. Healthcare aides should help the patient avoid potential risks, rather than teaching and reteaching.

CHAPTER 17

1. d
2. b
3. d
4. b
5. e
6. c
7. b
8. c
9. e
10. c
11. d
12. b
13. c
14. d
15. d
16. b
17. b
18. b
19. b
20. d
21. Brudzinski
22. concussion
23. neuromuscular junction
24. Guillain-Barré syndrome
25. multiple sclerosis

Case Study Analysis and Application

Mrs. B. exhibits risk factors for a CVA. She smokes cigarettes, is overweight, has used estrogen for 20 years, and is hypertensive. Her mother and siblings each had a history of diabetes, CVA, and hypertension; all of these indicate a family history that increases the risk for CVA.

Mrs. B.'s symptoms and signs suggest a *thrombotic stroke* with ischemia rather than a hemorrhagic or embolic stroke. Her elevated blood pressure is likely caused by atherosclerosis, which can lead to a thrombus formation. The absence of blood CSF rules out a hemorrhagic stroke. Because there was no fibrillation on the electrocardiogram, the heart was an unlikely source for emboli, thus excluding the possibility of an embolic stroke.

CHAPTER 18

1. f
2. f
3. a
4. c
5. c
6. e
7. b
8. f
9. a
10. c

11. a
12. d
13. f
14. f
15. a
16. f
17. g
18. a
19. d
20. e
21. d
22. b, d
23. e
24. d
25. f

Case Study Analysis and Application

Ms. B. is experiencing *major (unipolar) depression.* Causes for the disorder expressed during this episode likely include a family predisposition, previous episodes, the psychosocial trauma of losing a close friend, and the guilt associated with allowing the friend to drive under the influence of alcohol. Signs and symptoms of the episode include a lack of concentration at work, excessive crying, extreme sadness, lack of appetite, weight loss, and sleep disturbances.

CHAPTER 19

1. T
2. F
3. T
4. T
5. F
6. T
7. T
8. T
9. T
10. F
11. F
12. Reye, hepatic
13. posterior
14. anterior
15. meningitis
16. Craniosynostosis
17. i
18. h
19. g
20. f
21. e
22. d
23. c
24. b
25. a

Case Study Analysis and Application

Radiographs will most likely reveal an absence of spinal processes on the vertebrae from L3 to L5. An MRI will then be ordered, which will reveal a *meningomyelocele* at the same level, with tethering of the cord. A neurosurgical consultation is ordered, and surgery is planned. However, 1 week before surgery, some loss of bladder control is noted. This is a rather unusual presentation for a meningomyelocele, but it illustrates that these problems may be fairly obscure and only become apparent later in childhood.

CHAPTER 20

1. a
2. c
3. c
4. b
5. d
6. b
7. a
8. c
9. d
10. d
11. e
12. c
13. d
14. d
15. e
16. b
17. d
18. e
19. a
20. c
21. e
22. d
23. f
24. a, c
25. b, d

CHAPTER 21

1. c
2. a
3. a
4. d
5. b
6. a
7. d
8. a, e
9. a
10. d
11. a
12. b
13. b
14. b
15. c
16. c
17. a, d
18. c
19. c
20. b
21. d
22. c
23. e

24. d
25. b

Case Study 1 Analysis and Application

Scott's symptoms, signs, and laboratory values are classic for *diabetic ketoacidosis*. The serum values indicate metabolic acidosis with some accompanying respiratory compensation. His elevated glycosylated hemoglobin shows that he likely has been hyperglycemic for several months. This is type 1 diabetes and will require insulin administration and personal instructions about the recognition of future signs and symptoms of hyperglycemia and hypoglycemia, self–blood glucose monitoring, insulin therapy, diet, and exercise.

Case Study 2 Analysis and Application

Initial laboratory tests require a random glucose and a urine dipstick. Subsequent laboratory tests could include a fasting glucose, a glycosylated hemoglobin analysis, a fasting lipid profile, an electrocardiogram, and an electromyogram.

Repeat BP (152/100 mmHg) is hypertensive. Random glucose (262 mg/dl), fasting glucose (171 mg/dl), and high quantities of glycosylated hemoglobin exceed the criteria for diagnosis of diabetes. Microalbuminuria indicates early nephropathy and an increased risk for renal and cardiovascular disease. The fasting lipid profile indicates diabetic dyslipidemia with increased cardiovascular risk. ECG indicates left ventricular hypertrophy and suggests the existence of hypertension for some time, and the presence of peripheral neuropathy is validated by the EMG.

CHAPTER 22

1. b
2. b
3. e
4. d
5. c
6. d
7. a
8. b
9. e
10. b
11. a
12. b
13. b
14. c
15. a
16. c
17. d
18. c
19. a
20. a
21. a
22. c
23. b
24. e
25. a

CHAPTER 23

1. a
2. d
3. c
4. d
5. e
6. d
7. e
8. d
9. b
10. c
11. d
12. e
13. e
14. b
15. d
16. d
17. d
18. a
19. d
20. d
21. b
22. e
23. d
24. c
25. b

Case Study 1 Analysis and Application

A transabdominal and transvaginal pelvic ultrasound is necessary.

Result: *Indistinct right ovary: grossly normal; 7.6 × 9.0 × 3.3 cm left adnexal mass; ill-defined left ovary*

Next, a MRI of the pelvis with contrast is required.

Result: *Left adnexal mass; no free pelvic fluid; no significant adenopathy; right ovary: grossly normal; sigmoid colon: diverticulosis*

These diagnostic tests dictated a diagnostic laparoscopy with excision of the mass with frozen cytologic examination of any suspicious lesions. *Frozen sections: malignancy.* The presence of malignancy requires a total abdominal hysterectomy and a bilateral salpingo-oophorectomy and staging of the extent of the malignancy. The surgery and staging was completed with specimens, including a resected section of the descending colon, were submitted for cytological evaluation. The *final diagnosis is papillary carcinoma consistent with serous carcinoma of uterine tube (flavored), or serous carcinoma of both ovaries and metastatic papillary carcinoma of descending colon.*

The standard treatment protocol for this particular case of ovarian cancer is chemotherapy; then, complete debulking surgery followed by more chemotherapy.

Case Study 2 Analysis and Application

Mrs. B.'s history and examination are indicative of *breast cancer* in her left breast. A positive familial history of breast cancer has a strong and confirmed causal link to breast cancer. A chromosome 17 defect has also been implicated as a genetic causal factor in breast cancer. Other associated risk factors for breast cancer that Mrs. B. exhibits include late age at first delivery, early menarche, history of taking birth control pills, and benign breast tumors.

The cardinal manifestation of breast cancer was a hard, fixed mass that was palpable in Mrs. B.'s left breast. The freely moveable, soft masses of the right breast likely are benign, because they display different and fluctuating patterns of tissue proliferation as compared with the left breast. The palpation of the axillary lymph node indicated that cancer cells have metastasized throughout the lymphatic channels that surround the breast.

CHAPTER 24

1. c
2. e
3. f
4. h
5. i
6. ophthalmia neonatorum
7. dark-field microscopy
8. protozoa
9. painful blister-like lesions
10. placental barrier
11. ectopic pregnancy
12. malodorous
13. 50% to 80%
14. asymptomatic
15. skin rash
16. *Neisseria gonorrhoeae,* anaerobic
17. Acyclovir
18. Condylomata acuminata
19. Pruritus
20. liver
21. cervical, penile
22. DNA probe
23. epididymitis
24. epigastric
25. death

Case Study Analysis and Application

Cervicitis is common in the STIs of gonorrhea, Chlamydia, and herpes. No blisters are observed, so herpes is unlikely. The vaginal discharge indicates gonorrhea or chlamydial infection. The absence of diplococci inside neutrophils rules out gonorrhea and leads to a presumptive diagnosis of *Chlamydia trachomatis* as the cause of this STI. A test on a sample of cervical discharge could be used to establish a definitive diagnosis of chlamydial infection. Such a test would use fluorescein-labeled monoclonal antibody against *Chlamydia trachomatis.* The test would be read microscopically.

CHAPTER 25

1. e
2. b
3. e

4. e
5. a
6. c
7. c
8. c
9. d
10. e
11. d
12. d
13. b
14. d
15. d
16. a
17. a
18. b
19. tissue factor (TF)
20. TF-FVIIa
21. Tissue plasminogen activator (t-PA)
22. fibrin
23. fibrinolysis
24. b
25. c

CHAPTER 26

1. e
2. d
3. c
4. a
5. a
6. b
7. b
8. a
9. b
10. b
11. e
12. b
13. a
14. b
15. c
16. a
17. b
18. a
19. c
20. c
21. c
22. c
23. b
24. b
25. c

Case Study Analysis and Application

Three anemias have erythrocytes that are microcytic and hypochromic: iron deficiency anemia, sideroblastic anemia, and thalassemia. A.'s history has factors that could contribute to anemia from blood loss. The menorrhagia causes more iron loss than is normal with each menstrual period, and excessive aspirin intake irritates the gastrointestinal mucosa and can precipitate chronic mucosal microhemorrhage.

An *iron deficiency anemia* is likely and can be verified by providing oral iron replacement and checking A.'s hemoglobin values in 1 month. If the hemoglobin deficit is corrected, it is likely that the correct diagnosis was made. The source of bleeding should be corrected, if possible; a substitute for aspirin should be used; and iron supplementation should be used for at least 1 year.

A.'s homeostatic mechanisms are trying to compensate in several ways, including shunting blood to more critical organs, increasing erythropoiesis, increasing the heart rate to handle increased venous return, and increasing breathing to make oxygen available to the remaining erythrocytes. The last two signs are relevant compensation efforts in A.'s circumstance.

CHAPTER 27

1. d
2. c
3. e
4. c
5. d
6. c
7. b
8. b
9. c
10. a
11. d
12. d
13. e
14. a
15. e
16. b
17. d
18. a
19. a
20. b
21. d
22. d
23. a
24. b
25. c

Case Study Analysis and Application

The nurse practitioner would likely believe that L.L. has *acute lymphocytic leukemia*. The pale skin with petechiae and ecchymoses is abnormal, and so is the gingival bleeding from minor trauma. Although the abnormal values for RBCs, hemoglobin, total leukocyte count, and platelet count have many possible causes, the presence of blastocysts in peripheral blood indicates a bone marrow dysfunction. At this time, the nurse practitioner likely will refer L.L. to a pediatric oncologist for extensive diagnostic tests and treatment.

CHAPTER 28

1. F
2. T
3. T

4. F
5. T
6. F
7. F
8. a
9. b
10. a
11. d
12. c
13. a
14. d
15. b
16. b
17. e
18. a
19. a
20. b
21. e
22. c
23. d
24. c
25. d

Case Study Analysis and Application

S.C. has the typical manifestations of *idiopathic thrombocytopenia purpura (ITP)*, although it has come to medical attention in a very roundabout manner. Corticosteroid therapy reduces ITP severity. Intravenous anti D (gamma globulin) is effective for Rh-positive individuals with ITP.

CHAPTER 29

1. b
2. b
3. b
4. c
5. b
6. e
7. a
8. c
9. e
10. a
11. a
12. c
13. d
14. a
15. c
16. d
17. a
18. d
19. b
20. e
21. b
22. b, c
23. b, d, e
24. d, b, c, a, e
25. d, b, a, e, c

CHAPTER 30

1. d
2. e
3. c
4. b
5. a
6. b
7. d
8. c
9. c
10. c
11. a
12. c
13. d
14. b
15. c
16. b
17. d
18. d
19. b
20. c
21. c
22. b
23. c
24. e
25. f

Case Study 1 Analysis and Application

Mr. T. likely has *hypertension* or is at risk for it. Appropriate questions are: Do you eat much fatty food and/or salt, do you drink alcohol, do you regularly exercise, and do you check your blood pressure regularly? Laboratory tests to confirm the presence of hypertension include blood chemistries including BUN, creatinine, fasting glucose, calcium and magnesium, CBC, a lipid profile, and an ECG.

The diagnosis of *stage 1 HTN* is confirmed by the initial and subsequent blood pressure measurements of mid 150s over mid 90s. Laboratory results showed all blood chemistries and CBC normal, total cholesterol and LDL elevated, and HDL low. ECG showed increased QRS waves. The laboratory studies rule out secondary causes HTN. Left ventricular hypertrophy observed on the ECG indicates long-standing HTN adding to Mr. T.'s risk for CHF. If conventional therapy is ineffective, specialized tests are required to determine the cause of secondary hypertension.

Case Study 2 Analysis and Application

Alterable myocardial infarction risk factors for W.S. are essential hypertension and cigarette smoking. Unalterable risk factors for W.S. include advancing age, male sex, and family history of early cardiac death. Atherosclerosis in the anterior descending branch of the left coronary artery was the beginning process that led to this infarction. The location of infarction was verified by electrocardiogram.

The precipitating event in this myocardial infarction was complete occlusion of the coronary artery. Dysrhythmias are common complications of myocardial infarctions rather than the cause. The history of hypertension also supports occlusion of the coronary artery as the cause for this myocardial infarction.

Pulmonary thromboembolism is a common cause of death from myocardial infarction, because emboli disseminate from debris or clots from the infarcted endocardium. Prophylactic heparin therapy decreases the risk of pulmonary embolism by interfering with the conversion of prothrombin to thrombin, thereby making thrombi less likely to form.

CHAPTER 31

1. F
2. T
3. F
4. T
5. F
6. shunt
7. left, right
8. right, left
9. oxygenated, unoxygenated
10. equal
11. left, right
12. first weeks
13. pulmonary stenosis
14. afterload, congestive heart failure
15. coarctation of the aorta
16. e
17. a
18. a
19. b
20. c
21. c
22. e
23. d
24. d
25. a

Case Study Analysis and Application

After consultation, D.M.'s echocardiogram demonstrates a moderate *coarctation of the aorta* in the aortic arch. The discrepancy in the quality of upper and lower extremity pulses is because of well-developed collateral circulation to the descending aorta; the femoral pulses will be decreased as blood fills the collateral vessels. Although this boy is presently asymptomatic, the degree of coarctation will cause symptoms such as headache, hypertension, and epistaxis later in life

CHAPTER 32

1. d
2. d
3. c
4. d
5. d
6. b
7. d
8. c

358

9. a
10. a
11. c
12. d
13. b
14. d
15. a
16. b
17. a
18. a
19. a
20. a
21. b
22. d
23. b
24. c
25. c

CHAPTER 33

1. c
2. e
3. d
4. e
5. a
6. e
7. b
8. d
9. e
10. b
11. a
12. a, b
13. a, b, d
14. b
15. d
16. Kussmaul respiration
17. hemoptysis
18. cyanosis
19. Cheyne-Stokes respiration
20. pleural space atelectasis
21. bronchiectasis
22. pneumoconiosis
23. flail chest
24. pneumothorax
25. lobar pneumonia

Case Study Analysis and Application

Mr. S. presents the classic symptoms and signs of *emphysema*. His long-term, extensive smoking is consistent with most cases of emphysema, and so is his dyspnea on exertion that progressed to dyspnea even at rest. Hyperinflation of the lungs causes the anteroposterior chest diameter to increase. Mr. S.'s chest radiograph is consistent with findings in emphysema. Prolonged forced expiratory volume, decreased tidal volume, and increased total lung capacity are also present in emphysema. These tests indicate that the walls of alveoli have been destroyed and that the lungs have become more distended or less compliant and that they have less elastic recoil; therefore, air is trapped, and expiration flow is diminished.

CHAPTER 34

1. flexibility, compliance
2. increased resistance
3. 20 to 24 weeks
4. atelectasis
5. Asthma
6. metabolic rates, oxygen consumption
7. b
8. d
9. d
10. a
11. c
12. c
13. c
14. e
15. d
16. c
17. a, b, d
18. a, b
19. f
20. d, f
21. e
22. c
23. d
24. c
25. a

Case Study Analysis and Application

T.C. has classic manifestations of *bronchiolitis*. The most likely etiologic agent in T.C.'s illness is respiratory syncytial virus, to which his parents likely exposed him during their "colds." He is displaying the classic signs of respiratory distress in an infant and is unable to feed because of this respiratory distress. His lethargy is probably due to mild hypoxia and hypercapnia, and his general fatigue is from prolonged ventilatory effort. He may experience respiratory failure if left untreated. Hospitalization for oxygen therapy, rehydration, and respiratory therapy should support him through the worst of his illness, and he should improve within a few days.

CHAPTER 35

1. f, d, b, a, c, e
2. a
3. d
4. a
5. d
6. b
7. b
8. c
9. b
10. c
11. e
12. b
13. b
14. d
15. b
16. d

359

17. a
18. c
19. d
20. a
21. b
22. c
23. c
24. d
25. d

CHAPTER 36

1. d
2. b
3. a
4. a
5. e
6. d
7. b
8. b
9. d
10. a
11. d
12. d
13. d
14. d
15. a
16. d
17. c
18. b
19. b
20. c
21. a
22. c
23. d
24. a
25. e

Case Study 1 Analysis and Application

E.C.'s history of sore throat and back pain and his laboratory values suggest *poststreptococcal glomerulonephritis*. Proteinuria is a sensitive indicator of glomerular dysfunction. In glomerulonephritis, the glomerulus is injured, and its permeability is increased enough to permit protein to enter into the filtrate and urine. Blood and red blood cell casts also are seen in glomerulonephritis. BUN and creatinine are excreted entirely by the kidneys and therefore are directly related to renal excretion. E.C.'s pediatrician will most likely place him on penicillin and may prescribe an antihypertensive medication; E.C.'s blood pressure, electrolyte balance, and BUN and creatinine levels will also be monitored.

Case Study 2 analysis and application

Ms. J. has either a recurrent UTI (cystitis) or pyelonephritis. All of the historical evidence, the physical examination, and the laboratory results support a final diagnosis of a lower tract UTI *(cystitis)* rather than and upper tract UTI (pyelonephritis), because she does not have a fever nor

any atypical symptoms or signs. The antibiotic therapy used should be effective against *E. coli*.

CHAPTER 37

1. third
2. Wilms tumor gene 1
3. 30% to 50%
4. metanephrogenic blastema
5. metabolic acidosis
6. secondary enuresis
7. dysplastic
8. Utereropelvic junction obstruction
9. Hypospadias
10. exstrophy of the bladder
11. dominant
12. fatal
13. primary vesicoureteral reflux
14. Chronic glomerulonephritis
15. nephrotic syndrome
16. a
17. d
18. c
19. d
20. d
21. b
22. d
23. c
24. b, c, a
25. b

Case Study Analysis and Application

The laboratory values reveal an anemia and thrombocytopenia; the child is losing red blood cells and platelets. Because she has not voided any urine, acute renal failure is very likely. These results suggest the diagnosis of *hemolytic uremic syndrome*. This child will require hospitalization for blood transfusions and dialysis.

CHAPTER 38

1. d
2. d
3. b
4. e
5. e
6. d
7. d
8. a
9. d
10. b
11. d
12. b
13. a
14. c
15. c
16. d
17. a
18. b

19. a
20. c
21. b
22. c
23. gastrin
24. 1.0 mg/dl
25. *Helicobacter pylori*

CHAPTER 39

1. b
2. b
3. a
4. e
5. a
6. d
7. c
8. e
9. a
10. b
11. b
12. c
13. b
14. a
15. a
16. d
17. e
18. e
19. a
20. c
21. c
22. d
23. a
24. d
25. a

Case Study 1 Analysis and Application

A *gastric ulcer* is likely. Factors associated with these ulcers include smoking, stress, and use of aspirin or other ulcerogenic drugs. Although the clinical manifestations of gastric ulcers are similar to those of duodenal ulcers, the pain of gastric ulcers is more likely to occur immediately after eating. Also, gastric ulcers tend to be chronic rather than to alternate between periods of remission and exacerbation. An upper gastrointestinal study using barium sulfate as a contrasting medium and endoscopy can detect the location of the ulcer and confirm that Dr. R. has a gastric ulcer.

Case Study 2 Analysis and Application

Laboratory values should include a CBC with a differential for evidence of infection; liver function tests to assess the liver's metabolism, storage, filtration, and excretion; chemistries to evaluate renal function; and serologic analysis to reveal the presence or absence of HBsAg, anti-HAV, anti-HCV, and anti-HIV. D.K. is at risk for HIV as well as hepatitis because of possible shared, contaminated needles with other IV drug users.

D.K.'s history by itself does little to suggest a particular diagnosis. The absence of ascites, occult or rectal blood, or confusions during the physical examination tend to rule out hepatic failure. An elevated WBC count with increased lymphocytes indicates a viral infection. Normal coagulation and albumin values indicate insignificant hepatic and renal dysfunction. Unremarkable increases in bilirubin and alkaline phosphatase tend to exclude biliary disease. The serologic analysis of antigen and antibodies implicates HBV but not HAV, HCV, nor HIV. D.K. has *hepatitis B.*

CHAPTER 40

1. Pyloric stenosis
2. Tracheoesophageal fistula
3. Wilson disease
4. Intussusception
5. kernicterus
6. gastrin secretion
7. cystic fibrosis
8. gluten-sensitive enteropathy
9. Congenital aganglionic megacolon
10. Kwashiorkor
11. nonorganic FTT
12. necrotizing enterocolitis
13. biopsy
14. decrease
15. paranasal sinuses, middle ear
16. Rectal prolapse
17. a
18. c
19. b
20. a
21. e
22. d
23. d
24. c
25. b, c

Case Study Analysis and Application

Baby B.'s problem was somewhat diagnosed when an attempt to pass a catheter from his mouth into his stomach failed. Radiography shows a "kink" in the esophagus. Both observations are fairly characteristic manifestations of *esophageal atresia.* Baby B. is transferred to a pediatric surgeon for surgical correction.

CHAPTER 41

1. d
2. b
3. b
4. d
5. b
6. d
7. d
8. a
9. a

10. b
11. d
12. b
13. c
14. d
15. e
16. e
17. c
18. b
19. c, a, b, d, e
20. c
21. a
22. d
23. d
24. e
25. b

CHAPTER 42

1. a
2. b
3. d
4. c
5. c
6. c
7. e
8. a
9. a
10. e
11. b
12. d
13. d
14. a
15. e
16. b
17. d
18. e
19. a
20. c
21. b
22. d
23. d
24. c
25. e

Case Study 1 Analysis and Application

Mrs. B's presenting symptoms are compatible with either osteoarthritis or rheumatoid arthritis. The laboratory studies support a diagnosis of *rheumatoid arthritis* because of the presence of rheumatoid factor; this is a positive finding in about 80% of individuals who have rheumatoid arthritis. Although other diseases may produce a positive test result, osteoarthritis will not. Synovial fluid analysis that shows poor mucin precipitates and inflammatory exudates satisfies the diagnostic criteria for rheumatoid arthritis. The radiograph is more representative of rheumatoid arthritis than osteoarthritis. In osteoarthritis, deformity of articular cartilage, bone sclerosis, cystic areas, and bony spurs would be likely observations.

Case Study 2 Analysis and Application

The osteopenia is the result of *menopausal osteoporosis.* The fracture must be stabilized with a back brace, and then the goal is to prevent future fractures and disability. Management requires regular, moderate weightbearing exercise; dietary supplements of calcium, vitamin D, and magnesium; selective estrogen receptor modulators; intranasal calcitonin; and bisphosphonates to encourage osteocyte survival.

CHAPTER 43

1. dominant
2. abduction
3. collagen
4. Metatarsus abductus
5. Trendelenburg gait
6. Osteomyelitis
7. Ponseli
8. benign
9. creatine phosphokinase
10. brain
11. femoral ischemia
12. asymmetric
13. dystrophin
14. abduction, flexion
15. tumor suppressor gene
16. b
17. f
18. e
19. f
20. d
21. e
22. d
23. c
24. b
25. a

Case Study Analysis and Application

Bobby displays the clinical manifestations of *Duchenne muscular dystrophy*. The diagnosis can be confirmed by the measurement of serum creatine phosphokinase (CPK) levels, electromyography, and muscle biopsy. The CPK level in Duchenne muscular dystrophy will be increased to more than 10 times normal. Histologic examination of the biopsy will show muscle degeneration, with fat and connective tissue replacing muscle fibers.

CHAPTER 44

1. c
2. a
3. a
4. d
5. d
6. e
7. d
8. b

9. e
10. c
11. e
12. d
13. d
14. b
15. c
16. c
17. a
18. b
19. d
20. e
21. f
22. c
23. a
24. b
25. d

Case Study Analysis and Application

Mr. E. should be concerned about the changing appearance of his mole, because moles are precursor lesions for *malignant melanomas*. He is at risk for melanoma because he has fair skin and exposes himself regularly to ultraviolet light. Additionally, his mole is subjected to irritation by his rubbing belt.

The changing appearance of Mr. E.'s mole makes his lesion a candidate for a full-thickness excisional biopsy. Such a biopsy permits the accurate measurement of the lesion's thickness if it is a melanoma, and it also indicates the best treatment. If the lesion is benign, the excisional biopsy constitutes treatment.

Mr. E.'s prognosis depends on the thickness of the lesion. Lesions on the trunk have the poorest prognosis. If the thickness of his lesion is greater than 1.5 mm, his prognosis would not be good because of prior or likely metastasis.

CHAPTER 45

1. sebum production
2. human-to-human
3. contagious
4. eczema
5. upper respiratory
6. systemic antifungal
7. fade
8. do not fade
9. vesicular
10. *Staphylococcus aureus*
11. f
12. c
13. e
14. b
15. i
16. f
17. h
18. j
19. g
20. a
21. d

22. c
23. k
24. a
25. d

Case Study Analysis and Application

This is a fairly classic case of *bullous impetigo* caused by a *Staphylococcus aureus* infection in L.D.'s nasopharynx. Abrasion from blowing his nose frequently has opened the skin and allowed the bacteria to enter the skin and cause the lesions. The infection spread to L.D.'s arm because he has been wiping his nose on his arm. L.D. is treated with antibiotics, and the infection resolves.

CHAPTER 46

1. a
2. c
3. e
4. b
5. d
6. d
7. a
8. c
9. d
10. d
11. metabolism
12. organ failure
13. vasodilation
14. anaerobic glycolysis
15. kidneys
16. hypovolemic
17. intracellular Na, H_2O
18. endothelium
19. peripheral pooling
20. MODS
21. oliguria
22. cool, clammy
23. intravascular
24. clot
25. Sepsis, septic shock

Case Study 1 Analysis and Application

It is likely K.S.'s appendectomy "nicked" the colon allowing colonic bacterial and fecal contents to escape into the abdominal/pelvic cavity. He is progressing, if not already, into MODS. An exploratory surgery to validate the suspicion of "nicked" colon and débride necrotic tissue and drain infectious fluid is needed. Then, a combination of effective, powerful antibiotics, continuous oxygenation, fluid and electrolyte therapy, and enteral feeding is required.

Case Study 2 Analysis and Application

Adults with burns that involve 20% to 40% of the TBSA require cardiovascular support through intravenous fluid, because *hypovolemic shock* develops quickly after a major burn injury. Within minutes of a major burn injury, the capillary bed not only at the site of the burn but throughout the entire body becomes more permeable to water, sodium, and proteins. This leads to fluid loss from the intravascular spaces into the interstitial spaces and massive edema; the blood volume and cardiac output diminish. Nasotracheal intubation is required to avoid edematous obstruction of the upper airway. The infusion of intravenous fluid or burn shock resuscitation for the first 24 hours must be faster than the rate of loss or circulatory volume. To determine adequate levels of infusion, urine output must be measured, so Mr. E. will require a catheter placement into his bladder.

Although hypovolemic shock is the immediate concern for major burn patients, other alterations are very important; monitoring and maintenance of electrolytes is required. Circulation to burned extremities may be impaired, because the circumferential nature of the burns and the edema may act as a tourniquet; therefore, a surgical cut through the circumferential area may be required to restore adequate blood supply to the limbs. Cleansing and hydrotherapy of burned areas should not draw vital electrolytes from cells because of altered toxicity. The hypermetabolic rate of burned individuals requires adequate nutrition to provide a positive nitrogen balance. Finally, excision and grafting procedures require meticulous care.

CHAPTER 47

1. decompensated
2. high
3. compensated
4. proinflammatory, anti-inflammatory
5. Hypovolemic
6. Tachycardia
7. cool
8. delayed
9. decreased
10. mottled
11. vasodilation
12. capillary permeability
13. septic
14. Neurogenic, vascular space
15. lactic acidosis, oliguria, altered mental states
16. blood pressure
17. cardiogenic, ventricular
18. Acidosis
19. Reperfusion
20. Scald
21. thinner, susceptible
22. full-thickness
23. respiratory excursions
24. dehydration
25. collagen, vascularity

Case Study Analysis and Application

Dehydration is a common cause of *hypovolemic* shock in children. When intravascular fluid or plasma is lost through diarrhea, the interstitial fluid shifts into the vascular bed in an attempt to maintain circulating blood volume. Fluid loss in K.H. caused peripheral vasoconstriction to compensate for her fluid loss; this resulted in weak peripheral pulses and mottled or grayish skin color. Her elevated heart rate and respirations also are compensatory attempts to assist the perfusion of tissues with oxygen and nutrients.

The hospital therapy likely will involve a first phase of appropriate electrolyte intravenous fluid replacement for the dehydration. Improvement in K.H.'s physical signs, including her urine output and laboratory values, will determine when oral feeding and discharge are appropriate.